Circadian Medicine

Circadian Medicine

Edited by

Christopher S. Colwell
*Laboratory of Circadian and Sleep Medicine, Department of Psychiatry
and Biobehavioral Sciences, University of California Los Angeles,
Los Angeles, CA, USA*

WILEY Blackwell

Published by John Wiley & Sons, Inc., Hoboken, New Jersey
Published simultaneously in Canada

For general information on our other products and services or for technical support, please contact our Customer Care Department within the United States at (800) 762-2974, outside the United States at (317) 572-3993 or fax (317) 572-4002.

Wiley also publishes its books in a variety of electronic formats. Some content that appears in print may not be available in electronic formats. For more information about Wiley products, visit our web site at www.wiley.com.

Library of Congress Cataloging-in-Publication Data:

Circadian medicine / edited by Christopher S. Colwell.
     p. ; cm.
   Includes bibliographical references and index.
   ISBN 978-1-118-46778-7 (paper)
I. Colwell, Christopher S., editor.
[DNLM: 1. Circadian Clocks–physiology.   2. Circadian Rhythm–physiology.
3. Chronobiology Disorders–etiology.   QT 167]
   QP84.6
   612′.022–dc23

                                                        2015004403

Printed in Singapore by C.O.S. Printers Pte Ltd

Set in 9.5/11.5pt Warnock by SPi Global, Pondicherry, India

10 9 8 7 6 5 4 3 2 1

1   2015

Contents

List of Contributors

Kandis Adams
Department of Neurobiology and Neuroscience
Institute, Morehouse School of Medicine
Atlanta, GA, USA

Urs Albrecht
Dept of Biology, Unit of Biochemistry, University
of Fribourg
Fribourg, Switzerland

Michael Antle
Departments of Psychology, Physiology &
Pharmacology, Hotchkiss Brain Institute,
University of Calgary
Calgary, AB, Canada

Gene D. Block
Laboratory of Circadian and Sleep Medicine,
Department of Psychiatry and Biobehavioral
Sciences, University of California Los Angeles
Los Angeles, CA, USA

David R. Bonsall
Neuroscience Program, Smith College
Northampton, MA, USA

Steven A. Brown
Institute of Pharmacology and Toxicology,
University of Zürich
Zürich, Switzerland

Oscar Castanon-Cervantes
Department of Neurobiology and Neuroscience
Institute, Morehouse School of Medicine
Atlanta, GA, USA

Christopher S. Colwell
Laboratory of Circadian and Sleep Medicine,
Department of Psychiatry and Biobehavioral
Sciences, University of California Los Angeles
Los Angeles, CA, USA

Alec J. Davidson
Department of Neurobiology and Neuroscience
Institute, Morehouse School of Medicine
Atlanta, GA, USA

Elizabeth Devore
Channing Division of Network Medicine,
Department of Medicine, Brigham
and Women's Hospital and Harvard
Medical School
Boston, MA, USA

Masao Doi
Department of Systems Biology, Graduate School
of Pharmaceutical Sciences
Kyoto University, Sakyo-ku, Kyoto, Japan

Russell G. Foster
Nuffield Department of Clinical Neurosciences
(Nuffield Laboratory of Ophthalmology), John
Radcliffe Hospital
Oxford, UK

Jean-Michel Fustin
Department of Systems Biology, Graduate School
of Pharmaceutical Sciences
Kyoto University, Sakyo-ku, Kyoto, Japan

Mary E. Harrington
Neuroscience Program, Smith College
Northampton, MA, USA

Michael H. Hastings
Division of Neurobiology, Medical Research
Council Laboratory of Molecular Biology
Cambridge, UK

Akihiro Kanematsu
Department of Urology, Hyogo College of
Medicine
Nishinomiya, Hyogo, Japan

Alexei Leliavski
Circadian Rhythms Group, Max Planck
Institute for Biophysical Chemistry
Göttingen, Germany;
Medical Department I,
University of Lübeck
Lübeck, Germany

Aleksey V. Matveyenko
Department of Physiology and Biomedical
Engineering, Mayo Clinic
Rochester, MN, USA;
Department of Medicine, University of
California Los Angeles
Los Angeles, CA, USA

Colleen A. McClung
Department of Psychiatry, University of
Pittsburgh School of Medicine
Pittsburgh, PA, USA

Johanna H. Meijer
Department of Molecular Cell Biology,
Leiden University Medical Center
Leiden, The Netherlands

Stephan Michel
Department of Molecular Cell
Biology, Leiden University Medical
Center
Leiden, The Netherlands

Ralph Mistlberger
Department of Psychology, Cognitive and
Neural Sciences Area, Simon Fraser
University
Burnaby, BC, Canada

A. Jennifer Morton
Department of Physiology, Development
and Neuroscience, University of Cambridge
Cambridge, UK

Hiromitsu Negoro
Department of Urology, Graduate School of
Medicine, Kyoto University
Sakyo, Kyoto, Japan

Hitoshi Okamura
Department of Systems Biology,
Graduate School of Pharmaceutical Sciences
Kyoto University, Sakyo-ku, Kyoto, Japan

John S. O'Neill
Division of Cell Biology, Medical Research
Council Laboratory of Molecular Biology,
Cambridge, UK

Henrik Oster
Circadian Rhythms Group, Max Planck Institute
for Biophysical Chemistry
Göttingen, Germany;
Medical Department I, University of Lübeck
Lübeck, Germany

An Pan
School of Public Health, Tongji Medical College,
Huazhong University of Science and
Technology, Wuhan,
Hubei Province, China

Stuart N. Peirson
Nuffield Department of Clinical Neurosciences
(Nuffield Laboratory of Ophthalmology), John
Radcliffe Hospital
Oxford, UK

R. Daniel Rudic
Pharmacology and Toxicology, Georgia Regents
University
Augusta, GA, USA

Eva S. Schernhammer
Department of Epidemiology, Harvard School
of Public Health, Boston,
MA, USA;
Department of Epidemiology, Centre for Public
Health, Medical University of Vienna,
Austria

Analyne M. Schroeder
Laboratory of Circadian and Sleep Medicine,
Department of Psychiatry and Biobehavioral
Sciences, University of California Los Angeles
Los Angeles, CA, USA

Shigenobu Shibata
Department of Electrical Engineering and
Bioscience, Waseda University
Tokyo, Japan

Rae Silver
Silver Neurobiology Laboratory, Department of
Psychology, Columbia University
New York, NY, USA

Roxanne Sterniczuk
Department of Psychology and Neuroscience,
Dalhousie University
Halifax, NS, Canada

Yu Tahara
Department of Electrical Engineering and
Bioscience, Waseda University
Tokyo, Japan

T. Katherine Tamai
Centre for Cell and Molecular Dynamics,
Department of Cell and Developmental Biology,
University College London
London, UK

David Whitmore
Centre for Cell and Molecular Dynamics,
Department of Cell and Developmental Biology,
University College London
London, UK

Paul Witkovsky
Department of Neuroscience and Physiology,
New York University
New York, NY, USA;
Silver Neurobiology Laboratory,
Department of Psychology, Columbia
University
New York, NY, USA

Miho Yasuda
Department of Systems Biology,
Graduate School of Pharmaceutical
Sciences
Kyoto University, Sakyo-ku, Kyoto, Japan

Preface

It is becoming increasingly clear that robust daily rhythms of sleep and wake are essential to good health. A wide range of studies have demonstrated that disruption of the circadian system leads to a cluster of symptoms, including metabolic deficits, cardiovascular problems, immune dysfunction, difficulty sleeping and cognitive deficits. Many people, including patients with psychiatric and neurological diseases, exhibit disturbances in their daily sleep–wake cycle as part of their daily life. These people have difficulty sleeping at night and staying awake during the day, which has a profound impact on the quality of life not only for those not sleeping but also for their family members. The last decades have brought much progress in terms of understanding the mechanistic underpinnings of circadian rhythms at the molecular, cellular and circuit levels. Still, a major gap remains in our ability to translate these discoveries into therapies or even lifestyle recommendations. This book focuses on the question of how we can move from understanding disease mechanisms towards the translation of this knowledge into therapeutics. Given the widespread impact of circadian rhythms on health and disease, I have decided to call this book "Circadian Medicine" to emphasize the practical implications of these biological rhythms.

There is a set of core ideas that underlies all of the chapters in this book. Some of these ideas have been rigidly tested while others are more hypotheses at the moment. The first core idea is that circadian timekeeping is important for the proper functioning of cells, physiological systems, and behavior. The second core idea is that the disruption of the circadian system leads to a cluster of symptoms, including metabolic deficits, cardiovascular problems, immune dysfunction, and cognitive deficits. Thirdly, many diseases cause disruption of the circadian system and this disruption appears to be especially prevalent in neurological and psychiatric disorders. Disruption of the sleep–wake cycle appears to be a very sensitive, although not specific, marker of deteriorating health. Finally, treating the sleep–wake disturbance may both improve the quality of life of the patient and also delay the onset of some of the symptoms. This core idea is the most speculative and also the most exciting. The costs of diseases associated with circadian disruption (including type 2 diabetes, cardiovascular disease, and neurodegenerative diseases) are steep and there is an urgent need for new therapeutic approaches.

The book itself has been divided into three main sections. The first set of five chapters focuses on fundamental concepts, including a description of the molecular and cellular mechanisms that generate circadian oscillations by Drs Hastings and O'Neill (MRC, University of Cambridge, UK) and Dr Brown (University of Zurich, Switzerland) focusing on applying this understanding to human clocks. The circuitry of the central clock in the suprachiasmatic nucleus (SCN) is covered by Drs Silver, Witkovsky, and Colwell (Columbia University, University of California, Los Angeles, USA), the discussion of sleep by Dr Mistlberger (Simon Fraser University, Canada) and fatigue by Drs Bonsall and Harrington (Smith College, USA).

The second set of chapters focuses on the circadian regulation of key physiological systems in our body, including the liver by Leliavski and Oster (Max-Planck Institute, Germany) as well as Tahara and Shibata (Waseda University, Japan) with the latter chapter focusing on the role of nutrition and diet. The cardiovascular clock is described by Dr Rudic (Georgia Health Science University, USA) with Drs Okamura, Yasuda, Fustin, and Doi (Kyoto University, Japan) describing how circadian dysfunction may be linked to hypertension. One of the areas that most of us do not think about is the daily changes in the bladder. Yet difficulty sleeping at night due to the need to urinate is common with circadian dysfunction, as explained by Drs Kanematsu and Negoro (Hyogo College, Kyoto University, Japan). The links between circadian rhythms and type 2 diabetes are discussed by Dr Matveyenko (University of California, Los Angeles; Mayo Clinic, USA). The circadian regulation of the cell cycle and how dysfunction could increase risks for cancer is covered by Drs Tamai and Whitmore (University College London, UK). Drs Pan, Devore, and Schernhammer (Harvard University, USA) summarize the evidence that shift work can increase risk for type 2 diabetes and cancer. The role of circadian timing in the regulation of immune function is covered by Drs Adams, Castanon-Cervantes, and Davidson (Morehouse University, USA).

The third set of chapters focuses on the role of circadian timing in the central nervous system as well as diseases of the nervous system. For this section, we start off with a chapter by Dr Albrecht (University of Fribourg, Switzerland) on circadian clocks, reward and addictive behaviors. These behaviors can be considered a form of learning and in the next chapter, Dr Colwell (University of California, Los Angeles, USA) discusses the evidence generally linking circadian disruption with learning and memory deficits. The close association between affective disorders and sleep disruption is well known to psychiatrists. Dr McClung (University of Pittsburgh, USA) will discuss the more mechanistic evidence linking circadian rhythms and mood disorders. Another psychiatric disorder in which disrupted rhythms has been proposed as a biomarker is schizophrenia, as discussed by Drs Peirson and Foster (University of Oxford, UK). Considered then is a set of neurodegenerative disorders in order of prevalence, including Alzheimer's disease by Drs Sterniczuk (Dalhousie University, Canada) and Antle (University of Calgary, Canada), Parkinson's disease by Dr Colwell (University of California, Los Angeles, USA), and Huntington's disease by Dr Morton (University of Cambridge, UK). While Huntington's disease is rare, it has become an important model for examining the interplay between disease and circadian dysfunction. Finally, Drs Michel, Meijer, and Block discuss our current understanding of how age impacts the circadian system, with an emphasis on the impact on central nervous system.

All of these chapters have been written by experts in these areas and I am extremely grateful for their contributions. The authors are an international group which brings a breadth of perspective and a multidisciplinary set of approaches. Many of the ideas in this book were germinated in a workshop held at the Lorentz Center in Leiden, the Netherlands, on "Clinical Relevance of Circadian Rhythms" and I am grateful for the fruitful discussions held during this workshop. I would also like to acknowledge the careful editing provided by UCLA (University of California, Los Angeles, USA) students Tamara Cutler and Shaina Sedighim who helped me see the work through the eyes of the intended audience. I apologize to the authors for the delays in getting this project off the ground and particularly those who wrote their chapters in a timely manner. It is my sincere hope that this book will stimulate further work in this important research area.

January, 2015

Christopher S. Colwell
University of California Los Angeles,
Los Angeles, CA, USA

Fundamental Concepts

Cytosolic and Transcriptional Cycles Underlying Circadian Oscillations

1

Michael H. Hastings[1] and John S. O'Neill[2]

[1] *Division of Neurobiology, Medical Research Council Laboratory of Molecular Biology, Cambridge, UK*
[2] *Division of Cell Biology, Medical Research Council Laboratory of Molecular Biology, Cambridge, UK*

1.1 Introduction

Circadian (*circa-* approximately, *-dian* a day) clocks are the internal pacemakers that drive the daily rhythms in our physiology and behavior that adapt us to the 24-hour world (Duffy *et al.*, 2011). They thereby maintain temporal coherence in our core metabolism, even when individuals are held in isolation, experimentally deprived of external timing cues such as light–dark (LD) cycles. As a result of this ability of our endogenous circadian system to define internal time and use it to drive daily rhythms, our brains and bodies can be viewed as 24-hour machines, alternating between states of wakefulness and sleep, catabolism and anabolism, growth/repair and physical activity. It is now widely recognized that disturbance of this daily program can carry significant costs for morbidity and even mortality (Hastings *et al.*, 2003). Some personal insights into this can come from the subjective experiences of jet lag. More insidiously, however, the disturbance of nocturnal sleep, and consequent disaffected mood, loss of mental capacity and social disruption, is a common element of neurodegenerative and psychiatric conditions (Hatfield *et al.*, 2004; Wulff *et al.*, 2010; Bliwise *et al.*, 2011) (This volume, several chapters). Moreover, epidemiological evidence now associates increased risk of cancer as well as cardiovascular and metabolic diseases with extensive experience of rotational shift-work (Knutsson, 1989; Viswanathan *et al.*, 2007; Huang *et al.*, 2011) (This volume, Chapter 13), a life-style that will inevitably compromise circadian coherence, and which represents a major and growing hazard to public health. Evolution has programmed us to live by a 24-hour day and where genetic, pathological, environmental or social factors drive us against this program, we pay a heavy price. Conversely, the recognition that our body is a 24-hour machine, with different metabolic and physiological states across day and night, provides a route into enhancing therapeutic efficacy by administering medicines on a schedule that maximizes their bioavailability and by targeting disease states at their most critical and vulnerable phases of the day (Levi and Schibler, 2007).

Key to appreciating the role of the circadian clock in both health and illness, and thereby identifying novel therapeutic strategies, is the unravelling of its molecular and cellular bases. Whilst the formal properties of circadian clocks have been understood for over 60 years, and the identification in 1972

Circadian Medicine, First Edition. Edited by Christopher S. Colwell.
© 2015 John Wiley & Sons, Inc. Published 2015 by John Wiley & Sons, Inc.

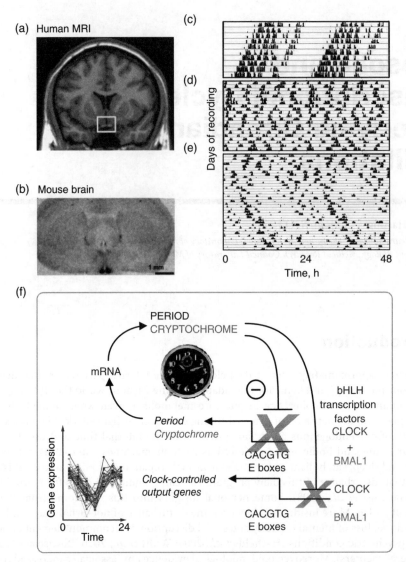

Fig. 1.1 The suprachiasmatic nucleus (SCN) as circadian pacemaker. (a) Frontal MRI view of human brain to identify location of SCN (boxed) in anterior hypothalamus at junction of third ventricle and optic chiasm (courtesy of Dr Adrian Owen, MRC CBU, Cambridge UK). (b) Comparable view of mouse brain labelled auto-radiographically to reveal SCN in ventral hypothalamus. (c) Recording of wheel-running activity of mouse (double-plotted on 48-h time base) free-running in continuous dim red light, with a sustained circadian period of slightly less than 24 h (King *et al.*, 2003). (d) Behavior of same mouse following ablation of SCN – note total loss of circadian organization in absence of SCN, but no change in overall activity level. (e) Behavior of same SCN-lesioned mouse following intracerebral graft of SCN from a Clock^delta19 mouse. Note modest restoration of circadian patterning to behavior, but with a period longer than 24 h as determined by graft genotype. This genetic specification of circadian period proves that the rhythm is controlled by the grafted SCN and, thus, the SCN is the definitive pacemaker to circadian behavior. (f) Schematic representation of conventional TTFL at the heart of the SCN circadian pacemaker. (See text for details.)

of the suprachiasmatic nucleus (SCN) as the brain's principal pacemaker provided a neuroanatomical focus to circadian biology (Weaver, 1998; Chapter 3) (Fig. 1.1a–e), proper mechanistic under-standing of the timing process proved to be elusive. This changed dramatically from the late 1970s onwards, when "circadian clock genes" and their mechanisms of action were identified: firstly in *Drosophila*, then in *Neurospora*, and more recently in mouse (Takahashi *et al.*, 2008). The outcome of these studies was to reveal that an autoregulatory negative feedback oscillator, based on sequential transcriptional and posttranslational processes, lies at the heart of the circadian timepieces of these divergent groups. Even though the molecular components may differ, the "logic" of the mechanism is conserved. But things move on, and there is growing realization that these transcriptionally based clocks do not operate in isolation; rather, they are mutually dependent upon intrinsically rhythmic cytosolic signals (cAMP, Ca^{2+}, kinases), such that the cell as a whole has a resonant structure, tuned to 24-hour operation (Hastings et al., 2008). Finally, the most recent development has been to show that even in cells lacking transcriptional apparatus (most notably mammalian erythrocytes), circadian cycles of metabolic state can be sustained (O'Neill and Reddy, 2011). The purpose of this chapter is to review the development of this molecular and cellular model of the circadian clockwork of mammals.

1.2 Assembling the transcriptional feedback loop

1.2.1 Discovering clock genes and their actions in lower species

The idea that a complex behavioral trait such as the circadian cycle of rest and activity could be understood from the viewpoint of single gene actions was, for some time, contentious in both the circadian field and also more widely. Nevertheless, the creation by Ron Konopka and Seymour Benzer of mutant Drosophila with atypically short or long periods to their circadian behavior, and the subsequent cloning of the Period gene as the molecular target of these mutations, initiated a revolution in clock biology (Konopka, 1987). Alongside the Frq (Frq) gene of Neurospora, cloned by Jay Dunlap and colleagues (Loros et al., 1989), Period (Per) provided an entry point into the molecular mechanisms of clocks: changes in the encoded proteins could make the clock run faster, or slower or not at all. They therefore MUST be an intrinsic part of the clockwork. Moreover, it became apparent that the key action of the encoded proteins was to inhibit the expression of their cognate genes. Given that there is an inevitable time lag between transcriptional activation and nuclear entry of the fully formed protein, an oscillation is bound to ensue, as in any other delayed negative feedback system (Hardin et al., 1990; Aronson et al. 1994). Indeed, autoregulation of this type is well recognized in molecular biology, with oscillations commonly occurring over a couple of hours. The critical property here, however, is that the dynamics of the contributory stages (gene activation, protein synthesis, intracellular transport, protein degradation) are extended such that the cycle runs for approximately 24 hours. Subsequent mutational and biochemical studies revealed that Per and Frq are components of dynamic, multiprotein complexes, the assembly of which is facilitated in part by their protein interaction domains (Hardin, 2005; Crosthwaite et al., 1997). Of particular note were the so-called PAS (Per–Arnt–Sim) interaction domains of Per. The positive drives to the feedback loops that stimulate expression of Per and Frq, comes from additional PAS-containing proteins: CLOCK and CYCLE in flies (Allada et al., 1998; Rutila et al., 1998), and WHITE COLLAR 1 and 2 in Neurospora (Crosthwaite et al., 1997; de Paula et al., 2007). After forming heteromers, these positive factors activate transcription via specific regulatory sequences in the enhancer regions of Per and Frq, respectively. Thus, positive factors drive the expression of negative factors, which in turn oppose the positive drive leading to a decline in negative factor abundance, which allows the cycle to start again approximately 24 hours after the previous point of initiation.

Although both systems are light sensitive – a prerequisite for synchronization with solar cycles and, thereby, environmental time, their molecular basis to entrainment is different. In flies, the stability of PER is dependent on association with another circadian protein, TIMELESS (Myers et al., 1996; Koh et al., 2006), which in turn is subject to degradation by CRY, a light-dependent factor with similarity to photolyase DNA repair proteins (Cashmore, 2003). Consequently, PER protein can only accumulate in the night, thereby stably entraining the entire molecular cycle to solar time. In contrast, the light-sensitive component in the Neurospora loop is the positive factor White Collar-1, which binds FAD (flavin adenine dinucleotide) as a chromophore (Crosthwaite et al., 1997; de Paula et al., 2007). Thus, expression of Frq is activated at the start of the day, again linking the phase of the molecular cycle to environmental (solar) time.

1.2.2 Discovering clock genes and their actions in mammals

Knowledge of the clock in flies and fungus played a large role in deciphering the mammalian clockwork (Fig. 1.1f). Homology cloning or sequence alignment of novel transcripts, based heavily on knowledge of the PAS domains of *Drosophila Period*, led ultimately to the discovery of three *Per* genes in mammals (Tei *et al.*, 1997; Reppert and Weaver, 2002). Mammalian *Cryptochromes* (*Cry1* and *Cry2*) had previously been studied in the context of DNA repair, but findings from flies focused attention on their potential circadian role, which was confirmed by the demonstration that *Cry*-deficient mice cannot exhibit circadian behavior (van der Horst *et al.*, 1999). Initial description of a mammalian *Timeless* gene was subsequently shown to be misleading, as the mammalian gene in question is, in fact, a homologue to *Timeout*, a different, noncircadian fly gene. A further difference, consistent with the absence of *Timeless*, is that mammalian CRY proteins are not the light-sensitive component of the cycle: resetting in mammals is mediated by the activation of *Per1* and *Per2* expression (see below) (Shigeyoshi *et al.*, 1997; Albrecht *et al.*, 1997), an echo of the light-dependent induction of *Frq* expression in *Neurospora*. Critically, both *Per* and *Cry* mRNA and proteins are expressed rhythmically in the SCN, with respective phases that are consistent with negative feedback action (Field *et al.*, 2000). But what of the positive factors that would drive such a negative feedback system? The identification of mammalian *Clock*, by mutagenesis and subsequent transgenic rescue, was a landmark achievement by the laboratory of Joe Takahashi – it preceded the discovery of *Drosophila Clock*, and was dependent upon classical positional cloning, pre-dating the mouse genome era (King *et al.*, 1997). As in flies, CLOCK forms heteromeric complexes to activate expression of *Per* and other circadian genes, including *Cry*. The partner to CLOCK is BMAL1, a homologue of *Drosophila Cycle*, which was initially identified by co-expression screens (Hogenesch *et al.*, 1998).

Both CLOCK and BMAL1 contain PAS dimerization domains, but only CLOCK carries a poly-Q transactivation domain. Loss of BMAL1 leads to circadian incompetence at both molecular and behavioral levels, whereas loss of CLOCK has mixed effects that vary between tissues, depending upon whether or not NPAS2, a paralogue of CLOCK, can compensate (DeBruyne *et al.*, 2007). Nevertheless, the original Clock[delta19] mutation generated by Takahashi has compromised transactivation; consequently, circadian period is lengthened in the heterozygote and completely disorganized in homozygous mutants because of insufficient transcriptional drive to the *Per* and *Cry* genes. Finally, the negative feedback loop has been closed experimentally by the demonstration that CLOCK/BMAL1 heterodimers can acutely activate E-box mediated transcription and that this effect is suppressed by co-expression with PER and CRY (Kume *et al.*, 1999). The details of this transcriptional repression are unclear, but both PER and CRY contribute (see below). In the established transcriptional model in mammals, therefore, the start of circadian day sees CLOCK/BMAL1 activation of *Per* and *Cry* expression via their E-box regulatory sequences (Fig. 1.1f). The accumulating mRNAs are translated into protein and by the end of circadian day SCN neurons have high levels of nuclear PER and CRY proteins. This is followed by a progressive decline in mRNA levels, reflecting the negative feedback action of the accumulated PER/CRY complexes. By late circadian night the existing PER/CRY complexes, no longer replenished in the absence of mRNA, are finally cleared from the nucleus such that CLOCK/BMAL1 activity is de-repressed and the cycle starts anew at circadian dawn. The application of this basic model to humans is described in Chapter 2.

1.2.3 Imaging the transcriptional clock in real time: a multitude of cellular oscillators appears

Circadian timing is an intrinsically dynamic process and major advances in analyzing circadian gene expression have come about with the development of real-time reporter genes in which circadian regulatory sequences are coupled to bioluminescent (firefly luciferase) or fluorescent proteins. Although recording of circadian rhythms of intrinsic bioluminescence in unicellular organisms has a long pedigree in clock research (Hastings, 2007), this approach found greater application when directed towards the newly discovered clock genes, firstly in plants and flies and more recently in mammals. Early examples are transgenic lines of mouse and rat in which upstream sequences of *Per1* (carrying five E-boxes) are used to drive luciferase. Organotypic slice cultures of SCN from such animals express robust, clearly defined bioluminescence rhythms arising from individual neurons (Fig. 1.2a–c), the phases of which are synchronized but exhibit a complex, wave-like progression across the SCN (Yamaguchi *et al.*, 2003),

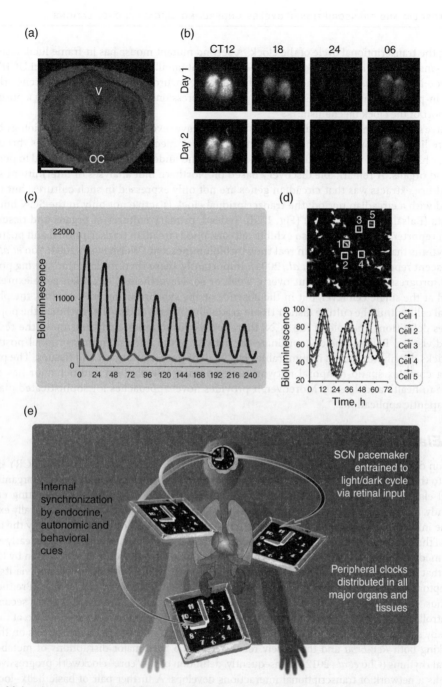

Fig. 1.2 Molecular pacemaking in SCN and other tissues and cells. (a) View of PER2::LUC SCN organotypic slice culture under phase illumination. V = third ventricle, oc = location of optic chiasm, scale bar = 500 um. (b) Serial bioluminescent images from same field of view as in (a), collected for 1 h every 6 h over 2 days in culture. Note stable and synchronized circadian oscillation in both SCN, with regionally specific phases of PER2 expression. CT = circadian time, CT12 = projected time of lights off. (c) Graphical plots of circadian bioluminescence from PER2::LUC organotypic SCN slices that are wild type (dark) or homozygote VIP-null (pale). Note stable molecular oscillation (with progressively smaller peaks due to luciferin substrate utilization) in wild type slices, but rapid loss of circadian organization in SCN lacking VIP. (d) Representative image of bioluminescent PER2::lUC fibroblasts (above) and plots of circadian rhythms of bioluminescence from individual cells in the culture (below). Note very stable molecular pacemaking, but no synchrony between cells. (e) Schematic representation of the internal circadian hierarchy in mammals, whereby local circadian clocks distributed across all major organs are governed by a variety of synchronizing cues ultimately derived from the SCN. In this way, daily rhythms across the body are synchronized to each other and also to solar time.

reflecting the transcriptional cycle of the clock. A second mutant mouse has in-frame luciferase coding sequences inserted into the endogenous *Per2* locus to generate an allele encoding a PERIOD::LUCIFERASE fusion protein (Yoo *et al.*, 2004), and again individual SCN neurons express bioluminescence rhythms, this time in-phase with predicted native PER2 protein expression and, thereby, providing a posttranslational report of the clock mechanism.

Extensive studies using these and other reporter lines have revolutionized circadian biology because they, quite literally, provide a "window" on the SCN clock mechanism as it progresses through real time. They have, however, provided an even more profound understanding when applied to peripheral tissues and organs. A remarkable discovery based on Northern blot analyses of intermittent samples of cell culture extracts was that circadian genes are not only expressed in such cultures, but they are expressed with a circadian period: the transcriptional clock is active not only in the SCN but also in fibroblasts (Balsalobre *et al.*, 1998) (Fig. 1.2d). Indeed, primary cultures of organs and tissues from circadian reporter animals could also exhibit self-sustained circadian transcriptional and posttranslational rhythms that can be imaged in real time by bioluminescent (Welsh *et al.*, 2004; Yoo *et al.*, 2004) or fluorescent reporters (Nagoshi *et al.*, 2004). Importantly, these rhythms lack the "staying power" of the SCN, progressively damping out over a week or so. Nevertheless, circadian gene expression is sustained at the single cell level, but in the absence of any synchronising cues *in vitro*, the phases of individual cells within the culture dish or tissue gradually disperse and so the rhythm at the population level loses definition. The role of the SCN, therefore, is not to impose rhythms upon the rest of the brain and viscera. Rather, it is to coordinate the activity of the intrinsic transcriptional/posttranslational clocks distributed across innumerable cells in all of the major organs and tissues. The presence of such a complex spatio-temporal network underpinning metabolism and behavior has obvious relevance to health and disease. Moreover, it provides novel approaches for sophisticated diagnostic and therapeutic applications.

1.2.4 Elaborating the core transcriptional clockwork

Elucidation of the feedback actions mediated by PER/TIM in flies, FRQ in fungi and PER/CRY in mammals led to the idea of the "core" feedback loop, but developments in all three of the model organisms saw a gradual elaboration, adding additional rhythmic components and identifying rate-limiting enzymes. Importantly, in all three systems it became evident that some positive factors were rhythmically expressed due to the influence of their targets. In the case of mammals, this advance was facilitated by the tractable analysis of the transcriptional clockwork of peripheral tissues and cell lines, and the strongest early evidence came from identification of *Rev-Erbα*. This is a highly rhythmic circadian output gene driven by CLOCK/BMAL1 that encodes an orphan nuclear receptor that, in turn, inhibits *Bmal1* expression via its retinoic acid receptor-related orphan receptors response elements (RORE) regulatory sequences (Preitner *et al.*, 2002). Thus, output of the "core" loop becomes its input. Further elaboration showed how a second circadian-controlled gene, *Rora*, acts as a positive factor to *Bmal1*, opposing the effect of *Rev-Erbα* at the RORE and thereby sculpting *Bmal1* expression. Whereas single-mutant mice show limited effects on the clock, mice lacking both *Rev-Erbα* and the closely related *Rev-Erbβ* have major disruptions of metabolic and behavioral rhythms (Cho *et al.*, 2012). Consequently, definition of the "core" clockwork progressively loses its focus as a network of transcriptional interactions develops. A further pair of basic helix–loop–helix transcription factors, DEC-1 and DEC-2, has also been implicated in the clock, insofar as they are expressed rhythmically in the SCN and also interfere with CLOCK/BMAL1 mediated transactivation. A final auxiliary loop consists of *Dbp* and *E4BP4*, which respectively activate and suppress transcription mediated by so-called D-boxes present in the *Per*, *Rev-Erβ* and *Rora* genes. The clock-driven, rhythmic activities of DBP/E4BP4 will, therefore, feed back to influence the clock, generating a further autoregulatory group. The significance of this architecture of internested transcriptional loops is twofold (Ueda *et al.*, 2005). First, it confers robustness to the overall behavior of the molecular oscillator and likely also boosts its amplitude. Second, because of the time constants of the various interlocking stages, the network establishes a phase map defined by serial episodes of activation and suppression of a number of genes, thereby providing more precise and definitive temporal resolution within the composite oscillation.

The discovery that cells and tissues contain transcriptional clocks very similar to those of the SCN was transformational for the experimental analysis of their regulatory mechanisms. The utility of cell cultures as a proxy for SCN pacemaking and the use of abundant tissues such as liver for biochemical analysis have made it possible to conduct studies that would be extremely difficult to perform on SCN. This has allowed a more comprehensive decoding of the molecular events associated with transcriptional activation. For example, with the description of the CLOCK/BMAL1 heterodimer to 2.3 Å it is now possible to define the roles of the basic helix–loop–helix and PAS domains in dimerization and DNA binding, and reveal key residues in the protein interfaces, mutations of which can alter transcriptional activity and the period of circadian pacemaking in fibroblasts (Huang *et al.*, 2012). ChIP-seq and other biochemical analyses of liver have been able to track the various components of the CLOCK/BMAL1 complex (including RNA polymerase II, CRY, PER and associated factors) as it progresses through activated and suppressed states, associating with E-box-containing (and other) sequences (Koike *et al.*, 2012). This cycle is accompanied by pronounced rhythms of histone modifications, including differentially phased cycles of methylation and acetylation as the oscillation progresses through times of transcriptional activation and suppression. Careful analysis of this molecular procession will likely provide important information regarding the general mechanisms of transcriptional coordination, with relevance well beyond the field of circadian clocks.

1.3 Keeping the transcriptional clockworks in tune

1.3.1 Entrainment of the SCN transcriptional clockwork

Retinal innervation of the SCN, carried via the retino-hypothalamic tract (RHT) is the means by which the transcriptional program of the SCN is synchronized to solar and seasonal time, as represented by the cycle of light and darkness (Reppert and Weaver, 2002). This pathway is described in detail in Chapter 3. The RHT consists of the axons of retinal ganglion cells (RGCs) and enters the ventro-lateral subdivision of the SCN, which contains neurons that express the neuropeptides vasoactive intestinal peptide (VIP) and gastrin-releasing peptide (GRP). The nonretinorecipient zone surrounding the core, termed the shell, is characterized by neurons expressing arginine vasopressin (AVP). Until recently it was assumed that conventional rods and cones are the circadian photoreceptors but a remarkable recent discovery was that a subclass of RGCs expresses a novel invertebrate-like opsin, melanopsin, that confers upon them intrinsic photoreceptivity (Rollag *et al.*, 2003) (This volume, Chapter 3). These intrinsically photoreceptive RGCs (iPRGCs) are sufficient for circadian entrainment of the SCN, and they also mediate numerous other subliminal aspects of vision (Guler *et al.*, 2008). They have broad receptive fields and act as luminance detectors rather than feature detectors: properties clearly adapted to their circadian role.

The principal neurotransmitter of RGCs is glutamate and the terminals of the RHT act upon the NMDA- and AMPA-type glutamate receptors expressed by retinorecipient SCN neurons. The subsequent influx of Ca^{2+} mediated by NMDAR increases the rate of firing of the neurons, which is otherwise low in circadian night (Kuhlman *et al.*, 2003). It also activates a signaling cascade leading to increased gene expression mediated by the cAMP/Ca^{2+} response element (CRE) regulatory sequences in target genes (Obrietan *et al.*, 1999; Schurov *et al.*, 1999). Importantly, both *Per1* and *Per2* carry CREs, additional to their E-boxes (Travnickova-Bendova *et al.*, 2002), so nocturnal light pulses acutely induce *Per* expression in the core SCN at a circadian time when it is otherwise very low (Albrecht *et al.*, 1997; Shigeyoshi *et al.*, 1997). This can be followed a few hours later by an increase in *Per* expression in the shell – likely triggered by the increased firing of action potentials by the core neurons and subsequent release of VIP, GRP and other transmitters onto the shell. These neuropeptides act via G-protein coupled receptors to activate cAMP and Ca^{2+} signaling, so will, in turn, increase *Per* expression via the CREs.

Thus, during circadian night, when spontaneous E-box-mediated expression of *Per* in the SCN is low, a light pulse will activate it and the additional pulse of PER protein will feed through the core loop and reset it to a new phase. If this occurs in the early subjective night when PER levels are falling, progression of the SCN molecular cycle is delayed, whereas light delivered in late circadian night when *Per* expression is beginning to rise, will accelerate the rise and shift the molecular cycle forwards. During circadian day-time, when *Per* expression is already high, light has little impact on the molecular cycle. Thus, in the "real world," small phase adjustments to the molecular cycle at dusk (delay) and dawn (advance) will keep it synchronized to, and predictive of, the solar cycle, thereby ensuring appropriate phasing of the behavioral and physiological rhythms it controls. It is important to note that this entrainment by photic-induction of *Per* expression is equally applicable to both diurnal and nocturnal species because the cycle of *Per* expression in the SCN is the same in both: high in circadian day, low in circadian night, regardless of the animal's behavioral habits (Maywood and Mrosovsky, 2001). This transcriptional effect of light upon the SCN clock also enables the molecular cycle to encode season – the longer days of summer drive a broader peak of *Per* expression (Messager *et al.*, 1999; Nuesslein-Hildesheim *et al.*, 2000), which is ultimately decoded by brain and pituitary to engage adaptive seasonal changes such as altered appetite and nutrient utilization, reproductive status and migratory behavior (Dardente *et al.*, 2010). The SCN can also be synchronized by cues other than light, principally behavioral arousal mediated by serotoninergic and neuropeptidergic cues from the brain stem (Hastings *et al.*, 1997). In this case, the clock is most sensitive during circadian daytime, when *Per* expression is high and the cycle is acutely reset (advanced) by early suppression of *Per* – the mirror image of the effect of light. Indeed, because they have convergent but opposite molecular actions, light can block the resetting effect of arousal on the SCN and vice versa (Mead *et al.*, 1992; Maywood *et al.*, 2002).

1.3.2 Entrainment of transcriptional clocks in peripheral tissues

In contrast to the relatively limited number of mechanisms serving the SCN, the entrainment of the clocks within other brain regions, peripheral organs and cells is dependent upon a kaleidoscope of stimuli, some general and others specific to the cell types involved (Fig. 1.2e). The starting point is the SCN efferent innervation, which is distributed to a variety of target nuclei in the hypothalamus, brain stem and beyond, indirectly, to spinal cord and pituitary. The intrinsic clockwork of the SCN will enable it to convey time cues encoded as firing rate and very probably changes in the neurotransmitter types being released onto target cells. Although a small number of SCN neuropeptides have been implicated in transmitting circadian cues to the brain, we are far away from understanding how, at a systems-level such information is used to time fundamental neural processes, not least the alternation between states of sleep and wakefulness. In coordinating rhythms across the body, three general mechanisms are evident: behavior and the consequential cycle of feeding and fast; endocrine cues, especially the daily surge of corticosteroid hormones from the adrenal glands; and cues derived from the autonomic nervous system, such as the daily cycle of body temperature (Fig. 1.2e). Taking the liver clock as an example, under normal circumstances the SCN will determine the phases of feeding, core body temperature and corticosteroid secretion, which, in turn, will affect the local molecular pacemakers in the liver to ensure its various functions are appropriately timed to match the needs of the animal across day and night. This internal phasing can be altered experimentally by, for example, restricting the time of food availability or by injecting exogenous corticosteroids. Under such experimental conditions, the SCN remains phase-locked to solar time but the liver clockwork can be advanced or delayed by the new cues, thereby interfering with internal temporal coordination and, thus, metabolic efficiency.

The molecular basis of such entrainment is inevitably varied, although in the case of corticosteroid hormones (which are secreted at the start of the respective activity phase of nocturnal and diurnal species) the presence of glucocorticoid-response elements in *Per*, *Cry* and *Bmal1* genes provides a direct entry point to shifting the core clockwork. In contrast, entrainment by temperature cycles can involve transcriptional effects of heat shock factor (HSF 1), acting via response elements in the *Per2* gene, and posttranscriptionally via cold-inducible RNA-binding protein (CIRP), which appears to be necessary for normal expression and function of CLOCK protein. Indeed, the pivotal role of *Per2* as a sensor of entraining cues to the liver is demonstrated by the fact that in mice with a genetically compromised liver clock, *Per2* expression nevertheless continues to oscillate under the influence of systemic cues.

One clear demonstration of the functional importance of internal circadian tuning comes from the observation that mice lacking a liver clock but with otherwise normal circadian behavior are prone to daily episodes of hypoglycemia because they are unable to perform the usual circadian up-regulation of hepatic gluconeogenesis to maintain glucose homeostasis during the fasting day. Notwithstanding these successes in identifying molecular pathways that entrain the local hepatic clock, the scale of the remaining problem remains enormous: the complexities of intercellular signaling between different tissues are already evident anatomically and biochemically, but now it must be taken to a new level by factoring in biological time. Solving this problem, however, will provide new therapeutic opportunities by the exploitation of circadian-based cues to regulate vital functions. One immediate example comes from the circadian morning surge in cardiovascular output (Fig. 1.3). Under normal circumstances this is adaptive, preparing the individual to engage with the world, but in those suffering from cardiovascular disease it represents a point of vulnerability – as reflected in the increased incidence of sudden cardiac death in hours immediately after awakening. Knowledge of the circadian signaling cascades from SCN to brain stem, to myocardium and to vascular endothelium that generate the morning surge could be used to develop time-based therapies to ameliorate the point of vulnerability without affecting baseline ongoing cardiovascular regulation (This volume, Chapters 8 & 9). This principle of circadian targeting applies to any number of systemic illnesses, not least metabolic syndrome and diabetes (This volume, Chapter 11).

1.3.3 Local tissue clocks direct local transcriptional and posttranscriptional programs

The relevance of transcription to circadian coordination extends far beyond the core feedback loops. A variety of DNA microarray studies and, more recently, RNA sequencing have shown that (depending on the algorithms used to detect significant rhythms) between 5 and 20% of the local transcriptome is subject to circadian modulation. Importantly in tissues such as the liver, this circadian modulation is most pronounced for transcripts involved in metabolic and signaling pathways (Akhtar et al., 2002; Koike et al., 2012; Menet et al., 2012), as well as cell cycle regulators. Characteristically, it is the enzymatic components of the cell that are clock-regulated rather than structural genes, such that the clock up- and down-regulates the "software" of the tissue, rather than its "hardware". The most immediate point of regulation of the circadian transcriptome is provided by the rhythmic activity of the proteins of the core oscillation, which periodically activates/suppresses the expression of target genes carrying E-boxes, D-boxes and ROREs. Recent ChIP-seq studies have established the genome-wide extent of such circadian control (and also highlighted the numerous targets of "clock" genes that are not circadian in their activity). Furthermore, some of the rhythmic targets of the core loop factors are themselves transcriptional regulators, for example, PPAR and HNF4a, so further tiers of circadian gene expression will be driven in a cascading effect. In addition, cues that entrain the core clock can also act upon clock-controlled genes directly, most obviously corticosteroids, which may act via glucocorticoid response elements (GREs) either independently or in concert with E-boxes, ROREs and other "circadian motifs." The transcriptome can, therefore, be viewed as a resonant network, enabling tissues to prepare to perform night- and day-specific metabolic and other functions in a timely manner, thereby supporting the individual's daily cycle of rest and activity.

The control of transcription is not, however, the only means to achieve temporal adaptation. Analysis of the cytosolic proteome of liver and SCN has revealed numerous proteins that are regulated at the level of protein abundance but not at steady-state transcript level. Furthermore, several isoforms of the same protein can be rhythmic but with contrasting phases of peak abundance, and recent RNA-sequencing studies suggest that only about 20% of rhythmically expressed genes in the liver are driven by de novo transcription. Clearly, posttranscriptional and posttranslational modifications are also important avenues for the clock to sculpt the functions of a tissue. Many RNA-binding proteins are circadian in their expression, and for example in liver and lung the clock and clock-related cues can influence the splicing of primary transcripts into different isoforms with contrasting temporal profiles. Posttranslational modifications, not least phosphorylation, are an additional circadian influence on the proteome, generating temporal diversity in cellular function. The prevailing view, however, remains one in which circadian cycles of gene expression drive rhythmic regulation of metabolism and signaling networks.

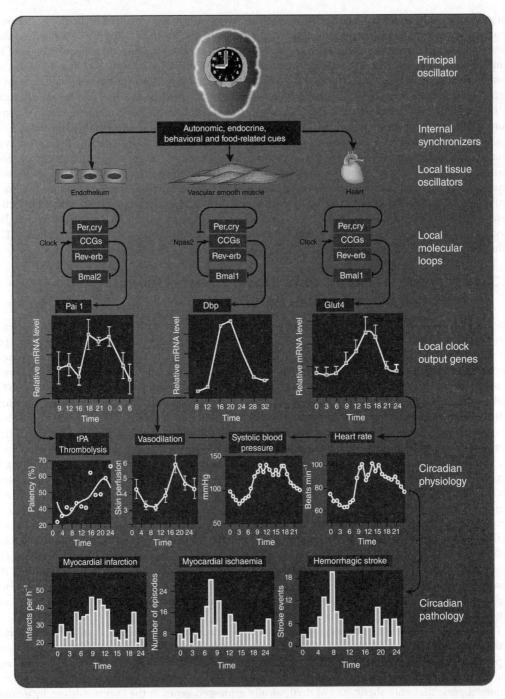

Fig. 1.3 Schematic view of systems-level circadian organization. Schematic view of circadian coordination across the individual in which the primary pacemaker of the SCN, entrained to solar time by retinal afferents, maintains and synchronises tissue-based clocks in the major organ systems by a blend of endocrine, autonomic and behavioral (feeding-related) cues. Disruption of these timing cues can result in pathology throughout the body. In this way, a robust circadian system contributes to our health and well-being while disrupting these rhythms as wide-ranging negative consequences. Redrawn with permission from Hastings *et al.* 2003.

1.4 Building posttranslational mechanisms into the circadian pacemaker

1.4.1 Posttranslational control of the clock: localization and stability of clock proteins

The obvious sophistication of posttranscriptional mechanisms in coordinating clock outputs raises the question of their potential role in the core pacemaking loop itself. For the nested transcriptional loops to oscillate effectively it is necessary for them to incorporate delays, which cannot be generated by the (inherently noisy) process of transcription itself (Suter *et al.*, 2011). Rather, they can arise from regulation of the localization, activity and stability of the transcription factors that exert rhythmic transcriptional regulation (Hastings *et al.*, 2007; Zheng and Sehgal, 2008; Asher and Schibler, 2011). These properties are themselves points of regulation by such mechanisms as phosphorylation and ubiquitinylation, and a conserved feature of the clock in fungi, flies and mammals is the role that dynamic protein phosphorylation plays in supporting rhythmicity *per se* and setting the clock's period (Hastings *et al.*, 2008).

A good example is the ubiquitously expressed, highly conserved, and multifunctional serine/threonine-phosphorylating CASEIN KINASE 1 (CK1). In mammals both CK1e and CK1d (which are encoded by different genes) complex with and phosphorylate the PER proteins, directing their nuclear localization and stability. In the absence of both enzymes PER cannot be degraded, so the core transcriptional oscillation ceases (Etchegaray *et al.*, 2010; Meng *et al.*, 2010). Pharmacological inhibition of the enzymes slows down the rate of PER degradation, so progressively lengthens the period of the core loop and, thereby, slows down the behavioral activity rhythm. Conversely the gain-of-function *Tau* mutation in CK1e destabilizes PER protein and accelerates the pacemaker to 20 hours in homozygous mice and hamsters (Meng *et al.*, 2008; Lowrey *et al.*, 2000). In humans, mutations in both CK1d and the CK1 binding domain of PER2 are associated with a pronounced sleep disturbance, specifically advanced sleep phase, which is indicative of an accelerated circadian cycle consistent with the observations in rodents (Toh *et al.*, 2001). The importance of CK1-dependent phosphorylation of PER is in its dual roles of licensing nuclear localization and yet also targeting the protein for ubiquitinylation by bTRCP and proteasomal degradation (Eide *et al.*, 2005; Shirogane *et al.*, 2005). In the case of CRY, stability is regulated in part by AMP kinase-mediated phosphorylation, which in turn licenses it for ubiquitinylation by the ligase FBXL3 (Godinho *et al.*, 2007; Lamia *et al.*, 2009). Various pharmacological and genetic manipulations of bTRCP and FBXL3 in mice, SCN and cell cultures can enhance PER and CRY stability, respectively, and thereby lengthen circadian period both *in vitro* and *in vivo* (Hirota *et al.*, 2012).

Casein kinase 2 (CK2) and glycogen synthase kinase 3 (GSK3) are other well-known examples of ubiquitously expressed, multifunctional, highly conserved eukaryotic serine/threonine kinases that, in addition to their other established roles in the biology of the cell, have been shown to play critical roles in determining the cellular localization and/or stability of circadian transcription factors across a wide range of eukaryotes – even though the transcription factors themselves are not conserved (Yin *et al.*, 2006; Hastings *et al.*, 2008; Maier *et al.*, 2009; O'Neill *et al.*, 2011). As might be expected, the role of protein phosphatases, for example, PP1, is equally well conserved (Yang *et al.*, 2004; Gallego *et al.*, 2006; Fang *et al.*, 2007; Schmutz *et al.*, 2011). In the context of the transcriptional/translational feedback loop (TTFL) that has been proposed to account for cellular circadian rhythms, current data support a general model wherein a dynamic interplay between clock protein phosphorylation and de-phosphorylation by these ubiquitous enzymes acts as an interval timer to regulate the kinetics of complex formation, protein degradation and nuclear entry. Certain specific serine/threonine residues on each clock protein substrate are implicated in tipping the balance between degradation and nuclear localization (Reischl and Kramer, 2011).

1.4.2 Metabolic regulation of the transcriptional clockwork

An important question, therefore, is whether the posttranslational mechanisms discussed above are themselves circadian in nature or whether they are constitutively active and modify PER and CRY proteins as these proteins are generated. Although the expression level of most of these enzymes does not appear to be circadian, it remains possible that their activity is controlled in a rhythmic fashion and they act coordinately, as in WNT signaling (Del Valle-Perez et al., 2011), to facilitate rhythmic intracellular localization and degradation of PER and CRY. In support of this possibility is the observation that the phosphorylation status, and therefore activity, of GSK3β is spontaneously rhythmic in cultured fibroblasts (Iitaka et al., 2005). Indeed the ubiquitin ligase FBXL21, which also targets CRY for degradation, is expressed in the SCN with high amplitude (Dardente et al., 2008). Even more intriguing is the fact that the kinase activity of AMPK is itself subject to the ratio of AMP and ADP:ATP in the cell (Oakhill et al., 2011). Thus, the ability of the cell to degrade CRY may vary as a function of the metabolic state of the cell, which in the case of the SCN, with its rhythm of electrical activity, is highly circadian. From this perspective a clock output (metabolic state) can be viewed as a clock input, and thus becomes part of the oscillator mechanism.

More generally it has been observed in several contexts that cellular metabolism is intrinsically rhythmic, for example, in mouse liver in vivo (Kaminsky et al., 1984; Eckel-Mahan et al., 2012; Fustin et al., 2012) and isolated mammalian cells in vitro (Radha et al., 1985; O'Neill and Reddy, 2011). This becomes of particular interest in light of observations that the cell's metabolic state can directly regulate transcription factor activity. For example, the DNA-binding activities of the CLOCK/BMAL1 and NPAS2/BMAL1 complexes is directly regulated by the redox state of nicotinamide adenine dinucleotide (NAD and NADP) cofactors, in vitro (Rutter et al., 2001).

In a still broader context, gene expression at loci bound by many clock gene transcription factors is associated with chromatin remodeling via recruitment of assorted histone methyl- and acetyl-transferases (Etchegaray et al., 2003; Ripperger and Schibler, 2006; Hosoda et al., 2009; Katada and Sassone-Corsi, 2010), all of which are ultimately reliant on the availability of their respective 1- and 2-carbon substrates (S-adenosylmethionine and Acetyl-CoA, respectively). These are generated by primary metabolism, and therefore also probably rhythmic, since intermediates in the pathways that generate them are (Eckel-Mahan et al., 2012). By the same token, the stability of PER2 and activity of BMAL1, are additionally regulated by dynamic lysine acetylation (Asher et al., 2008; Nakahata et al., 2008) and are deacetylated via specific recruitment of deacetylase SIRT1, which also targets histone H3, in an NAD^+-dependent manner. This facilitates the transition to transcriptionally repressive/inactive clock protein complexes later in the circadian cycle, again in a manner dependent on primary metabolism, in this case NAD^+ availability – which is also clock-regulated (Kaminsky et al., 1984; Ramsey et al., 2009). Finally, it is highly significant that several of the identified "clock gene" transcription factors are heme-binding proteins and exhibit reciprocal regulation between rhythmic heme metabolism and the heme protein's redox/ligand status, for example, heme-binding and, thus, activity of the nuclear receptor REV-ERBβ is governed by a redox-sensitive cysteine (Kaasik and Lee, 2004; Gupta and Ragsdale, 2011).

1.4.3 Cause versus effect in circadian transcriptional regulation

There are far more interactions between circadian timekeeping and metabolism than are discussed above; these are covered at length in some excellent reviews (Green et al., 2008; Asher and Schibler, 2011). In the latter, Asher and Schibler make the insight that "the discrimination between metabolic and circadian oscillations may be somewhat arbitrary." At the level of circadian timekeeping in cell culture or organotypic slice, therefore, there is an issue of cause and effect. The prevailing view is that circadian cycles of gene expression drive cellular rhythms of metabolism; however, as much evidence exists to support the contrary view that circadian cycles of metabolism drive rhythms of gene expression.

Certainly overexpression of clock gene transcription factors does not result in a major detriment to cellular timekeeping (Fan et al., 2007; Yamanaka et al., 2007; Asher and Schibler, 2011) and even gene knock-out does not completely abolish time-keeping in SCN slices (Liu et al., 2007; Ko et al., 2010; Maywood et al., 2011). Thus, whilst it is clear that circadian regulation of transcriptional circuits is essential for normal mammalian physiology and rhythmic behavior, at the cellular level rhythmic gene expression cannot be accounted for without delegating the majority of timekeeping function to rhythmic posttranslational regulation of clock protein localization, stability and activity. These are, in turn, determined by rhythmic enzyme activities and metabolic status – many of which are regulated at the level of transcription or translation: Catch 22 – or seemingly so.

1.5 Is the transcriptional clock paramount?

1.5.1 Cytosolic rhythms and the SCN pacemaker

To be effective as a central timekeeper, individual SCN neurons have to synchronize their molecular cycles, one to another and also to the light–dark cycle. When dispersed in cell culture, SCN neurons obviously lose synchrony as expected, but they are also less effective circadian pacemakers than when embedded in the usual SCN circuit – the transcriptional rhythms of individual cells lose amplitude and coherence. This dependence upon coupling is even more marked when the cells lack individual *Per* or *Cry* genes – single gene mutations that do not affect coherence at the level of the SCN ensemble. Clearly, intercellular signaling is a critical aspect not only in synchronizing the SCN cellular transcriptional clocks but also in maintaining them. Consistent with this, interference with electrophysiological signaling by tetrodotoxin (TTX) not only causes SCN neurons to become desynchronized but also to lose amplitude and definition to their transcriptional cycle (Yamaguchi *et al.*, 2003; Maywood *et al.*, 2007). There are several ways in which altering electrical communication across the circuit may affect the transcriptional clockwork. Suppression of action potential firing may alter intracellular Ca^{2+} signaling in both pre- and post-synaptic neurons, which in turn will alter transcriptional activation of *Per* and other genes via their CREs. In addition, the consequently reduced secretion of neuropeptides, including AVP, VIP and GRP, across the SCN will attenuate intracellular cues mediated via their G-protein coupled receptors, dis-regulating, *inter alia*, Ca^{2+}, cAMP and kinase cascades. Again this will compromise CRE-mediated transcription of *Per* and, thereby, undermine the core loops. A clear example of this is seen in mice lacking VIP or its cognate receptor, VPAC2. Not only are they behaviorally arrhythmic, but cellular transcriptional cycles in the SCN are also desynchronized and of low amplitude and coherence. These transcriptional cycles in the mutant SCN can be re-activated by paracrine cues, including AVP and VIP, derived from wild-type SCN grafted onto the mutant slice *in vitro* (Maywood *et al.*, 2011). These peptides act via receptors that activate Gq and Gs signaling respectively, thereby driving Ca^{2+}, cAMP and kinase cascades to "rescue" the transcriptional loop. Under normal circumstances, the core loop drives the circadian rhythms of action potential firing, cAMP and Ca^{2+} levels, neuropeptide synthesis and secretion. Consequently, nontranscriptional outputs of the core loop within the SCN neuron are also its sustaining inputs, acting both within a neuron and between neurons. It can, therefore, be argued that this intercellular coupling is what makes the SCN special as a sustained pacemaker: the first amongst equals (Liu *et al.*, 2007). Whereas bioluminescence recordings of other tissues (perhaps with the exception of the retina) progressively damp out as component, non-communicative cells lose phase coordination, that of the SCN slice will continue indefinitely (literally for many months, subject to an adequate supply of culture medium) with high amplitude and astonishing precision, as cells drive each other in reciprocal dependence. There is also a converse to this paramount competence – when dissociated from each other, SCN neurons may oscillate actually worse than individual fibroblasts do (Liu *et al.*, 2007; Webb *et al.*, 2009). The dependence upon coupling and intracellular signaling is, therefore, hardwired into the SCN as a condition of its pre-eminent role, and thus under contrived experimental conditions the SCN clockwork appears more vulnerable than that of a simple fibroblast.

The interdependence of intercellular cues, signaling cascades and the expression of clock genes blurs the distinction of a core loop. This distinction is further challenged by the observation that pharmacological manipulations of intracellular cAMP levels can change the canonical oscillatory properties of the transcriptional loop: its phase, amplitude and period (O'Neill *et al.*, 2008). The case can be made, therefore, that the "real" pacemaker consists of both transcriptional and cytosolic components that are mutually dependent and act in concert. Some evidence for autonomous function of the cytosolic components comes from studies in *Cry*-null and *Bmal1*-null SCN, where the transcriptional loops are compromised but circadian cycles of *Per*-driven bioluminescence can still be observed in SCN neurons, albeit with shortened period and poor coherence (Ko *et al.*, 2010; Maywood *et al.*, 2011). This suggests that some capacity for cytosolic oscillation: a "cytoscillator," can exist independently of the transcriptional timer. Indeed, when transcription of nascent mRNA is compromised by treatment with alpha-amanitin oleate (a potent transcriptional inhibitor), SCN slices can exhibit at least one and sometimes two further cycles of PER2::LUC- reported bioluminescence (O'Neill *et al.*, 2013).

The possibility of a self-sustained cytosolic clock that normally couples with, but can run in the absence of, cycling clock genes has received further attention following recent observations made using undifferentiated embryonic stem cells (ESCs). ESCs were previously thought not to possess any intrinsic timekeeping because there is is no detectable cycling gene expression until differentiation. Paulose *et al.* report, however, a self-sustained rhythm in ESC glucose uptake prior to, and following, differentiation (Paulose *et al.*, 2012). This again implies the existence of intrinsic timekeeping that is not reliant on any known transcriptional clock mechanism.

These observations reiterate earlier experiments in diverse model organisms that also addressed whether nascent transcription was necessary for cellular timekeeping, the earliest being in the alga *Acetabularia mediterranea*, where circadian rhythms of chloroplast movement persisted when the nucleus of the cell was removed (Sweeney and Haxo, 1961; Woolum, 1991). The landmark observations, however, were performed in the cyanobacteria *Synechococcus elongatus*, a prokaryote. Here it was shown that the approximately 24-hour rhythm of KaiA/B/C protein phosphorylation and complex formation that occurs in living cells, and which normally interacts reciprocally with genome-wide transcriptional regulation (Johnson *et al.*, 2008), could be reconstituted *in vitro* using just the three recombinant proteins (KaiA, B and C) with ATP (Nakajima *et al.*, 2005). Bacterial expression systems tend to work on a 1 protein = > 1 function principle, whilst mammalian proteins tend to possess multiple domains with multiple, context-dependent cellular functions. We therefore think it unlikely that a directly equivalent experiment can be performed for mammalian timekeeping. It does raise the possibility, however, that the smallest functional circadian timekeeping unit in mammals may not include the nucleus.

1.5.2 Totally transcription-free pacemaking

Recently the absolute requirement for nascent gene expression in mammalian cells was investigated *in vitro*. The ultimately cytotoxic effects of chronic inhibition of gene expression often confound pharmacological approaches to this question. To circumvent this, preparations of human red blood cells (which are naturally anucleate) were employed (O'Neill and Reddy, 2011). A rhythmic posttranslational modification of the peroxiredoxin (PRX) family of anti-oxidant proteins, first observed in mouse liver (Reddy *et al.*, 2006), was used as a rhythmic marker. Briefly, the PRX family constitutes a major part of the cellular defense against reactive oxygen species (ROS), specifically H_2O_2, which are an unavoidable byproduct of aerobic metabolism. Erythrocytes express PRX at high levels (approximately 1% total protein), presumably due to the high ROS generation resulting from hemoglobin auto-oxidation. 2-Cys PRXs exist primarily as dimers that catalyze their own oxidation by H_2O_2 at conserved peroxidatic cysteine residues. The resultant sulfenic acid (Cys_P-SOH) may be reduced by a resolving cysteine on the opposing monomer (Cys_P-S-S-Cys_R), and ultimately reduced to the free thiol (SH) by the thioredoxin system. The kinetics of the resolving cysteine attack is quite slow, however, and in the presence of additional H_2O_2 overoxidation to the sulfenic (Cys_P-SO_2H) or even sulfonic (Cys_P-SO_3H) form, occurs (reversible through sulfiredoxin-catalyzed, ATP-dependent mechanisms). By performing anti-2-Cys PRX-$SO_{2/3}$ immunoblots on time-courses of erythrocytes, isolated in a minimal glucose/salt buffer under constant conditions, circadian rhythms of PRX oxidation were observed. These rhythms were temperature-compensated, entrainable by temperature cycles, and (predictably) robust to inhibitors of gene expression. In addition, the concentrations of several cellular metabolites ([ATP], [NADH], [NADPH]) appeared to be rhythmically modulated, as did an indirect fluorescence assay for hemoglobin multimeric state (O'Neill and Reddy, 2011).

As a marker for circadian timekeeping, the PRX oxidation rhythm appears to be highly conserved, being observable in representative organisms from across all three domains of life (Bacteria, Archeaea, Eukaryota), unlike any TTFL component (Edgar *et al.*, 2012). Whilst PRX itself does not appear to play a critical timekeeping role, the redox rhythm it reports persists (albeit perturbed) in organisms that are deficient in "core" TTFL components. It is thus plausible that this remarkable conservation reflects either some underlying and ancient metabolic oscillation, which remains deeply embedded in the cellular machinery, or an evolutionary convergence upon rhythmic redox regulation to facilitate temporal segregation of mutually antagonistic metabolic processes.

1.5.3 A general model for mammalian cellular circadian timekeeping

Nascent transcription (cycling or otherwise) is not required for cellular circadian timekeeping (Tomita *et al.*, 2005; O'Neill *et al.*, 2011) but metabolism and signal transduction are required since they sustain life. In "normal" cells and organisms, however, circadian cycles of gene expression are observed and many of these cycling genes influence cell signaling and metabolism; ultimately facilitating rhythmic control of physiology. The activities of most known clock-relevant transcription factors are reliant upon metabolism and redox state, whereas their localization and stability, and in some cases acute induction, are determined posttranslationally and regulated by intracellular signaling systems. Furthermore, there are many established reciprocal pathways connecting redox balance and cellular metabolism with the activity of the various signaling mechanisms discussed above (Cheong and Virshup, 2011; Dickinson and Chang, 2011; Hardie, 2011; Sethi and Vidal-Puig, 2010; Metallo and Vander Heiden, 2010; Montenarh, 2010; Vander Heiden *et al.*, 2009). In order to integrate these observations into a coherent framework (Fig. 1.4), therefore, we speculate that circadian rhythms in the cytoplasm persist through cyclical,

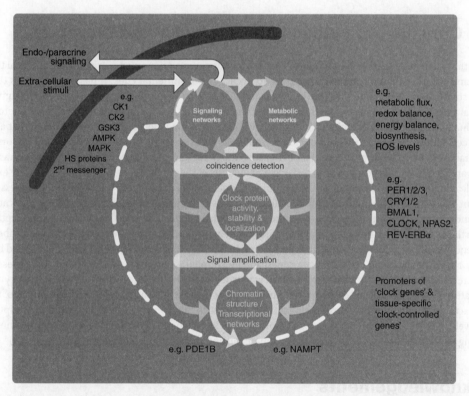

Fig. 1.4 A general model for mammalian cellular circadian timekeeping. Circadian timekeeping is functionally distributed within the cell's metabolic and signaling networks (top level) independently of nascent gene expression. In most (nucleated) cells, however, the integrated output from transcriptional networks (lower level) is manifest in the circadian cycles of protein activity/stability/localization (middle level) observed, for example, in canonical clock protein transcription factors which act as coincidence-detecting substrate effectors for network state. Rhythmically modulated chromatin structure facilitates coordinated temporal regulation of downstream networks of gene expression, including their own cognate clock gene circuitry, resulting in signal amplification. Rhythmic modulation of "clock-controlled genes" facilitates coordinated temporal regulation of physiology, and feeds forward into metabolic/signaling networks (right-hand flow), modulating expression of some component mechanisms, e.g., rhythmic NAMPT expression facilitates rhythmic activity of the NAD+ salvage pathway (Ramsey *et al.*, 2009), PDE1B degrades cAMP and affects rhythmic amplitude (Zhang *et al.*, 2009). The circadian state of the signaling network modulates communication with local and distant targets, whilst selectively and temporally gating the capacity of relevant extracellular signals to affect circadian phase (left-hand flow).

distributed cross-talk between multiple metabolic and signaling networks, with transcriptional clock components acting as coincidence-detecting, substrate effectors. They thereby integrate the state of the network as a whole to coordinate genome-wide temporal, and cell type-specific, programs of gene expression. In this context, irrelevant network perturbations would be ignored but appropriate extracellular cues responded to in a phase-dependent fashion. Rhythmic licensing of transcription, with its slower kinetics, would impart robustness to the "cytoscillator" by rhythmic modulation of component protein/transcript levels. Critically, a rhythmic transcriptional contribution would not be required for oscillator competence but the additional repression of clock protein activity upon its cognate gene and CCGs would facilitate signal amplification. Similarly, rhythmic protein degradation is not required for cellular timekeeping (fibroblast rhythms are relatively insensitive to proteasomal inhibition) (Stratmann *et al.*, 2012) but where present, it would increase the signal-to-noise ratio and amplify any transcriptional/translational contribution to the following cycle (Fig. 1.3). In essence, we suggest that, in contrast to the discreet clock mechanism in cyanobacteria, circadian timekeeping in mammalian (and by inference all eukaryotic) cells is functionally distributed amongst its component systems, which seem to have been coopted into the clock as soon as, or shortly after, they arose evolutionarily (Edgar *et al.*, 2012).

1.6 Conclusion: cytoscillators, clocks and therapies

Since the acceptance that circadian rhythms are truly endogenous phenomena, driven by an internal timing mechanism rather than a response to undefined cyclical environmental cues, it has been obvious that an understanding of their nature and the mechanisms that govern them would provide a deeper insight into normal physiology and behavior, and thus identify new avenues for therapeutic intervention. There have been many surprises as the clock mechanisms have been unraveled; perhaps the greatest being that almost every cell has the potential to act as a circadian oscillator. This revelation brings complexity and opportunity in equal measure to biology and medicine. Because the paradigm of biology for the last decades has been genes and genomes, it is perhaps unsurprising that analysis of the clock mechanism focused on gene expression, leading to the development of the canonical model of TTFLs. Indeed, transcriptional processes are evident at all levels of the mammalian circadian system – from the core feedback loop, to entrainment by gene induction to orchestration of outputs and ultimate physiological rhythms by circadian transcriptomes. Nevertheless, the idea that the cellular environment within which the feedback loops are embedded influences their behavior has gained ground, leading to the view that transcriptional pacemaking and intrinsically rhythmic cytosolic oscillations are inescapably coupled, conferring precision and robustness. The latest revelations of transcription-free clocks in erythrocytes push this model further to show that cytosolic oscillations can exist independently of the nucleus: an echo of work on *Acetabularia* 50 years ago. Given the tractable "drugability" of cytosolic signaling in contrast to the dangers of meddling with transcription, it may well be that elucidation of the cytoscillator will provide the best entry point for future chronotherapies seeking to address diseases with a circadian dimension and, hence, circadian vulnerability (Fig. 1.3).

Acknowledgements

The work of the authors' laboratories is supported by the Medical Research Council (UK) (MC_UP_1201/4) and the Wellcome Trust (Grant 093734/Z/10/Z, JSO'N). The authors are indebted to Mr P. Margiotta, LMB Visual Aids Department, for expert assistance with the figures.

References

Akhtar RA, Reddy AB, Maywood ES, *et al.* 2002. Circadian cycling of the mouse liver transcriptome, as revealed by cDNA microarray, is driven by the suprachiasmatic nucleus. *Curr Biol* **12**: 540–50.
Albrecht U, Sun Z, Eichele G, Lee C. 1997. A differential response of two putative mammalian circadian regulators, mper1 and mper2 to light. *Cell* **91**: 1055–64.

Allada R, White NE, So WV, et al. 1998. A mutant Drosophila homolog of mammalian clock disrupts circadian rhythms and transcription of period and timeless. *Cell* **93**: 791–804.

Aronson BD, Johnson KA, Loros JJ, Dunlap JC. 1994. Negative feedback defining a circadian clock: autoregulation of the clock gene Frq. *Science* **263**: 1578–84.

Asher G, Schibler U. 2011. Crosstalk between components of circadian and metabolic cycles in mammals. *Cell Metab* **13**: 125–37.

Asher G, Gatfield D, Stratmann M, et al. 2008. SIRT1 regulates circadian clock gene expression through PER2 deacetylation. *Cell* **134**: 317–28.

Balsalobre A, Damiola F, Schibler U. 1998. A serum shock induces circadian gene expression in mammalian tissue culture cells. *Cell* **93**: 929–37.

Bliwise DL, Mercaldo ND, Avidan AY, et al. 2011. Sleep disturbance in dementia with Lewy bodies and Alzheimer's disease: a multicenter analysis. *Dement Geriatr Cogn Disord* **31**: 239–46.

Cashmore AR. 2003. Cryptochromes: enabling plants and animals to determine circadian time. *Cell* **114**: 537–43.

Cheong JK, Virshup DM. 2011. Casein kinase 1: Complexity in the family. *Int J Biochem Cell Biol* **43**: 465–9.

Cho H, Zhao X, Hatori M, et al. 2012. Regulation of circadian behavior and metabolism by REV-ERB-alpha and REV-ERB-beta. *Nature* **485**: 123–7.

Crosthwaite SK, Dunlap JC, Loros JJ. 1997. Neurospora wc-1 and wc-2: transcription, photoresponses, and the origins of circadian rhythmicity. *Science* **276**: 763–9.

Dardente H, Mendoza J, Fustin JM, et al. 2008. Implication of the F-Box Protein FBXL21 in circadian pacemaker function in mammals. *PLoS One* **3**: e3530.

Dardente H, Wyse CA, Birnie MJ, et al. 2010. A molecular switch for photoperiod responsiveness in mammals. *Curr Biol* **20**: 2193–8.

DeBruyne JP, Weaver DR, Reppert SM. 2007. CLOCK and NPAS2 have overlapping roles in the suprachiasmatic circadian clock. *Nat Neurosci* **10**: 543–5.

Del Valle-Perez B, Arques O, Vinyoles M, et al. 2011. Coordinated action of CK1 isoforms in canonical Wnt signaling. *Mol Cell Biol* **31**: 2877–88.

Dickinson BC, Chang CJ. 2011. Chemistry and biology of reactive oxygen species in signaling or stress responses. *Nat Chem Biol* **7**: 504–11.

Duffy JF, Cain SW, Chang AM, et al. 2011. Sex difference in the near-24-hour intrinsic period of the human circadian timing system. *Proc Natl Acad Sci USA* **108** (Suppl 3): 15602–8.

Eckel-Mahan KL, Patel VR, Mohney RP, et al. 2012. Coordination of the transcriptome and metabolome by the circadian clock. *Proc Natl Acad Sci USA* **109**: 5541–6.

Edgar RS, Green EW, Zhao Y, et al. 2012. Peroxiredoxins are conserved markers of circadian rhythms. *Nature* **485**: 459–64.

Eide EJ, Woolf MF, Kang H, et al. 2005. Control of mammalian circadian rhythm by CKIepsilon-regulated proteasome-mediated PER2 degradation. *Mol Cell Biol* **25**: 2795–807.

Etchegaray JP, Lee C, Wade PA, Reppert SM. 2003. Rhythmic histone acetylation underlies transcription in the mammalian circadian clock. *Nature* **421**: 177–82.

Etchegaray JP, Yu EA, Indic P, et al. 2010. Casein kinase 1 delta (CK1delta) regulates period length of the mouse suprachiasmatic circadian clock in vitro. *PLoS One* **5**: e10303.

Fan Y, Hida A, Anderson DA, et al. 2007. Cycling of CRYPTOCHROME proteins is not necessary for circadian-clock function in mammalian fibroblasts. *Curr Biol* **17**: 1091–100.

Fang Y, Sathyanarayanan S, Sehgal A. 2007. Posttranslational regulation of the Drosophila circadian clock requires protein phosphatase 1 (PP1). *Genes Dev* **21**: 1506–18.

Field MD, Maywood ES, O'Brien JA, et al. 2000. Analysis of clock proteins in mouse SCN demonstrates phylogenetic divergence of the circadian clockwork and resetting mechanisms. *Neuron* **25**: 437–47.

Fustin JM, Doi M, Yamada H, et al. 2012. Rhythmic nucleotide synthesis in the liver: temporal segregation of metabolites. *Cell Rep* **1**: 341–9.

Gallego M, Kang H, Virshup DM. 2006. Protein phosphatase 1 regulates the stability of the circadian protein PER2. *Biochem J* **399**: 169–75.

Godinho SI, Maywood ES, Shaw L, et al. 2007. The after-hours mutant reveals a role for Fbxl3 in determining mammalian circadian period. *Science* **316**: 897–900.

Green CB, Takahashi JS, Bass J. 2008. The meter of metabolism. *Cell* **134**: 728–42.

Guler AD, Ecker JL, Lall GS, et al. 2008. Melanopsin cells are the principal conduits for rod-cone input to non-image-forming vision. *Nature* **453**: 102–5.

Gupta N, Ragsdale SW. 2011. Thiol-disulfide redox dependence of heme binding and heme ligand switching in nuclear hormone receptor rev-erb{beta}. *J Biol Chem* **286**: 4392–403.

Hardie DG. 2011. AMP-activated protein kinase: an energy sensor that regulates all aspects of cell function. *Genes Dev* **25**: 1895–908.

Hardin PE. 2005. The circadian timekeeping system of Drosophila. *Curr Biol* **15**: R714–22.

Hardin PE, Hall JC, Rosbash M. 1990. Feedback of the *Drosophila* period gene product on circadian cycling of its messenger RNA levels. *Nature* **343**: 536–40.

Hastings JW. 2007. The Gonyaulax clock at 50: translational control of circadian expression. *Cold Spring Harb Symp Quant Biol* **72**: 141–4.

Hastings MH, Duffield GE, Ebling FJ, *et al.* 1997. Non-photic signalling in the suprachiasmatic nucleus. *Biol Cell* **89**: 495–503.

Hastings MH, Reddy AB, Maywood ES. 2003. A clockwork web: circadian timing in brain and periphery, in health and disease. *Nat Rev Neurosci* **4**: 649–61.

Hastings MH, O'Neill JS, Maywood ES. 2007. Circadian clocks: regulators of endocrine and metabolic rhythms. *J Endocrinol* **195**: 187–98.

Hastings MH, Maywood ES, O'Neill JS. 2008. Cellular circadian pacemaking and the role of cytosolic rhythms. *Curr Biol* **18**: R805–15.

Hatfield CF, Herbert J, Van Someren EJ, *et al.* 2004. Disrupted daily activity/rest cycles in relation to daily cortisol rhythms of home-dwelling patients with early Alzheimer's dementia. *Brain* **127**(5): 1061–74.

Hirota T, Lee JW, St John PC, *et al.* 2012. Identification of small molecule activators of cryptochrome. *Science* **337**: 1094–7.

Hogenesch JB, Gu YZ, Jain S, Bradfield CA. 1998. The basic-helix-loop-helix-PAS orphan MOP3 forms transcriptionally active complexes with circadian and hypoxia factors. *Proc Natl Acad Sci USA* **95**: 5474–9.

Hosoda H, Kato K, Asano H, *et al.* 2009. CBP/p300 is a cell type-specific modulator of CLOCK/BMAL1-mediated transcription. *Mol Brain* **2**: 34.

Huang N, Chelliah Y, Shan Y, *et al.* 2012. Crystal structure of the heterodimeric CLOCK:BMAL1 transcriptional activator complex. *Science* **337**: 189–94.

Huang W, Ramsey KM, Marcheva B, Bass J. 2011. Circadian rhythms, sleep, and metabolism. *J Clin Invest* **121**: 2133–41.

Iitaka C, Miyazaki K, Akaike T, Ishida N. 2005. A role for glycogen synthase kinase-3beta in the mammalian circadian clock. *J Biol Chem* **280**: 29397–402.

Johnson CH, Mori T, Xu Y. 2008. A cyanobacterial circadian clockwork. *Curr Biol* **18**: R816–R25.

Kaasik K, Lee CC. 2004. Reciprocal regulation of haem biosynthesis and the circadian clock in mammals. *Nature* **430**: 467–71.

Kaminsky YG, Kosenko EA, Kondrashova MN. 1984. Analysis of the circadian rhythm in energy metabolism of rat liver. *Int J Biochem* **16**: 629–39.

Katada S, Sassone-Corsi P. 2010. The histone methyltransferase MLL1 permits the oscillation of circadian gene expression. *Nat Struct Mol Biol* **17**: 1414–21.

King DP, Zhao Y, Sangoram AM, *et al.* 1997. Positional cloning of the mouse circadian Clock gene. *Cell* **89**: 641–53.

King VM, Chahad-Ehlers S, Shen S, *et al.* 2003. A hVIPR transgene as a novel tool for the analysis of circadian function in the mouse suprachiasmatic nucleus. *Eur J Neurosci* **17**: 822–32.

Knutsson A. 1989. Shift work and coronary heart disease. *Scand J Soc Med Suppl* **44**: 1–36.

Ko CH, Yamada YR, Welsh DK, *et al.* 2010. Emergence of noise-induced oscillations in the central circadian pacemaker. *PLoS Biol* **8**: e1000513.

Koh K, Zheng X, Sehgal A. 2006. JETLAG resets the Drosophila circadian clock by promoting light–induced degradation of TIMELESS. *Science* **312**: 1809–12.

Koike N, Yoo SH, Huang HC, *et al.* 2012. Transcriptional architecture and chromatin landscape of the core circadian clock in mammals. *Science* **338**: 349–54.

Konopka RJ. 1987. Genetics of biological rhythms in *Drosophila*. *Annu Rev Genet* **21**: 227–36.

Kuhlman SJ, Silver R, Le Sauter J, *et al.* 2003. Phase resetting light pulses induce Per1 and persistent spike activity in a subpopulation of biological clock neurons. *J Neurosci* **23**: 1441–50.

Kume K, Zylka MJ, Sriram S, *et al.* 1999. mCRY1 and mCRY2 are essential components of the negative limb of the circadian clock feedback loop. *Cell* **98**: 193–205.

Lamia KA, Sachdeva UM, DiTacchio L, *et al.* 2009. AMPK regulates the circadian clock by cryptochrome phosphorylation and degradation. *Science* **326**: 437–40.

Levi F, Schibler U. 2007. Circadian rhythms: mechanisms and therapeutic implications. *Annu Rev Pharmacol Toxicol* **47**: 593–628.

Liu AC, Welsh DK, Ko CH, *et al.* 2007. Intercellular coupling confers robustness against mutations in the SCN circadian clock network. *Cell* **129**: 605–16.

Loros JJ, Denome SA, Dunlap JC. 1989. Molecular cloning of genes under control of the circadian clock in Neurospora. *Science* **243**: 385–8.

Lowrey PL, Shimomura K, Antoch MP, *et al.* 2000. Positional syntenic cloning and functional characterization of the mammalian circadian mutation tau. *Science* **288**: 483–92.

Maier B, Wendt S, Vanselow JT, *et al.* 2009. A large-scale functional RNAi screen reveals a role for CK2 in the mammalian circadian clock. *Genes Dev* **23**: 708–18.

Maywood ES, Mrosovsky N. 2001. A molecular explanation of interactions between photic and non-photic circadian clock-resetting stimuli. *Brain Res Gene Expr Patterns* **1**(1): 27–31.

Maywood ES, Okamura H, Hastings MH. 2002. Opposing actions of neuropeptide Y and light on the expression of circadian clock genes in the mouse suprachiasmatic nuclei. *Eur J Neurosci* **15**: 216–20.

Maywood ES, O'Neill JS, Chesham JE, Hastings MH. 2007. Minireview: The circadian clockwork of the suprachiasmatic nuclei – analysis of a cellular oscillator that drives endocrine rhythms. *Endocrinology* **148**: 5624–34.

Maywood ES, Chesham JE, O'Brien JA, Hastings MH. 2011. A diversity of paracrine signals sustains molecular circadian cycling in suprachiasmatic nucleus circuits. *Proc Natl Acad Sci USA* **108**: 14306–11.

Mead S, Ebling FJ, Maywood ES, *et al.* 1992. A nonphotic stimulus causes instantaneous phase advances of the light-entrainable circadian oscillator of the Syrian hamster but does not induce the expression of c-fos in the suprachiasmatic nuclei. *J Neurosci* **12**: 2516–22.

Menet JS, Rodriguez J, Abruzzi KC, Rosbash M. 2012. Nascent-Seq reveals novel features of mouse circadian transcriptional regulation. *eLife* **1**: e00011.

Meng QJ, Logunova L, Maywood ES, *et al.* 2008. Setting clock speed in mammals: the CK1epsilontau mutation in mice accelerates circadian pacemakers by selectively destabilizing PERIOD proteins. *Neuron* **58**: 78–88.

Meng QJ, Maywood ES, Bechtold DA, *et al.* 2010. Entrainment of disrupted circadian behavior through inhibition of casein kinase 1 (CK1) enzymes. *Proc Natl Acad Sci USA* **107**: 15240–5.

Messager S, Ross AW, Barrett P, Morgan PJ. 1999. Decoding photoperiodic time through Per1 and ICER gene amplitude. *Proc Natl Acad Sci USA* **96**: 9938–43.

Metallo CM, Vander Heiden MG. 2010. Metabolism strikes back: metabolic flux regulates cell signaling. *Genes Dev* **24**: 2717–22.

Montenarh M. 2010. Cellular regulators of protein kinase CK2. *Cell Tissue Res* **342**: 139–46.

Myers MP, Wager-Smith K, Rothenfluh-Hifiker A, Young MW. 1996. Light-induced degradation of TIMELESS and entrainment of the Drosophila circadian clock. *Science* **85**: 1737–41.

Nagoshi E, Saini C, Bauer C, *et al.* 2004. Circadian gene expression in individual fibroblasts: cell-autonomous and self-sustained oscillators pass time to daughter cells. *Cell* **119**: 693–705.

Nakahata Y, Kaluzova M, Grimaldi B, *et al.* 2008. The NAD+-dependent deacetylase SIRT1 modulates CLOCK-mediated chromatin remodeling and circadian control. *Cell* **134**: 329–40.

Nakajima M, Imai K, Ito H, *et al.* 2005. Reconstitution of circadian oscillation of cyanobacterial KaiC phosphorylation *in vitro*. *Science* **308**: 414–5.

Nuesslein-Hildesheim B, O'Brien JA, Ebling FJ, *et al.* 2000. The circadian cycle of mPER clock gene products in the suprachiasmatic nucleus of the Siberian hamster encodes both daily and seasonal time. *Eur J Neurosci* **12**: 2856–64.

O'Neill JS, Reddy AB. 2011. Circadian clocks in human red blood cells. *Nature* **469**: 498–503.

O'Neill JS, Maywood ES, Chesham JE, *et al.* 2008. cAMP-dependent signaling as a core component of the mammalian circadian pacemaker. *Science* **320**: 949–53.

O'Neill JS, van Ooijen G, Dixon LE, *et al.* 2011. Circadian rhythms persist without transcription in a eukaryote. *Nature* **469**: 554–8.

O'Neill JS, Maywood ES, Hastings MH. 2013. Cellular mechanisms of circadian pacemaking: beyond transcriptional loops. In: *Handbook of Experimental Pharmacology: Circadian Clocks* (eds A Kramer, M Merrow). Springer, pp. 67–103.

Oakhill JS, Steel R, Chen ZP, *et al.* 2011. AMPK is a direct adenylate charge-regulated protein kinase. *Science* **332**: 1433–5.

Obrietan K, Impey S, Smith D, *et al.* 1999. Circadian regulation of cAMP response element-mediated gene expression in the suprachiasmatic nuclei. *J Biol Chem* **274**: 17748–56.

de Paula RM, Vitalini MW, Gomer RH, Bell-Pedersen D. 2007. Complexity of the Neurospora crassa circadian clock system: multiple loops and oscillators. *Cold Spring Harb Symp Quant Biol* **72**: 345–51.

Paulose JK, Rucker EB, 3rd, Cassone VM. 2012. Toward the beginning of time: circadian rhythms in metabolism precede rhythms in clock gene expression in mouse embryonic stem cells. *PLoS One* **7**: e49555.

Preitner N, Damiola F, Lopez-Molina L, *et al.* 2002. The orphan nuclear receptor REV-ERBalpha controls circadian transcription within the positive limb of the mammalian circadian oscillator. *Cell* **110**: 251–60.

Radha E, Hill TD, Rao GH, White JG. 1985. Glutathione levels in human platelets display a circadian rhythm *in vitro*. *Thromb Res* **40**: 823–31.

Ramsey KM, Yoshino J, Brace CS, *et al.* 2009. Circadian clock feedback cycle through NAMPT-mediated NAD+ biosynthesis. *Science* **324**: 651–4.

Reddy AB, Karp NA, Maywood ES, *et al.* 2006. Circadian orchestration of the hepatic proteome. *Curr Biol* **16**: 1107–15.

Reischl S, Kramer A. 2011. Kinases and phosphatases in the mammalian circadian clock. *FEBS Lett* **585**: 1393–9.

Reppert SM, Weaver DR. 2002. Coordination of circadian timing in mammals. *Nature* **418**: 935–41.

Ripperger JA, Schibler U. 2006. Rhythmic CLOCK-BMAL1 binding to multiple E-box motifs drives circadian Dbp transcription and chromatin transitions. *Nat Genet* **38**: 369–74.

Rollag MD, Berson DM, Provencio I. 2003. Melanopsin, ganglion-cell photoreceptors, and mammalian photoentrainment. *J Biol Rhythms* **18**: 227–34.

Rutila JE, Suri V, Le M, *et al.* 1998. CYCLE is a second bHLH-PAS clock protein essential for circadian rhythmicity and transcription of Drosophila period and timeless. *Cell* **93**: 805–14.

Rutter J, Reick M, Wu LC, McKnight SL. 2001. Regulation of clock and NPAS2 DNA binding by the redox state of NAD cofactors. *Science* **293**: 510–4.

Schmutz I, Wendt S, Schnell A, *et al.* 2011. Protein phosphatase 1 (PP1) is a posttranslational regulator of the mammalian circadian clock. *PLoS One* **6**: e21325.

Schurov IL, McNulty S, Best JD, *et al.* 1999. Glutamatergic induction of CREB phosphorylation and Fos expression in primary cultures of the suprachiasmatic hypothalamus *in vitro* is mediated by co-ordinate activity of NMDA and non-NMDA receptors. *J Neuroendocrinol* **11**: 43–51.

Sethi JK, Vidal-Puig A. 2010. Wnt signalling and the control of cellular metabolism. *Biochem J* **427**: 1–17.

Shigeyoshi Y, Taguchi K, Yamamoto S, *et al.* 1997. Light-induced resetting of a mammalian circadian clock is associated with rapid induction of the mPer1 transcript. *Cell* **91**: 1043–53.

Shirogane T, Jin J, Ang XL, Harper JW. 2005. SCFbeta-TRCP controls clock-dependent transcription via casein kinase 1-dependent degradation of the mammalian period-1 (Per1) protein. *J Biol Chem* **280**: 26863–72.

Stratmann M, Suter DM, Molina N, *et al.* 2012. Circadian Dbp transcription relies on highly dynamic BMAL1-CLOCK interaction with E boxes and requires the proteasome. *Mol Cell* **48**: 277–87.

Suter DM, Molina N, Gatfield D, *et al.* 2011. Mammalian genes are transcribed with widely different bursting kinetics. *Science* **332**: 472–4.

Sweeney BM, Haxo FT. 1961. Persistence of a photosynthetic rhythm in Enucleated Acetabularia. *Science* **134**: 1361–63.

Takahashi JS, Shimomura K, Kumar V. 2008. Searching for genes underlying behavior: lessons from circadian rhythms. *Science* **322**: 909–12.

Tei H, Okamura H, Shigeyoshi Y, *et al.* 1997. Circadian oscillation of a mammalian homologue of the Drosophila period gene. *Nature* **389**: 512–6.

Toh KL, Jones CR, He Y, *et al.* 2001. An hPer2 phosphorylation site mutation in familial advanced sleep phase syndrome. *Science* **291**: 1040–3.

Tomita J, Nakajima M, Kondo T, Iwasaki H. 2005. No transcription-translation feedback in circadian rhythm of KaiC phosphorylation. *Science* **307**: 251–4.

Travnickova-Bendova Z, Cermakian N, Reppert SM, Sassone-Corsi P. 2002. Bimodal regulation of mPeriod promoters by CREB-dependent signaling and CLOCK/BMAL1 activity. *Proc Natl Acad Sci USA* **99**: 7728–33.

Ueda HR, Hayashi S, Chen W, *et al.* 2005. System-level identification of transcriptional circuits underlying mammalian circadian clocks. *Nat Genet* **37**: 187–92.

Vander Heiden MG, Cantley LC, Thompson CB. 2009. Understanding the Warburg effect: the metabolic requirements of cell proliferation. *Science* **324**: 1029–33.

van der Horst GT, Muijtjens M, Kobayashi K, *et al.* 1999. Mammalian Cry1 and Cry2 are essential for maintenance of circadian rhythms. *Nature* **398**: 627–30.

Viswanathan AN, Hankinson SE, Schernhammer ES. 2007. Night shift work and the risk of endometrial cancer. *Cancer Res* **67**: 10618–22.

Weaver DR. 1998. The suprachiasmatic nucleus: a 25-year retrospective. *J Biol Rhythms* **13**: 100–12.

Webb AB, Angelo N, Huettner JE, Herzog ED. 2009. Intrinsic, nondeterministic circadian rhythm generation in identified mammalian neurons. *Proc Natl Acad Sci USA* **106**: 16493–8.

Welsh DK, Yoo SH, Liu AC, *et al.* 2004. Bioluminescence imaging of individual fibroblasts reveals persistent, independently phased circadian rhythms of clock gene expression. *Curr Biol* **14**: 2289–95.

Woolum JC. 1991. A re-examination of the role of the nucleus in generating the circadian rhythm in Acetabularia. *J Biol Rhythms* **6**: 129–36.

Wulff K, Gatti S, Wettstein JG, Foster RG. 2010. Sleep and circadian rhythm disruption in psychiatric and neurodegenerative disease. *Nat Rev Neurosci* **11**: 589–99.

Yamaguchi S, Isejima H, Matsuo T, *et al.* 2003. Synchronization of cellular clocks in the suprachiasmatic nucleus. *Science* **302**: 1408–12.

Yamanaka I, Koinuma S, Shigeyoshi Y, *et al.* 2007. Presence of robust circadian clock oscillation under constitutive over-expression of mCry1 in rat-1 fibroblasts. *FEBS Lett* **581**: 4098–102.

Yang Y, He Q, Cheng P, *et al.* 2004. Distinct roles for PP1 and PP2A in the Neurospora circadian clock. *Genes Dev* **18**: 255–60.

Yin L, Wang J, Klein PS, Lazar MA. 2006. Nuclear receptor Rev-erbalpha is a critical lithium-sensitive component of the circadian clock. *Science* **311**: 1002–5.

Yoo SH, Yamazaki S, Lowrey PL, *et al.* 2004. PERIOD2::LUCIFERASE real-time reporting of circadian dynamics reveals persistent circadian oscillations in mouse peripheral tissues. *Proc Natl Acad Sci USA* **101**: 5339–46.

Zhang EE, Liu AC, Hirota T, *et al.* 2009. A genome-wide RNAi screen for modifiers of the circadian clock in human cells. *Cell* **139**: 199–210.

Zheng X, Sehgal A. 2008. Probing the relative importance of molecular oscillations in the circadian clock. *Genetics* **178**: 1147–55.

Molecular Determinants of Human Circadian Clocks

2

Steven A. Brown

Institute of Pharmacology and Toxicology, University of Zürich, Zürich, Switzerland

This book is devoted to an explanation of the circadian clock, how it controls physiology, and the myriad of ways that it could influence health and disease. Much like other mammals, human beings have circadian clocks that are approximately but not exactly 24 hours in periodicity and adjust to the geophysical world principally via light cues. Nevertheless, infinite variations exist within this regime: not only can people be "larks" or "owls", but increasing evidence suggests that timing of specific circadian physiology can be divergent from behavior, with significant consequences for health.

For decades, the properties of the human circadian clock have been probed under strict laboratory conditions in order to understand the basic properties of the biological oscillator that entrains us to our environment. From fundamental experiments like these, basic human circadian properties have emerged that are largely conserved with other mammals: period length can determine the phase of interaction with the environment, with shorter period lengths associated with earlier timing of activity (Duffy *et al.*, 2001; Brown *et al.*, 2008). In the absence of strong external zeitgebers (for example, in blind individuals with no light perception), this clock will "free-run" if significantly different from 24 hours (Lockley *et al.*, 1997), or can entrain to weaker feeding or social timing cues if close to 24 hours (Klerman *et al.*, 1998). Finally, a clock entrained to a particular period length different from its endogenous one can show alterations of this period length for some time afterwards ("aftereffects") (Scheer *et al.*, 2007).

Fascinatingly, however, this consideration of circadian properties within the whole person probably gives only a part of the story. Careful examination of human physiology shows that multiple different timing systems are probably operative. For example, pioneering temporal isolation experiments showed that the circadian rhythm of human body temperature could have a period different from that of activity in the same person (Mills *et al.*, 1974). Similarly, phase relationships between different aspects of human circadian physiology can change according to the environment (Morris *et al.*, 2012). The origin of these observations is likely linked to the fact that *most cells of the human body contain independent cell-autonomous clocks controlling different aspects of circadian physiology*. It is the goal of this chapter to explain current knowledge about this elegant web of clocks and technologies by which they can be measured.

2.1 Molecular elements of human clocks: a brief review

Within mammals, the cell-autonomous mechanism of circadian clocks is almost universally conserved. As described in Chapter 1, it consists principally of interconnected feedback loops of transcription and translation of specialized clock transcription factors. One set of such factors, represented by the homologous factors CLOCK and NPAS2 and their dimerization partner BMAL1 (and possibly BMAL2), serves

---

Circadian Medicine, First Edition. Edited by Christopher S. Colwell.

© 2015 John Wiley & Sons, Inc. Published 2015 by John Wiley & Sons, Inc.

as transcriptional activators at cis-acting E-box elements. Among the genes regulated by these elements are the *Period* and *Cryptochrome* genes (*Per1–3; Cry1–2*), as well as the *Rev-Erb* family of orphan nuclear receptors (*Rev-Erbα and Rev-Erbβ*), encoding transcriptional repressors. The PER and CRY protein products form a protein complex that represses E-box mediated transcription including their own, and the REV-ERB proteins bind to RRE elements to repress the transcription of *Bmal1*, competing with antiphasically expressed RAR-related orphan receptor (ROR) nuclear receptor proteins that bind to the same elements. To delay this feedback process, an elaborate network of posttranscriptional modifications of these factors, including phosphorylation by the casein kinase and glycogen synthase kinase families, as well as regulated acetylation and deacetylation, continues during the day. The result is synchronous oscillations of transcription and protein accumulation in different phases by different classes of clock factors, loosely classified as the "negative limb" and "positive limb" of the circadian clock.

Interestingly, circadian output (i.e., the sum of physiology and behavior controlled by the circadian clock) is also in part regulated directly via the same transcriptional mechanisms. The cis-acting elements that control expression of core clock genes also control the circadian expression of many clock-controlled genes (CCGs) directing various aspects of cellular physiology. These elements include the E-boxes and RAR-related orphan receptor response elements (RREs) described above, and another element called a D-box that binds the antagonistic families of PAR-bZIP transcription factors (DBP/TEF/HLF) and DEC1/2. Most CCGs controlled directly by cellular circadian clocks contain combinations of these elements that fine tune gene expression to a particular phase (Ukai-Tadenuma *et al.*, 2011; Korencic *et al.*, 2012).

A second separate mechanism involves cascades of circadian transcription factors specific for classes of output genes. Such a cascade has been best elucidated in the liver, where some aspects of circadian metabolism are controlled by circadian expression of cytochrome P450 isoforms. Transcriptional control of these genes is directed by a circadian transcription factor, the constitutive androstane receptor (CAR), which in turn is controlled by the PAR-bZIP factors mentioned above (Gachon *et al.*, 2006). A more elaborate description of this cascade is described in Chapter 6.

Recent research strongly suggests that further control of circadian output genes by local cellular oscillators can happen posttranscriptionally. In some aspects, this regulation is probably widespread: in liver, circadian proteome analyses imply that the fraction of proteins showing circadian oscillations in abundance is nearly twice as great as that observed for transcripts (Reddy *et al.*, 2006). Similarly, posttranscriptional regulation of RNA may reinforce the diurnal oscillation of transcription on a global level (Koike *et al.*, 2012; Menet *et al.*, 2012), for example, by diurnal control of the degree of mRNA polyadenlyation (Kojima *et al.*, 2012) or of transcription termination (Padmanabhan *et al.*, 2012). Other posttranscriptional circadian processes may regulate gene expression more locally. For example, circadian control of alternative splicing is probably much more restricted (0.3% of genes by some estimates), and seems to happen in a tissue-specific fashion (McGlincy *et al.*, 2012).

From all of these mechanisms, a total of 10% of genes show circadian expression patterns in any given tissue (Panda *et al.*, 2002; Storch *et al.*, 2002). As described below, however, only a portion of this circadian gene expression is dependent upon local circadian clockwork in these cells. Another part arises from circadian signals from the central clock or the environment perceived directly in peripheral tissues, as is described below and summarized in Fig. 2.1.

2.2 Peripheral and central clocks

Since a separate molecular clockwork is present in most mammalian cells, the question of hierarchy and synchrony among clocks is perforce an important one in understanding circadian physiology. In the case of the "master clock" in the suprachiasmatic nucleus (SCN), which is discussed extensively in Chapter 3, synchrony is assured by coupling of adjacent cellular clocks through both neuropeptidergic and synaptic mechanisms (Granados-Fuentes and Herzog, 2013). To date, little evidence of locally enforced synchrony in peripheral oscillators outside the brain has been unearthed. Instead, these clocks appear to be synchronized by a number of redundant cues. One set of these cues comes via signals from

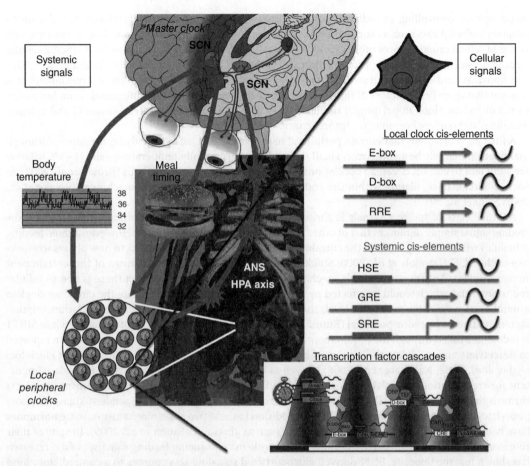

Fig. 2.1 Control of peripheral clocks. One set of signals controlling circadian physiology are systemic signals originating from the SCN or behaviors that it controls. These include meal timing, body temperature fluctuations, and activity of the autonomic nervous system (ANS) and hypothalamic–pituitary–adrenal (HPA) axis. These signals probably act upon clock- and clock-controlled gene expression via systemic cis-elements such as HSEs, GREs, and SREs. A second set of signals arises through local cell-autonomous circadian clocks and controls transcription through clock cis-elements such as E-boxes, D-boxes, and RRE elements. Other signals controlling circadian physiology, and in particular xenobiotic metabolism, arise via transcription factors cascades of PAR-bZIP family members. *(See insert for color representation of the figure.)*

the autonomous nervous system: both parasympathetic and sympathetic signals can be traced multi-synaptically to a number of organs, including thyroid, liver, pancreas, kidney, bladder, spleen, adrenal cortex, and heart (Bartness *et al.*, 2001). Their input influences circadian control of such diverse processes as heart rate (Scheer *et al.*, 2001), glucose homeostasis (Kalsbeek *et al.*, 2004), and corticosterone production (Ishida *et al.*, 2005). Interestingly, not only signals from the master pacemaker in the SCN, but also timing cues from the external world can be transmitted in this fashion. Thus, nighttime light induces *Per1* clock gene expression not only in the SCN via the retinohypothalamic tract (RHT) but also in the adrenal cortex via sympathetic efferents (Ishida *et al.*, 2005). It is currently unclear how widespread this type of photic regulation might be throughout the body.

A second major class of signals comes from hormones. Early landmark experiments in which a transplanted SCN "master clock" encased in porous plastic could rescue circadian behavior showed that diffusible signals played an important role in circadian timing (Silver *et al.*, 1996), even within the brain to control locomotor activity (a topic discussed in Chapter 3). More broadly, several hormones play a direct role in controlling circadian phase in various tissues, including those of the hypothalamic–pituitary–adrenal axis such as corticosteroids, and the pineal hormone melatonin. In experiments with cultured cells, a broad range of other cytokines have also been shown to be capable of influencing cellular circadian oscillators, including prostaglandins (Tsuchiya *et al.*, 2005), endothelin (Yagita *et al.*, 2001), and fibroblast and epidermal growth factors (Akashi and Nishida, 2000). From these experiments, it is thought that three broad classes of signaling pathways are capable of transducing signals from hormones to the circadian clock in peripheral tissues: cAMP and MAP kinases, protein kinase C and calcium signaling, and nuclear hormone receptors (Izumo *et al.*, 2006).

A final class of signals that entrain peripheral tissues is indirect, such as body temperature. Although mammals are largely homeothermic, small daily oscillations in body temperature exist (1–4 °C). These are sufficient to entrain circadian oscillations in both tissues and in cultured cells (Brown *et al.*, 2002), in part via circadian oscillation within the endogenous mammalian heat shock machinery (Reinke *et al.*, 2008; Saini *et al.*, 2012).

Another class of indirect signals is those furnished by feeding. Under normal circumstances, the feeding signal simply reinforces that of other more direct signals from the SCN. However, altered feeding schedules will ultimately result in the entrainment of peripheral circadian clocks to new phases irrespective of the SCN (Damiola *et al.*, 2000; Stokkan *et al.*, 2001). The exact mechanism of this entrainment remains unclear but several plausible mechanisms have been proposed. One of these is tied to cellular redox potential, which would be affected by metabolism and can directly regulate the circadian clock in a number of ways. At a molecular level, the dimerization potential of CLOCK:BMAL1 transcription factors is affected by redox potential (Rutter *et al.*, 2001). Similarly, the activity of the deacetylase SIRT1 is redox-controlled through the requirement for an NAD+ cofactor, and SIRT1 in turn has been reported to deacetylate and modulate the activity of both clock proteins themselves and chromatin at clock loci (Asher *et al.*, 2008; Nakahata *et al.*, 2008), as well as other enzymes such as poly-ADP ribosylase important for transcriptional regulation (Asher *et al.*, 2010). A second independent mechanism likely acts through the actual ratio of ATP/AMP, which controls the activity of AMP-dependent kinase to phosphorylate CRY proteins (Lamia *et al.*, 2009). In addition to these two main mechanisms, some hormones have been proposed to play specific roles as well, such as ghrelin (LeSauter *et al.*, 2009). In spite of their role in glucose metabolism, corticosteroids play no role in transducing feeding signals; in fact, research has shown just the opposite: SCN-derived glucocorticoid signaling acts counter to a contradictory food entrainment signal to slow the pace of re-entrainment (Le Minh *et al.*, 2001).

Another fascinating aspect of feeding signals to the circadian oscillator is food anticipation. In a fashion independent of the known circadian clock (Storch and Weitz, 2009), animals receiving regular feeding stimuli can quickly anticipate these signals (Mistlberger, 2011; Silver *et al.*, 2011).

2.3 Signaling to peripheral circadian clocks

Given the hierarchical organization of circadian oscillators in mammals, it would be logical to imagine a similarly structured cascade of signals controlling the circadian output genes that direct diurnal physiology and behavior – that is, environmental entrainment signals proceed to the "master clock" in the SCN, and then this clock, via the pathways mentioned above, entrains local clocks, which in turn direct circadian physiology. In fact, as foreshadowed above, reality has proven far more complicated … and far more interesting. Genetic disruption of cellular circadian clocks in a single tissue only disrupts a part of circadian gene expression in that tissue. Therefore, one portion of circadian physiology is driven by local cell-autonomous oscillators, and another component is systemically driven by external cues (Lamia *et al.*, 2008). For example, genetic disruption of circadian clocks specifically in liver tissue results in the elimination of 90% of circadian gene expression but another 10% remains rhythmic (Kornmann *et al.*, 2007). Comparable results are observed when clocks are specifically rescued in the brain of a clock-disrupted animal (Hughes *et al.*, 2012). Thus, a certain proportion of circadian gene expression in liver is independent of cell-autonomous clocks in liver cells, and is instead driven by external cues. These cues are likely the very same signals driving the entrainment of peripheral circadian oscillators: signals from the autonomous nervous system, hormones, rhythmic feeding, and body temperature variation. They in turn act upon transcription via independent sets of cis-acting elements, such as heat shock elements (HSEs) (Reinke *et al.*, 2008), glucocorticoid-responsive elements (GREs) (Surjit *et al.*, 2011), and serum-responsive elements (SREs) (Gerber *et al.*, 2013).

Recent experiments suggest that, for some genes, combinations of local and global circadian signals might be operative. Nuclear hormone receptor (NHR)-dependent genes provide an excellent example of such regulation. Circadian NHR-dependent signaling occurs in two principal fashions. The first is conventional: nuclear hormone receptors bind directly to cis-acting elements in target genes, thereby conveying circadian signals either because of diurnal differences in ligand concentrations (e.g., gluco-corticoids, a systemic signal) (Son *et al.*, 2008; Surjit *et al.*, 2011) or because of circadian fluctuation in abundance of the receptors themselves (REV ERBα/β and RORα/γ, local clock-dependent signals) (Guillaumond *et al.*, 2005). Moreover, a second less conventional mode comes via direct binding of PER proteins to nuclear receptors to regulate their activity (Schmutz *et al.*, 2010).

Such binding of clock factors to other proteins to regulate their activity is likely to prove a more general paradigm in the years ahead. For example, the PER proteins have been found to bind to the DBHS (Drosophila Behavior, Human Splicing) family of RNA-binding proteins, where they can regulate not only circadian transcription but also the expression of cell cycle genes in order to confer circadian regulation of the cell cycle (Kowalska *et al.*, 2012, 2013). Similarly, the clock protein REV-ERBα has been shown to bind to the oligophrenin protein at neuronal synapses to affect synaptic structure and function (Valnegri *et al.*, 2011). Overall, the reutilization of clock proteins in roles outside the clockwork itself has proven to be an oft-repeated mechanism, one that is crucial to many different aspects of circadian physiology.

2.4 Human peripheral and central clocks

Although much of the information cited so far about mammalian circadian clocks is derived from animal models, expression studies in human cells suggest that the same mechanisms are operative. For example, human U2OS osteosarcoma cells have been used extensively as a circadian model system, and RNA interference studies in these cells have demonstrated that the same genes important for circadian gene expression in mouse cells are also important in human ones (Maier *et al.*, 2009; Zhang *et al.*, 2009). Likewise, transcriptome-wide circadian expression studies have been conducted from cultured U2OS cells (Hughes *et al.*, 2009) and macrophages (Keller *et al.*, 2009), and additional more limited studies have been conducted in other primary cell types, such as adipocytes (Otway *et al.*, 2011). The overall picture that emerges is very similar to what has been shown in mouse, although circadian amplitude is often lower than *in vivo* and ultradian harmonics of transcription appear less prevalent.

2.5 Human genetics

Probably the best indication of the pertinence to humans of clock mechanisms unearthed in other mammals comes from genetic studies in humans: using families showing altered circadian behavior, multiple clock genes have been identified as playing crucial roles in human clocks. For example, one cause of Familial Advanced Sleep Phase Syndrome (FASPS) has been localized to a mutation in the *Per2* gene that eliminates a phosphorylation site in the encoded protein (Toh *et al.*, 2001). Another functional mutation has been identified in the casein kinase 1δ gene (CKID), whose protein product is one of a family of kinases that phosphorylate PER proteins at multiple positions (Xu *et al.*, 2005). The effects of these mutations, confirmed in cellular and mouse models (Vanselow *et al.*, 2006; Xu *et al.*, 2007), established strongly that one critical mechanism of determining circadian phase in humans is determined by the phosphorylation of "negative limb" proteins, which can either stabilize them or target them for proteasomal degradation.

In addition to familial mutations, a significant number of common polymorphisms in clock genes have been reported to affect circadian function. These include alleles of *Clock* and *Per3*, both conferring delayed phase (Katzenberg *et al.*, 1998; Ebisawa *et al.*, 2001; Archer *et al.*, 2003). For these genes, the circadian functional significance of the identified polymorphisms has been both contested and verified in other studies, so the penetrance of the phenotypes is uncertain. Recently, an additional polymorphism has also been identified near *Per1* that also associates with delayed phase (Lim *et al.*, 2012), and another silent mutation within the coding region that associates with early chronotype (Carpen *et al.*, 2006).

Genetic evidence further suggests that several of the same clock genes that are established as important to circadian function in humans also regulate sleep length via unknown mechanisms. For example, a mutation found in the *Dec2* gene (a transcriptional inhibitor at D-box elements) results in a familial short sleep syndrome (He *et al.*, 2009), while some alleles of the *Clock* gene are associated with longer sleep duration in multiple populations (Allebrandt *et al.*, 2010). Although sleep and circadian function are traditionally regarded as separately regulated phenomena, these human studies – as well as an extensive literature of sleep phenotypes in circadian clock mutant mice – suggest that the two processes are more extensively coregulated than one might suspect (Franken and Dijk, 2009).

2.6 Technologies for measurement of human circadian clocks

As outlined in this chapter, although a basic clock mechanism is present in most cells of the body, the control of circadian physiology and behavior is, in fact, a complex process involving clocks in different tissues. Therefore, in order to understand the impact of clock function upon health and disease, methods are required to analyze basic human circadian properties in different tissues and, to the extent possible, the phase relationship among these tissues.

Classically, human circadian clocks have been measured by prolonged observation of human subjects under controlled laboratory conditions. For example, human clocks can be measured either by putting individuals into a homogenous laboratory environment devoid of timing cues (a "constant routine") (Minors and Waterhouse, 1984) or else by placing them into a rhythmic environment with a period far longer or shorter than the normal 24-h day, so that the human clock cannot adequately adjust, and instead "free-runs" with a period close to its endogenous one (a "forced desynchrony") (Kleitman and Kleitman, 1953). Both of these methods suggest that the human clock usually runs with a period of slightly longer than 24-h (Czeisler *et al.*, 1999; Pagani *et al.*, 2010). Other experiments using light to change circadian phase in human subjects have established that the potential of light to phase-shift the circadian clock varies with time of day, but that there is no prolonged "dead zone" where bright light has no effect (Khalsa *et al.*, 2003). In these experiments, the phase and period of the human circadian clock is usually measured via the timing of the circadian hormone melatonin, or else by circadian variations in body temperature or sleep–wake timing.

Although these experiments have provided virtually all the information that is available about the basic properties of the circadian oscillator, it is also clear that such measurements provide only a partial picture of human circadian physiology. For example, ageing results in a change in phase angle between sleep–wake timing and circadian melatonin expression, suggesting that a complex adjustment of circadian phases within different tissues occurs during the ageing process (Duffy and Czeisler, 2002). Similarly, as already described, it is likely that feeding schedules can influence peripheral clocks in humans as in other animals.

2.7 Cellular methods

Another tool for investigating human circadian clocks at a molecular level involves reporter technologies to look directly at circadian promoter activity in real time. By introducing viral constructs into primary human cells such as fibroblasts, it is possible to obtain measures of circadian period based upon circadian

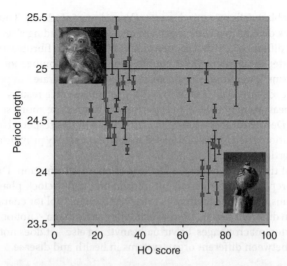

Fig. 2.2 Human owls on average had longer fibroblast circadian periods than larks. Y-axis: fibroblast circadian period length from individuals of self-reported extreme diurnal behavior; X axis: score of these subjects on the Horne–Ostberg morningness–eveningness questionnaire. Similar results were obtained using another questionnaire, the Munch Chronotype Questionnaire (Brown *et al.*, 2008).

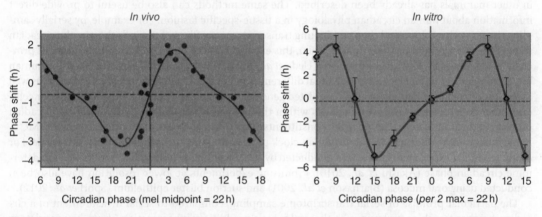

Fig. 2.3 Phase response curves (PRCs) *in vivo* and *in vitro* are qualitatively similar. Left, the phase response curve of human subjects to a single bright light pulse administered at different times of day (Khalsa *et al.*, 2003). X axis, time in hours, adjusted so that the midpoint of melatonin expression is 22 h. Right, the PRC of human fibroblast cells in response to a forskolin pulse to activate cAMP synthesis. X axis, circadian phase in hours, adjusted so that maximum expression of *Per2* occurs at 22 h (Dumas and Brown, unpublished observations). Dotted line, vertical midpoint of phase-shift curve.

oscillations of reporter expression (Brown *et al.*, 2005). From these studies, numerous basic properties of the human circadian oscillator could be confirmed at a molecular level. For example, it could be demonstrated that cells taken from individuals with self-reported early chronotypes ("larks") had on average shorter periods than those with late chronotypes ("owls") (Fig. 2.2). It could also be demonstrated that clock amplitude can have a direct effect upon entrained phase and sensitivity to phase-shifting (Brown *et al.*, 2008). Overall, these studies established that human cell-autonomous circadian clocks in peripheral tissues have very similar properties to those of the central oscillator in the SCN. For example, the phase-response curve (PRC) of human fibroblast cells in response to the adenyl cyclase stimulating agent forskolin nicely resembles the PRC of human clocks in response to light (Fig. 2.3), and mutations that affect human clocks *in vivo* (such as the FASPS mutation described in the previous paragraph) have similar effects upon fibroblast cells measured *in vitro* (Vanselow *et al.*, 2006). Thus, peripheral cells could be useful to identify clock defects in a wide spectrum of diseases, including sleep and mood disorders.

However, one critical difference exists between clocks measured in fibroblasts and those operative in the SCN: whereas the latter show intercellular coupling to maintain homogenous phase, the former lack these coupling mechanisms. Therefore, clock defects are often exaggerated in peripheral tissues relative to the SCN. For example, deletion of CLOCK or CRY proteins in mice results in only small changes in behavior, but *ex vivo* measurements show that peripheral tissues are more severely affected or even completely arrhythmic (DeBruyne *et al.*, 2007; Liu *et al.*, 2007). In this respect, based upon a wide variety of mouse circadian mutations, peripheral cell-based measures probably provide an exaggerated measure of abnormal clock properties (Brown *et al.*, 2005).

A second drawback of this method involves the loss of phase information. During the time required for cell cultivation and reporter introduction, all information about clock phase at the time that cells were removed is lost. Thus, while this method provides a powerful tool for characterizing genetic variations in clock function in different tissues from which cells can be taken – not only skin, but also adipose tissue, muscle, hepatocytes, macrophages, or virtually anything else – it does not provide a way to assess the phase relationships between different organ systems in health and disease.

2.8 Omics-based methods to analyze human clocks

How transcriptome analyses have helped to prove the basic similarity between human clocks and clocks in other mammals has already been described. The same methods can also be useful to provide direct information about human circadian physiology in a tissue-specific fashion. For example, by serially sampling tissues such as blood and then conducting transcriptome profiling of the cells therein, the circadian state of these cells could be determined. So far, this experiment has been conducted as a "proof of principle" using mouse livers with good success (Ueda *et al.*, 2004). However, actual experiments using human blood would likely suffer from interindividual differences not present in genetically identical mice, as well as the low circadian amplitude of clock-regulated gene expression in peripheral blood mononuclear cells, due either to lower synchrony among cells within the population or to lower amplitudes of circadian oscillations in B or T cells, the primary constituents of peripheral blood mononuclear cells (PBMCs). Nevertheless, clear information about human clock phase using this method is certainly attainable. For example, similar experiments have been conducted by serially sampling human hair root follicles to determine circadian phase (Akashi *et al.*, 2010). Promising experiments at lower resolution have also been conducted using oral mucosa (Bjarnason *et al.*, 2001) and suction blister epithelium (Sporl *et al.*, 2012).

The particular promise of serial transcriptome sampling, compared to serial measurement of a circadian hormone such as melatonin, is threefold. Firstly, additional information about key regulatory pathways can be obtained. For example, in the study of suction blister epithelium, pathway analysis permitted identification of the gene *Klf9* as a likely key player in circadian epithelial regulation (Sporl *et al.*, 2012). Secondly, analysis of peripheral gene expression gives a glimpse of peripheral circadian clocks, whereas melatonin is thought to reflect the timing of the central pacemaker in the SCN, whose multisynaptic cues direct melatonin synthesis. Finally, the large number of oscillating substances in different phases in a whole transcriptome could in principle permit single-timepoint identification of circadian phase by comparing levels of transcripts of different levels. So far, however, interindividual differences in transcript levels between different persons have made such analyses difficult: at best, two samplings have permitted phase identification with a precision of two hours (Akashi *et al.*, 2010).

In addition to transcriptome analyses, human metabolomics also offers significant promise for circadian discovery (Dallmann *et al.*, 2012). Like the transcriptome studies, analysis of the human metabolome – the sum of all small-molecule metabolites in a particular tissue or matrix – can allow identification of circadian phase, albeit with the same aforementioned limitations in precision for this type of technology (Minami *et al.*, 2009). In addition, however, metabolite analyses offer the further promise of simultaneous circadian characterizations of a number of different tissues or physiological processes, because various classes of metabolites are byproducts of multiple physiological processes in different tissues (Eckel-Mahan *et al.*, 2012). Finally, circadian metabolomics can be conducted upon easy-to-access matrices, such as saliva (Dallmann *et al.*, 2012) or even breath (Sinues *et al.*, 2013), far less invasive than serial blood sampling.

2.9 Summary and outlook

Doubtless, the technologies outlined above represent only the beginnings of molecular circadian investigations in humans. From pioneering studies of human clock properties, both in the laboratory and in daily life, circadian research has begun to turn to questions of how daily clocks are important to all aspects of human physiology, from mood to metabolism and obesity. These questions are explicitly addressed in subsequent chapters of this book. Because of the complex hierarchy of circadian clocks affecting human physiology, however, the analysis of this question is not as simple as initially hoped. Not only must the question of clock synchrony with the environment be considered – as in the case of jetlag or shiftwork – but also the question of internal clock synchrony and amplitude. These questions are only now being addressed and new noninvasive molecular technologies, including the ones described above, will be critical to these endeavors.

References

Akashi, M. and E. Nishida (2000). Involvement of the MAP kinase cascade in resetting of the mammalian circadian clock. *Genes Dev* **14**(6): 645–649.

Akashi, M., H. Soma, T. Yamamoto, *et al.* (2010). Noninvasive method for assessing the human circadian clock using hair follicle cells. *Proc Natl Acad Sci USA* **107**(35): 15643–15648.

Allebrandt, K.V., M. Teder-Laving, M. Akyol, *et al.* (2010). CLOCK gene variants associate with sleep duration in two independent populations. *Biol Psychiatry* **67**(11): 1040–1047.

Archer, S.N., D.L. Robilliard, D.J. Skene, *et al.* (2003). A length polymorphism in the circadian clock gene Per3 is linked to delayed sleep phase syndrome and extreme diurnal preference. *Sleep* **26**(4): 413–415.

Asher, G., D. Gatfield, M. Stratmann, *et al.* (2008). SIRT1 regulates circadian clock gene expression through PER2 deacetylation. *Cell* **134**(2): 317–328.

Asher, G., H. Reinke, M. Altmeyer, *et al.* (2010). Poly(ADP-ribose) polymerase 1 participates in the phase entrainment of circadian clocks to feeding. *Cell* **142**(6): 943–953.

Bartness, T.J., C.K. Song and G.E. Demas (2001). SCN efferents to peripheral tissues: implications for biological rhythms. *J Biol Rhythms* **16**(3): 196–204.

Bjarnason, G.A., R.C. Jordan, P.A. Wood, *et al.* (2001). Circadian expression of clock genes in human oral mucosa and skin: association with specific cell-cycle phases. *Am J Pathol* **158**(5): 1793–1801.

Brown, S.A., G. Zumbrunn, F. Fleury-Olela, *et al.* (2002). Rhythms of mammalian body temperature can sustain peripheral circadian clocks. *Curr Biol* **12**(18): 1574–1583.

Brown, S.A., F. Fleury-Olela, E. Nagoshi, *et al.* (2005). The period length of fibroblast circadian gene expression varies widely among human individuals. *PLoS Biol* **3**(10): e338.

Brown, S.A., D. Kunz, A. Dumas, *et al.* (2008). Molecular insights into human daily behavior. *Proc Natl Acad Sci USA* **105**(5): 1602–1607.

Carpen, J.D., M. von Schantz, M. Smits, *et al.* (2006). A silent polymorphism in the PER1 gene associates with extreme diurnal preference in humans. *J Hum Genet* **51**(12): 1122–1125.

Czeisler, C.A., J.F. Duffy, T.L. Shanahan, *et al.* (1999). Stability, precision, and near-24-hour period of the human circadian pacemaker. *Science* **284**(5423): 2177–2181.

Dallmann, R., A.U. Viola, L. Tarokh, *et al.* (2012). The human circadian metabolome. *Proc Natl Acad Sci USA* **109**(7): 2625–2629.

Damiola, F., N. Le Minh, N. Preitner, *et al.* (2000). Restricted feeding uncouples circadian oscillators in peripheral tissues from the central pacemaker in the suprachiasmatic nucleus. *Genes Dev* **14**(23): 2950–2961.

DeBruyne, J.P., D.R. Weaver and S.M. Reppert (2007). Peripheral circadian oscillators require CLOCK. *Curr Biol* **17**(14): R538–539.

Duffy, J.F. and C.A. Czeisler (2002). Age-related change in the relationship between circadian period, circadian phase, and diurnal preference in humans. *Neurosci Lett* **318**(3): 117–120.

Duffy, J.F., D.W. Rimmer, and C.A. Czeisler (2001). Association of intrinsic circadian period with morningness-eveningness, usual wake time, and circadian phase. *Behav Neurosci* **115**(4): 895–899.

Ebisawa, T., M. Uchiyama, N. Kajimura, *et al.* (2001). Association of structural polymorphisms in the human period3 gene with delayed sleep phase syndrome. *EMBO Rep* **2**(4): 342–346.

Eckel-Mahan, K.L., V.R. Patel, R.P. Mohney, *et al.* (2012). Coordination of the transcriptome and metabolome by the circadian clock. *Proc Natl Acad Sci USA* **109**(14): 5541–5546.

Franken, P. and D.J. Dijk (2009). Circadian clock genes and sleep homeostasis. *Eur J Neurosci* **29**(9): 1820–1829.

Gachon, F., F.F. Olela, O. Schaad, *et al.* (2006). The circadian PAR-domain basic leucine zipper transcription factors DBP, TEF, and HLF modulate basal and inducible xenobiotic detoxification. *Cell Metab* **4**(1): 25–36.

Gerber, A., C. Esnault, G. Aubert, *et al.* (2013). Blood–Borne Circadian Signal Stimulates Daily Oscillations in Actin Dynamics and SRF Activity. *Cell* **152**(3): 492–503.

Granados-Fuentes, D. and E.D. Herzog (2013). The clock shop: Coupled circadian oscillators. *Exp Neurol* **243**:21–27.

Guillaumond, F., H. Dardente, V. Giguere, and N. Cermakian (2005). Differential control of Bmal1 circadian transcription by REV-ERB and ROR nuclear receptors. *J Biol Rhythms* **20**(5): 391–403.

He, Y., C.R. Jones, N. Fujiki, *et al.* (2009). The transcriptional repressor DEC2 regulates sleep length in mammals. *Science* **325**(5942): 866–870.

Hughes, M.E., L. DiTacchio, K.R. Hayes, *et al.* (2009). Harmonics of circadian gene transcription in mammals. *PLoS Genet* **5**(4): e1000442.

Hughes, M.E., H.K. Hong, J.L. Chong, *et al.* (2012). Brain-specific rescue of Clock reveals system-driven transcriptional rhythms in peripheral tissue. *PLoS Genet* **8**(7): e1002835.

Ishida, A., T. Mutoh, T. Ueyama, *et al.* (2005). Light activates the adrenal gland: timing of gene expression and glucocorticoid release. *Cell Metab* **2**(5): 297–307.

Izumo, M., T.R. Sato, M. Straume, and C.H. Johnson (2006). Quantitative analyses of circadian gene expression in mammalian cell cultures. *PLoS Comput Biol* **2**(10): e136.

Kalsbeek, A., S. La Fleur, C. Van Heijningen, and R.M. Buijs (2004). Suprachiasmatic GABAergic inputs to the paraventricular nucleus control plasma glucose concentrations in the rat via sympathetic innervation of the liver. *J Neurosci* **24**(35): 7604–7613.

Katzenberg, D., T. Young, L. Finn, *et al.* (1998). A CLOCK polymorphism associated with human diurnal preference. *Sleep* **21**(6): 569–576.

Keller, M., J. Mazuch, U. Abraham, *et al.* (2009). A circadian clock in macrophages controls inflammatory immune responses. *Proc Natl Acad Sci USA* **106**(50): 21407–21412.

Khalsa, S.B., M.E. Jewett, C. Cajochen, and C.A. Czeisler (2003). A phase response curve to single bright light pulses in human subjects. *J Physiol* **549**(Pt 3): 945–952.

Kleitman, N. and E. Kleitman (1953). Effect of non-twenty-four-hour routines of living on oral temperature and heart rate. *J Appl Physiol* **6**(5): 283–291.

Klerman, E.B., D.W. Rimmer, D.J. Dijk, *et al.* (1998). Nonphotic entrainment of the human circadian pacemaker. *Am J Physiol* **274**(4 Pt 2): R991–996.

Koike, N., S.H. Yoo, H.C. Huang, *et al.* (2012). Transcriptional architecture and chromatin landscape of the core circadian clock in mammals. *Science* **338**(6105): 349–354.

Kojima, S., E.L. Sher-Chen, and C.B. Green (2012). Circadian control of mRNA polyadenylation dynamics regulates rhythmic protein expression. *Genes Dev* **26**(24): 2724–2736.

Korencic, A., G. Bordyugov, R. Kosir, *et al.* (2012). The interplay of cis-regulatory elements rules circadian rhythms in mouse liver. *PLoS One* **7**(11): e46835.

Kornmann, B., O. Schaad, H. Bujard, *et al.* (2007). System-driven and oscillator-dependent circadian transcription in mice with a conditionally active liver clock. *PLoS Biol* **5**(2): e34.

Kowalska, E., J.A. Ripperger, D.C. Hoegger, *et al.* (2013). NONO couples the circadian clock to the cell cycle. *Proc Natl Acad Sci USA* **110**(5): 1592–1599.

Kowalska, E., J.A. Ripperger, C. Muheim, *et al.* (2012). Distinct roles of DBHS family members in the circadian transcriptional feedback loop. *Mol Cell Biol* **32**(22): 4585–4594.

Lamia, K.A., K.F. Storch and C.J. Weitz (2008). Physiological significance of a peripheral tissue circadian clock. *Proc Natl Acad Sci USA* **105**(39): 15172–15177.

Lamia, K.A., U.M. Sachdeva, L. DiTacchio, *et al.* (2009). AMPK regulates the circadian clock by cryptochrome phosphorylation and degradation. *Science* **326**(5951): 437–440.

Le Minh, N., F. Damiola, F. Tronche, *et al.* (2001). Glucocorticoid hormones inhibit food-induced phase-shifting of peripheral circadian oscillators. *EMBO J* **20**(24): 7128–7136.

LeSauter, J., N. Hoque, M. Weintraub, *et al.* (2009). Stomach ghrelin-secreting cells as food-entrainable circadian clocks. *Proc Natl Acad Sci USA* **106**(32): 13582–13587.

Lim, A.S., A.M. Chang, J. M. Shulman, *et al.* (2012). A common polymorphism near PER1 and the timing of human behavioral rhythms. *Ann Neurol* **72**(3): 324–334.

Liu, A.C., D.K. Welsh, C.H. Ko, *et al.* (2007). Intercellular coupling confers robustness against mutations in the SCN circadian clock network. *Cell* **129**(3): 605–616.

Lockley, S.W., D.J. Skene, J. Arendt, *et al.* (1997). Relationship between melatonin rhythms and visual loss in the blind. *J Clin Endocrinol Metab* **82**(11): 3763–3770.

Maier, B., S. Wendt, J.T. Vanselow, *et al.* (2009). A large-scale functional RNAi screen reveals a role for CK2 in the mammalian circadian clock. *Genes Dev* **23**(6): 708–718.

McGlincy, N.J., A. Valomon, J.E. Chesham, *et al.* (2012). Regulation of alternative splicing by the circadian clock and food related cues. *Genome Biol* **13**(6): R54.

Menet, J.S., J. Rodriguez, K.C. Abruzzi and M. Rosbash (2012). Nascent-Seq reveals novel features of mouse circadian transcriptional regulation. *Elife* **1**: e00011.

Mills, J.N., D.S. Minors and J.M. Waterhouse (1974). Proceedings: Dissociation between different components of circadian rhythms in human subjects deprived of knowledge of time. *J Physiol* **236**(1): 51P–52P.

Minami, Y., T. Kasukawa, Y. Kakazu, *et al.* (2009). Measurement of internal body time by blood metabolomics. *Proc Natl Acad Sci USA* **106**(24): 9890–9895.

Minors, D.S. and J.M. Waterhouse (1984). The use of constant routines in unmasking the endogenous component of human circadian rhythms. *Chronobiol Int* **1**(3): 205–216.

Mistlberger, R.E. (2011). Neurobiology of food anticipatory circadian rhythms. *Physiol Behav* **104**(4): 535–545.

Morris, C.J., D. Aeschbach, and F.A. Scheer (2012). Circadian system, sleep and endocrinology. *Mol Cell Endocrinol* **349**(1): 91–104.

Nakahata, Y., M. Kaluzova, B. Grimaldi, *et al.* (2008). The NAD + -dependent deacetylase SIRT1 modulates CLOCK-mediated chromatin remodeling and circadian control. *Cell* **134**(2): 329–340.

Otway, D.T., S. Mantele, S. Bretschneider, *et al.* (2011). Rhythmic diurnal gene expression in human adipose tissue from individuals who are lean, overweight, and type 2 diabetic. *Diabetes* **60**(5): 1577–1581.

Padmanabhan, K., M.S. Robles, T. Westerling, and C. J. Weitz (2012). Feedback regulation of transcriptional termination by the mammalian circadian clock PERIOD complex. *Science* **337**(6094): 599–602.

Pagani, L., E.A. Semenova, E. Moriggi, *et al.* (2010). The physiological period length of the human circadian clock in vivo is directly proportional to period in human fibroblasts. *PLoS One* **5**(10): e13376.

Panda, S., M.P. Antoch, B.H. Miller, *et al.* (2002). Coordinated transcription of key pathways in the mouse by the circadian clock. *Cell* **109**(3): 307–320.

Reddy, A.B., N.A. Karp, E.S. Maywood, *et al.* (2006). Circadian orchestration of the hepatic proteome. *Curr Biol* **16**(11): 1107–1115.

Reinke, H., C. Saini, F. Fleury-Olela, *et al.* (2008). Differential display of DNA-binding proteins reveals heat-shock factor 1 as a circadian transcription factor. *Genes Dev* **22**(3): 331–345.

Rutter, J., M. Reick, L.C. Wu and S.L. McKnight (2001). Regulation of clock and NPAS2 DNA binding by the redox state of NAD cofactors. *Science* **293**(5529): 510–514.

Saini, C., J. Morf, M. Stratmann, *et al.* (2012). Simulated body temperature rhythms reveal the phase-shifting behavior and plasticity of mammalian circadian oscillators. *Genes Dev* **26**(6): 567–580.

Scheer, F.A., G.J. Ter Horst, J. van Der Vliet, and R.M. Buijs (2001). Physiological and anatomic evidence for regulation of the heart by suprachiasmatic nucleus in rats. *Am J Physiol Heart Circ Physiol* **280**(3): H1391–1399.

Scheer, F.A., K.P. Wright, Jr, R.E. Kronauer, and C.A. Czeisler (2007). Plasticity of the intrinsic period of the human circadian timing system. *PLoS One* **2**(8): e721.

Schmutz, I., J.A. Ripperger, S. Baeriswyl-Aebischer, and U. Albrecht (2010). The mammalian clock component PERIOD2 coordinates circadian output by interaction with nuclear receptors. *Genes Dev* **24**(4): 345–357.

Silver, R., J. LeSauter, P.A. Tresco, and M.N. Lehman (1996). A diffusible coupling signal from the transplanted suprachiasmatic nucleus controlling circadian locomotor rhythms. *Nature* **382**(6594): 810–813.

Silver, R., P.D. Balsam, M.P. Butler, and J. LeSauter (2011). Food anticipation depends on oscillators and memories in both body and brain. *Physiol Behav* **104**(4): 562–571.

Sinues, P.M., M. Kohler, and R. Zenobi (2013). Monitoring diurnal changes in exhaled human breath. *Anal Chem* **85**(1): 369–373.

Son, G.H., S. Chung, H.K. Choe, *et al.* (2008). Adrenal peripheral clock controls the autonomous circadian rhythm of glucocorticoid by causing rhythmic steroid production. *Proc Natl Acad Sci USA* **105**(52): 20970–20975.

Sporl, F., S. Korge, K. Jurchott, *et al.* (2012). Kruppel-like factor 9 is a circadian transcription factor in human epidermis that controls proliferation of keratinocytes. *Proc Natl Acad Sci USA* **109**(27): 10903–10908.

Stokkan, K.A., S. Yamazaki, H. Tei, *et al.* (2001). Entrainment of the circadian clock in the liver by feeding. *Science* **291**(5503): 490–493.

Storch, K.F., O. Lipan, I. Leykin, *et al.* (2002). Extensive and divergent circadian gene expression in liver and heart. *Nature* **417**(6884): 78–83.

Storch, K.F. and C.J. Weitz (2009). Daily rhythms of food-anticipatory behavioral activity do not require the known circadian clock. *Proc Natl Acad Sci USA* **106**(16): 6808–6813.

Surjit, M., K.P. Ganti, A. Mukherji, *et al.*(2011). Widespread negative response elements mediate direct repression by agonist-liganded glucocorticoid receptor. *Cell* **145**(2): 224–241.

Toh, K.L., C.R. Jones, Y. He, *et al.* (2001). An hPer2 phosphorylation site mutation in familial advanced sleep phase syndrome. *Science* **291**(5506): 1040–1043.

Tsuchiya, Y., I. Minami, H. Kadotani ,and E. Nishida (2005). Resetting of peripheral circadian clock by prostaglandin E2. *EMBO Rep* **6**(3): 256–261.

Ueda, H.R., W. Chen, Y. Minami, *et al.* (2004). Molecular-timetable methods for detection of body time and rhythm disorders from single-time-point genome-wide expression profiles. *Proc Natl Acad Sci USA* **101**(31): 11227–11232.

Ukai-Tadenuma, M., R.G. Yamada, H. Xu, *et al.* (2011). Delay in feedback repression by cryptochrome 1 is required for circadian clock function. *Cell* **144**(2): 268–281.

Valnegri, P., M. Khelfaoui, O. Dorseuil, *et al.* (2011). A circadian clock in hippocampus is regulated by interaction between oligophrenin-1 and Rev-erbalpha. *Nat Neurosci* **14**(10): 1293–1301.

Vanselow, K., J.T. Vanselow, P.O. Westermark, *et al.* (2006). Differential effects of PER2 phosphorylation: molecular basis for the human familial advanced sleep phase syndrome (FASPS). *Genes Dev* **20**(19): 2660–2672.

Xu, Y., Q.S. Padiath, R.E. Shapiro, *et al.* (2005). Functional consequences of a CKIdelta mutation causing familial advanced sleep phase syndrome. *Nature* **434**(7033): 640–644.

Xu, Y., K.L. Toh, C.R. Jones, *et al.* (2007). Modeling of a human circadian mutation yields insights into clock regulation by PER2. *Cell* **128**(1): 59–70.

Yagita, K., F. Tamanini, G.T. van Der Horst, and H. Okamura (2001). Molecular mechanisms of the biological clock in cultured fibroblasts. *Science* **292**(5515): 278–281.

Zhang, E.E., A.C. Liu, T. Hirota, *et al.* (2009). A genome-wide RNAi screen for modifiers of the circadian clock in human cells. *Cell* **139**(1): 199–210.

The Suprachiasmatic Nucleus (SCN): Critical Points

3

Christopher S. Colwell[1], Paul Witkovsky[2,3], and Rae Silver[3]

[1] Laboratory of Circadian and Sleep Medicine, Department of Psychiatry and Biobehavioral Sciences, University of California Los Angeles, Los Angeles, CA, USA
[2] Department of Neuroscience and Physiology, New York University, New York, NY, USA
[3] Silver Neurobiology Laboratory, Department of Psychology, Columbia University, New York, NY, USA

3.1 SCN is site of master circadian pacemaker in mammals

One of the fundamental goals of neuroscience research is to link specific brain regions to specific functions. While in many cases this goal has proven elusive, an overwhelming body of evidence shows that the suprachiasmatic nuclei (SCN) of the anterior hypothalamus are the site of the master circadian pacemaker in mammals (Fig. 3.1). Whole books have been devoted to describing this evidence (Klein et al., 1991); this body of literature will not be restated here. To briefly lay out the argument, if the SCN is destroyed, the circadian patterning of behaviors (activity, sleep, drinking), hormones (melatonin, cortisol) and other physiological parameters (body temperature, heart rate) are lost forever (Moore and Eichler, 1972; Stephan and Zucker, 1972; Rusak, 1977; Klein and Moore, 1979). The SCN are rhythmic in vivo, as determined by extracellular recording of action potential frequency as well as metabolically, as measured with ^{14}C-2-deoxyglucose (Schwartz et al., 1987; Newman et al., 1992), with peak activity occurring in the day regardless of whether the organism is nocturnal or diurnal. In an elegant set of experiments, Inouye and Kawamura (1979) recorded rhythms in neural activity in the SCN and a motor control region (striatum) in vivo. They then surgically isolated the SCN from the rest of the brain. When they resumed the recordings, the SCN region continued to show a circadian rhythm with high neural activity during the day whereas the striatum lost the daily pattern. The ability of the SCN to generate rhythms in the frequency of action potentials when the tissue is isolated in a brain slice has been demonstrated many times and has become a standard preparation in the field (Green and Gillette, 1982; Groos and Hendriks, 1982; Shibata et al., 1982).

Finally, the SCN can be transplanted from one animal to another and this transplanted tissue will both restore rhythmicity (Drucker-Colin et al., 1984; Sawaki et al., 1984; Lehman et al., 1987; DeCoursey and Buggy, 1989) and determine the cycle length of the behavioral rhythm in the host organism (Ralph et al., 1990). To provide a striking example, Silver and colleagues restored rhythmicity in a wild-type (WT) hamster with the cycle length of the behavioral rhythm determined by the genotype of the donor tissue (Silver et al., 1996). This restoration of rhythmic behavior occurred even when the SCN was encased in

Circadian Medicine, First Edition. Edited by Christopher S. Colwell.

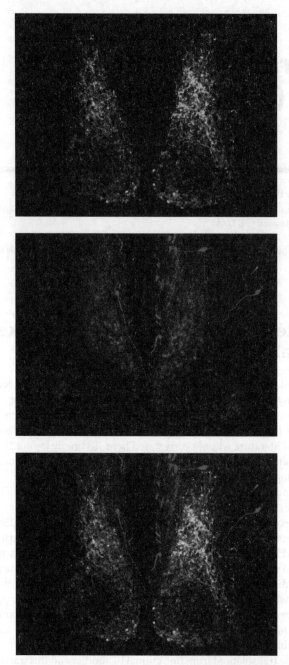

Fig. 3.1 The SCN is the master circadian clock in mammals. Neural cell populations within the SCN are defined by the expression of neuropeptides. The top panel shows expression of the peptide vasoactive intestinal peptide (VIP, green). The cell bodies of these neurons are located close to the optic chiasm. These neurons then project to the more dorsal cell populations and outward toward the subparaventrical zone (sPVZ) and other targets. The middle panel shows expression of the peptide arginine vasopressin (AVP, red). The bottom panel shows the merged image with yellow indicating the area of co-expression. The data are collected from adult male C57 mice using the technique of immunohistochemistry. The data are courtesy of Dr T. Kudo. *(See insert for color representation of the figure.)*

a polymer that blocked neural outgrowth for the implanted tissue. Together, this compelling body of work allows us to conclude that the SCN is the master circadian clock in mammals and provides a level of confidence for a localization of function which is unusual in the nervous system.

3.2 SCN receives photic information through a specialized light detection pathway

Light is the most potent environmental cue for the circadian system, predictably adjusting the phase of the circadian system through synchronization of the SCN clock. Even in visually blind animals, light and dark can also have a direct effect on behavior, apparently through an SCN-mediated circuit. In each case, the light signal is detected by specialized intrinsically photosensitive retinal ganglion cells (ipRGCs) containing melanopsin. This photopigment is most sensitive to blue/green wavelengths but is relatively insensitive to red shifted fluorescent lighting. The ipRGCs are both directly light sensitive and receive information from rods and cones (Panda, 2007; Ecker *et al.*, 2010; Lall *et al.*, 2010). These ipRGCs thus encode ambient lighting (Berson, 2003) and generate action potentials that travel down the retinohypothalamic tract (RHT) and innervate the SCN. In fact, the SCN was first described by laboratories that used tract tracing techniques to follow anatomical projections along the RHT from the eye to the hypothalamus (Hendrickson *et al.*, 1972; Moore and Lenn, 1972). More recent work has elaborated these initial studies (Canteras *et al.*, 2011; Chen *et al.*, 2011; Morin 2013). This intimate association between photoreceptors and the circadian clock, as demonstrated by the monosynaptic connection between photoreceptive ipRGCs and the SCN, is one of special features of this timing system.

The fundamental role of the RHT is to signal the onset of daytime to the SCN, resetting its cycle to local daytime. When animals are placed in complete darkness, this "dawn" signal is lacking and animals revert to an intrinsic circadian rhythm. At dawn, the spiking activity of the RHT increases, thus providing SCN neurons with a wakeup call signaling onset of day. Additionally, light signals that are presented during the nighttime have the potential to reset the clock: signals arriving in early night delay the clock; those arriving near the end of night advance the clock.

The RHT terminals release glutamate and, under certain conditions, the neuropeptide PACAP (Ding *et al.*, 1994; Hannibal *et al.*, 2002). During the night, SCN neurons are normally silent but they do respond to photic stimulation transduced by ipRGCs to generate action potentials up to 20Hz (Meijer *et al.*, 1998; Irwin and Allen, 2007). This light-induced increase in neural activity drives synaptic communication with the rest of the cells in the circuit. The retinal recipient cells use GABA and peptide transmitters such as gastrin-releasing peptide (GRP) and vasoactive intestinal peptide (VIP) to communicate with the rest of the circuit. The impact of GRP and VIP is to produce long term increases (lasting hours) in excitability in SCN neurons (Gamble *et al.*, 2011; LeSauter *et al.*, 2011; Kudo *et al.*, 2013). These changes in electrical activity also trigger intracellular signaling cascades in SCN neurons.

RHT stimulation during the night and the resulting increase in the frequency of action potentials produce a robust increase in Ca^{2+} in SCN neurons. In dendrites, the Ca^{2+} influx is likely mediated by NMDA receptors, with a major contribution from the NR2B subunit (Wang *et al.*, 2008), whereas in the cell body the L-type voltage sensitive Ca^{2+} channels are the main contributor (Irwin and Allen, 2007). The concentration of intracellular Ca^{2+} in neurons is tightly controlled by various channels, pumps and buffers. In addition, ryanodine receptors have a role in mediating the effects of light- and glutamate-induced phase delays of the circadian system (Ding *et al.*, 1998) and in regulation of the electrical activity of SCN neurons (Aguilar-Roblero *et al.*, 2007). Thus, RHT-evoked Ca^{2+} influx within SCN neurons is likely to be a major transducer of light information to the circadian system.

The signal transduction events following the influx of Ca^{2+} induced by RHT stimulation during the night are beginning to be understood and include a number of signaling pathways (Antle *et al.*, 2009; Golombek and Rosenstein, 2010). The specific roles of each pathway in regulating the molecular clockwork however, are not yet clear, although there is evidence that the relative importance of each signaling cascade may vary between early and late night (Gillette and Mitchell, 2002). There is no doubt that other signaling pathways are also involved and that the role of phosphatase cascades in counterbalancing these kinase cascades has not been adequately examined in the SCN. The kinase signaling pathways converge on cyclic AMP response element binding protein (CREB) phosphorylation at Ser133 and Ser142 (Ginty et al., 1993; Ding et al., 1997; Gau et al., 2002; Tischkau et al., 2003). For example, transgenic mice in which phosphorylation at Ser142 cannot take place (Gau et al., 2002) or that express a CREB repressor (Lee et al., 2010) show attenuated light-induced gene expression in the SCN and a reduced behavioral response to light exposure. Phosphorylated CREB is translocated into the nucleus, where it binds to cyclic AMP response elements (CREs) that act on the promoter regions of Per1 and Per2 (Travnickova-Bendova et al., 2002). The net result is an increase in Per1 and Per2 mRNA and protein that occurs within the SCN network over the next couple of hours (Yan and Silver, 2002, 2004). This suggests that increasing the transcription of Period genes in the early night delays the molecular clockwork, whereas increasing the transcription of these genes in the late night speeds up the beginning of the next cycle, although this has not been explicitly tested (see also Chapter 1).

3.3 SCN neurons are endogenous single cell oscillators that generate rhythms in neural activity

A unique property of central clock neurons and one that is essential to the function of the circadian timing system is the ability to generate circadian rhythms in electrical activity. The SCN has been shown to generate neural activity rhythms in vivo (Inouye and Kawamura, 1979; Meijer et al., 1998; Nakamura et al., 2008), in brain slice preparations (Schaap et al., 2003), and in cell cultures made from SCN tissue (Welsh et al., 1995; Herzog et al., 1998; Honma et al., 1998). These findings are consistent with the idea that many SCN neurons are stable, self-sustained oscillators that have the intrinsic capacity to generate circadian rhythms in electrical activity (Fig. 3.2). Regardless of whether the animal is diurnal or nocturnal in terms of behavior, cells in the SCN are electrically active in the day and show circadian rhythms in action potential firing rates, with peaks of around 6–10 Hz in the middle of the day (Kuhlman and McMahon, 2006; Colwell, 2011). Even when isolated from the circuit, single SCN neurons can exhibit a rhythm in firing rate, with most estimates placing the number of SCN neurons that exhibit such a rhythm at about 60–70% of the total SCN neuron population (Aton et al., 2005; Webb et al., 2009). Individual neurons do not appear to spend a full 12 hours firing action potentials, however; it is estimated that single neurons may be active for 4–6 hours per day (VanderLeest et al., 2007; Meijer et al., 2010). In this electrically active state, the neurons do not respond strongly to excitatory stimulation but do respond to synaptic input that reduces their firing. During the night, the cells are electrically inactive and are most responsive to excitatory or depolarizing stimulation.

Given that SCN neurons generate action potentials in the absence of synaptic drive, they can, therefore, be considered endogenously active neurons. To maintain spontaneous activity, a set of intrinsic currents must interact to depolarize the cell membrane to threshold, elicit an action potential, and return the membrane to negative potentials from which the next spike can be initiated. This "spontaneous" firing arises from specific combinations of intrinsic membrane currents (Bean, 2007). Some progress has been made in identifying the specific ion channels that drive spontaneous activity in the SCN (Colwell, 2011). Conceptually, it can be useful to divide the ionic mechanisms into: firstly, currents that are responsible for providing the excitatory drive required for all spontaneously active neurons; secondly, currents that translate this excitatory drive into a regular pattern of action potentials; and thirdly, currents that are responsible for the nightly silencing of firing due to the hyperpolarization of the membrane.

The best evidence that the molecular clockwork in the SCN can drive the rhythms in electrical activity – and, by extension, in behavior and physiology – comes from several studies that have explored the impact of mutations in the core clockwork on electrical activity rhythms recorded in the SCN (Fig. 3.2). The Tau (casein kinase 1ε) mutation in hamsters shortens the period of wheel-running activity and neural activity rhythms (Liu et al., 1997). Similarly, homozygote Clock mutant mice are behaviorally arrhythmic, whereas heterozygote animals show lengthened behavioral rhythms, findings that are

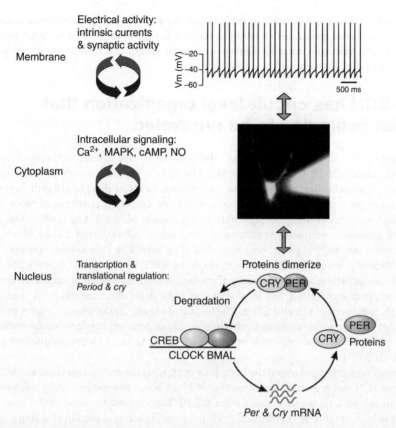

Fig. 3.2 SCN neurons generate rhythms of neural activity that peak in the day. The neural activity regulates Ca²⁺ as well as other signaling pathways via voltage-sensitive currents and the release of neurotransmitters. In the SCN, and perhaps other neurons, many of these signaling networks, including Ca²⁺ and cAMP, nitric oxide (NO), casein kinases and ras-dependent (MAP) kinases, are strongly rhythmic in levels and activity. The balance between the activity of kinases and phosphatases at the end of these pathways regulates the transcription and translation of genes. Finally, within many cells in the body, a transcription/translational negative feedback loop drives rhythms in gene expression. At the beginning of the cycle, CLOCK and BMAL1 protein complexes bind DNA at specific promoter regions (E-box) to activate the transcription of a family of genes including the *Period* (*Per1/Per2/Per3*) and Cryptochrome (*Cry1/Cry2*) genes. The levels of the *Per* and *Cry* transcripts reach their peak during mid to late day while the PER and CRY proteins peak in the early night. The PERs, CRYs, and other proteins form complexes that translocate back into the nucleus and turn off the transcriptional activity driven by CLOCK–BMAL1 with a delay (due to transcription, translation, dimerization, nuclear entry). The proteins would be degraded by ubiquitation, allowing the cycle to begin again. Thus, in its simplest form, many cells contain this molecular feedback loop that regulates the rhythmic transcription of a number of genes. Other feedback loops within the cells serve to contribute to the precision and robustness of the core oscillation. In the nervous system, many of the genes involved in control of excitability and secretion are rhythmically regulated by this molecular feedback loop. To produce a functional cellular oscillator within SCN neurons, there must be reciprocal signaling between membrane, cytosolic, and nuclear processes. Figure adapted from Colwell, 2011.

paralleled by physiological recordings from the SCN (Herzog *et al.*, 1998; Nakamura *et al.*, 2002). Furthermore, *Cry1/2* double mutants show behavioral arrhythmicity and loss of rhythms in SCN neural activity (Albus *et al.*, 2002). These findings suggest that clock gene rhythms are translated into daily patterns of action potential activity in the SCN. Together, these studies provide clear evidence that the molecular clockwork can drive neural activity as an output. It is not yet understood how these ion channels are regulated by the molecular clockwork and it must be emphasized that this is a major gap in our knowledge. To date, the data support two general conclusions: (i) multiple ionic mechanisms exist for controlling SCN neuronal spike rates and may be specific to subpopulations of SCN neurons; (ii) at least some ionic channels exhibit circadian rhythms in expression and function, illustrating that SCN neuronal excitability is under circadian control.

3.4 The SCN has circuit level organization that is just beginning to be unraveled

While SCN neurons are single cell pacemakers, their properties are strongly influenced by circuit level organization (Liu *et al.*, 2007; Welsh *et al.*, 2010). The SCN is divisible into functional compartments based on three principal criteria: the location of terminal fields of diverse afferent inputs (Leak and Moore, 2001), the presence or absence of high amplitude circadian rhythms of clock gene/protein expression, electrical activity and phosphorylation (Hamada *et al.*, 2001; Lee *et al.*, 2003) and the peptide content of individual neurons (Abrahamson and Moore, 2001). Using these criteria, researchers have distinguished two SCN regions: core and shell (Fig. 3.3). The core region contains the neurons receiving the strongest input from the retina through the RHT. Core neurons express the peptides VIP, GRP, calbindin, somatostatin and neurotensin. Core neurons exhibit low amplitude rhythms in electrical activity or clock gene expression but they do show light-dependent increases in the expression of *Period 1* and *Period 2* genes (Yan and Silver, 2002; Hamada *et al.*, 2004). These sensory processing ventral cells exhibit relatively low amplitude rhythms in clock gene expression. Mathematical modeling supports the concept that low amplitude rhythms are easier to reset to environmental perturbations (Pulivarthy *et al.*, 2007).

The larger shell region wraps around the core, thus occupying the dorsal aspects of the SCN from anterior to posterior SCN and extending to the ventral SCN surface at the borders of the nucleus. Neurons in the shell region exhibit a diminished input from the RHT, compared to those of the core region. Shell neurons express high amplitude rhythms of clock gene oscillation and electrical activity. Shell neurons express the peptides arginine vasopressin (AVP), angiotensin II and met-enkephalin (Abrahamson and Moore, 2001). Some progress has been made in understanding why the dorsomedial shell region is the earliest to turn on in the daily cycle of rhythmic activity. This SCN area is known to have a high concentration of AVP+ neurons as well as the co-expression of a regulator of G-protein activity (RGS16). In the early day, this cell population is the first to exhibit activation of clock gene expression, which then spreads like a wave throughout the rest of the SCN circuit (Doi *et al.*, 2011). In mice lacking this regulator, both rhythmic gene expression and cAMP-dependent processes were attenuated, including activation of extracellular signal-regulated kinase (ERK) and c-Fos expression. These data provide a rationale for understanding why the dorsomedial zone is uniquely constituted to initiate the daily cycle of activity. Given the importance of cAMP to intracellular signaling within SCN neurons, the idea that the timing of responsiveness of the cAMP pathway is under local control is intriguing.

Track tracing studies suggest that the core projects massively to the shell, whereas the reverse projection is sparse (Leak and Moore, 2001). While careful fluorescent microscopy finds evidence for abundant and reciprocal contacts between the SCN cell populations (Romijn *et al.*, 1997), this method does not prove the presence of synapses. When core and shell regions of SCN are separated surgically and then cultured, the shell region rapidly loses its ability to maintain circadian rhythmicity (Yamaguchi *et al.*, 2003). Complementary studies on intact hamster demonstrated that small lesions that destroyed the core region but spared the shell abolished multiple rhythms of behavior and physiology (Kriegsfeld *et al.*, 2004). These experiments indicate that signaling from the core to the shell is required to maintain synchronicity among the individual SCN neurons.

There are conditions in which the SCN has to exhibit plasticity in its function. Perhaps the best studied example is the response to changes in the photoperiod, that is, the number of hours of daylight in a 24-h cycle. In response to the changes in day length that occur over the course of the year, many animals undergo strong alterations in their anatomy, physiology, and behavior. Migratory and seasonal breeding organisms provide dramatic examples of photoperiod-driven changes in behavior and physiology. For

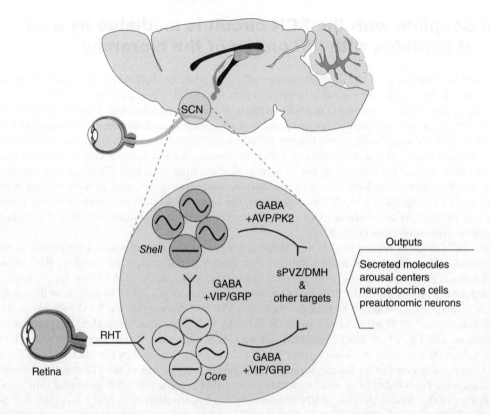

Fig. 3.3 Schematic of SCN circuit responsible for circadian behavior. (A) The SCN is small nucleus of perhaps 10,000 neurons located in the anterior hypothalamus. It is located immediately dorsal to optic chiasm and receives a direct projection from the retina known as the retinohypothalamic track (RHT). (B) Broadly speaking, anatomical studies generally support the division of the SCN into at least two subdivisions including a ventrolateral (Core) and dorsomedial (Shell). The Core neurons are thought to act as an integrator of external input, receiving light information from RHT as well as modulatory information from the thalamus and midbrain structures such as the Raphe nucleus. The outputs of both the Core and Shell SCN largely travel to other hypothalamic regions including the sPVZ and the dorsal medial hypothalamus. These hypothalamic relay nuclei send projections throughout the central nervous system and endocrine system, providing multiple pathways by which the SCN can convey temporal information to the brain and body. The HPA axis and the autonomic nervous system are strongly rhythmic. At least some of the Shell neurons are neurosecretory cells that rhythmically release signaling molecules including AVP into the third ventricle. Within this general framework, many questions remain about cellular communication and anatomical organization. Figure adapted from Colwell, 2011.

many seasonal breeders, a long duration of melatonin is equivalent to winter while a short duration of melatonin is the cue for summer. The SCN plays an important role in the seasonal encoding processes, including driving the duration of the melatonin signal. The electrical activity profile of the SCN is also strongly altered under influence of long and short days, as shown by *in vivo* recordings of the SCN, or by *in situ* analysis of clock gene expression (Brown and Piggins, 2009; Meijer *et al.*, 2010). The peak width appears to serve as an internal representation of the length of the day. The electrical activity and gene expression profiles become compressed (narrow peak) in short days, and decompressed (broad peak) in long days. Importantly, the photoperiod-driven changes in the SCN waveform and activity patterns are maintained for weeks even when the animal is released back into constant conditions. Photoperiod changes primarily the phase distribution but not the duration of electrical activity within individual cells. Even in humans, the numbers of AVP-expressing neurons in the SCN vary seasonally, being higher during autumn compared to late spring/early summer (Kalsbeek *et al.*, 2010). Thus, photoperiodic-driven changes in circadian rhythmicity provide a clear example of plasticity within the SCN circuit.

3.5 Coupling with the SCN circuit is mediated by a set of peptides with VIP on top of the hierarchy

Although SCN neurons are circadian pacemakers that can generate rhythms in neural activity in isolation from other neurons, they normally function as part of a circuit. These neurons communicate via the binding, by postsynaptic neurons, of peptides released by presynaptic terminals. Transfer of information may occur at anatomically defined synapses, but may also result from diffusion of the neuroactive substance to multiple target cells, a mechanism called paracrine signaling. Whatever the mechanism of information transfer, release of peptides and synaptic communication between cells in the SCN circuit appears to be critical for rhythms in neural activity. For example, treating SCN slices with botulinum toxin A or dynasore to block exocytosis or endocytosis compromises circadian gene expression as measured by PER2::LUC (Deery *et al.*, 2009). Similarly, the targeted deletion of secretory vesicle proteins IA-2 and IA-2β alters the rhythms in a variety of circadian outputs, including SCN neural activity and clock gene expression (Kim *et al.*, 2009).

Most SCN neurons release GABA, and blocking synaptic transmission would be expected to block this signaling; however, some studies indicate that GABA is not critical for coupling the circadian oscillations in gene expression between neurons (Aton *et al.*, 2006). Rather, GABA may function to actually reduce the synchrony of the SCN cell population (Freeman *et al.*, 2013). In fact, most data suggest that SCN neurons are coupled by peptides including VIP and its receptor VIPR2 (Vosko *et al.*, 2007). Mice deficient in VIPR2 exhibit low amplitude PER2::LUC rhythms that resemble those seen with the application of TTX, which blocks neuronal spiking (Maywood *et al.*, 2006). Importantly, this loss of amplitude in the molecular clockwork in the VIPR2 KO mice was "rescued" by the addition of media high in K$^+$ that broadly depolarizes the membrane. This suggests that one role of the VIP may be to maintain the membrane potential of SCN neurons within a range that is consistent with molecular timekeeping. In support of this model, the loss of VIPR2 results in the hyperpolarization of the membrane of SCN neurons (Pakhotin *et al.*, 2006). So, the effect of treatments that block synaptic transmission within the SCN can be rationalized by assuming that they are blocking peptide signaling between SCN neurons.

In one of the more interesting studies in this area, Maywood, Hastings and colleagues used a co-culture technique in which a circadian deficient "host" SCN slice carrying a bioluminescence reporter (PER2::LUC) is coupled with nonreporter "graft" SCN (Maywood *et al.*, 2011). They demonstrate that paracrine signaling is sufficient to restore cellular synchrony and amplitude of clock gene expression in SCN circuits lacking VIP. By combining pharmacological with genetic manipulations, the author's data convincingly show that a hierarchy of neuropeptidergic signals underpins this communication, with a dominant role for VIP along with AVP and GRP. This peptide signaling was sufficiently powerful to maintain circadian gene expression even in an arrhythmic Cry-null SCN. Thus, neuropeptidergic signals determine key cellular and circuit-level properties of circadian clockwork in the SCN (Fig. 3.4).

3.6 SCN outputs

The finding that molecular circadian oscillators are widely distributed throughout the body has completely changed the conversation about the nature of SCN output (Fig. 3.5). Conceptually, the SCN is now thought of as the central clock which sits at the apex of a hierarchy of oscillators found in each of the major organ systems (Dibner *et al.*, 2010). When speaking of "SCN output," we are really talking about potentially distinct processes. Firstly, how the SCN synchronizes these different oscillators found throughout the body has to be considered. The local tissue-specific molecular oscillators would regulate the transcription/translation of key genes that are components of locally important gene networks (see also Chapters 1 and 2). The molecular clockwork appears to be reset by a large number of signaling pathways. At least when isolated in culture, circadian oscillators appear to be synchronized by anything that gives a strong kick to the cAMP signaling cascade. Secondly, broadly speaking, the nervous system makes use of both the autonomic nervous system (ANS) and the endocrine systems to regulate the body.

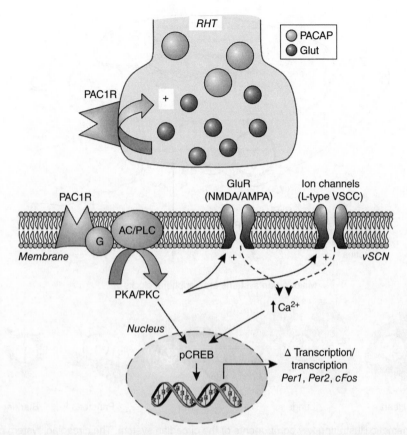

Fig. 3.4 Schematic of RHT/SCN synaptic connection illustrating the signaling events between the release of neurotransmitters and the transcriptional/translational regulation of *Per1*. The intrinsically photosensitive melanopsin-expressing retinal ganglion cells (ipRGC) encode ambient lighting and generate action potentials that travel down the RHT and innervate the SCN. The RHT terminals release glutamate and, under certain conditions, the neuropeptide pituitary adenylate cyclase activating peptide (PACAP). The glutamate release is detected by both AMPA and NMDA glutamate receptors (GluR). GluR induced membrane depolarization can be amplified by intrinsic voltage gated ion channels like the L-type calcium (Ca^{2+}) channel. The net result of RHT stimulation is an increase in firing rate and Ca^{2+} increase in SCN neurons. A number of signaling pathways are then activated and apparently converge to alter transcriptional and/or translational regulators, including CREB. Phosphorylated CREB is translocated into the nucleus where it can bind to CREs that in the promoter regions of *Per1* and *Per2* and drives transcription of these genes over the course of hours. *(See insert for color representation of the figure.)*

As discussed below, the SCN circuit directly regulates the temporal patterning of ANS function as well as the secretion of critical hormones. Finally, the SCN circuit drives the temporal patterning of key behaviors such as activity, sleep and the consumption of food through polysynaptic connections. These critical CNS-driven behaviors have broad impact on most processes in the body. Thus, the SCN circuit uses a variety of outputs to provide temporal patterning and partitioning of key biological processes found throughout the body.

3.6.1 SCN neurons are directly neurosecretory cells

The SCN is adjacent to the third ventricular space and some of its neurons are directly neurosecretory. One study estimated that as many as 35 neuropeptides are being rhythmically secreted into the cerebral spinal fluid (Kramer *et al.*, 2005), thereby potentially gaining access to the central nervous

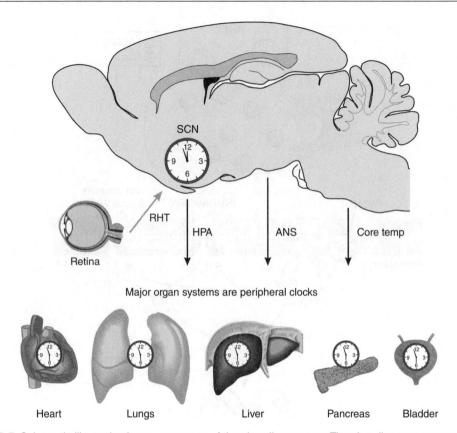

Fig. 3.5 Schematic illustrating key components of the circadian system. The circadian system consists of a network of circadian oscillators. The central clock is located in the SCN. Neurons in this cell population receive light information from ipRGCs found in the retina. The axons of these ganglion cells make a direct synaptic connection onto cells in the SCN. These SCN neurons integrate this photic information with other timing cues to generate robust circadian oscillations that are synchronized to the environment. Signals from the SCN travel out via the hypothalamic–pituitary–adrenal (HPA) axis, the autonomic nervous system (ANS) as well as through the SCN regulation of core body temperature to coordinate and regulate the independent circadian oscillations found throughout the body.

system. Mass spectrometry-based discovery of circadian peptides also indicates that numerous peptides are released from the SCN over circadian time and following retinal stimulation (Hatcher *et al.*, 2008). Perhaps the best example of the role of SCN as a neurosecretory structure comes from the case of AVP. AVP is a well-known regulator of blood pressure in the periphery where it is sometimes described as the "antidiuretic hormone." In the CNS, less is known about this peptide's function, although is it clear that the concentration of AVP in the cerebrospinal fluid varies with a daily cycle that peaks in the morning. This rhythm is abolished by SCN lesions (Schwartz and Reppert, 1985). AVP is also released from the SCN rhythmically in culture (Earnest and Sladek, 1986). While the rhythm in secretion is presumably driven by action potential dependent secretory mechanisms, there is also evidence that the molecular clock regulates the transcription of AVP as the CLOCK/BMAL complex activates AVP expression through E-boxes in the promotor region (Jin *et al.*, 1999). While the function of AVP rhythms as a SCN output is still unclear, recent work has refocused attention on the role of AVP within the SCN circuit itself. For example, mice lacking AVP receptors actually reset faster to changes in the light/dark cycle and by this measure can be viewed as "resistant to jet lag" (Yamaguchi *et al.*, 2013).

3.6.2 Body temperature rhythms as an output

At first thought, the idea that body temperature rhythms could be an important timing cue for organisms that homeostatically regulate body temperature appears counterintuitive. Still there is some good evidence that is at least consistent with this possibility. Firstly, mammals undergo a daily rhythm in body temperature with perhaps a two degree difference from peak to trough. This rhythm is SCN-regulated through neural connections between the SCN and the hypothalamic preoptic nucleus responsible for body temperature homeostasis. In addition, by gating activity and arousal levels, the SCN partitions most physical activity to daytime hours for diurnal animals, a mechanism which would also influence body temperature. Even though the circadian period is temperature compensated, the phase of circadian oscillations in cultured fibroblasts and other peripheral tissues can be entrained by temperature (Brown *et al.*, 2002; Buhr *et al.*, 2010). While the mechanisms are not yet clearly understood, the role of heat shock proteins (Buhr *et al.*, 2010) as well as thermosensitive transient receptor potential (TRP) channels has been suggested. While it is not yet clear whether body temperature is an output that can influence behavior and gene expression, the observation that people have a strong tendency to fall asleep during the falling phase of the body temperature cycle is at least suggestive (Wright *et al.*, 2002). Therefore, there is support for the model that body temperature is one of the systemic timing cues used by the SCN to align peripheral clocks. These systemic cues would need to be adjusted by local cues to allow the range of phases in oscillations observed throughout the body.

3.6.3 SCN regulates the autonomic nervous system

The ANS consists of circuitry that controls the body's physiology and is broadly under circadian regulation (Kalsbeek *et al.*, 2006). Autonomic adjustments are often fast and work in the background to maintain homeostasis. The day/night cycle is a major challenge to homeostasis but the circadian regulation of the ANS and endocrine systems allows the body to anticipate daily perturbations. There are three divisions to the ANS: the sympathetic (SNS), parasympathetic (PSNS), and enteric nervous system. The classic example for sympathetic function has been the "fight or flight" response, in which the body is quickly prepared for intense activity. More broadly, the SNS prepares the body for energy use, and thus sympathetic tone is normally higher during the active portion of the daily cycle. In contrast, the PSNS is organized to prepare the body for energy conservation and repair functions. The parasympathetic tone is normally higher during sleep. While less is known about the temporal patterning of the enteric nervous system, there is good reason to suspect that this branch is also regulated by the circadian network.

The general organization of the ANS includes the preganglionic neurons found in the CNS with cell bodies mostly located in brain stem and spinal cord. These neurons project to a cell population of autonomic ganglia located between the CNS and the targets in the periphery. This organization gives rise to flexible and tonically active circuitry that can respond to homeostatic challenges. The circadian system can regulate this circuit at more than one location. Firstly, the SCN sends neural connections to the hypothalamic paraventricular nucleus (PVN), where the preganglionic neurons are located. Anatomical studies have provided evidence that the PVN receives VIP-positive innervation from the SCN. It is believed that this pathway enables the SCN to broadly modulate the balance between SNS and PSNS. The SCN gates complementary endocrine output, such as the strong circadian regulation of the hypothalamic–pituitary–adrenal (HPA) axis, as well as secretion of hormones like melatonin.

3.6.4 Melatonin is a key hormone under circadian regulation

Melatonin is one of the strongest outputs of the circadian system and the increase in melatonin under dim light conditions in the evening has been found to be a useful marker for the phase of the human rhythm (Chapter 2). Whether the species is diurnal or nocturnal, melatonin levels are high during the night and low during the day. The rhythms observed under natural conditions are driven by a combination of circadian regulation along with acute light-induced suppression of levels of this hormone. Both the acute and circadian regulation are mediated by the SCN, which controls the synthesis and release of this

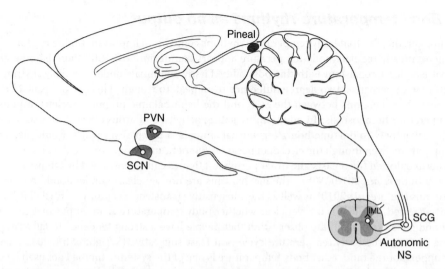

Fig. 3.6 Circadian regulation of the pineal gland. The synthesis and secretion of melatonin is one of the best understood pathways by which the SCN can regulate the secretion of a hormone. Light is detected in the retina by an array of photoreceptors. The light information is transmitted through ipRGC which project to the SCN. Neurons from the SCN (likely both VIP and AVP+) project to the paraventricular nucleus (PVN) which in turn project to the intermediolateral cell column of the thoracic cord (IML). The IML innervates sympathetic neurons in the superior cervical ganglion (SCG) which directly innervate the pineal. In humans, the pineal is located centrally in the brain causing the philosopher Descartes to suggest it might be the "seat of the soul". Figure modified from Moore, 1996.

hormone through a multisynaptic pathway (Fig. 3.6). In humans and other mammals, the pineal production of melatonin is a driven output. The pineal still has a molecular clock that gates transcription (Nishide *et al.*, 2014) but this clock is not directly tied to the production of rhythmic melatonin. A great deal is known about the control of melatonin synthesis and secretion due to pioneering work of Drs Axelrod and Klein at the US National Institutes of Health, which used the noradrenergic regulation of melatonin as a test case to understand how neurotransmitters regulate hormone secretion. For his work on catecholamine neurotransmitters, Dr Axelrod was honored with the Nobel Prize in Physiology or Medicine in 1970. In nonmammalian vertebrates, the pineal is itself a circadian oscillator that plays a critical role in the regulation of behavior and the SCN (Cassone and Menaker, 1984).

Circadian signals, which control the pattern of melatonin synthesis and other aspects of pineal function, originate in the SCN. As described above, light acts to reset the clock on a daily basis through the ipRGCs and also acutely regulate the output from the SCN to the pineal gland. The pathway from the SCN to the pineal gland passes through the PVN, down the brain stem and the spinal cord to the sympathetic intermediolateral cell column in the upper thoracic segments of the spinal cord. From there, nerve fibers project to the cervical sympathetic trunk to innervate neurons in the superior cervical ganglion (SCG). Projections from the SCG travel to the pineal gland (Klein 1985; Møller and Baeres, 2002). Anyone who wants to argue for intelligent design should consider this pathway. In mammals, the pineal gland is in the center of the brain and located close to the hypothalamus. From an engineering point of view, there could be a short, direct pathway connecting the SCN with this circadian target. Instead, the circuit controlling melatonin goes from the hypothalamus to the peripheral nervous system before heading back inside the CNS to innervate the pineal. From a mammalian-centric point of view, this pathway is needlessly complicated. From a broader perspective, this circuit makes evolutionary sense since in nonmammalian vertebrates the pineal is outside of the CNS and sits on top of the skull as the "third eye".

In the pineal, the enzyme in the melatonin synthesis pathway that exhibits a large daily rhythm is arylalkylamine N-acetyltransferase (Aanat) (Klein, 2007), which converts serotonin to the melatonin precursor, N-acetylserotonin. This enzyme has been extensively studied because of its essential role in controlling melatonin synthesis. Its activity is controlled in all vertebrates through posttranslational phosphorylation driven by the timed release of norephinephrine. In addition to Aanat, expression of the gene encoding the cofactor synthesizing enzyme Mat2a (methionine adenosyltransferase 2a) increases at night (Kim *et al.*, 2005). Melatonin production is low during the day because both Aanat activity and Mat2a are low. At night, the situation changes, and N-acetylserotonin is converted to melatonin. In this manner, the whole melatonin biosynthetic pathway is rhythmic through the temporal control of one key enzyme and a cofactor. The other components of the pathway do not appear to be rhythmic. Melatonin signaling is detected by two classes of high affinity G-protein coupled receptors (MT1; MT2) (Dubocovich, 2007; Slominski *et al.*, 2012). The melatonin receptors are widely distributed in the CNS, heart, endocrine and immune system, where their activation has been reported to have wide ranging effects. The nightly surge in melatonin levels likely aids in mediating entrainment of other peripheral tissues.

3.6.5 HPA axis is another important endocrine network regulated by the circadian system

While cortisol may be best known as a marker of acute stress, the glucocorticoid (GC) hormones are well known to be secreted with a daily rhythm that peaks before the start of the activity cycle. Lesions of the SCN cause the loss of these rhythms, which are not restored by transplantation of SCN tissue. Transneuronal and retrograde viral tracing shows multisynaptic pathways between the SCN and the adrenal glands (Buijs *et al.*, 1999, 2003). The SCN regulation of the HPA axis is thought to be a critical output of the circadian system, as gluctocorticoids regulate both peripheral organs as well as many CNS structures. For example, there has been a great deal of work examining the impact of cortisol on neural structure and physiology in the hippocampus and other brain regions (McEwen, 2007). Surprisingly, the SCN are one of the few brain regions that do not express GC receptors. The circadian regulation of the HPA axis is covered in detail in Chapter 6.

3.6.6 The SCN regulates the arousal of the central nervous system

The SCN regulates the major CNS arousal centers (see Chapter 5). The circadian system controls the timing of arousal through the regulation of electrical activity in a network of neurotransmitter systems including noradrenergic (locus coeruleus), serotonergic (raphe), dopaminergic (ventral tegmental area) and histaminergic components (tubelomammillary nucleus) (Siegel, 2009; Saper *et al.*, 2010). Among these rhythmically regulated cell populations are those expressing the neuropeptide orexin (hypocretin). This hypothalamic peptide plays a critical role in promoting arousal and the loss of these neurons is associated with the sleep disorder narcolepsy (Mieda and Sakurai, 2012). The SCN send polysynaptic connections to regulate the neural activity level of these different cell populations. This has been best studied in the noradrenergic locus coeruleus (Aston-Jones, 2005). The locus coeruleus neurons modulate cortical circuits and cognitive performance through their release of norephinephrine. The neuromodulatory neurons exhibit a diurnal/circadian rhythm in neural activity with peak firing rates during wake behavioral states. Anatomical studies suggest that the SCN projects to the dorsomedial hypothalamus (DMH) and that these orexin expressing neurons, in turn, project to the locus coeruleus (Aston-Jones *et al.*, 2001). Lesion studies or pharmacological blockade of orexin receptors decreased the daytime firing of locus coeruleus neurons (González and Aston-Jones, 2006; Gompf and Aston-Jones, 2008). Thus, the SCN influences the activity and function of cortical circuits through the timed release of norephinephrine. Neural regulation of arousal centers by the SCN is a general regulatory theme. Rhythms in neural activity have been reported in the dopamine (DA) cell population in the ventral tegmental area (VTA) as well as 5HT expressing cells in the Raphe. Some possible consequences of the rhythmic regulation of DA for addition are described in Chapter 14. Under normal conditions, peak circadian drive of arousal in humans is thought to occur in the afternoon to counteract growing fatigue as the homeostatic drive to sleep increases (Czeisler and Gooley, 2007).

3.6.7 The SCN circuit controls the temporal patterning behaviors (activity, sleep, feeding) with widespread implications for our bodily function

Circadian rhythms in behavior have widespread regulatory consequences through the body. The daily cycle of feeding/fasting as well as activity/sleep has profound consequences on all cells in our body. The circadian system has reciprocal neural connections to the brain regions that regulate sleep (Chapter 4) and activity, as described above. Through the SCN and CNS connections described above, the SCN controls the temporal patterning of behavior. Interestingly, this communication appears to be bidirectional, as feeding, sleep and activity-dependent circuits all provide feedback to the SCN. Thus, the exact contributions of the direct and indirect circadian control to a particular cell population can be difficult to fully differentiate. To provide one example, humans and other animals exhibit robust rhythms in cardiovascular parameters such as heart rate and blood pressure. The daily increase in activity causes an increase in these parameters, but the circadian system itself can influence these parameters through its daily increase in cortisol and sympathetic tone. One approach to disentangle these direct and indirect regulatory streams involves holding people under long cycles of light and dark (e.g., light:dark 14:14). Human sleep will follow the dark while the underlying circadian system may be unable to remain synchronized (Blatter and Cajochen, 2007). Under these special conditions, subjects still show endogenous circadian rhythms in heart rate and blood pressure, but the amplitude of the rhythms are lower than under freely moving conditions (Morris *et al.*, 2012). The temporal patterning of activity is an output regulated by the circadian system, but studies demonstrate that stimulated activity or exercise can also feed back to the circadian system and alter its function. Thus, by regulating the temporal patterning of sleep and activity, the circadian system can indirectly influence a wide range of processes.

In summary, the SCN sits at the peak of a hierarchy of clocks found throughout the body. The central clock has to coordinate these molecular clocks and also to regulate directly the temporal patterning of physiology and behavior. The SCN have a wide range of rhythmic outputs that function to regulate both other CNS regions as well as peripheral organs. Centrally, the SCN secrete neuropeptides directly and SCN neurons project through multisynaptic pathways to arousal and sleep control centers. Through these neural and hormonal pathways, the SCN can direct the temporal patterning of the ANS and hormonal secretions that constitute the main ways the nervous system communicates with the rest of the body. Furthermore, by regulating the timing of behaviors such as sleep, activity, and feeding, the circadian circuit will indirectly have a major impact on every cell in our body. At this point, it can be assumed that there is redundancy in the signaling mechanisms involved. This redundancy no doubt protects against the misalignment of the peripheral clocks but also make the experiments in this area more challenging! It also seems likely that the relative importance of the players will vary with the specific tissues. The SCN-driven factors regulating rhythmic gene expression in the liver seem likely to have a different weighting than the factors driving rhythmic heart rate and blood pressure in the cardiovascular system. Still, the net result should be a body prepared for energy conservation and system repair during sleep as well as energy mobilization and system function during periods of wakefulness.

3.7 SCN in aging and disease

While SCN dysfunction is not directly implicated in any single disease, a decline in circadian output appears to be a common feature in aging (Chapter 19) as well as in a number of other diseases of the nervous system (Chapters 15–18). Sleep and circadian disruption appears to be a sensitive but perhaps not selective symptom of nervous system dysfunction and ill health. To provide one example, African sleeping sickness is characterized by disruption of the sleep/wake cycle (Kristensson *et al.*, 2010). The underlying mechanisms have been studied using rats infected by the Trypanosoma parasite. In this model, circadian behaviors as well as neural activity rhythms in the SCN are disrupted (Lundkvist *et al.*, 1998). While there is some effect on clock gene expression in the SCN, a more profound impact is found in the gene expression rhythms in peripheral organs such as pituitary and spleen (Lundkvist *et al.*, 2010).

Interestingly, these effects may be mediated by the proinflammatory cytokine interferon (IFN-gamma) that has also been shown to alter neural activity within the SCN (Kwak *et al.*, 2008). As the release of this compound is part of the response of immune cells to infections, cyctokine-induced changes in SCN neural activity could be part of the mechanism underlying the loss of a coherent sleep/wake rhythm that is so characteristic of our body's response to infectious disease.

Based on this body of work, we propose that the neural activity rhythms in the SCN may be the "weak link" of the circadian system. With aging and diseases of the nervous system, there is a weakening of the neural output at times at which the molecular clock work is still fairly normal. Importantly, the maintenance of neural activity is extremely metabolically demanding. 2DG studies have revealed robust rhythms in energy metabolism in the SCN with peaks in daytime (Schwartz *et al.*, 1987; Newman *et al.*, 1992). Perhaps due to this demand, neural activity may be a critically sensitive output of the SCN. The disruption of circadian neural activity rhythms is likely to have profound consequences on patient health. It is becoming increasing clear that robust daily sleep/wake rhythms are essential to good health. A wide range of studies have demonstrated that disruption of the circadian system leads to a cluster of symptoms, including metabolic deficits, cardiovascular problems, difficulty sleeping and cognitive deficits. Many of these same symptoms are seen in aging and diseases. These relationships will be covered in the remaining chapters.

References

Abrahamson E.E., Moore R.Y. 2001. Suprachiasmatic nucleus in the mouse: retinal innervation, intrinsic organization and efferent projections. *Brain Res* **916**(1–2):172–91.

Aguilar-Roblero R., Mercado C., Alamilla J., *et al.* 2007. Ryanodine receptor Ca^{2+}-release channels are an output pathway for the circadian clock in the rat suprachiasmatic nuclei. *Eur. J. Neurosci* **26**:575–82.

Albus H., Bonnefont X., Chaves I., *et al.* 2002. Cryptochrome-deficient mice lack circadian electrical activity in the suprachiasmatic nuclei. *Curr Biol* **12**:1130–3.

Antle M.C., Smith V.M., Sterniczuk R., *et al.* 2009. Physiological responses of the circadian clock to acute light exposure at night. *Rev Endocr Metab Disord* **10**(4):279–91.

Aston-Jones G. 2005. Brain structures and receptors involved in alertness. *Sleep Med* **6**(Suppl 1):S3–7.

Aston-Jones G., Chen S., Zhu Y., Oshinsky M.L. 2001. A neural circuit for circadian regulation of arousal. *Nat Neurosci* **4**(7):732–8.

Aton S.J., Colwell C.S., Harmar A.J., *et al.* 2005. Vasoactive intestinal polypeptide mediates circadian rhythmicity and synchrony in mammalian clock neurons. *Nat Neurosci* **8**(4):476–83.

Aton S.J., Huettner J.E., Straume M., Herzog E.D. 2006. GABA and Gi/o differentially control circadian rhythms and synchrony in clock neurons. *Proc Natl Acad Sci USA* **103**(50):19188–93.

Bean B.P. 2007. The action potential in mammalian central neurons. *Nat Rev Neurosci* **8**(6):451–65.

Berson D.M. 2003. Strange vision: ganglion cells as circadian photoreceptors. *Trends Neurosci.* **26**(6):314–20.

Blatter K., Cajochen C. 2007. Circadian rhythms in cognitive performance: methodological constraints, protocols, theoretical underpinnings. *Physiol Behav* **90**(2–3):196–208.

Brown T.M., Piggins H.D. 2009. Spatiotemporal heterogeneity in the electrical activity of suprachiasmatic nuclei neurons and their response to photoperiod. *J Biol Rhythms* **24**(1):44–54.

Brown S.A., Zumbrunn G., Fleury-Olela F., *et al.* 2002. Rhythms of mammalian body temperature can sustain peripheral circadian clocks. *Curr Biol* **12**:1574.

Buijs R.M., Wortel J., Van Heerikhuize J.J., *et al.* 1999. Anatomical and functional demonstration of a multisynaptic suprachiasmatic nucleus adrenal (cortex) pathway. *Eur J Neurosci* **11**(5):1535–44.

Buijs, R., La Fleur, S., Wortel, J., *et al.* 2003. The suprachiasmatic nucleus balances sympathetic and parasympathetic output to peripheral organs through separate preautonomic neurons. *J Comp Neurol* **464**:36–48.

Buhr, E.D., Yoo, S.H., Takahashi, J.S., 2010. Temperature as a universal resetting cue for mammalian circadian oscillators. *Science* **330**:379–85.

Canteras, N.S., Ribeiro-Barbosa, E.R., Goto, M., *et al.* 2011. The retinohypothalamic tract: comparison of axonal projection patterns from four major targets. *Brain Res Rev* **65**:150–83.

Cassone V.M., Menaker M. 1984. Is the avian circadian system a neuroendocrine loop? *J Exp Zool* **232**(3):539–49.

Chen, S.K., Badea, T.C., Hattar, S., 2011. Photoentrainment and pupillary light reflex are mediated by distinct populations of ipRGCs. *Nature* **476**: 92–4.

Colwell C.S. 2011. Linking neural activity and molecular oscillations in the SCN. *Nat Rev Neurosci* **12**(10):553–69.

Czeisler C.A., Gooley J.J. 2007. Sleep and circadian rhythms in humans. *Cold Spring Harb Symp Quant Biol* **72**:579–97.

DeCoursey P.J., Buggy J. 1989. Circadian rhythmicity after neural transplant to hamster third ventricle: Specificity of suprachiasmatic nuclei. *Brain Res* **500**:263–75.

Deery M.J., Maywood E.S., Chesham J.E., *et al.* 2009. Proteomic analysis reveals the role of synaptic vesicle cycling in sustaining the suprachiasmatic circadian clock. *Curr Biol* **19**(23):2031–6.

Dibner C., Schibler U., Albrecht U. 2010. The mammalian circadian timing system: organization and coordination of central and peripheral clocks. *Annu Rev Physiol* **72**:517–49.

Ding J.M., Chen D., Weber E.T., *et al.* 1994. Resetting the biological clock: mediation of nocturnal circadian shifts by glutamate and NO. *Science* **266**(5191):1713–7.

Ding J.M., Faiman L.E., Hurst W.J., *et al.* 1997. Resetting the biological clock: mediation of nocturnal CREB phosphorylation via light, glutamate, and nitric oxide. *J. Neurosci* **17**: 667–75.

Ding J.M., Buchanan G.F., Tischkau S.A., *et al.* 1998. A neuronal ryanodine receptor mediates light-induced phase delays of the circadian clock. *Nature* **394**(6691):381–4.

Doi M., Ishida A., Miyake A., *et al.* 2011. Circadian regulation of intracellular G-protein signalling mediates intercellular synchrony and rhythmicity in the suprachiasmatic nucleus. *Nat Commun* **2**:327.

Drucker-Colin R., Aquilar-Roblero R., Garcia-Fernandez F., *et al.* 1984. Fetal suprachiasmatic nucleus transplants: Diurnal rhythm recovery of lesioned rats. *Brain Res* **311**:353–7.

Dubocovich M.L. 2007. Melatonin receptors: role on sleep and circadian rhythm regulation. *Sleep Med* **8**(Suppl 3): 34–42.

Earnest D.J., Sladek C.D. 1986. Circadian rhythms of vasopressin release from individual rat suprachiasmatic explants in vitro. *Brain Res* **382**(1):129–33.

Ecker J.L., Dumitrescu O.N., Wong K.Y., *et al.* 2010. Melanopsin-expressing retinal ganglion-cell photoreceptors: cellular diversity and role in pattern vision. *Neuron* **67**(1):49–60.

Freeman G.M. Jr, Krock R.M., Aton S.J., *et al.* 2013. GABA networks destabilize genetic oscillations in the circadian pacemaker. *Neuron* **78**(5):799–806.

Gamble K.L., Kudo T., Colwell C.S., McMahon D.G. 2011. Gastrin-releasing peptide modulates fast delayed rectifier potassium current in Per1-expressing SCN neurons. *J Biol Rhythms* **26**(2):99–106.

Gau D., Lemberger T., Von Gall C., *et al.* 2002. Phosphorylation of CREB Ser142 regulates light-induced phase shifts of the circadian clock. *Neuron* **34**:245–53.

Gillette M.U., Mitchell J.W. 2002. Signaling in the suprachiasmatic nucleus: selectively responsive and integrative. *Cell Tissue Res* **309**(1):99–107.

Ginty D.D., Kornhauser J.M., Thompson M.A., *et al.* 1993. Regulation of CREB phosphorylation in the suprachiasmatic nucleus by light and a circadian clock. *Science* **260**(5105):238–41.

Golombek D.A., Rosenstein R.E. 2010. Physiology of circadian entrainment. *Physiol Rev* **90**(3):1063–102.

Gompf H.S., Aston-Jones G. 2008. Role of orexin input in the diurnal rhythm of locus coeruleus impulse activity. *Brain Res* **1224**:43–52.

González M.M., Aston-Jones G. 2006. Circadian regulation of arousal: role of the noradrenergic locus coeruleus system and light exposure. *Sleep* **29**(10):1327–36.

Green D.J., Gillette R. 1982. Circadian rhythm of firing rate recorded from single cells in the rat suprachiasmatic slice. *Brain Res* **245**:283–8.

Groos G., Hendriks J. 1982. Circadian rhythms in electrical discharge of rat suprachiasmatic neurones recorded in vitro. *Neurosci Lett* **34**:283–8.

Hannibal J., Hindersson P., Knudsen S.M., *et al.* 2002. The photopigment melanopsin is exclusively present in pituitary adenylate cyclase-activating polypeptide-containing retinal ganglion cells of the retinohypothalamic tract. *J. Neurosci* **22**:RC191.

Hamada T., LeSauter J., Venuti J.M., Silver R. 2001. Expression of Period genes: rhythmic and nonrhythmic compartments of the suprachiasmatic nucleus pacemaker. *J Neurosci* **21**(19):7742–50.

Hamada T., Antle M.C., Silver R. 2004. Temporal and spatial expression patterns of canonical clock genes and clock–controlled genes in the suprachiasmatic nucleus. *Eur J Neurosci* **19**:1741–8.

Hatcher N.G., Atkins N. Jr., Annangudi S.P., *et al.* 2008. Mass spectrometry-based discovery of circadian peptides. *Proc Natl Acad Sci USA* **105**(34):12527–32.

Herzog E.D., Takahashi J.S.., Block G.D. 1998. Clock controls circadian period in isolated suprachiasmatic nucleus neurons. *Nat Neurosci* **1**:708–13.

Hendrickson A.E., Wagoner N., Cowan W.M.1972. An autoradiographic and electron microscopic study of retino-hypothalamic connections. *Z Zellforsch* **135**:1–26.

Honma S., Shirakawa T., Katsuno Y., *et al.* 1998. Circadian periods of single suprachiasmatic neurons in rats. *Neurosci Lett* **250**(3):157–60.

Inouye S.T., Kawamura H. 1979. Persistence of circadian rhythmicity in a mammalian hypothalamic "island" containing the suprachiasmatic nucleus. *Proc Natl Acad Sci USA* **76**:5962–6.

Irwin R., Allen C. 2007. Calcium response to retinohypothalamic tract synaptic transmission in suprachiasmatic nucleus neurons. *J Neurosci* **27**:11748–57.

Jin X., Shearman L.P., Weaver D.R., *et al.* 1999. A molecular mechanism regulating rhythmic output from the suprachiasmatic circadian clock. *Cell* **96**(1):57–68.

Kalsbeek A., Palm I.F., La Fleur S.E., *et al.* 2006. SCN outputs and the hypothalamic balance of life. *J Biol Rhythms* **21**:458–69.

Kalsbeek A., Fliers E., Hofman M.A., *et al.* 2010. Vasopressin and the output of the hypothalamic biological clock. *J Neuroendocrinol* **22**(5):362–72.

Kim J.S., Coon S.L., Blackshaw S., *et al.* 2005. Methionine adenosyltransferase:adrenergic-cAMP mechanism regulates a daily rhythm in pineal expression. *J Biol Chem* **280**:677–84.

Kim S.M., Power A., Brown T.M., *et al.* 2009. Deletion of the secretory vesicle proteins IA-2 and IA-2beta disrupts circadian rhythms of cardiovascular and physical activity. *FASEB J* **23**(9):3226–32.

Klein D.C. 1985. Photoneural regulation of the mammalian pineal gland. *Ciba Found Symp* **117**:38–56.

Klein D.C. 2007. Arylalkylamine N-acetyltransferase: "the Timezyme". *J Biol Chem* **282**(7):4233–7.

Klein D.C., Moore R.Y. 1979. Pineal N-acetyltransferase and hydroxyindole-O-methyltransferase: Control by the retinohypothalamic tract and the suprachiasmatic nucleus. *Brain Res* **174**:245–62.

Klein D.C., Moore R.Y., Reppert S.M. 1991. *Suprachiasmatic Nucleus: The Mind's Clock*. Oxford University Press, New York.

Kramer A., Yang F.C., Kraves S., Weitz C.J. 2005. A screen for secreted factors of the suprachiasmatic nucleus. *Methods Enzymol* **393**:645–63.

Kriegsfeld L.J., LeSauter J., Silver R. 2004. Targeted microlesions reveal novel organization of the hamster suprachiasmatic nucleus. *J Neurosci* **24**(10):2449–57.

Kristensson K., Nygård M., Bertini G., Bentivoglio M. 2010. African trypanosome infections of the nervous system: parasite entry and effects on sleep and synaptic functions. *Prog Neurobiol* **91**(2):152–71.

Kudo T., Tahara Y., Gamble K.L., *et al.* 2013. Vasoactive intestinal peptide produces long-lasting changes in neural activity in the suprachiasmatic nucleus. *J Neurophysiol* **110**(5):1097–106.

Kuhlman S., McMahon D. 2006. Encoding the ins and outs of circadian pacemaking. *J Biol Rhythms* **21**:470–81.

Kwak Y., Lundkvist G.B., Brask J., *et al.* 2008. Interferon-gamma alters electrical activity and clock gene expression in suprachiasmatic nucleus neurons. *J Biol Rhythms* **23**(2):150–9.

Lall G.S., Revell V.L., Momiji H., *et al.* 2010. Distinct contributions of rod, cone, and melanopsin photoreceptors to encoding irradiance. *Neuron* **66**(3):417–28.

Leak R.K., Moore R.Y. 2001. Topographic organization of suprachiasmatic nucleus projection neurons. *J Comp Neurol* **433**:312–34.

Lee H.S., Billings H.J., Lehman M.N. 2003. The suprachiasmatic nucleus: a clock of multiple components. *J Biol Rhythms* **18**:435–49.

Lee B., Li A., Hansen K.F., *et al.* 2010. CREB influences timing and entrainment of the SCN circadian clock. *J Biol Rhythms* **25**(6):410–20.

Lehman M.N., Silver R., Gladstone W.R., *et al.* 1987. Circadian rhythmicity restored by neural transplant: Immunocytochemical characterization of the graft and its integration with the host brain. *J Neurosci* **7**:1626–38.

LeSauter J., Silver R., Cloues R., Witkovsky P. 2011. Light exposure induces short- and long-term changes in the excitability of retinorecipient neurons in suprachiasmatic nucleus. *J Neurophysiol* **106**: 576–88.

Liu C., Weaver D.R., Strogatz S.H., Reppert S.M. 1997, Cellular construction of a circadian clock: period determination in the suprachiasmatic nuclei. *Cell* **91**:855–60.

Liu A.C., Welsh D.K., Ko C.H., *et al.* 2007. Intercellular coupling confers robustness against mutations in the SCN circadian clock network. *Cell* **129**:605–16.

Lundkvist G.B., Christenson J., ElTayeb RA., *et al.* 1998. Altered neuronal activity rhythm and glutamate receptor expression in the suprachiasmatic nuclei of Trypanosoma brucei-infected rats. *J Neuropathol Exp Neurol* **57**(1):21–9.

Lundkvist G.B., Sellix M.T., Nygård M., *et al.* 2010. Clock gene expression during chronic inflammation induced by infection with Trypanosoma brucei brucei in rats. *J Biol Rhythms* **25**:92–102.

Maywood E.S., Reddy A.B., Wong G.K., *et al.* 2006. Synchronization and maintenance of timekeeping in suprachiasmatic circadian clock cells by neuropeptidergic signaling. *Curr Biol* **16**:599–605.

Maywood E.S., Chesham J.E., O'Brien J.A., *et al.* 2011. A diversity of paracrine signals sustains molecular circadian cycling in suprachiasmatic nucleus circuits. *Proc Natl Acad Sci USA* **108**:14306–11.

McEwen B.S. 2007. Physiology and neurobiology of stress and adaptation: central role of the brain. *Physiol Rev* **87**(3):873–904.

Meijer J., Watanabe K., Schaap J., *et al.* 1998. Light responsiveness of the suprachiasmatic nucleus: long-term multiunit and single-unit recordings in freely moving rats. *J Neurosci* **18**:9078–87.

Meijer J., Michel S., Vanderleest H.T., Rohling J.H. 2010. Daily and seasonal adaptation of the circadian clock requires plasticity of the SCN neuronal network. *Eur J Neurosci* **32**(12):2143–51.

Mieda M., Sakurai T. 2012. Overview of orexin/hypocretin system. *Prog Brain Res* **198**:5–14.

Møller M., Baeres F.M. 2002. The anatomy and innervation of the mammalian pineal gland. *Cell Tissue Res* **309**:139–50.

Nishide S.Y., Hashimoto K., Nishio T., *et al.* 2014. Organ specific development characterizes circadian clock gene Per2 expression in rats. *Am J Physiol Regul Integr Comp Physiol* **306**(1):R67–74.

Moore R.Y. 1996. Neural control of the pineal gland. *Behav Brain Res* **73**(1–2):125–30.

Moore R.Y., Eichler V.B. 1972. Loss of a circadian adrenal corticosterone rhythm following suprachiasmatic lesions in the rat. *Brain Res* **42**:201–6.

Moore R.Y., Lenn N.J. 1972. A retinohypothalamic projection in the rat. *J Comp Neurol* **146**:1–14.

Morin L.P. 2013. Neuroanatomy of the extended circadian rhythm system. *Exp Neurol* **243**:4–20.

Morris C.J., Yang J.N., Scheer F.A. 2012. The impact of the circadian timing system on cardiovascular and metabolic function. *Prog Brain Res* **199**:337–58.

Nakamura W., Honma S., Shirakawa T., Honma K. 2002. Clock mutation lengthens the circadian period without damping rhythms in individual SCN neurons. *Nat Neurosci* **5**:399–400.

Nakamura W., Yamazaki S., Nakamura T.J., *et al.* 2008. In vivo monitoring of circadian timing in freely moving mice. *Curr Biol* **18**(5):381–5.

Newman G.C., Hospod F.E., Patlak C.S., Moore R.Y. 1992. Analysis of in vitro glucose utilization in a circadian pacemaker model. *J Neurosci* **12**(6):2015–21.

Pakhotin P., Harmar A.J., Verkhratsky A., Piggins H. 2006. VIP receptors control excitability of suprachiasmatic nuclei neurones. *Pfluegers* **452**:7–15.

Panda S. 2007. Multiple photopigments entrain the mammalian circadian oscillator. *Neuron* **53**(5):619–21.

Pulivarthy S.R., Tanaka N., Welsh D.K., *et al.* 2007. Reciprocity between phase shifts and amplitude changes in the mammalian circadian clock. *Proc Natl Acad Sci USA* **104**(51):20356–61.

Ralph M.R., Foster R.G., Davis F.C., Menaker M. 1990. Transplanted suprachiasmatic nucleus determines circadian period. *Science* **247**:975–8.

Romijn H.J., Sluiter A.A., Pool C.W., *et al.* 1997. Evidence from confocal fluorescence microscopy for a dense, reciprocal innervation between AVP-, somatostatin-, VIP/PHI-, GRP-, and VIP/PHI/GRP-immunoreactive neurons in the rat suprachiasmatic nucleus. *Eur. J. Neurosci* **9**:2613–23.

Rusak B. 1977. The role of the suprachiasmatic nuclei in the generation of circadian rhythms in the golden hamster, Mesocricetus auratus. *J Comp Physiol* **118**:145–64.

Saper C.B., Fuller P.M., Pedersen N.P., *et al.* 2010. Sleep state switching. *Neuron* **68**:1023–42.

Sawaki Y., Nihonmatsu I., Kawamura H. 1984. Transplantation of the neonatal suprachiasmatic nuclei into rats with complete bilateral suprachiasmatic lesions. *Neurosci Res* **1**:67–72.

Schaap J., Pennartz C., Meijer J. 2003. Electrophysiology of the circadian pacemaker in mammals. *Chronobiol Int* **20**:171–88.

Schwartz W.J., Reppert S.M. 1985. Neural regulation of the circadian vasopressin rhythm in cerebrospinal fluid: a pre-eminent role for the suprachiasmatic nuclei. *J Neurosci* **5**(10):2771–8.

Schwartz W.J., Gross R.A., Morton M.T. 1987. The suprachiasmatic nuclei contain a tetrodotoxin-resistant circadian pacemaker. *Proc Natl Acad Sci USA* **84**(6):1694–8.

Shibata S., Oomura Y., Kita H., Hattori K. 1982. Circadian rhythmic changes in neuronal activity in the suprachiasmatic nucleus of the rat hypothalamic slice. *Brain Res* **247**:154–8.

Siegel, J.M. 2009. The neurobiology of sleep. *Semin Neurol* **29**:277–96.

Silver R., LeSauter J., Tresco P.A., Lehman M.N. 1996. A diffusible coupling signal from the transplanted suprachiasmatic nucleus controlling circadian locomotor rhythms. *Nature* **382**:810–3.

Slominski R.M., Reiter R.J., Schlabritz-Loutsevitch N., *et al.* 2012. Melatonin membrane receptors in peripheral tissues: distribution and functions. *Mol Cell Endocrinol* **351**:152–66.

Stephan F.K., Zucker I. 1972. Circadian rhythms in drinking and locomotor activity of rats are eliminated by hypothalamic lesions. *Proc Natl Acad Sci USA* **69**:1583–6.

Tischkau S.A., Mitchell J.W., Tyan S.H., *et al.* 2003. Ca2+/cAMP response element-binding protein (CREB)-dependent activation of Per1 is required for light-induced signaling in the suprachiasmatic nucleus circadian clock. *J Biol Chem* **278**:718–23.

Travnickova-Bendova Z., Cermakian N., Reppert S.M., Sassone-Corsi P. 2002. Bimodal regulation of mPeriod promoters by CREB-dependent signaling and CLOCK/BMAL1 activity. *Proc Natl Acad Sci USA* **99**:7728–33.

VanderLeest H.T., Houben T., Michel S., *et al.* 2007. Seasonal encoding by the circadian pacemaker of the SCN. *Curr Biol* **17**(5):468–73.

Vosko A.M., Schroeder A., Loh D.H., Colwell C.S. 2007. Vasoactive intestinal peptide and the mammalian circadian system. *Gen Comp Endocrinol* **152**:165–75.

Wang L.M., Schroeder A., Loh D., *et al.* 2008. Role for the NR2B subunit of the N-methyl-D-aspartate receptor in mediating light input to the circadian system. *Eur J Neurosci* **27**(7):1771–9.

Webb A.B., Angelo N., Huettner J.E., Herzog E.D. 2009. Intrinsic, nondeterministic circadian rhythm generation in identified mammalian neurons. *Proc Natl Acad Sci USA* **106**(38):16493–8.

Welsh D.K., Logothetis D.E., Meister M., Reppert S.M. 1995. Individual neurons dissociated from rat suprachiasmatic nucleus express independently phased circadian firing rhythms. *Neuron* **14**:697–706.

Welsh D., Takahashi J., Kay S. 2010. Suprachiasmatic nucleus: cell autonomy and network properties. *Annu Rev Physiol* **72**:551–77.

Wright K.P. Jr, Hull J.T., Czeisler C.A. 2002. Relationship between alertness, performance, and body temperature in humans. *Am J Physiol Regul Integr Comp Physiol* **283**(6):R1370–7.

Yamaguchi S., Isejima H., Matsuo T., *et al.* 2003. Synchronization of cellular clocks in the suprachiasmatic nucleus. *Science* **302**(5649):1408–12.

Yamaguchi Y., Suzuki T., Mizoro Y., *et al.* 2013. Mice genetically deficient in vasopressin V1a and V1b receptors are resistant to jet lag. *Science* **342**(6154):85–90.

Yan L., Silver R. 2002. Differential induction and localization of mPer1 and mPer2 during advancing and delaying phase shifts. *Eur J Neurosci* **16**(8):1531–40.

Yan L., Silver R. 2004. Resetting the brain clock: time course and localization of mPER1 and mPER2 protein expression in suprachiasmatic nuclei during phase shifts. *Eur J Neurosci* **19**(4):1105–9.

Sleep and Circadian Rhythms: Reciprocal Partners in the Regulation of Physiology and Behavior

4

Ralph Mistlberger

Department of Psychology, Cognitive and Neural Sciences Area, Simon Fraser University, Burnaby, BC, Canada

4.1 Introduction

Human behavior, physiology and biochemistry are regulated by circadian clocks located in the brain and in most other tissues and organ systems. Circadian clocks are comprised of populations of coupled clock cells with the intrinsic capacity to oscillate by virtue of autoregulatory transcription-translation feedback loops involving so-called clock genes and their protein products, or by nontranscriptional, biochemical processes (Chapters 1 and 2). The role of circadian clocks in health and disease is the subject of intensive basic and translational research. A primary goal of basic research is to elucidate the pathways by which circadian clocks confer temporal organization on physiological processes, to reveal how disruptions of circadian timing might precipitate, exacerbate or predispose to disease processes.

Clock output pathways to physiology are diverse and may involve intracellular, intercellular and behavioral components. Intracellular pathways are illustrated by circadian clock proteins that function as transcription factors (via binding to E-boxes on gene promotors) (Jin *et al.*, 1999) or that modulate other transcription factors (e.g., via actions on nuclear receptors) (Schmutz *et al.*, 2010), thereby regulating expression of genes critical to cellular functions. Cellular functions include regulation of neuronal membrane potential, firing rate, and the synthesis and release of signaling molecules (neurotransmitters and hormones) that transmit timing signals from neuronal clock cells to other cells in the brain or in peripheral tissues (Dibner *et al.*, 2010; Colwell, 2011; Kalsbeek *et al.*, 2011). Some of these timing signals are transmitted to neural systems that regulate sleep–wake states. The daily sleep–wake cycle, in turn, gates the expression of locomotor and ingestive behaviors and exposure to environmental stimuli such as light and social cues. These photic and nonphotic stimuli can directly drive daily rhythms of physiology or act on clock genes to entrain circadian oscillators in the brain and in peripheral organ systems. The circadian sleep–wake cycle is, therefore, both a clock output and a modulator of clock inputs. Neural or endocrine correlates of sleep–wake states may also function directly as clock inputs, independent of light exposure, food intake and other stimuli (Fig. 4.1).

The role of behavioral state in the cascade from cycling clock genes to circadian physiology raises the possibility that disruptions of the daily sleep–wake cycle may be causal to adverse health outcomes associated with chronic disturbances of circadian rhythms (e.g., with rotating shiftwork) (Knutson, 2000). Effects

Circadian Medicine, First Edition. Edited by Christopher S. Colwell.
© 2015 John Wiley & Sons, Inc. Published 2015 by John Wiley & Sons, Inc.

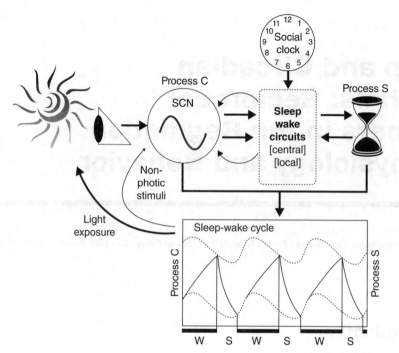

Fig. 4.1 A simplified representation of sleep–wake regulation in mammals. The box labeled "sleep–wake circuits" represents those central and local neuronal populations that are the effectors for electrophysiological and behavioral phenomena that define the sleep–wake states. Neuronal activity within these circuits is continuously modulated by inputs from circadian clocks (Process C; most notably the light-entrainable SCN, with oscillators elsewhere in the brain possibly also involved) and by recent sleep–wake history, which determines the level of wake-dependent sleep drive (Process S) that only sleep can reverse. The level of Process S depends on the duration of prior wake and prior sleep, and thus can be represented visually by an hourglass clock. Sleep–wake circuits are also affected by environmental stimuli, some of which are imposed by social schedules (e.g., alarm clocks). Integration of circadian, hourglass and social clocks determines sleep characteristics, including its timing, duration, sleep stage content, and cortical electrophysiology (EEG waves). In the lower panel, Process C is represented by two skewed sine waves, one representing an upper threshold for sleep onset and the second representing a lower threshold for wake onset. The wake-dependent drive for sleep (Process S) increases exponentially during waking until it meets the clock-dependent threshold for sleep onset. During sleep, Process S dissipates exponentially until meeting the clock-dependent threshold for wake onset. The kinetics of Process S have been derived from the number and/or amplitude of EEG slow waves (~0.5–4 Hz) observed during sleep following varying durations of prior waking. The sleep–wake regulatory system includes numerous direct and indirect feedback loops. For example, the behavioral sleep–wake cycle determines daily patterns of exposure to environmental light, which is the primary stimulus controlling the phase of the master circadian clock (The SCN). The sleep–wake cycle also gates the expression of locomotor activity, food intake, social stimuli and other nonphotic factors that may also modulate the phase or period of circadian clocks in the brain and body. There may also be more direct feedback from clock-controlled sleep–wake mechanisms to circadian clocks, which may be responsible for variations in neural activity that have been observed within the SCN in association with variations in sleep–wake states.

of such disturbances on other parameters of sleep, including its duration, consolidation, intensity or ultradian sleep stage architecture, may also be important. Indeed, there is now considerable evidence linking sleep with health and mortality. Epidemiological studies have uncovered significant associations between habitual sleep duration (both long and short) and cardiovascular disease, metabolic disorders, cancer and all-cause mortality (Hasler *et al.*, 2004; Gallicchio and Kalesan, 2008; Altman *et al.*, 2012; Faraut *et al.*, 2012; Grandner *et al.*, 2012; but see Kurina *et al.*, 2013). An important research agenda going forward will be to disentangle the contributions made by disruptions of circadian timing and sleep *per se* to disease processes.

If circadian timekeeping and sleep make significant, independent contributions to physiological functioning, the health impacts of circadian and sleep disruptions will be compounded to the extent that circadian processes and sleep are reciprocally regulated. The objective of this chapter is to examine how circadian clocks and sleep–wake states interact at the systems, cellular, and molecular genetic levels.

4.2 What is sleep

Across the animal kingdom, daily rhythms of rest and activity are ubiquitous. However, the presence of "rest" behavior at the species or individual organism levels does not necessarily imply "sleep". The correspondence between rest and sleep depends on how these states are defined. Definitions can be based on phenomenology (what they look like), mechanism (how they are controlled), and function (what they are "for"). Ultimately, establishing homology between rest in nonmammalian species and sleep as defined in humans and laboratory rodents will require a deep understanding of the physiological and behavioral functions that are achieved by being asleep. At present, a consensus on these functions is lacking. Therefore, although rest states are evident behaviorally across a wide range of phylogeny, homology with mammalian sleep at the functional level remains to be established.

Sleep is recognized as a behavioral state of quiescence distinguished from "rest" by an elevated arousal threshold and from torpor, hibernation and death by rapid reversibility (Flanigan *et al.*, 1973). In many species, sleep behavior is preceded by preparatory behavior (building or retiring to a nest or shelter) and exhibits a characteristic posture. Sleep is further distinguished from rest by a "history dependence" consistent with homeostatic regulation (Tobler, 2011). Homeostasis in physiology is inferred when physiological systems employ sensors and corrective mechanisms to maintain regulated variables within an operational range conducive to life. Corrective mechanisms may include autonomic and behavioral responses (e.g., food deprived animals mobilize stored glycogen to maintain blood glucose levels, engage in foraging behavior, and eat more when food is obtained). In control systems terminology, the corrective response is proportional in some way to the magnitude of the error between the current and the desired state. Sleep exhibits similar self-regulatory properties. If sleep behavior is acutely prevented or chronically restricted, efforts ("drive") to engage in sleep increase and subsequent free sleep is more consolidated (fewer brief awakenings), has a higher arousal threshold (suggesting increased "depth"), and may be increased in duration ("rebound" increase).

Typically, the increments in sleep duration following sleep deprivation amount to only a small fraction of total sleep time lost. The lack of proportionality between sleep debt accrued and sleep recovered is attributed, in part, to variations in sleep intensity. In mammals, the membrane properties and parallel alignment of neocortical pyramidal neurons generate electric fields that can be detected by electrodes fixed to the scalp or threaded into the skull. The resulting "electroencephalogram" (EEG) exhibits waves of varying frequency and amplitude that, together with muscle tone and eye movements, distinguish sleep from wake, and define stages of sleep.

The presence of rapid eye movements (REMs) during sleep is associated with muscle atonia and a low voltage EEG similar to waking. This REM sleep stage in humans occurs at intervals of about 90 minutes, alternating with "nonrapid eye movement" (NREM) sleep. NREM sleep can be divided into sequential stages based on the presence of low voltage EEG with slow rolling eye movements (stage N1), sleep spindles and K complexes (stage N2), or high amplitude, low frequency (~ 0.5–$4.5\,Hz$) "slow" or "delta" waves (stage N3, also called slow wave sleep, SWS, or NREM stages 3 and 4 in the traditional Rechtschaffen and Kales sleep staging system). SWS is normally concentrated early in the night, and decreases exponentially across the night, while the proportion of each 90-minute NREM/REM cycle occupied by REM sleep (REMS) increases across the night. Following acute sleep deprivation or chronic restriction, it is SWS that is preferentially increased, and the amount of SWS lost (unlike sleep duration) may be fully recovered. Stages N1 and N2 are typically decreased during sleep restriction and recovery, while REMS may be unchanged, increased late in the night, or increased on the second night of recovery.

The level of slow wave activity (SWA, synonymous with delta waves) at sleep onset increases as a saturating exponential function of prior wake duration (Tobler and Borbely, 1986; Dijk *et al.*, 1987).

Following a daytime nap, SWA at night is correspondingly decreased, so that total daily SWA may be conserved (Feinberg *et al.*, 1985). In humans, arousal thresholds are inversely related to SWA (Williams *et al.*, 1964). These characteristics of EEG SWA constitute the best evidence that sleep is regulated by an homeostatic process and suggest that homeostasis is achieved in large part by variations in sleep intensity, of which SWA is an electrophysiological correlate (by analogy, the "sleep hungry" eat "faster" rather than "longer"). Quantitative models of sleep regulation postulate joint control by two interacting processes, one homeostatic (a linear process by which sleep "need" or "pressure" accumulates with time awake and dissipates with time asleep) and the other circadian (a cyclic process that modulates sleep propensity according to circadian clock phase; Fig. 4.1). These have been denoted Process "S" and Process "C", respectively, in a two-process model of sleep regulation (Daan *et al.*, 1984; Achermann and Borbély, 2011).

To end this section where it began, despite the evidence for sleep homeostasis, and the compelling intuition that sleep reverses something that impairs waking functions, the nature of the regulated variable(s) (what is being sensed and what is being corrected by sleep) remains a major unresolved question in biology. There is no shortage of competing hypotheses (Scharf *et al.*, 2008; Siegel, 2009; Vassalli and Dijk, 2009; Krueger and Tononi, 2011; Vyazovskiy and Harris, 2013; Xie *et al.*, 2013). The next section examines circadian regulation of sleep–wake states at the behavioral, neural and molecular levels.

4.3 Circadian regulation of sleep

4.3.1 Behavioral studies: human sleep

Although sleep–wake states are regulated by powerful circadian and homeostatic processes, environmental factors can override, or "mask", circadian and homeostatic control. This is a common experience when social schedules (e.g., work hours) require an early wake-up relative to internal circadian time and homeostatic sleep "need" (inducing social jetlag) (Roenneberg *et al.*, 2007). An early sleep onset or delayed wake-up can be induced by confining subjects to long nights in complete darkness (Wehr *et al.*, 1993). In nocturnal animals, artificial light at night can suppress activity and promote sleep while darkness during the day can stimulate activity (Mrosovsky, 1999b; Morin and Studholme, 2009; Muindi *et al.*, 2013). Consequently, light–dark (LD) cycles can induce a daily sleep–wake rhythm in animals in which circadian regulation has been eliminated by brain lesions or clock gene knockouts. The daily sleep–wake rhythm is, therefore, shaped by endogenous and environmental factors. To characterize the circadian contribution to sleep control, it is necessary to remove environmental factors that constrain sleep timing. For human subjects, this may include knowledge of clock time.

Early studies exploited natural caves and concrete bunkers as temporal isolation environments to confirm that the daily sleep–wake cycle in humans, as in other animals, is endogenously generated and circadian in periodicity (Aschoff, 1965). Serial correlations between sleep episode duration and prior wake episode duration in humans "free-running" in temporal isolation were negative, indicating that the circadian clock has priority over the sleep homeostat in setting daily sleep duration (Wever, 1984). Within each sleep–wake cycle, it is the period of the circadian cycle that is conserved rather than the duration of the sleep phase (if sleep begins late in the circadian cycle, it will be truncated by a circadian wake-up process). Homeostasis of circadian period trumps homeostasis of sleep duration.

With prolonged exposure to a time-free environment (typically 3 weeks or longer), most subjects exhibit occasional very long sleep and wake bouts, inducing an apparent lengthening of the average sleep–wake cycle to a noncircadian 33 h or more (48 h "circabidian" cycles have been observed) (Aschoff and Wever, 1976). During this time, the circadian rhythm of core body temperature (Tb) persists with a periodicity of about 25 h. Consequently, across many weeks of recording, sleep bouts are initiated at different phases of the Tb cycle. This dissociation between the sleep–wake and Tb rhythms has been called spontaneous internal desynchrony. During internal desynchrony, sleep episodes are most often initiated just before the daily minimum of Tb and are terminated 6–8 h later, on the rising phase of the

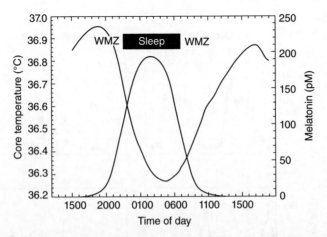

Fig. 4.2 The normal relationship between nocturnal sleep, evening and morning wake-maintenance zones (WMZs) and two variables (core body temperature and plasma melatonin) considered to be the most accurate physiological measures of circadian phase in humans. WMZs (also called "forbidden zones for sleep") are not absolute but have been detected in numerous experimental protocols, including time-free environments, forced desynchrony, and ultradian sleep–wake schedules (from Lack and Wright, 2007).

Tb rhythm (Czeisler *et al.*, 1980). A smaller number of episodes are initiated near the maximum of the Tb rhythm, which is normally the middle of the wake phase, and some of these also terminate spontaneously after the Tb minimum, on the rising phase of Tb. Sleep bout length is, therefore, predicted by the circadian phase of sleep onset. Sleep episodes initiated near the Tb maximum are often very long, while episodes initiated near the Tb minimum are short, and sleep episodes of both lengths usually terminate at the same phase of the Tb cycle, defining a daily circadian wake-onset phase.

The variability of sleep and wake bout duration during internal desynchrony provides a further opportunity to explore homeostatic regulation of spontaneous sleep bout duration. Homeostasis predicts that longer sleep bouts should be preceded by longer wake bouts. Surprisingly, when average sleep and wake bout duration for each phase of the Tb rhythm is subtracted from each observed sleep and wake bout, statistically removing the circadian contribution to bout duration, the residual sleep and wake bout lengths are uncorrelated (Strogatz *et al.*, 1986). Thus, sleep duration in a time-free environment appears to be determined by the circadian clock and random factors, with little or no contribution made by prior wake duration.

Sleep timing during internal desynchrony also reveals two phases of the circadian Tb rhythm when sleep is rarely initiated (Strogatz *et al.*, 1987). These "wake-maintenance zones" occur just after the Tb maximum, as Tb begins to fall (an "evening" zone, just before sleep would normally be initiated), and again 2–3 h after the Tb min, on the rising phase of Tb (a "morning" zone, after sleep would normally terminate) (Fig. 4.2). The evening wake-maintenance zone has also been observed in studies of sleep on short and ultra-short sleep–wake schedules in which subjects receive a 30 min or 7 min sleep opportunity every 90 or 21 min, respectively (Carskadon and Dement, 1975; Lavie, 2001). Subjects in the ultrashort sleep–wake protocol exhibit an approximately two-hour zone in the evening when sleep is difficult to obtain and easy to resist (if instructed).

These experiments reveal that sleep propensity is lowest near the end of the circadian wake phase, just after the Tb max, and is highest at the Tb min, which is normally near the end of the circadian sleep phase (Fig. 4.3). The daily rhythm of sleep propensity is thus markedly phase delayed relative to the daily rhythm of sleep onset and termination. This phase relationship is paradoxical when viewed from a homeostatic perspective; if sleep is a response to prior waking, then the need and thus propensity for sleep should increase with prior wake duration and decrease with prior sleep duration. The seeming paradox reflects a primary function of the circadian clock in humans, which is to promote wake near the end of the circadian "day", and sleep near the end of the circadian "night", opposing the sleep homeostat

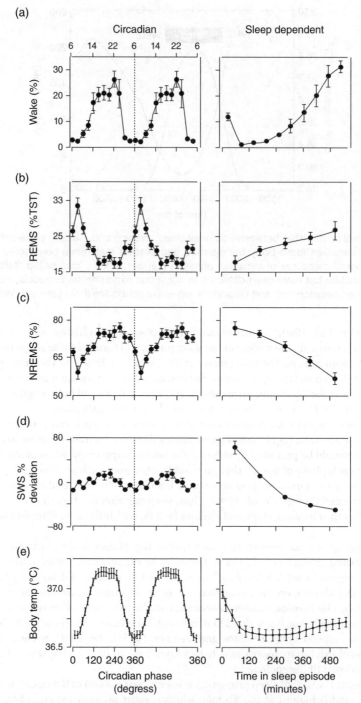

Fig. 4.3 Circadian and sleep-dependent variations in sleep–wake parameters derived from studies of human sleep in the forced desynchrony protocol (Dijk and Czeisler, 1995). The panels forming the left-hand column represent wake percentage (A), REMS percentage (B), NREM sleep percentage (C), and EEG slow wave variation (as a percentage of the daily mean; D) as a function of the phase of the circadian body temperature rhythm (E). The panels forming the right-hand column represent the same variables replotted as a function of time from the beginning of a sleep episode.

and, thereby, creating a monophasic sleep–wake cycle within which humans stay awake and alert during daytime hours and remain asleep throughout the night (Dijk and Czeisler, 1994, 1995).

Among sleep stages, REMS is the most strongly gated by circadian phase and remains concentrated near the Tb minimum (normally late in the sleep phase) under a variety of experimental protocols (Carskadon and Dement, 1980; Czeisler *et al.*, 1980; Dijk and Czeisler, 1995). SWS, by contrast, does not show strong clock control. This is clearly shown in forced desynchrony studies, in which subjects live on a 20-h or 28-h sleep–wake schedule for several weeks. The circadian clock cannot entrain to forced sleep–wake (and light exposure) schedules that far removed from 24 h, thus each scheduled sleep episode is initiated at a progressively earlier or later circadian phase (tracked by measuring the Tb cycle).

Under these conditions, SWA is always highest at sleep onset and decreases exponentially during the sleep period, regardless of the circadian phase at which sleep onset is initiated (Dijk and Czeisler, 1995) (**Fig.** 4.3). The amount of SWA may vary slightly with circadian phase of sleep onset, but this is likely due to variations in how much sleep subjects obtained during the previous sleep episode, which is determined by circadian phase; the less sleep obtained during a scheduled sleep episode, the more SWA during the next scheduled sleep episode (r = −0.90) (Dijk and Czeisler, 1995). These observations have been taken as evidence that the circadian clock in humans does not directly modulate sleep homeostasis or intensity independent of sleep timing. This assumption that circadian and homeostatic processes make separate, independent contributions to sleep regulation is a core feature of the original two-process quantitative model of sleep regulation (Daan *et al.*, 1984). Analyses of SWA and sleep in rats with SCN-ablation, in mice with clock gene mutations, and in humans with certain clock gene variants, has produced evidence challenging the assumption, which is discussed further later.

Although SWA predominantly (if not entirely) reflects sleep homeostasis, sleep propensity and other sleep parameters (onset time, latency to onset, wakeup, duration, REMS timing) are all jointly controlled by circadian and homeostatic processes. During extended sleep deprivation, the interaction between these processes is nonlinear. Thus, as subjective sleepiness and sleep propensity increase over the course of a three-day sleep deprivation, the magnitude of the daily variation also increases (Akerstedt and Gillberg, 1990). A similar nonlinearity is evident in behavioral measures of cognitive function. Performance on tasks designed to assess attention, executive function and memory is progressively impaired during sleep deprivation. Impairments are accentuated at the body temperature minimum and are attenuated, and in some cases absent, during the evening "wake-maintenance zone" (Dijk *et al.*, 1992; Cajochen *et al.*, 1999; Van Dongen and Dinges, 2003; Lo *et al.*, 2012). This interaction creates circadian phases of enhanced vulnerability and resistance to performance failure during overnight or continuous operations.

4.3.2 Behavioral studies: rodent models

Sleep in nocturnal rats and mice also exhibits joint circadian and homeostatic control. Circadian regulation is evident by the concentration of sleep during the day and wake at night and the persistence of this rhythm in constant dark or dim light, with a circadian periodicity characteristic of the species or strain. As in humans, SWA is maximal early in the sleep period and REMS later in the sleep period (Rosenberg *et al.*, 1976). Homeostatic regulation is revealed by sleep deprivation studies (Borbély and Neuhaus, 1979; Mistlberger *et al.*, 1983; Trachsel *et al.*, 1986). Following 24 hours of total sleep deprivation, SWA and REMS show an immediate rebound, while total sleep time lost is minimally recovered (e.g., about 30% of sleep lost during a 24-h deprivation was recouped over three recovery days) (Mistlberger *et al.*, 1983). This is partly due to circadian constraints on sleep time, as revealed in conflict experiments in which sleep deprivation ends at the beginning of the night (wake phase). At this circadian phase, sleep deprived rats fall asleep within 15 min and show significantly increased total sleep time relative to baseline for that phase, but total sleep accumulated during the first 12 hours of recovery is less than half the amount accumulated during the 12-h light period (Mistlberger *et al.*, 1983).

Sleep in nocturnal rats and mice can be distinguished from sleep in humans by its polyphasic distribution. Sleep bouts occur in every hour of the 24-h LD cycle, at least under laboratory conditions. Bouts at night are less frequent and significantly shorter, but still account for about 35% of total daily sleep time

(Mistlberger *et al.*, 1983). This suggests less strict control of behavioral state by the circadian clock in these species. Consistent with this interpretation, NREMS and REMS show little or no circadian variation, respectively, in rats forced to stay awake for two hours of every four hours for 48 hours (a 2 h:2 h ultradian sleep–wake schedule) (Yasenkov and Deboer, 2010). In this protocol, rats were able to sleep at all circadian phases and thus sustained only a minor decrease in total daily sleep time.

A study of selective REMS deprivation in rats showed that attempts to enter REMS were higher during the sleep phase of the circadian cycle (Wurts and Edgar, 2000) but evidently there is little circadian constraint on the expression of REMS during a sleep opportunity in sleep restricted rats (Yasenkov and Deboer, 2010). Humans, by contrast, show strong circadian gating of REMS and a significant reduction in total daily sleep under similar ultradian sleep–wake schedule protocols (Maron *et al.*, 1964; Carskadon and Dement, 1975; Lavie, 2001). Flexibility in the timing of rest-activity rhythms in rats is further evident when food availability is limited to the daytime (Mistlberger and Antle, 2011) or requires a high workload (Hut *et al.*, 2011). Under these conditions, the activity of nocturnal rats and mice becomes increasingly diurnal. "Temporal niche switching" of this sort may involve resetting of circadian oscillators downstream from the master circadian pacemaker located in the suprachiasmatic nucleus (SCN, Chapter 3), which in the general case is not reset by these procedures.

Comparisons between humans and laboratory rodents are complicated by the dissimilar recording conditions under which they are typically studied. Rodents in polysomnographic sleep studies are usually tethered to a recording cable and socially isolated in a small cage. A comparable recording condition for a human would be continuous bed rest or confinement to a small recording room with no external stimulation (e.g., no social interactions, computers, books, music, video, etc.). Under such conditions, sleep in humans is significantly less consolidated and occurs more frequently in the circadian day (Campbell and Zulley, 1989; Lavie, 2001). Conversely, sleep in rodents may be more consolidated in natural environments, where the costs of being awake, active and making noise at the "wrong" time of day can be high, and where foraging activities would likely promote longer, consolidated nocturnal wake bouts than are evident under laboratory conditions. Dramatic differences between sleep in the laboratory and in the wild have been noted in other species (e.g., the sloth) (Rattenborg *et al.*, 2008).

4.3.3 Neural mechanisms

A pandemic of viral encephalitus characterized by severe sleep disturbances provided the first clues to the location of brain mechanisms regulating sleep and wake (Von Economo, 1930). Post mortem inspection of brain tissue revealed anterior hypothalamic damage associated with insomnia, and posterior hypothalamic damage associated with hypersomnia. Experimental reproduction of these effects by lesions in animals supported a "dual-center" concept of sleep–wake regulation (Ranson, 1939; Nauta, 1946).

More refined lesions, electrophysiological recordings, cellular markers of activity (e.g., immediate early gene expression) and tract tracing with neurochemical phenotyping have identified sleep active, NREMS-promoting GABA neurons in the ventrolateral preoptic area (VLPO), median preoptic nucleus (MnPN) and basal forebrain (McGinty and Szymusiak, 2003, 2011; Jones, 2004). Wake-promoting neurons releasing orexin, acetylcholine or monoamines (histamine, serotonin, norepinephrine, dopamine) are found in the basal forebrain, perifornical and lateral hypothalamus, tuberomammilary nuclei (TMN), midbrain and pontine reticular formation (McGinty and Szymusiak, 2003, 2011; Brown *et al.*, 2012). Sleep active cells in the VLPO and wake active cells in the TMN, raphe and locus coeruleus exchange inhibitory projections, a design feature that, in principle, should facilitate rapid "switching" between two stable states characteristic of sleep and wake (McGinty and Szymusiak, 2000). In its latest iteration, the reciprocal inhibition model is conceptualized as a neural "flip-flop" circuit critical for sleep–wake transitions and state consolidation (Saper *et al.*, 2001). While the concept has appeal, the role of a central executive circuit in sleep–wake control may be overstated (Krueger *et al.*, 2013; Section 4.3.4) and details of the model may require revision (Zecharia *et al.*, 2012).

Neural efferents from the SCN circadian pacemaker project to sleep active and wake active components of this system, both directly (Novak and Nunez, 2000; Deurveilher *et al.*, 2002; Deurveilher and

Semba, 2003) and indirectly, primarily via synapses in the subparaventricular zone and the dorsomedial hypothalamic nucleus (Watts, 1991; Sun *et al.*, 2000, 2001; Deurveilher *et al.*, 2002; Deurveilher and Semba, 2003; Canteras *et al.*, 2011). This projection pattern provides a basis for continuous modulation of sleep–wake states by SCN pacemaker outputs alternately promoting sleep and wake, a model suggested by circadian modulation of sleep propensity in humans as discussed above.

A critical role for the SCN in circadian regulation of sleep–wake was confirmed by SCN ablation, which eliminates the circadian sleep–wake cycle in nocturnal rodents (Ibuka *et al.*, 1980; Mistlberger *et al.*, 1983; Tobler *et al.*, 1983; Trachsel *et al.*, 1992) and diurnal primates (Edgar *et al.*, 1993). SCN lesions have no significant effect on total daily sleep time in rats (Mistlberger *et al.*, 1983; Wurts and Edgar, 2000; Trachsel *et al.*, 1986) and have either little (about 7% increase) (Easton *et al.*, 2004) or no effect (Ibuka *et al.*, 1980) on sleep time in mice. There is one report of a marked increase (about 50%) in sleep duration after SCN-ablation in a diurnal primate, the squirrel monkeys (Edgar *et al.*, 1993). Quantitative models accurately simulate sleep in intact and SCN-ablated rodents if the SCN is assumed to alternately promote (or inhibit) both sleep and wake at different circadian phases, but not if the SCN stimulates (or inhibits) only one state or the other (Fleshner *et al.*, 2011). The squirrel monkey data suggest that the circadian clock in that species has a critical role in wake maintenance, at least under laboratory conditions of temporal and social isolation. It is not known if the hypersomnia might be remediated by social housing (e.g., sloths in the laboratory sleep 50% more than sloths free-ranging in their natural habitat) (Rattenborg *et al.*, 2008). Truly comparative data on the effects of SCN damage on sleep in humans are not available. Tumors in the SCN area have been associated with both daytime hypersomnia (Cohen and Albers, 1991) and nocturnal insomnia (Borgers *et al.*, 2011, 2012), but anatomical specificity in such cases is lacking, and the effects may be more accurately described as an impaired ability to maintain state continuity as opposed to a change in total daily sleep time.

Consistent with the lack of effect on daily sleep duration, SCN ablation in rats and mice also does not impair the homeostatic response to acute sleep loss, as indicated by large immediate increases in SWA and REMS following sleep deprivation (Mistlberger *et al.*, 1983, 1987; Tobler *et al.*, 1983; Trachsel *et al.*, 1992). Notably, during the first 12 hours of recovery from 24 hour sleep deprivation, the total amount of NREM and REMS obtained by SCN-ablated rats is significantly higher by comparison with intact rats when recovery is initiated at the beginning of the night (wake phase), but significantly lower than nondeprived intact rats during the day (sleep phase). These results can only be explained if the circadian clock in nocturnal rodents, as in humans, exerts a continuous influence on sleep expression, actively promoting sleep in the day and wake at night (Mistlberger *et al.*, 1983; Mistlberger, 2005).

SCN neural activity at the population level exhibits a daily rhythm in freely moving rodents and in explants isolated from the rest of the brain *in vitro* (Gillette *et al.*, 1995; Meijer *et al.*, 1997). Single and multiple unit recordings exhibit some heterogeneity in the phase of the daily rhythm maximum (Saeb-Parsy and Dyball, 2003; Schaap *et al.*, 2003), but the integrated population rhythm is approximately sinusoidal and peaks in the middle of the light period, in nocturnal and diurnal species alike. Other measures of SCN circadian phase, including daily rhythms of SCN metabolic activity, clock gene expression and the response to phase resetting stimuli (as described by phase-response curves to light) are similarly invariant across chronotypes (Smale *et al.*, 2003). The neural basis of the inversion of sleep–wake relative to SCN phase and the solar day in nocturnal and diurnal species remains to be explained. The inversion may involve interneurons downstream from the SCN, differences in coupling between SCN circadian oscillators and circadian oscillators elsewhere in the brain (see below), or other mechanisms (Smale *et al.*, 2003).

The inverted phasing of the daily sleep–wake rhythm relative to the SCN pacemaker does provide clues to SCN output pathways regulating sleep. For example, in nocturnal and diurnal species, the pineal hormone melatonin is secreted only at night, under control of SCN neural outputs. Melatonin at pharmacological doses has modest efficacy in promoting sleep onset in humans, possibly by damping SCN outputs that promote alertness (Lavie, 1997; Liu *et al.*, 1997; Wyatt *et al.*, 2006). However, a role for melatonin in sleep induction cannot apply to nocturnal species, which are predominantly awake when melatonin is secreted and asleep when it is absent. Consistent with this phase relation between the daily rhythms of melatonin secretion and sleep–wake, pinealectomy has no effect on sleep parameters in rats (Fisher and Sugden, 2010).

Preservation of homeostatic sleep "rebounds" following sleep deprivation in arrhythmic, SCN-ablated rats constitutes direct evidence supporting the assumption that circadian and homeostatic processes regulate sleep in parallel and via separate neural substrates. One effect of SCN ablation in rats that has received little attention is the significant decrease in the incidence, amplitude and spectral power of slow waves in NREMS (Bergmann *et al.*, 1987; Trachsel *et al.*, 1992). The absence of extended spontaneous wake bouts during baseline sleep in SCN-ablated rats presumably contributes to reduced SWA, reflecting constant low homeostatic sleep drive. However, SWA in SCN-ablated rats is not normalized by 24 hours of sleep deprivation (Mistlberger *et al.*, 1987), suggesting that SCN outputs contribute to sleep intensity, at least as defined by SWA within NREMS. This would lead to the prediction that after sleep deprivation, SCN-ablated rats should require more sleep than intact rats, because of reduced sleep intensity. This does not appear to be true, as there is no significant difference between SCN-ablated and intact rats in total daily sleep time for up to three recovery days after 24 hours of sleep deprivation. From this it can be concluded that sleep intensity and homeostasis are reflected in relative but not absolute levels of SWA in NREMS. The reduced levels of SWA following SCN ablation remain to be explained.

4.3.4 Molecular mechanisms, local oscillators and local sleep

Sleep research and chronobiology are independent disciplines with distinct histories and subject matters that intersect in the study of sleep as a biological rhythm. Both fields are undergoing similar paradigm shifts by which early concepts of brain "centers" exerting top-down control over sleep and daily rhythms, respectively, are being replaced by new evidence for highly distributed systems and local control. In circadian biology, the metaphor of multicellular organisms as a "shop of clocks" has been validated in the last decade by the discovery that self-sustaining circadian oscillators exist in many, if not all, organs and tissues (Herzog and Tononi, 2001; Yoo *et al.*, 2004; Guilding and Piggins, 2007; Dibner *et al.*, 2010). Similarly, conceptual models of sleep control have evolved from sleep "centers" and anatomically distributed sleep "switching circuits" that impose sleep "from the top-down", to local circuits such as cortical columns within which sleep states emerge as a consequence of local activity and promote the emergence of global sleep "from the bottom-up" (Krueger and Tononi, 2011; Krueger *et al.*, 2013; Vyazovskiy and Harris, 2013).

Models that emphasize centralized top-down control of sleep are challenged by long-standing observations that no single brain lesion can permanently eliminate sleep, without also eliminating wake. In addition, elements of sleep can occur in otherwise waking organisms, as a result of sleep deprivation (e.g., microsleeps in cortical EEG, lapses of attention), sleep inertia (impaired waking functions following waking), unihemispheric sleep (marine mammals and birds) and sleep disorders (e.g., sleep walking, talking and leg movements). Sleep, therefore, appears to be a property of local circuits that can go "off-line" independently (Leemburg *et al.*, 2010; Rattenborg *et al.*, 2012; Vyazofskiy and Harris, 2013). Neural correlates of sleep in local circuits may modulate activity in central sleep–wake circuits (e.g., the VLPO and TMN), to promote appropriate switching of diffusely projecting modulatory systems (e.g., monoaminergic, cholinergic, orexinergic) and facilitate global state transitions.

Circadian clock genes are also expressed locally in numerous brain regions outside of the SCN pacemaker, including areas that exhibit state-dependent variations in neural activity or local sleep (Guilding and Piggins, 2007). Clock cells in the central SCN pacemaker generate timing signals that directly drive daily rhythms or coordinate local oscillators with each other and the solar day. The role of clock genes in local functions is not yet well understood and little is known about interactions with local sleep processes. Sleep homeostasis does not require an intact SCN or circadian organization of behavioral state, but that does not rule out the possibility that clock genes expressed in tissues and brain regions outside of the SCN influence the sleep process at the cellular level. If clock genes do participate in sleep homeostasis, then animal models and humans with clock gene mutations or polymorphisms should exhibit changes in average daily sleep duration, sleep intensity (EEG SWA) and/or the response to sleep deprivation. The absence of such effects would be consistent with the assumption that circadian and homeostatic regulation are independent processes. Evidence for such effects would raise the possibility that clock genes participate more directly in sleep homeostasis.

Of course, interpretation of any observed effects may not be straightforward. If sleep parameters reflect the operation of a sleep somnostat that "senses" sleep need and adjusts sleep propensity, duration and intensity accordingly, changes in sleep parameters could be caused by altered inputs, setpoint or outputs. The metaphor of a central somnostat may be no more than a convenient fiction but it does help illustrate the interpretive complexity. Clock genes could participate in processes, such as metabolic and immune functions, that may be upstream from the somnostat. Clock genes could act as sensors for prior wake time (e.g., if wake time alters expression of clock genes). Clock genes, as part of the clock mechanism, are certainly important for consolidating sleep and wake states, and the loss of a clock dependent alerting or sleep promoting signal may affect daily sleep duration and intensity secondary to fragmentation of behavioral states, an effect downstream from the somnostat. The first step is to determine if clock gene manipulations do affect sleep parameters other than circadian timing. The more difficult task will be to understand the mechanism causal to any sleep phenotypes, to determine whether clock genes participate in the sleep process directly, or via indirect pathways. The following is a summary of the available evidence, with some interpretive issues highlighted.

Sleep states have now been characterized in mice with mutations of the clock genes *Per1*, *Per2*, *Per 3*, *Cry1*, *Cry2*, *Clock*, *Bmal1*, *Npas2*, *CKe*, *Cbp*, and *Dec2* (reviewed in Franken and Dijk, 2009; Landgraf *et al.*, 2012) (Chapters 1 and 2). Sleep duration and the homeostatic response to sleep deprivation appear to be normal in 129/sv mice with single or double knockouts of *per1* and *per2* or single knockout of *per3* (Kopp *et al.*, 2002; Shiromani *et al.*, 2004). These mice exhibit changes in the phase of entrainment to LD cycles (single KOs) or loss of rhythmicity (double KOs). A more recent study of *Per3* KO mice on a C57BL/6j genetic background reported accelerated buildup of SWA across the daily wake phase, and increased sleep at lights-on, although again no change in total daily sleep time (Hasan *et al.*, 2011). This illustrates a limitation of the available literature; most clock gene KO have not yet been evaluated in multiple laboratories, and sleep phenotypes of specific mutations may vary with genetic background and other factors.

Cry1/2 double knockouts are also arrhythmic but exhibit an apparent intensification of NREMS processes, as indicated by increased NREMS bout length, NREM delta wave power and total daily NREMS duration (Wisor *et al.*, 2002). Paradoxically, although the baseline phenotype suggests increased homeostatic sleep drive (as if the mice are living under higher sleep pressure), a rebound response to sleep deprivation is absent in NREMS time and attenuated in EEG delta power, which implies increased resistance to sleep loss. This could reflect a ceiling effect (further increases in NREMS duration may be prevented by competing essential needs). Alternatively, the KO mice may be less tolerant to sleep deprivation, resulting in more microsleeps during deprivation (the greater the sleep pressure, the more prevalent are microsleeps) and a less complete sleep deprivation relative to wild-type (WT) mice. Consistent with this interpretation, double *Cry* KO mice exhibited markedly elevated EEG delta power during sleep deprivation (Wisor *et al.*, 2002). Microsleeps may have functional value, as suggested by the negative correlation between EEG microsleeps during chronic sleep restriction and the magnitude of subsequent rebound sleep in WT mice (Leemburg *et al.*, 2010). Whatever the explanation, comparing sleep in arrhythmic *Per1/2* KO mice with sleep in arrhythmic *Cry1/2* KO mice indicates that loss of rhythmicity at the cellular level does not predict changes in sleep homeostasis. This implies a pleiotropic function for *cry* genes independent of their role in circadian clock gene transcriptional/translational feedback loops (TTFLs).

Mice bearing a null mutation of *Bmal1* lose circadian rhythmicity in both LD and DD (constant dark), and exhibit a sleep phenotype similar to that of double *Cry* KO mice, with more NREMS, increased delta power in NREMS and a reduced homeostatic response to six-hour sleep deprivation (smaller increments of NREMS and slow wave activity) (Laposky *et al.*, 2005). Unlike *Cry* KO mice, sleep bouts in *Bmal1* null mice were shorter. The mice were noted to be more difficult to sleep deprive. Increased fragmentation of baseline sleep and difficulty staying awake during sleep deprivation suggest a primary impairment of state consolidation. Fragmented sleep may be less restorative, resulting in a chronically elevated sleep pressure, as suggested by increased NREMS delta power. Difficulty staying awake may result in more microsleeps during sleep deprivation, which again could explain the smaller increments of sleep duration and intensity during recovery sleep.

Mice homozygous for the *Clock* mutation retain circadian rhythms of sleep–wake in LD but exhibit about two hours less sleep per day than WT mice, due to a selective reduction in NREMS (Naylor *et al.*, 2000).

NREM SWA, REMS duration and NREMS rebounds following sleep deprivation were not affected. Reduced NREMS duration without increased NREMS intensity (at least as defined by SWA; see Rechtschaffen *et al.*, 1999 for an alternative view) implies a reduced need for NREMS (SWA should be intensified if NREMS duration is insufficient). If average daily sleep duration reflects a physiological setpoint in a control system, this may represent the best case so far for a clock gene mutation that affects sleep need (where "need" is equivalent to an apparent setpoint). Consistent with a role for *Clock* in sleep duration, *Clock* polymorphisms were found to associate with sleep duration in two separate populations of humans (Allebrandt *et al.*, 2010). *Clock* mutant mice also exhibit metabolic dysfunction (e.g., obesity, hypoinsulinemia, and metabolic syndrome) (Turek *et al.*, 2005) and it is possible that the sleep changes are secondary to these metabolic defects. It will be of interest to assess metabolic variables associated with *Clock* polymorphisms in humans.

A significant albeit less marked reduction of NREMS was also reported in mice deficient in the CLOCK paralog NPAS2, which is normally expressed in some brain regions outside of the SCN (Dudley *et al.*, 2003; Franken *et al.*, 2006). Male (but not female) *Npas2* null mice exhibited an attenuated rebound of NREMS, REMS and NREMS SWA following eight-hour sleep deprivation (Franken *et al.*, 2006). Notably, this sleep phenotype in CLOCK and NPAS2 deficient mice is in the opposite direction to that exhibited by *Cry1/2* null mice. CRY proteins suppress CLOCK and NPAS2-mediated transcription. In the absence of CRY proteins, transcripts of genes activated by CLOCK:BMAL1 or NPAS2:BMAL1 are increased and these could be responsible for the sleep phenotype in *Cry1/2* null mice. *Per* genes are among those increased in *Cry1/2* null mice. As noted above, sleep homeostasis appears to be normal in mice lacking PER1 and PER2 proteins. However, *Per1* and *Per2* expression is increased in several regions of the mouse brain (excluding the SCN) in proportion to the duration of prior waking, and decreases to baseline levels after recovery sleep (Wisor *et al.*, 2002, 2008; Franken *et al.*, 2007). *Per1/2* gene expression in these regions can, therefore, be described as a molecular correlate of sleep need, and could conceivably function as a sensor of prior wake time in local circuits. This role may be masked in KO models by developmental compensation. Of interest is whether similar changes can be detected in central sleep–wake circuits in the hypothalamus, basal forebrain and brainstem.

Albumin D-binding protein (DBP) is a transcription factor that binds to the promoters for *Per1, 2 and 3, Rev-erbα* and other genes. *Dbp* KO mice retain circadian sleep–wake rhythms, but with a reduced amplitude and shorter sleep–wake bout lengths (Franken *et al.*, 2000). The amplitude of the wake-dependent rise of SWA was also attenuated, but this could be secondary to the increased amount of sleep in the usual wake phase of the circadian cycle. Intact sleep homeostasis was further indicated by a normal NREMS SWA rebound response following sleep deprivation. By contrast, REMS did not show a significant increment after sleep deprivation.

DEC2 is another clock-driven transcription factor that participates in clock cycling by regulating transcriptional activity of CLOCK/NPAS2 and BMAL1 (Noshiro *et al.*, 2005). A point mutation of *DEC2* in mice significantly decreases both NREMS and REMS in the light period, resulting in an approximately 10% decrease in total daily sleep time relative to WT mice (He *et al.*, 2009). Mutant mice also showed smaller percentage increments of sleep time and NREMS SWA following sleep deprivation, consistent with an effect of the mutation on sleep homeostasis. Two human family members bearing the same *DEC2* mutation exhibited a 22% decrease in total daily sleep time relative to noncarrier family members (He *et al.*, 2009). Although these individuals were early risers, sleep onset times were within normal range, indicating no change in the phase of entrainment to LD, consistent with the lack of effect of the mutation on the circadian period in mice. The reduced sleep rebound response to sleep deprivation in the mouse model suggests that the human subjects might have an increased tolerance of sleep deprivation.

In addition to polymorphisms of *Clock* noted above, several other clock gene polymorphisms have been found to associate with sleep parameters in humans (Toh *et al.*, 2001; Archer *et al.*, 2003; Xu *et al.*, 2005). The most dramatic effects are evident in preferred sleep and wake onset times, defining "evening" and "morning" chronotypes, which at the extremes are classified as delayed and advanced sleep phase disorder (DSPD and ASPD), respectively (Jones *et al.*, 1999). Genetic determination of chronotype is predictable given the role of clock genes in setting the period of the circadian cycle and the phase resetting response to clock inputs, which together determine the phase of entrainment to environmental zeitgebers (e.g., LD cycles). Changes in sleep timing could also be secondary to effects on sleep homeostasis

(Archer et al., 2003; Mongrain et al., 2004, 2006; Mongrain and Dumont, 2007). Sleep pressure appears to accumulate more rapidly in morning types, as suggested by an accelerated increase of theta activity in the waking EEG across the day, and enhanced SWA at sleep onset (Kerkhof, 1991; Kerkhof and Lancel, 1991; Tallaird et al., 2003). This could result in earlier sleep onset relative to circadian pacemaker phase in some morning types (Mongrain et al., 2004).

Length polymorphisms of PER3 have been found to associate with chronotype, with a $Per3^{5/5}$ variant associated with advanced sleep, and $Per3^{4/4}$ with delayed sleep. Individuals homozygous for $Per3^{5/5}$, by contrast with $Per3^{4/4}$ carriers, appear to live under higher homeostatic sleep pressure. Sleep latency is shorter, NREMS bouts are longer, NREMS SWA is increased and cognitive impairment appears earlier during sleep deprivation (Archer et al., 2003, 2008; Viola et al., 2007). As noted above, a similar accelerated buildup of SWA has been reported in one study of Per3 KO mice (Hasan et al., 2011). Given the unremarkable circadian phenotype of Per3 null mice (Bae et al., 2001), the sleep phenotype is unlikely to be secondary to an alteration in the clock mechanism, and is consistent with a role for Per3 in sleep homeostasis.

What does this collection of observations mean for the two-process model of sleep regulation? In this model, circadian and homeostatic processes are treated as independent; the homeostatic Process S describes an effect of time awake and time asleep on sleep duration and intensity (EEG SWA), while the circadian Process C describes an effect of "time of day" (more accurately, circadian phase) on thresholds for sleep and wake onset. The circadian process attempts to limit sleep to a characteristic phase but accounts for little or no variance in the expression of slow waves (the marker for Process S) when time awake is controlled. Evidence for effects of clock gene mutations and polymorphisms on sleep duration, sleep intensity and the response to sleep deprivation invites revision of the two-process model, to incorporate a circadian clock influence on the homeostatic sleep process (Franken and Dijk, 2009; Dijk and Archer, 2010). The nature of the influence at the cellular and molecular level remains unspecified. This is not surprising, given that the cellular and molecular basis of Process S is also uncertain. Clock genes may represent a new window into that process, or several windows, if different clock genes affect sleep homeostasis in different ways. Some clock gene sleep phenotypes could be entirely independent of the role of the gene in circadian timing. In such cases, the phenotype would not be rescued by restoring circadian organization. Other clock gene effects on sleep homeostasis could be dependent on circadian modulation of cellular functions, conferred by inputs from the SCN pacemaker, or by clock genes cycling in non-SCN oscillators. Studies are needed in which SCN lesions are combined with clock gene knockouts, and knockouts are confined to specific brain structures, including the SCN, areas involved in central regulation of sleep and wake (e.g., VLPO and TMN), and areas that exhibit local sleep (e.g., cortical columns). It remains possible that sleep phenotypes in clock gene mutants do not reflect a primary role for these genes in sleep homeostasis, but rather are secondary to effects of the mutations on other processes that affect sleep (e.g., metabolism and immune signaling). Thus, even if clock gene mutations alter sleep parameters independently of circadian timing, until the mechanisms by which clock gene mutations affect sleep are clarified, there is a degree of uncertainty as to whether and how circadian modulation of sleep homeostasis should be incorporated into two-process models.

The two-process model in its original form also did not include modulation of the circadian process by sleep homeostasis. However, there is by now considerable evidence that clock-controlled sleep–wake states provide feedback that alters cellular and molecular processes in the SCN pacemaker, thereby altering SCN output and parameters of the circadian cycle.

4.4 Reciprocity: sleep–wake feedback to the circadian clock

4.4.1 Feedback from waking states

The flow of information through the circadian system was originally conceptualized as one way, with zeitgebers providing inputs to a central clock, which emitted timing signals to directly drive circadian rhythms or entrain secondary circadian oscillators in other brain regions and peripheral structures. The role of the central pacemaker in this hierarchical model was to coordinate behavior and physiology with environmental cycles. Feedback from clock-controlled processes was considered not only unnecessary but potentially destabilizing and, thus, maladaptive. The model was largely unopposed by evidence during the 1960s and 1970s when circadian pacemakers were being localized in various species. Neuroanatomical studies of afferent connections of the SCN circadian pacemaker in mammals revealed that this structure receives multiple inputs, only two of which (the retina and thalamic intergeniculate leaflet) are known to convey information about LD cycles (Morin and Allen, 2006). Many of the inputs arise from brain structures that exhibit marked behavioral state-dependent variations in activity (e.g., basal forebrain and midbrain monoamine systems). Neural pathways by which clock-driven sleep–wake states could feed back to the SCN pacemaker are clearly present, and many more such pathways to local circadian oscillators in other brain regions must also exist. Do these inputs alter the phase, period, amplitude and output of SCN and other neural circadian oscillators? Do any of these inputs encode sleep homeostasis and, if so, with what consequences for pacemaker function?

Empirical evidence for an effect of behavioral states on circadian clocks in mammals was discovered in two independent lines of work exploring the effects of activity recording devices on circadian pacemaker period in rats (Yamada *et al.*, 1986) and the effects of cage litter changes on circadian pacemaker phase in Syrian hamsters (Mrosovsky, 1988). Activity of a rat housed in a small cage, monitored using a motion sensor, exhibits a circadian rhythm that free-runs with a stable period usually longer than 24 hours in constant dark. If the rat is then provided with a running wheel, the period of the free-running rhythm shortens over the next few cycles, and assumes a new stable periodicity often less than 24 hours (Yamada *et al.*, 1986). If the wheel is removed, the circadian rest–activity cycle lengthens again. This effect is evident in sighted and blind rats, so was independent of light input (Yamada *et al.*, 1988). Some physiological correlate of a clock-controlled behavior (running) must alter the motion of the circadian clock. Lengthening of the circadian period by wheel running also occurs in mice (Edgar *et al.*, 1991; Mistlberger *et al.*, 1998) and Syrian hamsters (Mrosovsky, 1999a). The initial discovery using rats did not have an immediate impact on the field, likely because the results did not fit contemporary thinking that a master clock responsive to environmental cycles should be largely impervious to time-varying signals related to the animal's own behavior and physiology.

In a parallel line of work, an observant chronobiologist noticed that daily wheel running rhythms in the Syrian hamster sometimes exhibited annoying, unplanned, small phase shifts following routine cage cleaning (Mrosovsky, 1988). Hamsters run almost exclusively at night and continue to restrict activity to a "subjective night" when maintained in constant dark or light. The onset of activity is highly predictable by regression from previous cycles. A phase shift was determined if activity onset began early or late, and subsequent onsets were predictable from this new time (again by regression through activity onsets). The hamster wheel running circadian rhythm is remarkably precise, and even small shifts are unmistakable to visual inspection of graphs. Similar examples of presumed (and therefore ignored) "noise" in the timing of rest–activity cycles can be seen in older published records. Treating the noise as "signal", the now curious chronobiologist conducted a systematic "phase response" experiment, in which the stimulus (cage litter changing) was scheduled at different phases of the rest–activity cycle in Syrian hamsters in constant dark. Phase advance shifts (activity occurs earlier than usual as the clock is reset forward) followed litter changes in the usual rest period (the subjective day in nocturnal animals), and smaller delays or no responses followed litter changes in the usual active phase (subjective night) (Mrosovsky, 1988). The effect generalized to other arousing stimuli, including brief social interactions, confinement to a novel wheel (which induces near continuous running in most hamsters), and gentle handling, a method borrowed from the sleep research field to sleep deprive hamsters without stimulating stress or excessive activity (Mrosovsky, 1996; Antle and Mistlberger, 2000; Mistlberger *et al.*, 2000).

The effect was further generalized to rats and mice, although in these species, phase shifts induced by a single arousal session were not prevalent. Instead the arousal procedure (running stimulated by a wheel or forced on a treadmill) was scheduled at a fixed time of day for several weeks in DD or LL (constant light), and was found to entrain free-running rhythms, which requires a daily phase shift (Edgar and Dement, 1991; Mistlberger, 1991; Marchant *et al.*, 1997; Yamanaka *et al.*, 2013). Not all sources of arousal are effective. In Syrian hamsters (Webb *et al.*, 2010) and rats (Meerlo *et al.*, 1997), acute exposure to a stress stimulus does not shift circadian phase, despite strong behavioral activation.

Behavioral effects on circadian rhythms were discovered by manipulating behavior and measuring circadian period and phase in the absence of daily LD cycles. Behavioral inputs to the clock are of sufficient magnitude to modify the phase of entrainment to LD cycles, and the response of the circadian system to LD shifts. In mice entrained to LD 12:12, if running wheels are available only during the first or last six hours of the night, the circadian clock is advanced or delayed, respectively (Mistlberger and Holmes, 2000; Schroeder *et al.*, 2012). Modification of entrained phase may reflect integration of separate photic and nonphotic inputs to the clock, alteration of pacemaker period by wheel running (Mistlberger and Holmes, 2000) or modulation of the pacemakers' response to light. Other work has shown that behavioral arousal stimulated just before, during or after brief light exposure during the subjective night inhibits the phase shift normally induced by light at that circadian phase (Ralph and Mrosovsky, 1992; Mistlberger *et al.*, 1997, 1998; Burgess, 2010). Evening light normally phase delays the circadian clock, while morning light advances the clock. Early night running could thereby advance the clock by attenuating the phase delaying effect of evening light exposure. Late night running would do the reverse, to the extent that neural effects of running outlast the running stimulus. Nonlinear interactions between light and behavioral stimuli are suggested by the marked potentiation of the rate at which circadian rhythms adjust to an eight-hour phase advance of LD when hamsters are behaviorally aroused during the first few hours of the first new nighttime (Mrosovsky and Salmon, 1987).

Subsequent work has identified neural inputs to the SCN pacemaker that mediate behavioral effects on circadian rhythms. The period shortening effect of wheel running is absent in mice lacking serotonergic (5HT) innervation of the SCN, which is a dense terminal field arising from the midbrain median raphe (Mistlberger *et al.*, 1998). The phase shifting effect of waking hamsters in their usual sleep period is absent in hamsters with lesions of the IGL, which as noted is a retinorecipient thalamic structure that contains peptidergic neurons releasing NPY, enkephalons, GABA and other neurotransmitters from terminals in the SCN (Janik and Mrosovsky, 1994). This structure is also innervated by a 5HT projection from the dorsal raphe. 5HT neurons, while heterogeneous in their inputs, are active during waking, quiescent in NREMS and virtually silent during REMS (Jacobs and Fornal, 1999). IGL lesions in mice eliminate entrainment of free-running rhythms to daily running schedules, while 5HT lesions markedly reduce the efficacy of these schedules (Marchant *et al.*, 1997). Pharmacology and *in vivo* microdialysis have further established NPY and 5HT signaling as critical components of behavioral input pathways to the circadian clock (Mrosovsky, 1996; Glass *et al.*, 2010). Both of these transmitters also attenuate the response of SCN neurons to photic inputs, and thus presumably mediate the inhibitory effect of arousal on light-induced phase shifts (Challet and Pevet, 2003). Other neurotransmitters (e.g., acetylcholine, enkephalin, histamine, orexin) from other brain regions (cholinergic neurons in 6 different brain regions project to the SCN) may also participate.

4.4.2 Feedback from sleep states

The animal data indicate that known neural correlates of the wake state (e.g., activity of 5HT neurons) exert both feedforward (associated with externally stimulated waking) and feedback (associated with clock-controlled waking) effects on the clockworks, with a functional outcome (clock shifting or modulation of LD entrained phase). What about sleep; is it possible that neural, endocrine or other correlates of NREMS and REMS also impinge on and regulate the circadian clockworks? Any procedure that affects the timing of waking must per force affect the timing of sleep, so logic dictates a considered look.

An experimental approach to this question might follow that used to explore the effect of arousal on the phase of rest–activity rhythms in rodents. However, there is no behavioral procedure by which to induce an acute episode of sleep, without first stimulating arousal. An alternative approach is to stimulate sleep pharmacologically. Benzodiazepines, a sleep promoting class of GABA receptor agonists, can induce phase shifts in Syrian hamsters (Turek and Losee-Olson,, 1986) but paradoxically do so by stimulating "drunken" activity (shifts mimic those induced by arousal, and are absent if activity is prevented by confinement to a small box or restraint tube) (Mrosovsky and Salmon, 1990). Phase shifts have also been observed in a diurnal primate, the squirrel monkey, following injections of triazolam at doses that rapidly induce sleep (Mistlberger *et al.*, 1991). The phase-response shift profile was similar to that observed for behavioral arousal in hamsters (phase advances when drug was administered in the mid-subjective day, when squirrel monkeys are normally awake). This finding has not been extended to humans.

Sleep induction may also be involved in phase advance shifts induced by the adenosine receptor A1 agonist N6-cyclohexyladenosine (N-CHA) microinjected directly to the SCN in Syrian hamsters (Antle *et al.*, 2001). Adenosine exhibits properties of an endogenous, activity-dependent local sleep factor. It is a byproduct of cellular metabolism that in some brain regions increases in the extracellular compartment during waking, and decreases during sleep (Porkka-Heiskanen and Kalinchuk, 2011). Adenosine infusions in these areas induce sleep, while systemic adenosine antagonists (most famously caffeine) suppress sleep. Infusions of N-CHA into the SCN during the mid-subjective day in hamsters induced behavioral rest and mimicked the phase shifting effects of arousal. It is conceivable that when hamsters are behaviorally stimulated during the mid-subjective day when they should be asleep, adenosine accumulates in the SCN, and this causes the phase shifts induced by the arousal procedure. Consistent with this interpretation, the adenosine receptor antagonist caffeine induces arousal during the day but does not induce phase shifts, and suppresses phase shifts in response to stimulated running (Antle *et al.*, 2001). What remains to be confirmed is the site of action of systemic caffeine and intra-SCN N-CHA (diffusion to sleep-related preoptic nuclei is possible), and whether adenosine accumulates in the SCN during sleep deprivation procedures. Whether induction of sleep by adenosine injections in the VLPO induces phase shifts has also not been tested.

Another approach to the question of whether sleep states affect the circadian clock is to measure neuronal activity within the SCN pacemaker during natural sleep and wake states. This has been accomplished using extracellular recordings of actions potentials from multi-unit electrodes implanted within the SCN of freely behaving nocturnal rodents. Several studies first showed that SCN neural firing rates (multiple unit activity, MUA) in rats and Syrian hamsters decrease during spontaneous locomotor activity (Meijer *et al.*, 1997; Yamazaki *et al.*, 1998), consistent with other observations that basal levels of *c-Fos* expression (a marker of neural activity) in SCN neurons are decreased by a three-hour bout of arousal stimulated in the mid-subjective day (Mrosovsky, 1996; Antle and Mistlberger, 2000). Spontaneous and evoked locomotor activity also inhibits SCN neural activity in mice (van Oosterhout *et al.*, 2012). The population firing rate of SCN neurons varies sinusoidally, with a peak of MUA in the mid-subjective day (nocturnal rodent sleep phase), and a trough in the mid-subjective night (wake phase). The inhibitory feedback effect of spontaneous locomotor activity, which is maximal at night in nocturnal rodents, presumably reinforces this daily oscillation (the firing rate rhythm persists with high amplitude *in vitro*, so behavioral feedback does not cause the rhythm) (Meijer *et al.*, 1997).

More recent studies of mice show an apparently opposite effect, with SCN MUA decreasing during NREMS in proportion to EEG SWA, and then increasing during emergence from NREMS to REMS or waking (Deboer *et al.*, 2003, 2007). NREMS sleep homeostasis, therefore, does appear to be encoded in SCN neural activity. Given that nocturnal mice sleep in the day, when SCN MUA is high, feedback from clock-controlled sleep would seem to oppose the daily MUA rhythm. However, NREMS SWA is maximal at lights-on, when the daily sleep phase begins, and then declines monotonically throughout the day. SCN MUA is low early in the sleep phase and peaks in the middle of the day, thereby varying inversely with NREMS EEG SWA. It appears that the daily rhythm of SCN MUA reflects circadian regulation of neuronal properties (e.g., membrane potential) combined with feedback from clock-controlled behavioral states, with high intensity NREMS suppressing MUA early in the day, REMS increasing MUA later in the day, and active waking suppressing MUA at night. Not all SCN MUA recordings exhibit these behavioral correlates; phenotyping of behaviorally responsive cell types has not yet been done. A functional (admittedly speculative) interpretation of these data is that some SCN neurons promote waking, and these are inhibited during high intensity NREMS, while other SCN neurons promote sleep, and these are inhibited when animals are awakened in the middle of the day (it could be something dangerous), and/or by clock-driven activity at night (when sustained alert waking is required for foraging and other activities). Locomotor-induced changes in SCN neural activity presumably also explain phase shifts to acute arousal in the mid-day, and modification of circadian period by spontaneous wheel running in the subjective night.

4.5 Conclusions: Circadian clocks and sleep are intertwined processes

Epidemiological and experimental studies support an important role for sleep and circadian rhythms in health and disease. This chapter has explored how circadian clocks and sleep interact, to evaluate the potential for cross-talk to serve as a conduit for propagating disease cascades. Early conceptual models emphasized a one-way, limited interaction, with circadian clocks (Process C) directly regulating sleep timing, via modulation of thresholds for sleep and wake onset. In these models, a separate and privileged homeostatic Process S regulated sleep intensity (NREMS SWA) according to prior wake time and independent of circadian phase. The discovery of circadian clock genes in mammals permitted evaluation of sleep in clock mutants and naturally occurring clock gene polymorphisms. Clock gene variants that affect the period of the circadian clock are expected to alter the timing of sleep and wake onset. But more complex sleep phenotypes have been observed in some clock mutations and polymorphisms, marked by changes in average daily sleep duration, sleep intensity and the homeostatic response to sleep duration. It remains unclear whether these sleep phenotypes reflect noncircadian (pleiotropic) functions for clock genes or whether they are secondary to alterations in the circadian scaffolding of cellular functions or sleep–wake states. Pleiotropic effects could involve metabolic, immune or other pathways not specific to sleep. Further complexity is added by the distributed nature of circadian clocks in the brain and body. Clock cells mediating sleep phenotypes may be in the central SCN pacemaker, in central sleep–wake switching circuits, or in local circuits. Although details remain to be specified, disorders of circadian timekeeping devices have the potential to affect both the timing of sleep and the homeostatic process that is presumed to be at the heart of the restorative function(s) of sleep.

Early conceptual models did not envisage a role for sleep and wake in the regulation of functional parameters of the circadian clock (e.g., period, amplitude, phase and response to photic Zeitgebers). But the causal link between clock and behavioral state is clearly bidirectional. Neural correlates of either environmentally stimulated or clock-controlled waking can alter the phase and period of circadian rhythms in at least some species, and are presumably integrated with photic inputs to set the phase of circadian rhythms in natural entrainment. Yet to be defined neural and/or physiological correlates of sleep also regulate neural activity in the mammalian SCN pacemaker. To what end is not yet certain, but a reasonable line of speculation is that sleep–wake inputs to the circadian clock are functionally self-reinforcing, serving to promote sleep and wake states at the appropriate circadian phase, but also to permit sleep and wake expression at "wrong" phases, if accumulated sleep pressure or environmental conditions warrant. Sleep–wake states may well play an important role in maintaining high amplitude circadian organization of brain and peripheral functions. The circadian system thus represents a potential conduit for propagation of health effects associated with sleep–wake disruptions and chronic sleep disorders.

This analysis of reciprocal interactions between circadian clocks and sleep is relevant to other clock controlled functions, including eating and metabolism (Delezie and Challet, 2011). Circadian clocks and clock genes are likely embedded in multiple homeostatic systems with important implications for physiological functioning in health and disease.

References

Achermann, P. and Borbély, A.A. 2011. Sleep homeostasis and models of sleep regulation. In: *Principles and Practise of Sleep Medicine*, 5th edn (eds M.H. Kryger, T. Roth, and W.C. Dement). Saunders, MI, USA, pp. 431–4.

Akerstedt, T. and Gillberg, M. 1990. Subjective and objective sleepiness in the active individual. *International Journal of Neuroscience* 52(1–2):29–37.

Allebrandt, K.V., Teder-Laving, M., Akyol, M., *et al.* 2010. CLOCK Gene Variants Associate with Sleep Duration in Two Independent Populations. *Biological Psychiatry* 67:1040–7.

Altman, N.G., Izci-Balserak, B., Schopfer, E., *et al.* 2012. Sleep duration versus sleep insufficiency as predictors of cardiometabolic health outcomes. *Sleep Medicine* 13(10):1261–70.

Antle, M.C. and Mistlberger, R.E. 2000. Circadian clock resetting by sleep deprivation without exercise in the Syrian hamster. *Journal of Neuroscience* **20**(24):9326–32.

Antle, M.C., Steen, N.M., Mistlberger R.E. 2001. Adenosine and caffeine modulate circadian rhythms in the Syrian hamster *Neuroreport* **12**(13):2901–5.

Archer, S.N., Robilliard, D.L., Skene, D.J., *et al.* 2003. A length polymorphism in the circadian clock gene Per3 is linked to delayed sleep phase syndrome and extreme diurnal preference. *Sleep* **26**:413–5.

Archer, S.N., Viola, A.U., Kyriakopoulou, V., *et al.* 2008. Inter-individual differences in habitual sleep timing and entrained phase of endogenous circadian rhythms of BMAL1, PER2 and PER3 mRNA in human leukocytes. *Sleep* **31**:608–17.

Aschoff, J. 1965. Circadian rhythms in man. *Science* **148**(3676):1427–32.

Aschoff, J. and Wever, R. 1976. Human circadian rhythms: a multioscillatory system. *Federation Proceedings* **35**(12):236–32.

Bae, K., Jin, X., Maywood, E.S., *et al.* 2001. Differential functions of mPer1, mPer2, and mPer3 in the SCN circadian clock. *Neuron* **30**(2):525–36.

Bergman, B., Mistlberger, R.E. and Rechtschaffen, A. 1987. Period/amplitude analysis of EEG in the rat: Diurnal and stage variations and effects of suprachiasmatic nuclei lesions. *Sleep* **10**:523–36.

Borbely, A.A. and Neuhaus, H.U. 1979. Sleep deprivation: effects on sleep and EEG in the rat. *Progress in Neurobiology* **133**:71–87.

Borgers, A.J., Romeijn, N., van Someren E., *et al.* 2011. Compression of the optic chiasm is associated with permanent shorter sleep duration in patients with pituitary insufficiency. *Clinical Endocrinology (Oxford)* **75**:347–53.

Borgers, A.J., Fliers, E., Siljee, J.E., *et al.* 2012. Arginine vasopressin immunoreactivity is decreased in the hypothalamic suprachiasmatic nucleus of subjects with suprasellar tumors. *Brain Pathology* **23**:440–4.

Brown, R.E., Basheer, R., McKenna, J.T., *et al.* 2012. Control of sleep and wakefulness. *Physiological Reviews* **92**(3):1087–187.

Burgess, H.J. 2010. Partial sleep deprivation reduces phase advances to light in humans. *Journal of Biological Rhythms* **25**(6):460–8.

Campbell, S.S. and Zulley, J. 1989. Evidence for circadian influence on human slow wave sleep during daytime sleep episodes. *Psychophysiology* **26**(5):580–5.

Canteras, N.S., Ribeiro-Barbosa, E.R., Goto, M., *et al.* 2011. The retinohypothalamic tract: comparison of axonal projection patterns from four major targets. *Brain Research Reviews* **65**(2):150–83.

Cajochen, C., Khalsa, S.B., Wyatt, J.K., *et al.* 1999. EEG and ocular correlates of circadian melatonin phase and human performance decrements during sleep loss. *American Journal of Physiology* **277**:R640–9.

Carskadon, M.A. and Dement, W.C. 1975. Sleep studies on a 90-minute day. *Electroencephalography and Clinical Neurophysiology* **39**:145–55.

Carskadon, M.A. and Dement, W.C. 1980. Distribution of REM sleep on a 90 minute sleep–wake schedule. *Sleep* **2**:309–17.

Challet, E. and Pévet, P. 2003. Interactions between photic and nonphotic stimuli to synchronize the master circadian clock in mammals. *Frontiers in Bioscience* **8**:s246–57.

Cohen, R.A. and Albers, H.E. 1991.Disruption of human circadian and cognitive regulation following a discrete hypothalamic lesion: a case study, *Neurology* **41**:726–9.

Colwell, C.S. 2011. Linking neural activity and molecular oscillations in the SCN. *Nature Reviews Neuroscience* **12**:553–69.

Czeisler, C.A., Weitzman, E.D., Moore-Ede, M.C., *et al.* 1980. Human sleep: its duration and organization depend on its circadian phase. *Science* **210**(4475):1264–7.

Daan, S., Beersma, D.G. and Borbely, A.A. 1984. Timing of human sleep: recovery process gated by a circadian pacemaker, *American Journal of Physiology* **246**:R161–83.

Deboer, T., Vansteensel, M.J., Detari, L., and Meijer, J.H. 2003. Sleep states alter activity of suprachiasmatic nucleus neurons. *Nature Neuroscience* **6**:1086–90.

Deboer, T., Detari, L., and Meijer, J.H. 2007. Long term effects of sleep deprivation on the mammalian circadian pacemaker. *Sleep* **30**:257–62.

Delezie, J. and Challet, E. 2011. Interactions between metabolism and circadian clocks: reciprocal disturbances. *Annals of the New York Academy of Science* **1243**(1):30–46.

Deurveilher, S. and Semba, K. 2003. Indirect projections from the suprachiasmatic nucleus to the median preoptic nucleus in rat. *Brain Research* **987**:100–6.

Deurveilher, S., Burns, J. and Semba, K. 2002. Indirect projections from the suprachiasmatic nucleus to the ventrolateral preoptic nucleus: a dual tract-tracing study in rat. *European Journal of Neuroscience* **16**:1195–213.

Dibner, C., Schibler, U., Albrecht U. 2010. The mammalian circadian timing system: organization and coordination of central and peripheral clocks. *Annual Review of Physiology* **72**:517–49.

Dijk, D.J. and Archer, S.N. 2010. PERIOD3, circadian phenotypes, and sleep homeostasis. *Sleep Medicine Reviews* **14**:151–60.

Dijk, D.J. and Czeisler, C.A. 1994. Paradoxical timing of the circadian rhythm of sleep propensity serves to consolidate sleep and wakefulness in humans. *Neuroscience Letters* **166**(1):63–8.

Dijk, D.J. and Czeisler, C.A. 1995. Contribution of the circadian pacemaker and the sleep homeostat to sleep propensity, sleep structure, electroencephalographic slow waves, and sleep spindle activity in humans. *Journal of Neuroscience* **15**:3526–38.

Dijk, D.J., Beersma, D.G. and Daan, S. 1987. EEG power density during nap sleep: reflection of an hourglass measuring the duration of prior wakefulness *Journal of Biological Rhythms* **2**(3):207–19.

Dijk, D.J., Duffy, J.F., and Czeisler, C.A. 1992. Circadian and sleep/wake dependent aspects of subjective alertness and cognitive performance. *Journal of Sleep Research* **1**:112–7.

Dudley, C.A., Erbel-Sieler, C., Estill, S.J., *et al.* 2003. Altered patterns of sleep and behavioral adaptability in NPAS2-deficient mice, *Science* **301**:379–83.

Easton, A., Meerlo, P., Bergmann, B., and Turek, F.W. 2004. The suprachiasmatic nucleus regulates sleep timing and amount in mice. *Sleep* **27**:1307–18.

Edgar, D.M. and Dement, W.C. 1991. Regularly scheduled voluntary exercise synchronizes the mouse circadian clock. *American Journal of Physiology* **261**:R928–33.

Edgar, D.M., Martin, C.E., and Dement, W.C. 1991. Activity feedback to the mammalian circadian pacemaker: Influence on observed measures of rhythm period length. *Journal of Biological Rhythms* **6**:185–99.

Edgar, D.M., Dement, W.C., and Fuller, C.A. 1993. Effect of SCN lesions on sleep in squirrel monkeys: evidence for opponent processes in sleep–wake regulation. *Journal of Neuroscience* **13**:1065–79.

Faraut, B., Boudjeltia, K.Z., Vanhamme, L., and Kerkhofs, M. 2012.Immune, inflammatory and cardiovascular consequences of sleep restriction and recovery. *Sleep Medicine Reviews* **16**(2):137–49.

Feinberg, I., March, J.D., Floyd, T.C., *et al.* 1985. Homeostatic changes during post-nap sleep maintain baseline levels of delta EEG. *Electroencephalography and Clinical Neurophysiology* **1**:134–7.

Fisher, S.P. and Sugden, D. 2010. Endogenous melatonin is not obligatory for the regulation of the rat sleep–wake cycle *Sleep* **33**(6):833–40.

Flanigan, W.F. Jr., Wilcox, R.H., and Rechtschaffen, A. 1973. The EEG and behavioral continuum of the crocodilian, Caiman sclerops. *Electroencephalography and Clinical Neurophysiology* **34**(5):521–38.

Fleshner, M., Booth, V., Forger, D.B., and Diniz Behn, C.G. 2011. Circadian regulation of sleep–wake behavior in nocturnal rats requires multiple signals from suprachiasmatic nucleus. *Philosophical Transactions of the Royalty Society A* **369**:3855–83.

Frank, M.G. 2012. Erasing synapses in sleep: is it time to be SHY? *Neural Plasticity* **2012**:264378.

Franken, P. and Dijk, D.J. 2009. Circadian clock genes and sleep homeostasis. *European Journal of Neuroscience* **29**:1820–9.

Franken, P., Lopez-Molina, L., Marcacci, L., *et al.* 2000. The transcription factor DBP affects circadian sleep consolidation and rhythmic EEG activity. *Journal of Neuroscience* **20**(2):617–25.

Franken, P., Dudley, C.A., Estill, S.J., *et al.* 2006. NPAS2 as a transcriptional regulator of non-rapid eye movement sleep: Genotype and sex interactions. *Proceedings of the National Academy of Science USA* **103**:7118–23.

Franken, P., Thomason, R., Heller, H.C., and O'Hara, B.F. 2007. A non-circadian role for clock-genes in sleep homeostasis: a strain comparison. *BMC Neuroscience* **8**:87.

Gallicchio, L. and Kalesan, B. 2009. Sleep duration and mortality: a systematic review and meta-analysis. *Journal of Sleep Research* **18**(2):148–58.

Gillette, M.U., Medanic, M., McArthur, A.J., *et al.* 1995. Intrinsic neuronal rhythms in the suprachiasmatic nuclei and their adjustment. *Ciba Found Symp* **183**:134–44.

Glass, J.D., Guinn, J., Kaur, G., and Francl, J.M. 2010. On the intrinsic regulation of neuropeptide Y release in the mammalian suprachiasmatic nucleus circadian clock. *European Journal of Neuroscience* **31**(6):1117–26.

Grandner, M.A., Jackson, N.J., Pak, V.M., and Gehrman, P.R. 2012. Sleep disturbance is associated with cardiovascular and metabolic disorders. *Journal of Sleep Research* **21**(4):427–33.

Guilding, C. and Piggins, H.D. 2007. Challenging the omnipotence of the suprachiasmatic timekeeper: are circadian oscillators present throughout the mammalian brain? *European Journal of Neuroscience* **25**(11):3195–216.

Hasan, S., van der Veen, D.R., Winsky-Sommerer, R., *et al.* 2011. Altered sleep and behavioral activity phenotypes in PER3-deficient mice. *American Journal of Physiology* **301**(6):R1821–30.

Hasler, G., Buysse, D.J., Klaghofer, R., *et al.* 2004. The association between short sleep duration and obesity in young adults: a 13-year prospective study. *Sleep* **27**:661–6.

He, Y., Jones, C.R., Fujiki, N., *et al.* 2009. The transcriptional repressor DEC2 regulates sleep length in mammals. *Science* **325**(5942):866–70.

Herzog, E.D. and Tosini G. 2001. The mammalian circadian clock shop. *Seminars in Cell and Developmental Biology* **12**(4):295–303.

Hut, R.A., Pilorz, V., Boerema, A.S., *et al.* 2011. Working for food shifts nocturnal mouse activity into the day. *PLoS One* **6**(3):e17527.

Ibuka, N., Nihonmatsu, I. and Sekiguchi, S. 1980. Sleep–wakefulness rhythms in mice after suprachiasmatic nucleus lesions. *Waking and Sleeping* **4**(2):167–73.

Janik, D. and Mrosovsky, N. 1994. Intergeniculate leaflet lesions and behaviorally-induced shifts of circadian rhythms. *Brain Research* **651**(1-2):174–82.

Jin, X., Shearman, L.P., Weaver, D.R., *et al.* 1999. A molecular mechanism regulating rhythmic output from the suprachiasmatic circadian clock. *Cell* **96**(1):57–68.

Jacobs, B.L. and Fornal, C.A. 1999. Activity of serotonergic neurons in behaving animals. *Neuropsychopharmacology* **21**:9S–15S.

Jones, B.E. 2004. Arousal systems. *Frontiers in Bioscience* **8**:s438–51.

Jones, C.R., Campbell, S.S., Zone, S.E., *et al.* 1999. Familial advanced sleep-phase syndrome: a short-period circadian rhythm variant in humans. *Nature Medicine* **5**:1062–5.

Kalsbeek, A., Yi, C.X., Cailotto, C., *et al.* 2011. Mammalian clock output mechanisms. *Essays in Biochemistry* **49**(1):137–51.

Kerkhof, G.A. 1991. Differences between morning-types and evening-types in the dynamics of EEG slow wave activity during night sleep. *Electroencephalography and Clinical Neurophysiology* **78**:197–202.

Kerkhof, G.A. and Lancel, M. 1991. EEG slow wave activity, REM sleep, and rectal temperature during night and day sleep in morning-type and evening-type subjects. *Psychophysiology* **28**:678–88.

Knutson, A. 2000. Health disorders of shift workers. *Occupational Medicine (London)* **53**:103–8.

Kopp, C., Albrecht, U., Zheng, B., and Tobler, I. 2002. Homeostatic sleep regulation is preserved in mPer1 and mPer2 mutant mice. *European Journal of Neuroscience* **16**:1099–106.

Krueger, J.M. and Tononi, G. 2011. Local use-dependent sleep; synthesis of the new paradigm. *Current Topics in Medicinal Chemistry* **11**(19):2490–2.

Krueger, J.M., Huang, Y.H., Rector, D.M., and Buysse, D.J. 2013. Sleep: a synchrony of cell activity-driven small network states. *European Journal of Neuroscience* **38**:2199–209.

Kurina, L.M., McClintock, M.K., Chen, J.H., *et al.* 2013. Sleep duration and all-cause mortality: a critical review of measurement and associations. *Annals of Epidemiology* **23**:361–70.

Lack, L.C. and Wright, H.R. 2007. Chronobiology of sleep in humans. *Cellular and Molecular Life Sciences* **64**(10):1205–15.

Landgraf, D., Shostak, A., and Oster, H. 2012. Clock genes and sleep. *Pflugers Archives* **463**(1):3–14.

Laposky, A., Easton, A., Dugovic, C., *et al.* 2005. Deletion of the mammalian circadian clock gene BMAL1/Mop3 alters baseline sleep architecture and the response to sleep deprivation. *Sleep* **28**(4):395–409.

Lavie, P. 1997. Melatonin: role in gating nocturnal rise in sleep propensity. *Journal of Biological Rhythms* **12**(6):657–65.

Lavie, P. 2001. Sleep–wake as a biological rhythm. *Annual Review of Psychology* **52**:277–303.

Leemburg, S., Vyazovskiy, V. V., Olcese, U., *et al.* 2010. Sleep homeostasis in the rat is preserved during chronic sleep restriction. *Proceedings of the National Academy of Science USA* **107**:15939–44.

Liu, C., Weaver, D.R., Jin, X., *et al.* 1997. Molecular dissection of two distinct actions of melatonin on the suprachiasmatic circadian clock. *Neuron* **19**(1):91–102.

Lo, J.C., Groeger, J.A., Santhi, N., *et al.* 2012. Effects of partial and acute total sleep deprivation on performance across cognitive domains, individuals and circadian phase. *PLoS One* **7**(9):e45987.

Marchant, E.G., Watson, N.V. and Mistlberger, R.E. 1997. Both neuropeptide Y and serotonin are necessary for entrainment of circadian rhythms in mice by daily treadmill running schedules. *Journal of Neuroscience* **17**:7974–87.

Maron, L., Rechtschaffen, A., Wolpert, E.A. 1964. Sleep cycle during napping. *Archives of General Psychiatry* **11**:503–8.

McGinty, D. and Szymusiak, R. 2000. The sleep–wake switch: a neuronal alarm clock. *Nature Medicine* **6**:510–511.

McGinty, D. and Szymusiak, R. 2003. Hypothalamic regulation of sleep and arousal. *Frontiers in Bioscience* **8**:s1074–83.

McGinty, D. and Szymusiak, R. 2011. Neural control of sleep in mammals. In: *Principles and Practise of Sleep Medicine*, 5th edn (eds M.H. Kryger, T. Roth, and W.C. Dement). Saunders, MI, USA, pp. 76–91.

Meerlo, P., Van Den Hoofdakker, R.H., Koolhas, J.M., and Daan, S. 1997. Stress induced changes in circadian rhythms of body temperature and activity in rats are not caused by pacemaker changes. *Journal of Biological Rhythms* **12**(1):80–92.

Meijer, J.H., Schaap, J., Watanabe, K., and Albus, H. 1997. Multiunit activity recordings in the suprachiasmatic nuclei: in vivo versus in vitro models. *Brain Research* **753**(2):322–7.

Mistlberger, R.E. 1991. Effects of daily schedules of forced activity on free-running circadian rhythms in the rat. *Journal of Biological Rhythms* **6**:71–80.

Mistlberger, R. E. 2005. Circadian regulation of sleep in mammals: role of the suprachiasmatic nucleus. *Brain Research Reviews* **49**:429–54.

Mistlberger, R.E. and Antle, M.C. 2011. Entrainment of circadian clocks in mammals by arousal and food. *Essays in Biochemistry* **49**:119–36.

Mistlberger, R.E. and Holmes, M.M. 2000. Behavioral feedback regulation of circadian rhythm phase angle in light-dark entrained mice. *American Journal of Physiology* **279**:R813–21.

Mistlberger, R. E., Bergmann, B. M., Waldenar, W., and Rechtschaffen, A. 1983. Recovery sleep following sleep deprivation in intact and suprachiasmatic nuclei lesioned rats. *Sleep* **6**:217–33.

Mistlberger, R.E., Bergmann, B.M., and Rechtschaffen, A. 1987. Period/amplitude analysis of EEG in intact and suprachiasmatic nuclei lesioned rats: Effects of sleep deprivation and exercise. *Sleep* **10**:508–22.

Mistlberger, R.E., Bossert, J.M., Holmes, M.M., and Marchant, E.G. 1998. Serotonin and feedback effects of behavioral activity on circadian rhythms in mice. *Behavioural Brain Research* **96**:93–9.

Mistlberger, R.E., Houpt, T.A., and Moore-Ede, M.C. 1991. The benzodiazepine triazolam phase shifts circadian activity rhythms in a diurnal primate, the squirrel monkey (Saimiri sciureus). *Neuroscience Letters* **124**:27–30.

Mistlberger, R.E., Landry, G.J., and Marchant, E.G. 1997. Sleep deprivation can attenuate light-induced phase shifts of circadian rhythms in hamsters. *Neuroscience Letters* **238**: 5–8.

Mistlberger, R.E., Antle, M.C., Glass, J.D., and Miller, J.D. 2000. Behavioral and serotonergic regulation of circadian rhythms. *Biological Rhythm Research* **31**:240–83.

Mongrain, V. and Dumont, M. 2007. Increased homeostatic response to behavioral sleep fragmentation in morning types compared to evening types. *Sleep* **30**(6):773–80.

Mongrain, V., Lavoie, S., Selmaoui, B., *et al.* 2004. Phase relationships between sleep–wake cycle and underlying circadian rhythms in morningness–eveningness. *Journal of Biological Rhythms* **19**:248–57.

Mongrain, V., Carrier, J., and Dumont, M. 2006. Circadian and homeostatic sleep regulation in morningness–eveningness. *Journal of Sleep Research* **15**:162–6.

Morin, L.P. and Allen, C.N. 2006. The circadian visual system, 2005. *Brain Research Reviews* **51**(1):1–60.

Morin, L.P, and Studholme, K.M. 2009. Millisecond light pulses make mice stop running, then display prolonged sleep-like behavior in the absence of light. *Journal of Biological Rhythms* **24**(6):497–508.

Mrosovsky, N. 1988. Phase response curves for social entrainment. *Journal of Comparative Physiology* A **162**:35–46.

Mrosovsky, N. 1996. Locomotor activity and non-photic influences on circadian clocks. *Biological Reviews of the Cambridge Philosophical Society* **71**(3):343–72.

Mrosovsky, N. 1999a. Further experiments on the relationship between the period of circadian rhythms and locomotor activity levels in hamsters. *Physiology and Behavior* **66**(5):797–801.

Mrosovsky, N. 1999b. Masking: history, definitions, and measurement. *Chronobiology International* **16**(4):415–29.

Mrosovsky, N. and Salmon, P.A. 1987. A behavioural method for accelerating re-entrainment of rhythms to new light-dark cycles. *Nature* **330**(6146):372–3.

Mrosovsky, N. and Salmon, P.A. 1990. Triazolam and phase-shifting acceleration re-evaluated. *Chronobiology International* **7**(1):35–41.

Muindi, F., Zeitzer, J.M., Colas, D., and Heller, H.C. 2013. The acute effects of light on murine sleep during the dark phase: importance of melanopsin for maintenance of light-induced sleep. *European Journal of Neuroscience* **37**:1727–36.

Nauta, W.J. 1946. Hypothalamic regulation of sleep in rats; an experimental study. *Journal of Neurophysiology* **9**:285–316.

Naylor, E., Bergmann, B.M., Krauski, K., *et al.* 2000. The circadian clock mutation alters sleep homeostasis in the mouse. *Journal of Neuroscience* **20**(21):8138–43.

Noshiro, M., Furukawa, M., Honma, S., *et al.* 2005. Tissue-specific disruption of rhythmic expression of Dec1 and Dec2 in clock mutant mice. *Journal of Biological Rhythms* **20**(5):404–18.

Novak, C.M. and Nunez, A.A. 2000. A sparse projection from the suprachiasmatic nucleus to the sleep active ventro-lateral preoptic area in the rat. *Neuroreport* **11**:93–6.

Porkka-Heiskanen, T. and Kalinchuk, A.V. 2011. Adenosine, energy metabolism and sleep homeostasis. *Sleep Medicine Reviews* **15**(2):123–35.

Ralph, M.R. and Mrosovsky, N. 1992. Behavioral inhibition of circadian responses to light. *Journal of Biological Rhythms* **7**:353–359.

Ranson, S.W. 1939. Somnolence caused by hypothalamic lesions in the monkey. *Archives of Neurology and Psychiatry* **9**:285–316.

Rattenborg, N.C, Voirin, B., Vyssotski, A.L., *et al.* 2008. Sleeping outside the box: electroencephalographic measures of sleep in sloths inhabiting a rainforest. *Biological Letters* 4(4):402–5.

Rattenborg, N.C., Lima, S.L., and Lesku, J.A. 2012. Sleep locally, act globally. *Neuroscientist* 18:533–46.

Rechtschaffen, A., Bergmann, B.M., Gilliland, M.A., and Bauer, K. 1999. Effects of method, duration, and sleep stage on rebounds from sleep deprivation in the rat. *Sleep* 22(1):11–31.

Roenneberg, T., Kuehnle, T., Juda, M., *et al.* 2007. Epidemiology of the human circadian clock. *Sleep Med Reviews* 11(6):429–38.

Rosenberg, R.S., Bergmann, B.M. and Rechtschaffen, A. 1976. Variations in slow wave activity during sleep in the rat. *Physiology and Behavior* 17(6):931–8.

Saeb-Parsy, K. and Dyball, R.E. 2003. Defined cell groups in the rat suprachiasmatic nucleus have different day/night rhythms of single-unit activity in vivo. *Journal of Biological Rhythms* 18(1):26–42.

Saper, C.B., Chou, T.C., and Scammell, T.E. 2001. The sleep switch: hypothalamic control of sleep and wakefulness. *Trends in Neuroscience* 24:726–31.

Schaap, J., Albus, H., VanderLeest, H.T., *et al.* 2003. Heterogeneity of rhythmic suprachiasmatic nucleus neurons: implications for circadian waveform and photoperiodic encoding. *Proceedings of the National Academy of Science USA* 100(15):994–15.

Scharf, M.T., Naidoo, N., Zimmerman, J.E., and Pack, A.I. 2008. The energy hypothesis of sleep revisited. *Progress in Neurobiology* 86(3):264–80.

Schmutz, I., Ripperger, J.A., Baeriswyl-Aebischer, S., and Albrecht, U. 2010. The mammalian clock component PERIOD2 coordinates circadian output by interaction with nuclear receptors. *Genes and Development* 24(4):345–57.

Schroeder, A.M., Truong, D., Loh, D.H., *et al.* 2012. Voluntary scheduled exercise alters diurnal rhythms of behaviour, physiology and gene expression in wild-type and vasoactive intestinal peptide-deficient mice. *Journal of Physiology* 590(23):6213–26.

Shiromani, P.J., Xu, M., Winston, E.M., *et al.* 2004. Sleep rhythmicity and homeostasis in mice with targeted disruption of mPeriod genes. *American Journal of Physiology* 287:R47–57.

Siegel, J.M. 2009. Sleep viewed as a state of adaptive inactivity. *Nature Reviews Neuroscience* 10(10):747–53.

Smale, L., Lee, T., and Nunez, A.A. 2003. Mammalian diurnality: some facts and gaps. *Journal of Biological Rhythms* 18(5):356–66.

Strogatz, S.H., Kronauer, R.E., and Czeisler, C.A. 1986 Circadian regulation dominates homeostatic control of sleep length and prior wake length in humans. *Sleep* 9:353–64.

Strogatz, S., Kronauer, R., and Czeisler, C.A. 1987. Circadian pacemaker interferes with sleep onset at specific times each day: role in insomnia. *American Journal of Physiology* 253:R172–8.

Sun, X., Rusak, B., and Semba, K. 2000. Electrophysiology and pharmacology of projections from the suprachiasmatic nucleus to the ventromedial preoptic area in rat, *Neuroscience* 98:715–28.

Sun, X., Whitefield, S., Rusak, B., and Semba, K. 2001. Electrophysiological analysis of suprachiasmatic nucleus projections to the ventrolateral preoptic area in the rat. *European Journal of Neuroscience* 14:1257–74.

Tallaird, J., Philip, P., Coste, O., *et al.* 2003. The circadian and homeostatic modulation of sleep pressure during wakefulness differs between morning and evening chronotypes. *Journal of Sleep Research* 12:275–82.

Tobler I. 2011. Phylogeny of sleep regulation. In: *Principles and Practise of Sleep Medicine*, 5th edn (eds M.H. Kryger, T. Roth, and W.C. Dement). Saunders, MI, USA, pp. 112–125.

Tobler, I. and Borbély, A.A. 1986. Sleep EEG in the rat as a function of prior waking. *Electroencephalography and Clinical Neurophysiology* 64:74–6.

Tobler, I., Borbély, A.A., and Groos, G. 1983. The effect of sleep deprivation on sleep in rats with suprachiasmatic lesions. *Neuroscience Letters* 42(1):49–54.

Toh, K.L., Jones, C.R., He, Y., *et al.* 2001. An hPer2 phosphorylation site mutation in familial advanced sleep phase syndrome. *Science* 291:1040–3.

Trachsel, L., Tobler, I., and Borbély, A.A. 1986. Sleep regulation in rats: effects of sleep deprivation, light, and circadian phase. *American Journal of Physiology* 251(6 Pt 2):R1037–44.

Trachsel, L., Edgar, D.M., Seidel, W.F., *et al.* 1992. Sleep homeostasis in suprachiasmatic nuclei-lesioned rats: effects of sleep deprivation and triazolam administration. *Brain Research* 589:253–61.

Turek, F.W. and Losee-Olson, S. 1986. A benzodiazepine used in the treatment of insomnia phase-shifts the mammalian circadian clock. *Nature* 321(6066):167–8.

Turek, F.W., Joshu, C., Kosaka, A., *et al.* 2005. Obesity and Metabolic Syndrome in Clock Mutant Mice. *Science* 308(5724): 1043–5.

Van Dongen, H.P. and Dinges, D.F. 2003. Investigating the interaction between the homeostatic and circadian processes of sleep–wake regulation for the prediction of waking neurobehavioural performance. *Journal of Sleep Research* **12**:181–7.

van Oosterhout, F., Lucassen, E.A., Houben, T., *et al*. 2012. Amplitude of the SCN clock enhanced by the behavioral activity rhythm. *PLoS One* **7**(6):e39693.

Vassalli, A. and Dijk, D.J. 2009. Sleep function: current questions and new approaches. *European Journal of Neuroscience* **29**:1830–41.

Viola, A.U., Archer, S.N., James, L.M., *et al*. 2007. PER polymorphism predicts sleep structure and waking performance. *Current Biology* **17**:613–8.

Von Economo, E. 1930. Sleep as a problem of localization. *Journal of Nervous and Mental Disorders* **71**:249–59.

Vyazovskiy, V.V. and Harris, K.D. 2013. Sleep and the single neuron: the role of global slow oscillations in individual cell rest *Nature Reviews Neuroscience* **14**:443–51.

Watts A.G. 1991. The efferent projections of the suprachiasmatic nucleus: anatomical insights into the control of circadian rhythms, In: *Suprachiasmatic Nucleus: the Mind's Clock* (eds D.C. Klein, R.Y. Moore, and S.M. Reppert). Oxford Press, New York, pp. 77–106.

Webb, I.C., Patton, D.F., Landry, G.J., and Mistlberger, R.E. 2010. Circadian clock resetting by behavioral arousal: Neural correlates in the midbrain raphe nuclei and locus coeruleus. *Neuroscience* **166**(3):739–51.

Wehr, T.A., Moul, D.E., Barbato, G., *et al*. 1993. Conservation of photoperiod-responsive mechanisms in humans. *American Journal of Physiology* **265**:R846–57.

Wever, R.A. 1984. Properties of human sleep–wake cycles: parameters of internally synchronized free-running rhythms. *Sleep* **7**(1):27–51.

Williams, H.l., Hammack, J.T., Daly, R.L., *et al*. 1964. Responses to auditory stimulation, sleep loss and the EEG stages of sleep. *Electroencephalography and Clinical Neurophysiology* **16**:269–79.

Wisor, J.P., OHara, B.F., Terao, A., *et al*. 2002. A role for cryptochromes in sleep regulation. *BMC Neuroscience* **3**:20.

Wisor, J.P., Pasumarthi, R.K., Gerashchenko, D., *et al*. 2008. Sleep deprivation effects on circadian clock gene expression in the cerebral cortex parallel electroencephalographic differences among mouse strains. *Journal of Neuroscience* **28**:7193–201.

Wurts, S.W. and Edgar, D.M. 2000. Circadian and homeostatic control of rapid eye movement (REM) sleep: promotion of REM tendency by the suprachiasmatic nucleus, *Journal of Neuroscience* **20**:4300–10.

Wyatt, J.K., Dijk, D.J., Ritz-de Cecco, A., *et al*. 2006. Sleep-facilitating effect of exogenous melatonin in healthy young men and women is circadian-phase dependent. *Sleep* **29**(5):609–18.

Xie, L., Kang, H., Xu, Q., *et al*. (2013) Sleep drives metabolite clearance from the adult brain. *Science* **342**(6156): 373–7.

Xu, Y., Padiath, Q.S., Shapiro, R.E., *et al*. 2005. Functional consequences of a CKIdelta mutation causing familial advanced sleep phase syndrome. *Nature* **434**(7033):640–4.

Yamada, N., Shimoda, K., Takahashi, K., and Takahashi, S. 1986. Change in period of free-running rhythms determined by two different tools in blinded rats. *Physiology and Behavior* **36**:357–62.

Yamada, N., Shimoda, K., Ohi, K., *et al*. 1988. Free-access to a running wheel shortens the period of free-running rhythm in blinded rats. *Physiology and Behavior* **42**:87–91.

Yamanaka, Y., Honma, S., and Honma, K.I. 2013. Daily exposure to running-wheel entrains circadian rhythms in mice in parallel with development of pre-exposure increase in spontaneous movement. *American Journal of Physiology* **305**:R1367–75.

Yamazaki, S., Kerbeshian, M.C., Hocker, C.G., *et al*. 1998. Rhythmic properties of the hamster suprachiasmatic nucleus in vivo. *Journal of Neuroscience* **18**(24):10709–23.

Yasenkov, R. and Deboer, T. 2010. Circadian regulation of sleep and the sleep EEG under constant sleep pressure in the rat. *Sleep* **33**(5):631–41.

Yoo, S.H., Yamazaki, S., Lowrey, P.L., *et al*. 2004. PERIOD2::LUCIFERASE real-time reporting of circadian dynamics reveals persistent circadian oscillations in mouse peripheral tissues. *Proceedings of the National Academy of Science USA* **101**:5339–46.

Zecharia, A.Y., Yu, X., Götz, T., *et al*. 2012. GABAergic inhibition of histaminergic neurons regulates active waking but not the sleep-wake switch or propofol-induced loss of consciousness. *Journal of Neuroscience* **32**(38):13062–75.

Circadian Regulation of Arousal and its Role in Fatigue

5

David R. Bonsall and Mary E. Harrington

Neuroscience Program, Smith College, Northampton, MA, USA

In this chapter, how the circadian clock regulates our mental state is described. Although the circadian clock is often thought of as a gate for sleep–wake cycles, evidence suggests that circadian rhythms also sculpt our state of arousal. Thus, while we are awake we might be more or less alert, energetic, or mentally sharp. The dynamic neural networks shaping our inner state of arousal are being better understood. Here we will describe what is currently known, while also pointing toward future investigations necessary to advance this research into having a highly translational impact to begin to address disorders of arousal and, in particular, chronic fatigue.

This chapter begins with a brief overview of the neural system regulating arousal, describing both the brain regions that are currently thought to be involved and the neurochemicals utilized by these regions. It is beyond the scope of this chapter to provide anything more than an introduction to the field of arousal and its regulation by the circadian system. However, there are several extensive reviews published in recent years that provide further detail and insight into this area. Brown *et al.* (2012) discuss particularly thoroughly our current understanding of the arousal network and pathways that govern it. Colwell (2011) provides insight into the mechanisms controlling circadian rhythms at the level of the suprachiasmatic nucleus and its outputs. Finally, the neurobiological basis of fatigue, as a disorder of arousal is described in a review by Harrington (2012).

5.1 Defining arousal

Defining the term arousal for the purposes of this chapter is not a simple task. A subject's state of arousal describes not only their degree of consciousness (i.e., whether a subject is awake or sleeping) but also their level of vigilance and alertness, determining their ability to predict and react to different environmental stimuli effectively and appropriately (e.g., performance). Furthermore, arousal states receive input from other centrally governed biological phenomena, including emotional state, stress response, and circadian regulation. From this rather broad description, it is unsurprising that our state of arousal varies significantly throughout the day, from periods of minimal arousal during deep sleep, to highly alert wakefulness during the day. Intermediary states of arousal exist between these two extremes that allow for gentle transitions from sleep to wake or from highly alert to less alert states of wakefulness.

Circadian Medicine, First Edition. Edited by Christopher S. Colwell.
© 2015 John Wiley & Sons, Inc. Published 2015 by John Wiley & Sons, Inc.

One of the most effective tools used by researchers for tracking these transitions in humans and other mammals is electroencephalogram (EEG) recordings. The EEG can be used to detect multiple rhythmic waveforms of spontaneous neuronal activity occurring within different regions of the brain, each with a frequency distinct from other waveforms. Electrical signals with a frequency of 8–12 Hz for example are termed alpha activity, whereas delta activity typically oscillates at a frequency of 1–4 Hz. Different arousal states can be identified through the presence or absence of certain waveforms elicited in these EEG recordings and are classified into different stages: A1–A3, representing higher arousal and alertness, decreasing to drowsier stages B1–B3 (Fig. 5.1). During more vigilant states of wakefulness (A1), alpha activity is particularly prominent in recordings from more posterior brain regions. Alpha activity can be seen to migrate to the anterior electrode recordings as vigilance levels decrease (Olbrich *et al.*, 2009). The drowsier stages of B1-3 are characterized by the loss of alpha activity (Loomis *et al.*, 1937; Roth, 1961) during eye-closed periods and increasing delta (1–4 Hz) and theta (4–7 Hz) activity prior to the loss of wakefulness and onset of sleep.

The primary function of the arousal system is one of preparation. Throughout the day, the arousal system receives input from multiple stimuli, for example from dietary stimulants, social interactions and increasing internal sleep pressure (referred to as "Process S" in the commonly employed two-process model)(Borbely, 1982; Chapter 4). It is the role of the arousal system to anticipate and regulate appropriate behavioral and physiological responses to these different stimuli, ensuring wakefulness can be maintained when necessary (when working or driving, for example), but also permitting an easy transition into sleep during the night or when resting. It is common for most healthy individuals to cycle through multiple states of arousal throughout the day. Feelings of drowsiness are experienced not only during the transition from wake to sleep but are also commonly reported for brief periods during the early afternoon (Bes *et al.*, 2009). Daily rhythms of arousal transitions provide a clear example of how circadian regulation (referred to as "Process C") may act directly to affect our arousal systems. Shift workers working during the night present an example of when arousal pathways are capable of maintaining wakefulness despite circadian regulation of the drive for sleep. The point, therefore, is that while the

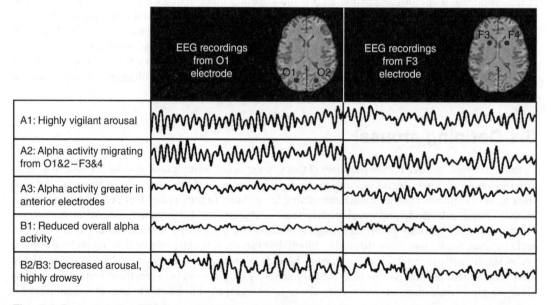

Fig. 5.1 Representative EEG trace recordings showing the transitions from a highly alert arousal state through to the lower, drowsy arousal state experienced prior to sleep onset. Traces recorded from electrodes in the O1 and F3 positions as indicated on transverse section of human brain (gray circles). (Adapted from Olbrich *et al.*, 2009, view of the transverse section of human brain from Allen Brain Atlas Resources [Internet]. Seattle (WA): Allen Institute for Brain Science ©2009. Available from: http://www.brain-map.org.)

arousal system is capable of receiving input from different internal and external environmental stimuli, the system remains highly adaptive and flexible.

It is often through the occurrence of different disease states and disorders that the importance of the arousal system in health becomes clear. In a number of disease states, patients may suffer symptoms such as insomnia, where there are phases of hyperarousal, preventing timely sleep onset and also sleep maintenance throughout the night. Conversely, but not entirely unrelated, patients may suffer from phases of hypoarousal during the day. In such cases, subjects may experience excessive daytime sleepiness (EDS) and/or fatigue, or in more extreme cases such as narcolepsy may lose consciousness altogether. The study of these disorders brings to light more than ever the complex nature of the arousal system, since similar disorders can arise from pathology of different brain structures associated with arousal, making study of the entire arousal pathway a critical area for future research.

5.2 Brain structures important for arousal

The arousal system is a collection of brain regions that send far-reaching interconnecting projections to various brain areas, implicated in the regulation of cortical excitability and stimulated responses. This neural network modifies excitability of neurons in response to changes in both the internal and the external environment, leading to adaptive responses related to long-term needs. The locations of the major brain regions thought to be involved in this network can be seen in Fig. 5.2.

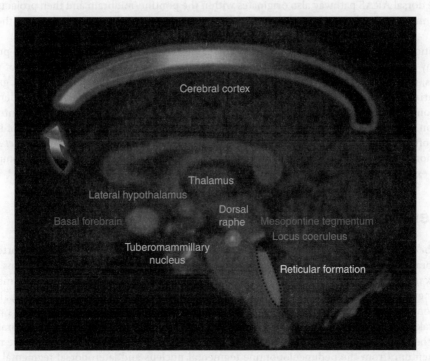

Fig. 5.2 The major structures of the arousal system. Cells in the reticular formation and other caudal regions, including noradrenergic neurons of the locus coeruleus, serotonergic raphe neurons, and dopaminergic neurons in the periaqueductal grey in the mesopontine tegmentum, project to more rostral areas via two pathways. A dorsal pathway via the thalamus provides input to the cerebral cortex. A ventral pathway provides input to the cerebral cortex via interconnected nuclei including orexigenic neurons in the lateral hypothalamus, histaminergic neurons in the tuberomammillary nucleus and cholinergic neurons in the basal forebrain. (View of the midline sagittal section of human brain from Allen Brain Atlas Resources [Internet]. Seattle (WA): Allen Institute for Brain Science ©2009. Available from: http://www.brain-map.org.) *(See insert for color representation of the figure.)*

Early work in this field involved studying the effects of isolating different brain regions on wake and sleep behavior in cats. Work by Bremer, isolating the brain from spinal cord input demonstrated control of sleep–wake behavior to be primarily maintained through the central nervous system localized within the brain (reviewed by Brown *et al.*, 2012). From these earlier studies, research in the field has expanded to identify several important brain regions involved in wakefulness behavior. In particular, regions within the midbrain and brainstem, including the reticular formation have been shown to project extensively into anterior areas such as the thalamus and cortex, where they are able to promote wakefulness within the brain. These projections from the **reticular formation** of the pontine/midbrain are termed the ascending reticular activating system (ARAS), relaying excitatory signals through several areas thought to govern wake regulation and also to areas capable of providing additional environmental information to the arousal system, including the hypothalamus as well as cortico-limbic areas (Siegel, 2004; Haas and Lin, 2012).

The ARAS network initiates signaling from the reticular formation and stimulates excitatory pathways projecting to the cerebral cortex through two separate pathways, one ventral, the other dorsal. The ventral ARAS projection extends from the reticular formation into the posterior hypothalamus. Two areas in the posterior hypothalamus, the orexin-expressing neurons within the perifornical region of the **lateral hypothalamus** and the histamine-expressing neurons in the **tuberomammillary nuclei**, appear to play important roles in maintaining wakefulness (Haas and Lin, 2012). Fibers from these areas project to a third region of focus, the **basal forebrain**. From here, the basal forebrain projects to the **cerebral cortex**, where it promotes wakefulness and neuronal activity in EEG recordings associated with the wake state. The dorsal ARAS pathway also originates within the pontine/midbrain and then projects through the **thalamus** to stimulate widespread activation of neocortical neurons, also promoting the wakeful state.

In addition to the reticular formation, both dorsal and ventral ARAS pathways receive projections from many other key regions present in the brainstem, including noradrenergic neurons of the **locus coeruleus**, serotonergic **raphe** neurons, and dopaminergic neurons in the periaqueductal grey in the **mesopontine tegmentum** (Brown *et al.*, 2012) (Fig. 5.2). Much work has been done to understand the specific contribution of each of these particular regions and those of the ARAS network. Interestingly, stimulation of individual elements is often capable of increasing arousal whereas ablation of individual elements often shows minimal or no effect on arousal and wakefulness (reviewed in Brown *et al.*, 2012). The ablation studies highlight the highly flexible nature of the arousal system with many compensatory pathways existing to adjust for any redundant signaling.

5.3 Neurochemicals signaling the states of arousal

As described above, the primary signaling pathways promoting activity within the cerebral cortex involve multiple brain regions. These regions are largely interconnected through neuronal projections that form a complex network. Many of the structures involved in signaling transitional arousal states make use of different neurotransmitters, some of which appear to play more situation-specific roles (e.g., histamine release from the tuberomammillary nuclei in response to stress or danger) whereas others play more general waking roles (neurons projecting from the mesopontine tegmentum and basal forebrain).

Neurochemical signals originating from the brainstem include cholinergic neurons of the mesopontine tegmentum (from the pedunculopontine tegmental nucleus and laterodorsal tegmental nucleus), glutamatergic neurons of the parabrachial nucleus, serotonergic neurons of the dorsal raphe nucleus, adrenergic neurons of the locus coeruleus, as well as dopaminergic neurons present in the midbrain (ventral tegmental area and periaqueductal grey) (Jones, 2005). While many of these regions are able to project directly to the cerebral cortex, they also innervate indirectly through the arousal network. The ventral ARAS pathway extends to the posterior hypothalamus, where it stimulates orexigenic lateral hypothalamic nuclei and histaminergic tuberomammillary nuclei. This pathway also directly stimulates the basal forebrain, resulting in further cholinergic signaling projecting directly into the cerebral cortex (Jones, 2005; Zant *et al.*, 2012). The projections of the dorsal ARAS feed into the midline and intralaminar

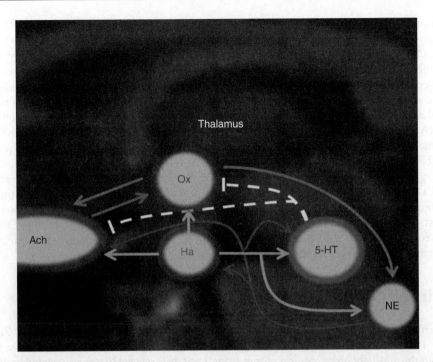

Fig. 5.3 Interactions of the main neuromodulatory systems that regulate wake within the arousal pathway. Cells in the basal forebrain producing acetylcholine (Ach) shown in green receive input from multiple regions. Excitatory projections from cells in the lateral hypothalamus expressing orexin (Ox) are shown in blue, projections from histamine (Ha)-producing cells in the tuberomammillary nucleus are shown in orange, projections from norepinephrine (NE)-containing cells in the locus coeruleus are shown in red. Inhibitory projections from cells in raphe nuclei expressing serotonin (5-HT) are shown by dashed lines. (Adapted from Brown *et al.*, 2012.) *(See insert for color representation of the figure.)*

nuclei of the thalamus. From here the dorsal ARAS broadly innervates areas of the cortex and neocortex to stimulate mental arousal (Newman and Ginsberg, 1994). Similar to the ventral ARAS, this pathway also receives input from the adrenergic, cholinergic and serotonergic regions described above.

The vast range of projections contained within the arousal network allows for a great number of neurotransmitter interactions within the system (Fig. 5.3). One example of this within the arousal network is the input to cholinergic neurons. The firing patterns of cholinergic neurons correlate closely with cortical activation associated with the wakeful brain (Manns *et al.*, 2003). These neurons, particularly those originating from the basal forebrain, receive significant input from virtually all other neurotransmitters of the arousal network. Histamine, for example, is able to promote increased wake and alertness, partially through stimulation of the cholinergic neurons of the basal forebrain. These effects of histamine on cortical activation and arousal behavior can be blocked through application of an H1 receptor antagonist in the region of the basal forebrain (Zant *et al.*, 2012). Similarly, orexin neurons of the lateral hypothalamus, which show changes in firing rate relative to levels of wake and alertness, are also able to exert excitatory effects on cholinergic firing (Espana, *et al.*, 2001). Like histamine, brainstem derived norepinephrine projections to the cholinergic neurons of the basal forebrain are thought to enhance alertness and wake in situations of stress and danger. One of the few inhibitory signals affecting cholinergic neurons arises from serotonergic firing from the dorsal raphe (Khateb *et al.*, 1993; Gasbarri *et al.*, 1999). Serotonergic activity is primarily attributed to relaxed wakefulness, with stimulatory effects within both the dorsal and ventral ARAS pathways. However, within the basal forebrain, serotonin is able to hyperpolarize cholinergic neurons. This inhibitory pathway is prevalent in stress arousal and has been suggested to play a homeostatic role in regulating the stress response to prevent excessively sustained hyperarousal (Monti, 2011).

In addition to these projections toward anterior areas, many brainstem regions involved in the arousal network also receive input from other regions, including those further forward in the ARAS signaling pathways. Orexin neurons for example, originating from the lateral hypothalamus, project not only anteriorly to the cortex and cholinergic neurons of the basal forebrain, but also strongly innervate norepinephrine-containing neurons of the locus coeruleus (Horvath *et al.*, 1999). Furthermore, orexin neurons are able to stimulate serotonergic activity within the dorsal raphe, dopaminergic neurons of the ventral tegmental area and have also been found to project to thalamo-cortical regions associated with the dorsal ARAS pathway (Korotkova *et al.*, 2003; Govindaiah and Cox, 2006; Kohlmeier *et al.*, 2008).

The idea, therefore, of solely ascending pathways of arousal as described through the ARAS projections is somewhat misleading. Instead of arousal signals being relayed in a unidirectional manner, with the signal being consolidated and strengthening as it passes through different regions, it is perhaps best viewed as a highly adaptive and receptive network. The promotion of arousal can indeed be consolidated by the interaction of many different neurotransmitters, providing a wide scope of transitions between different states of arousal and alertness. The adaptive network of arousal incorporates input from many environmental stimuli and maintains homeostatic control, utilizing both excitatory and inhibitory signals to retain an appropriate balance of sleep–wake control.

5.4 Circadian regulation of the arousal system

Circadian modulation of the arousal network arises from the suprachiasmatic nuclei (SCN) (Chapter 3). Neurons of the SCN spontaneously express a circadian rhythm in activity such that increased firing is observed in the mid-light phase. Neural output from the SCN is relayed to arousal-related brain regions via the dorsomedial hypothalamus, medial preoptic area, and subparaventricular zone (Deurveilher and Semba, 2005) (Fig.5.4). The SCN output signal is transduced by these structures immediately downstream, so that circadian modulation is altered according to the temporal niche (e.g., nocturnal, diurnal). Output of the SCN is also modified by photoperiod (Meijer *et al.*, 2012), locomotor activity (van Oosterhout *et al.*, 2012) and disease states. Neurodegenerative disorders, infectious disease, inflammation and metabolic disorders can all alter SCN neural output (Colwell, 2011). It is critical that future research explicate how the known changes in SCN output impact arousal network structures and neurotransmitters. This could provide novel inroads for the adjustment of levels of arousal in disease.

Some brain regions important in the arousal network can maintain a circadian rhythm for several cycles even when isolated *in vitro*, including the ventro-lateral preoptic area, lateral hypothalamus, and paraventricular nucleus of the hypothalamus (Abe *et al.*, 2002). Furthermore, many of the neurochemicals involved in the arousal network can sustain rhythmicity under conditions of constant darkness, including orexin, histamine, noradrenaline and serotonin, suggesting regulation of their activity by the circadian system (Cagampang *et al.*, 1993; Aston-Jones *et al.*, 2001; Zhang *et al.*, 2004). Input from the SCN likely synchronizes circadian rhythms among these cells and sets the phase. Some disorders of the arousal system might arise from poor coordination among these brain regions. For example, if select nodes within the network are normally synchronized in their signaling, boosting mental alertness, then temporal disorder due to problems in reception of the synchronizing input from the SCN could reduce the robustness of the downstream alerting signal. Conditions of chronic jet lag or rotating shift work desynchronize SCN neurons with dorsal and ventral groups of neurons resynchronizing at different rates (Davidson *et al.*, 2009). Downstream target areas that differentially receive input derived from dorsal versus ventral SCN neurons could be impacted differently (Schwartz *et al.*, 2009). Disruptive external signals, for example, through unpredictable daily mealtimes, can disturb the daily rhythms of circadian clock gene expression in certain brain regions (Verwey and Amir, 2012). Future research should address the impact of disruptive circadian cues on the circadian rhythmic activity of key structures within the arousal network.

The SCN are able to exert circadian influence not only through neuronal firing but also via the production of humoral outputs; substances able to pass into the circulatory system and drive circadian oscillations in tissues both local and distant to the SCN (Li *et al.*, 2012). While these humoral substances have yet to be fully identified, their ability to drive circadian rhythms in locomotor activity suggests future

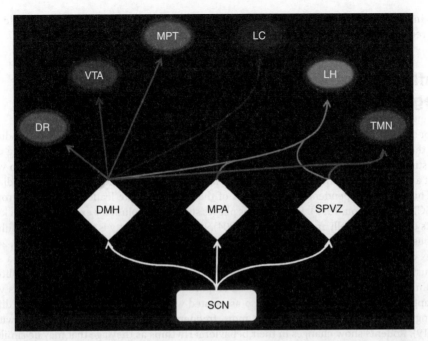

Fig. 5.4 Circadian signaling routes to govern regulation of sleep–wake and arousal pathways. Circadian pacemaker signals from the SCN project to three major relay nuclei, the dorsomedial nuclei of the hypothalamus (DMH), the medial preoptic area (MPA), and the subparaventricular zone (SPVZ). These areas then relay circadian information to areas within the arousal network including the dorsal raphe (DR), the ventral tegmental area (VTA), the mesopontine tegmentum (MPT), the locus coeruleus (LC), the lateral hypothalamus (LH) and the tuberomammillary nuclei (TMN). *(See insert for color representation of the figure.)*

research identifying these substances could provide useful tools for broad modulation of arousal. The circadian network provides redundant inputs so that circadian drive can come via multiple humoral or neural paths, as well as from circadian modulation of food, activity, or other inputs. Clinical use of daily routines restricting access to food, activity, light, and so on might allow nonpharmacological modulation of this system. Although chimera experiments (Vogelbaum and Menaker, 1992) suggest the SCN have both excitatory and inhibitory outputs, so far only substances associated with pathways that inhibit activity have been identified. These include prokineticin 2 and TGF-α; vasopressin provides output that largely seems to help synchronize hormonal rhythms (Li *et al.*, 2012).

A unified route for circadian drive over much of the arousal network could be mediated via circadian modulation of orexin-containing neurons. The SCN sends afferents to lateral hypothalamus orexinergic cells via all three relay nuclei typical for SCN efferents (Fig. 5.4). Additionally, some orexin neurons also receive direct input from the SCN (Yoshida *et al.*, 2006). Perifornical cells within the lateral hypothalamus that contain orexin are crucial elements within the arousal network. Optogenetic activation of these neurons increases the probability of a transition from sleep to wake (Adamantidis *et al.*, 2007). Orexin-containing neurons depolarize numerous regions including noradrenergic locus coeruleus neurons, serotonergic raphe neurons, tuberomammillary nuclei neurons, basal forebrain cholinergic neurons and neurons of the ventral tegmental area. Thus, it could be hypothesized that orexinergic cells mediate circadian drive for arousal.

However, the interconnected nature of the arousal network makes it unlikely that there is a single region through which all circadian input is mediated. Through the three potential relay nuclei (as well as direct innervations), the SCN communicate with multiple regions of the arousal network, present within both the ventral and dorsal routes of the ARAS pathway (Fig. 5.4). Each of these nodes is able, in turn, to project to others, consolidating the signals of arousal, but perhaps also reinforcing circadian synchronization.

With this in mind, a more effective research strategy may aim to elucidate a network-wide impact of circadian regulation/disruption on changing arousal states.

5.5 Influence of input pathways on circadian regulation of arousal

Locomotor activity is both an output of the circadian clock and can also serve as an input, modulating the output of the SCN. Research on this topic has often included presentation of a new running wheel to a rodent, a stimulus that can elicit several hours of vigorous exercise. Stimulating a rodent to voluntarily exercise at a time when the animal would normally be resting can alter the phase of the circadian activity rhythm. This effect is dependent upon neurons of the intergeniculate leaflet releasing neuropeptide Y onto the SCN (Harrington, 1997). During other phases stimulated voluntary exercise can block the resetting effects of light (Yannielli and Harrington, 2004). Locomotor activity is associated with inhibition of spontaneous firing of SCN neurons at all phases of the circadian cycle (van Oosterhout *et al.*, 2012).

Diseases can sometimes include changes in arousal state, such as persistent fatigue, as a symptom. Research using animal models has suggested that this may be associated with reduced amplitude firing rate rhythm from the SCN as well as decreased amplitude cycling of circadian clock genes within the SCN (Chapters 15–19). Advanced age is also associated with persistent fatigue as well as difficulty in maintaining arousal. Older humans report more frequent napping and more difficulty with fatigue (Chapter 19). Rodents show changes in their behavioral rhythms as they age that may be similar to this, in that they show less locomotor activity and shorter bouts of sleep or activity. This is associated with reduced amplitude firing rate rhythms apparent even at middle age in rodents (Nakamura *et al.*, 2011). Encouraging increased voluntary exercise by providing test rodents with running wheels can ameliorate some of the negative changes in the circadian system associated with age (Leise *et al.*, 2013).

These effects of exercise can be understood as coopting the ability of locomotor activity to directly alter SCN firing as well as clock resetting mechanisms. Exercise can increase the amplitude of SCN firing rate rhythm even when the SCN is isolated *in vitro* as a brain slice preparation (Leise *et al.*, 2013). It appears likely that this may be mediated by increasing the coupling among SCN neurons. This neuronal coupling may be mediated via signals derived from vasoactive intestinal polypeptide-containing SCN neurons, which are able to synchronize SCN neurons *in vitro* (Maywood *et al.*, 2011). Furthermore, knockout studies have revealed that this neuronal population is important for regulation of the SCN response to wheel-running activity (Schroeder *et al.*, 2012). Further research detailing more precisely how exercise can strengthen circadian rhythm signals would allow this potential pathway to be better harnessed to provide stronger input to the widespread arousal network.

5.6 Sustained states of fatigue: a disorder of the arousal network?

The experience of fatigue is common. Yet when this becomes a lasting condition, it can be debilitating, having a significant detrimental impact on our quality of life. Within the United Kingdom, data from the British National Survey of Psychiatric Morbidity reported a 15% prevalence of fatigue lasting at least six months (Watanabe *et al.*, 2008). Further, a second study reports nearly 38% of the United States workforce experienced fatigue within the two weeks prior to being interviewed (Ricci *et al.*, 2007). A complaint of fatigue includes a sensation of being tired for no apparent reason, with a reduced ability to function in everyday life. It is troubling in that it can come and go unpredictably, and can lead a person to feel vulnerable and frustrated. This symptom is associated with many disorders, most prominently with chronic fatigue syndrome and multiple sclerosis, but also with post-stroke, post-poliomyelitis, Parkinson's Disease, and traumatic brain injury, among others.

Commonly, populations of patients with fatigue display signs of a pro-inflammatory state. Some studies document increased inflammatory cytokines in serum samples, with the three most common cytokines being interleukin-6, interleukin-1β, and TGF-α. While it is easier to sample peripheral tissues, these serum markers likely indicate a coincident state of increased inflammation within the brain. There are multiple pathways by which peripheral inflammatory signals can alter the brain (reviewed by Dantzer *et al.*, 2008). Changes within the brain include activation of microglia, secretion of cytokines, altered excitability of brain circuits, and changes relevant to serotonergic transmission. There is an urgent need to better understand the myriad ways by which peripheral inflammation alters central nervous system function.

Researchers employ lipopolysaccharide, a component of bacterial cell walls, to simulate a bacterial infection without actually provoking an infection. Injection of lipopolysaccharide induces a range of behavioral changes, referred to as "sickness behavior", that include lethargy, decreased grooming, social withdrawal, and decreased food intake. Currently researchers are working to determine which brain circuits are mediating each of these behavioral changes and how inflammation can impact neural function. Administration of the pro-inflammatory cytokine IL-1β directly into the brain can induce sickness behavior, with suppression of feeding and reduced locomotor activity, demonstrating that cytokines alter behavior via central actions (Grossberg *et al.*, 2011).

Using the model of intracerebroventricular injection of IL-1β, researchers found that a subpopulation of the orexin-containing neurons in the lateral hypothalamus, those in the perifornical area, showed reduced activation as indicated by lower levels of the marker cFOS (Grossberg *et al.*, 2011). The reduced locomotor activity seen in response to IL-1β was blocked by knockdown of the IL-1β receptor in cerebrovascular endothelial cells (Ching *et al.*, 2007) and required the expression of TGF-β-activated kinase within brain endothelial cells (Ridder *et al.*, 2011).

The development of orexin knockout mice further supports the role of orexin as a target for induction of fatigue. These mice show significant reductions in voluntary running wheel activity, which appears to result from increased fatigability, whereby the duration of running bouts are shorter, as opposed to the total number of bouts which are similar to the wild-type mice (Espana *et al.*, 2007). Similarly, mice deficient in histamine (by targeted ablation of the synthetic enzyme histidine decarboxylase) show reduced voluntary wheel running (Abe *et al.*, 2004), possibly providing an alternative target for investigation. Interestingly, these mice showed reduced circadian rhythms in Per1 and Per2 expression in extra-SCN regions but no change in SCN gene expression, suggesting a reduction in the strength of circadian influence being relayed through output pathways.

Alterations in the projections of the SCN to different regions of the arousal network may play a role to induce a fatigued state. In addition to some direct projections, the SCN innervates three potential relay nuclei to indirectly influence several arousal nodes (Fig. 5.4). Disrupted circadian activity, therefore, can have effects spanning the entire arousal network. It is possible that an immunological challenge may well act either directly at the level of the SCN or through one of the SCN's relay nuclei to disrupt circadian regulation and bring about altered states of arousal. These altered states may subsequently increase the system's susceptibility to developing long term disorders, allowing the state of chronic fatigue to manifest itself (Fig. 5.5).

It is currently unclear what role the circadian system may play in the development or maintenance of lasting fatigue. The importance of exercise in coupling SCN neurons has been discussed above and it is possible that these deficits in locomotor activity, resulting from immunologically produced disruptions of the arousal network, may further aggravate the situation, leading to weaker SCN output and greater desynchrony of the arousal system. This would suggest that circadian disruption is not the primary inducer of fatigue but may have a role in sustaining the fatigued state once present (Fig. 5.5). If the circadian system is affected, either as an instigator or downstream consequence of the fatigued state, then inducing changes within this system could prove clinically beneficial. One example of how clinicians can improve circadian synchrony is via bright light therapy. Bright light therapy can help improve quality of life in women undergoing chemotherapy for breast cancer, apparently by reducing fatigue by resynchronization of the circadian system (Jeste *et al.*, 2012).

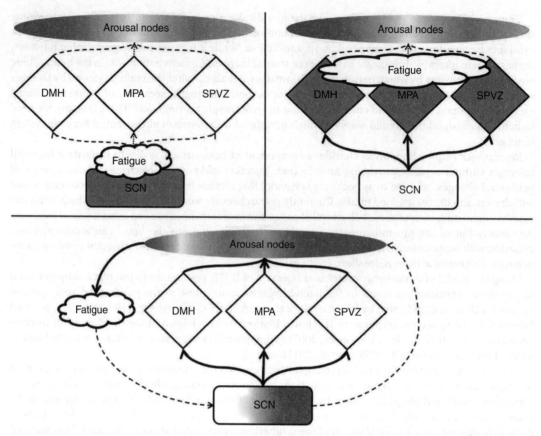

Fig. 5.5 Illustration highlighting the key areas impacted by disorders of arousal pathways and points where SCN regulation may either benefit or cause initial disorder. Top left: the induction of fatigue directly affects circadian regulation at the level of the SCN, resulting in impaired circadian output via the three major relay nuclei, the dorsomedial nuclei of the hypothalamus (DMH), the medial preoptic area (MPA), and the subparaventricular zone (SPVZ). Top right: the SCN is able to effectively signal circadian output to the three relay nodes; however, this signal is disrupted prior to innervation of the arousal network. Bottom: one or more nodes of the arousal network are directly affected by inducers of fatigue, reducing input to the circadian system and leading to subsequent declines in circadian output. *(See insert for color representation of the figure.)*

5.7 Conclusions

While it is clear that disruption of circadian rhythms may impact arousal, the neural pathways subserving this important impact are still under investigation. This is very important to clarify, given the expected cost to society.

We estimate that many people are currently experiencing pathological fatigue, either as an unexplained symptom or as a symptom of a diagnosed disease (for example, it is estimated that fatigue is a symptom in 75–95% of patients with multiple sclerosis). Fatigue impacts quality of life and the ability to hold a job. Insomnia, one of many causes of fatigue, has been estimated to cost US society $63.2 billion per year through reduced productivity related to fatigue (Kessler *et al.*, 2011). This is not so much from absenteeism but from "presenteeism", people reporting to work but being less efficient and effective at their jobs. Fatigue is correlated with levels of obesity and currently more than one-third of US adults are obese, a number that has been steadily increasing. Should the prevalence of fatigue follow this trend, the cost to society could rise dramatically in the near future.

Insight into circadian modulation of arousal may suggest treatments for chronic fatigue. Voluntary exercise has been shown to strengthen the circadian network and increase amplitude of the circadian pacemaker, as reviewed above. In fact, clinical studies have shown beneficial effects of increased exercise on symptoms of fatigue. Regularity of daily timing of exercise might add benefit. Clinicians could try to increase regularity of multiple entrainment cues such as light and dark, food, social interactions, and so on in an effort to better synchronize circadian system elements to a strong 24-h signal. Supplements of melatonin taken in the evening, when melatonin is normally higher, might also prove helpful. Bright light therapy has been shown to be helpful in a small sample of patients with cancer-related fatigue (Jeste *et al.*, 2012).

Study of the arousal network in the brain suggests that there could be multiple nodes by which arousal might be increased. Thus, for example, a stressful environment might stimulate noradrenaline release from the locus coeruleus, whereas a potent reward might instead activate dopaminergic release in the ventral tegmental area, but either input, if strong enough, might increase arousal in a fatigued patient.

Pharmacological tools might be developed by further research on this topic. Some clinical data suggest patients might benefit from either modafinil or methylphenidate. In fact, there might be many drugs that affect the arousal pathways that could lead to benefits for patients with fatigue. In addition, anti-inflammatory compounds or substances able to block the cascade initiated by inflammation might also be helpful (Harrington, 2012).

Future research targeted toward treatments for chronic fatigue should benefit from the basic scientific understanding of both the circadian system as well as the arousal network. It is our hope that soon we will have a wider array of therapies to suggest for the treatment of chronic fatigue, a widespread problem associated with an array of disease states as well as with obesity and following a variety of viral or neurological insults.

References

Abe, H., Honma, S., Ohtsu, H., and Honma, K. (2004) Circadian rhythms in behavior and clock gene expressions in the brain of mice lacking histidine decarboxylase. Brain Research. *Molecular Brain Research*, **124**(2), 178–187. doi: 10.1016/j.molbrainres.2004.02.015.

Abe, M., Herzog, E.D., Yamazaki, S., *et al.* (2002) Circadian rhythms in isolated brain regions. *The Journal of Neuroscience: The Official Journal of the Society for Neuroscience*, **22**(1), 350–356.

Adamantidis, A.R., Zhang, F., Aravanis, A.M., *et al.* (2007) Neural substrates of awakening probed with optogenetic control of hypocretin neurons. *Nature*, **450**(7168), 420–424. doi: 10.1038/nature06310.

Aston-Jones, G., Chen, S., Zhu, Y., and Oshinsky, M.L. (2001) A neural circuit for circadian regulation of arousal. *Nature Neuroscience*, **4**(7), 732–738. doi: 10.1038/89522.

Bes, F., Jobert, M., and Schulz, H. (2009) Modeling napping, post-lunch dip, and other variations in human sleep propensity. *Sleep*, **32**(3), 392–398.

Borbely, A.A. (1982) A two process model of sleep regulation. *Human Neurobiology*, **1**(3), 195–204.

Brown, R.E., Basheer, R., McKenna, J.T., *et al.* (2012) Control of sleep and wakefulness. *Physiological Reviews*, **92**(3), 1087–1187. doi: 10.1152/physrev.00032.2011.

Cagampang, F.R., Yamazaki, S., Otori, Y., and Inouye, S.I. (1993) Serotonin in the raphe nuclei: Regulation by light and an endogenous pacemaker. *Neuroreport*, **5**(1), 49–52.

Ching, S., Zhang, H., Belevych, N., *et al.* (2007) Endothelial-specific knockdown of interleukin-1 (IL-1) type 1 receptor differentially alters CNS responses to IL-1 depending on its route of administration. *The Journal of Neuroscience: The Official Journal of the Society for Neuroscience*, **27**(39), 10476–10486. doi: 10.1523/JNEUROSCI.3357-07.2007

Colwell, C.S. (2011) Linking neural activity and molecular oscillations in the SCN. *Nature Reviews. Neuroscience*, **12**(10), 553–569. doi: 10.1038/nrn3086;10.1038/nrn3086

Dantzer, R., O'Connor, J.C., Freund, G.G., *et al.* (2008) From inflammation to sickness and depression: When the immune system subjugates the brain. Nature Reviews. *Neuroscience*, **9**(1), 46–56. doi: 10.1038/nrn2297.

Davidson, A.J., Castanon-Cervantes, O., Leise, T.L., *et al.* (2009) Visualizing jet lag in the mouse suprachiasmatic nucleus and peripheral circadian timing system. *The European Journal of Neuroscience*, **29**(1), 171–180. doi: 10.1111/j.1460-9568.2008.06534.x.

Deurveilher, S. and Semba, K. (2005) Indirect projections from the suprachiasmatic nucleus to major arousal-promoting cell groups in rat: Implications for the circadian control of behavioural state. *Neuroscience*, **130**(1), 165–183. doi: 10.1016/j.neuroscience.2004.08.030.

Espana, R.A., Baldo, B.A., Kelley, A.E., and Berridge, C.W. (2001) Wake-promoting and sleep-suppressing actions of hypocretin (orexin): Basal forebrain sites of action. *Neuroscience*, **106**(4), 699–715.

Espana, R.A., McCormack, S.L., Mochizuki, T., and Scammell, T.E. (2007) Running promotes wakefulness and increases cataplexy in orexin knockout mice. *Sleep*, **30**(11), 1417–1425.

Gasbarri, A., Sulli, A., Pacitti, C., and McGaugh, J.L. (1999) Serotonergic input to cholinergic neurons in the substantia innominata and nucleus basalis magnocellularis in the rat. *Neuroscience*, **91**(3), 1129–1142.

Govindaiah, G. and Cox, C.L. (2006) Modulation of thalamic neuron excitability by orexins. *Neuropharmacology*, **51**(3), 414–425. doi: 10.1016/j.neuropharm.2006.03.030.

Grossberg, A.J., Zhu, X., Leinninger, G.M., *et al.* (2011) Inflammation-induced lethargy is mediated by suppression of orexin neuron activity. *The Journal of Neuroscience: The Official Journal of the Society for Neuroscience*, **31**(31), 11376–11386. doi: 10.1523/JNEUROSCI.2311-11.2011.

Haas, H.L. and Lin, J.S. (2012) Waking with the hypothalamus. *Pflugers Archiv: European Journal of Physiology*, **463**(1), 31–42. doi: 10.1007/s00424-011-0996-4

Harrington, M.E. (1997) The ventral lateral geniculate nucleus and the intergeniculate leaflet: Interrelated structures in the visual and circadian systems. *Neuroscience and Biobehavioral Reviews*, **21**(5), 705–727.

Harrington, M.E. (2012) Neurobiological studies of fatigue. *Progress in Neurobiology*, **99**(2), 93–105. doi: 10.1016/j.pneurobio.2012.07.004.

Horvath, T.L., Peyron, C., Diano, S., *et al.* (1999) Hypocretin (orexin) activation and synaptic innervation of the locus coeruleus noradrenergic system. *The Journal of Comparative Neurology*, **415**(2), 145–159.

Jeste, N., Liu, L., Rissling, M., *et al.* (2012) Prevention of quality-of-life deterioration with light therapy is associated with changes in fatigue in women with breast cancer undergoing chemotherapy. *Quality of Life Research: An International Journal of Quality of Life Aspects of Treatment, Care and Rehabilitation*, **22**(6), 1239–1244. doi: 10.1007/s11136-012-0243-2.

Jones, B.E. (2005) From waking to sleeping: Neuronal and chemical substrates. *Trends in Pharmacological Sciences*, **26**(11), 578–586. doi: 10.1016/j.tips.2005.09.009.

Kessler, R.C., Berglund, P.A., Coulouvrat, C., *et al.* (2011) Insomnia and the performance of US workers: Results from the america insomnia survey. *Sleep*, **34**(9), 1161–1171. doi: 10.5665/SLEEP.1230.

Khateb, A., Fort, P., Alonso, A., *et al.* (1993) Pharmacological and immunohistochemical evidence for serotonergic modulation of cholinergic nucleus basalis neurons. *The European Journal of Neuroscience*, **5**(5), 541–547.

Kohlmeier, K.A., Watanabe, S., Tyler, C.J., *et al.* (2008) Dual orexin actions on dorsal raphe and laterodorsal tegmentum neurons: Noisy cation current activation and selective enhancement of Ca2+ transients mediated by L-type calcium channels. *Journal of Neurophysiology*, **100**(4), 2265–2281. doi: 10.1152/jn.01388.2007.

Korotkova, T.M., Sergeeva, O.A., Eriksson, K.S., *et al.* (2003) Excitation of ventral tegmental area dopaminergic and nondopaminergic neurons by orexins/hypocretins. *The Journal of Neuroscience: The Official Journal of the Society for Neuroscience*, **23**(1), 7–11.

Leise, T.L., Harrington, M.E., Molyneux, P.C., *et al.* (2013) Voluntary exercise can strengthen the circadian system in aged mice. *Age*, **35**(6), 2137–2152. doi: 10.1007/s11357-012-9502-y.

Li, J.D., Hu, W.P., and Zhou, Q.Y. (2012) The circadian output signals from the suprachiasmatic nuclei. *Progress in Brain Research*, **199**, 119–127. doi: 10.1016/B978-0-444-59427-3.00028-9.

Loomis, A.L., Harvey, E.N., and Hobart, G.A. (1937) Cerebral states during sleep, as studied by human brain potentials. *Journal of Experimental Psychology*, **21**(2), 127–144.

Manns, I.D., Alonso, A., and Jones, B.E. (2003) Rhythmically discharging basal forebrain units comprise cholinergic, GABAergic, and putative glutamatergic cells. *Journal of Neurophysiology*, **89**(2), 1057–1066. doi: 10.1152/jn.00938.2002.

Maywood, E.S., Chesham, J.E., O'Brien, J.A., and Hastings, M.H. (2011) A diversity of paracrine signals sustains molecular circadian cycling in suprachiasmatic nucleus circuits. *Proceedings of the National Academy of Sciences of the USA*, **108**(34), 14306–14311. doi: 10.1073/pnas.1101767108.

Meijer, J.H., Colwell, C.S., Rohling, J.H., *et al.* (2012) Dynamic neuronal network organization of the circadian clock and possible deterioration in disease. *Progress in Brain Research*, **199**, 143–162. doi: 10.1016/B978-0-444-59427-3.00009-5.

Monti, J.M. (2011) Serotonin control of sleep–wake behavior. *Sleep Medicine Reviews*, **15**(4), 269–281. doi: 10.1016/j.smrv.2010.11.003.

Nakamura, T.J., Nakamura, W., Yamazaki, S., *et al.* (2011) Age-related decline in circadian output. *The Journal of Neuroscience: The Official Journal of the Society for Neuroscience*, **31**(28), 10201–10205. doi: 10.1523/JNEUROSCI.0451-11.2011.

Newman, D.B. and Ginsberg, C.Y. (1994) Brainstem reticular nuclei that project to the thalamus in rats: A retrograde tracer study. *Brain, Behavior and Evolution*, **44**(1), 1–39.

Olbrich, S., Mulert, C., Karch, S., *et al.* (2009) EEG-vigilance and BOLD effect during simultaneous EEG/fMRI measurement. *NeuroImage*, **45**(2), 319–332. doi: 10.1016/j.neuroimage.2008.11.014.

Ricci, J.A., Chee, E., Lorandeau, A.L., and Berger, J. (2007) Fatigue in the U.S. workforce: Prevalence and implications for lost productive work time. *Journal of Occupational and Environmental Medicine/American College of Occupational and Environmental Medicine*, **49**(1), 1–10. doi: 10.1097/01.jom.0000249782.60321.2a.

Ridder, D.A., Lang, M.F., Salinin, S., *et al.* (2011) TAK1 in brain endothelial cells mediates fever and lethargy. *The Journal of Experimental Medicine*, **208**(13), 2615–2623. doi: 10.1084/jem.20110398.

Roth, B. (1961) The clinical and theoretical importance of EEG rhythms corresponding to states of lowered vigilance. *Electroencephalography and Clinical Neurophysiology*, **13**, 395–399.

Schroeder, A.M., Truong, D., Loh, D.H., *et al.* (2012) Voluntary scheduled exercise alters diurnal rhythms of behavior, physiology and gene expression in WT and vasoactive intestinal peptide-deficient mice. *The Journal of Physiology*, **590**(Pt 23):6213–6226. doi: 10.1113/jphysiol.2012.233676.

Schwartz, M.D., Wotus, C., Liu, T., *et al.* (2009) Dissociation of circadian and light inhibition of melatonin release through forced desynchronization in the rat. *Proceedings of the National Academy of Sciences of the USA*, **106**(41), 17540–17545. doi: 10.1073/pnas.0906382106.

Siegel, J. (2004) Brain mechanisms that control sleep and waking. *Die Naturwissenschaften*, **91**(8), 355–365. doi: 10.1007/s00114-004-0541-9.

van Oosterhout, F., Lucassen, E.A., Houben, T., *et al.* (2012) Amplitude of the SCN clock enhanced by the behavioral activity rhythm. *PloS One*, **7**(6), e39693–. doi: 10.1371/journal.pone.0039693.

Verwey, M. and Amir, S. (2012). Variable restricted feeding disrupts the daily oscillations of Period2 expression in the limbic forebrain and dorsal striatum in rats. *Journal of Molecular Neuroscience: MN*, **46**(2), 258–264. doi: 10.1007/s12031-011-9529-z.

Vogelbaum, M.A. and Menaker, M. (1992) Temporal chimeras produced by hypothalamic transplants. *The Journal of Neuroscience: The Official Journal of the Society for Neuroscience*, **12**(9), 3619–3627.

Watanabe, N., Stewart, R., Jenkins, R., *et al.* (2008) The epidemiology of chronic fatigue, physical illness, and symptoms of common mental disorders: A cross-sectional survey from the second british national survey of psychiatric morbidity. *Journal of Psychosomatic Research*, **64**(4), 357–362. doi: 10.1016/j.jpsychores.2007.12.003.

Yannielli, P. and Harrington, M.E. (2004) Let there be "more" light: Enhancement of light actions on the circadian system through non-photic pathways. *Progress in Neurobiology*, **74**(1), 59–76. doi: 10.1016/j.pneurobio.2004.06.001.

Yoshida, K., McCormack, S., Espana, R.A., *et al.* (2006) Afferents to the orexin neurons of the rat brain. *The Journal of Comparative Neurology*, **494**(5), 845–861. doi: 10.1002/cne.20859.

Zant, J.C., Rozov, S., Wigren, H.K., *et al.* (2012) Histamine release in the basal forebrain mediates cortical activation through cholinergic neurons. *The Journal of Neuroscience: The Official Journal of the Society for Neuroscience*, **32**(38), 13244–13254. doi: 10.1523/JNEUROSCI.5933-11.2012

Zhang, S., Zeitzer, J.M., Yoshida, Y., *et al.* (2004) Lesions of the suprachiasmatic nucleus eliminate the daily rhythm of hypocretin-1 release. *Sleep*, **27**(4), 619–627.

Circadian Regulation of Major Physiological Systems

Physiology of the Adrenal and Liver Circadian Clocks

6

Alexei Leliavski[1,2] and Henrik Oster[1,2]

[1] Circadian Rhythms Group, Max Planck Institute for Biophysical Chemistry, Göttingen, Germany
[2] Medical Department I, University of Lübeck, Lübeck, Germany

6.1 Introduction

In most organisms, various aspects of physiology and behavior, including metabolic, endocrine and immune functions, show circadian rhythms that are governed by endogenous molecular clocks (Chapters 1 and 2). In mammals, it is assumed that (almost) every cell of the body contains its own circadian oscillator (Dibner *et al.*, 2010) based on interlocked transcriptional–translational feedback loops that are tightly coupled with the metabolic state of the cell (Zhang and Kay, 2010). Depending on tissue, the molecular clock orchestrates circadian oscillations of 5–10% of the cellular transcriptome, among them genes that encode key rate-limiting enzymes and regulatory proteins of cellular physiology (Ko and Takahashi, 2006).

Circadian clocks are able to sustain rhythmicity with a period close to 24 hours, even in constant conditions devoid of any external timing signals. Because this endogenous period differs slightly from 24 hours, under natural conditions synchronizing stimuli (*Zeitgeber*) such as light and food play an essential role in adjusting the period of endogenous clocks to geophysical time. To organize such *entrainment* at the organismal level, a hierarchy between different tissue clocks has developed. The hypothalamic *suprachiasmatic nuclei* (SCN; Chapter 3) are considered as a central circadian pacemaker that receives light input directly from a specific subpopulation of photosensitive ganglion cells in the retina and transmits this information downstream to synchronize single cell oscillators in various tissues (Dibner *et al.*, 2010). The SCN clock is necessary to maintain synchrony amongst tissue clocks under *Zeitgeber*-free conditions (Stephan and Zucker, 1972), but peripheral clocks can maintain rhythmicity in explants (Yoo *et al.*, 2004) or under entrained conditions (Oster *et al.*, 2006b). Light can modulate circadian clocks in certain peripheral tissues, including the adrenal gland and the liver. Much stronger peripheral synchronizers, however, are food intake, temperature changes or adrenal glucocorticoids (Dibner *et al.*, 2010).

The recent development of genetic tools allowing the tissue-specific deletion of clock genes has provided new insight into the contribution of peripheral clocks to the regulation of physiological rhythms. In this chapter, the circadian physiology of two organs heavily involved in metabolic regulation and energy homeostasis – the liver and the adrenal gland – is described. Both tissues harbor robust circadian clocks that possess partial autonomy from the SCN. Discussed are the functions of these oscillators, potential communication routes between them and the SCN, and how their disturbance may promote the development of diseases.

Circadian Medicine, First Edition. Edited by Christopher S. Colwell.

6.2 Circadian control of adrenal function

The adrenal gland is one of the eight major endocrine glands in mammals. Through its hormones – glucocorticoids (GCs), mineralocorticoids (MCs) and catecholamines (CAs) – it is heavily involved in the regulation of physiological processes such as stress responses, energy metabolism, blood pressure, learning and memory, and the immune system (Fig. 6.1). During development, adrenocortical precursor cells originate from the coelomic epithelium as part of the adrenogonadal primordia whilst the adrenal medulla is formed by neural crest cells, which subsequently invade the expanding population of cortical cells. The adrenal cortex of adult mammals has two clearly distinguished subregions – the *zona glomerulosa*, which produces mineralocorticoid aldosterone, and the *zona fasciculate*, responsible for glucocorticoid synthesis (mainly cortisol in humans and corticosterone in rodents). In primates, including humans, the adrenal cortex also contributes to the production of sex steroid precursors (dehydroepiandrosterone (DHEA) and DHEA-sulfate) synthesized in the third, most inner, cortical subregion, the *zona reticularis* (Havelock *et al.*, 2004). In contrast, the murine adrenal cortex lacks a clearly distinguished *zona reticularis* and cannot produce androgens due to the absence of 17α-hydroxylase. The medulla forms the core of the adrenal gland, where acetylcholine-responsive chromaffin cells synthesize the stress hormones epinephrine (70 % of cells) and norepinephrine (25 % of cells). In humans chromaffin cells synthesize both CAs, while in rodents the hormones are produced by two separate subpopulations of cells. A third subpopulation of medullar cells, small granule-containing cells (approximately 4 % in mice), produce further peptides such as met-enkephalin, substance P, neuropeptide Y, neurotensin and chromogranin A.

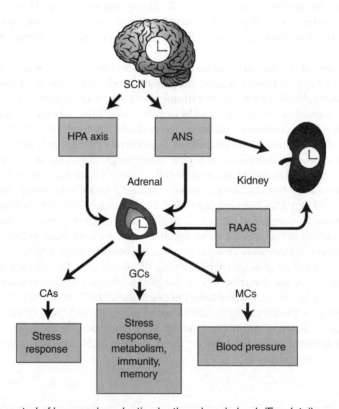

Fig. 6.1 Circadian control of hormonal production by the adrenal gland. (For details see text.)

6.2.1 Glucocorticoids (GCs)

Under basal conditions adrenocortical GC secretion follows robust circadian and ultradian (1–2 pulses/h) oscillations. The circadian peak of GC production is observed at the beginning of the activity phase, that is, during early morning in humans and other diurnal animals and the early night in nocturnal species such as most rodents. The SCN neurons seem to be indispensable for the generation of the circadian GC rhythm component (Stephan and Zucker, 1972), while ultradian GC pulses are preserved in SCN lesioned animals (Waite *et al.*, 2012). Timing signals from the SCN reach the adrenal gland via two confirmed modes, the hypothalamic–pituitary–adrenal (HPA) axis and the autonomic nervous system (ANS) (Fig. 6.1). The first node of the HPA axis is the hypothalamic paraventricular nucleus (PVN), which receives stress-driven signals from the brainstem structures and forebrain limbic circuits (Ulrich-Lai and Herman, 2009). The SCN sends indirect projections to PVN neurons, mainly via inhibitory projections to the subparaventricular zone and the dorsomedial hypothalamus (Buijs *et al.*, 1993). PVN neurons produce corticotropin-releasing hormone and vasopressin, which stimulate corticotropic cells in the pituitary to secrete adrenocorticotropic hormone (ACTH) from secretory granules. In adrenocortical cells, ACTH upregulates strereoidogenesis via steroidogenic acute regulatory protein (StAR)-mediated increase of cholesterol delivery to the inner mitochondrial membrane for conversion by cholesterol side-chain cleavage enzyme (CYP11A1). Long-term effects of ACTH include an increase in expression of other steroidogenic enzymes (CYP17, CYP21A1, CYP11B1) and improved cholesterol uptake via low and high density lipoprotein receptors. The system is kept under control via negative feedback: GCs suppress their own production acting through the glucocorticoid receptor at the level of the pituitary and the PVN. On the other hand, SCN neurons regulate rhythmic functioning of the adrenal gland through the ANS and hypophysectomy does ablate GC rhythms only in combination with adrenal denervation. The multisynaptic ANS pathway consists of pre-autonomic PVN neurons, sympathetic preganglionic intermediolateral neurons of the spinal cord, and splanchnic innervation of the adrenal gland (Buijs *et al.*, 1993). ANS signals can affect adrenal physiology via modulation of adrenal clock gene activity. A one-hour light pulse can activate *Per* gene expression in the adrenal gland and drive slow ACTH-independent GC release; this response requires intact adrenal innervation (Ishida *et al.*, 2005). SCN–adrenal neural connections are essential for maintaining circadian regulation of adrenal sensitivity to ACTH *in vivo* (Dallman *et al.*, 1978).

6.2.2 Mineralocorticoids (MCs)

The mineralocorticoid aldosterone, a key regulator of blood pressure, exhibits daily oscillations with a peak in the active phase. Aldosterone production is under control of the renin–angiotensin–aldosterone system (RAAS) (Bader, 2010). In brief, the peptidase renin released by renal juxtaglomerular cells in response to low blood volume converts its substrate, angiotensinogen, to angiotensin I (Ang I), which in turn is cleaved by the angiotensin-converting enzyme to liberate Ang II. Ang II stimulates aldosterone synthesis in the adrenal cortex. Aldosterone binding to the mineralocorticoid receptor in renal epithelial cells reduces extracellular fluid volume via stimulation of sodium reabsorption and potassium excretion by the kidneys, thus lowering blood pressure. Plasma renin activity, angiotensin-converting-enzyme (ACE) and Ang II levels display circadian variation both in rodents and humans, suggesting that circadian control of the RAAS by the SCN or renal clocks may contribute to aldosterone rhythmicity (Guo *et al.*, 2005).

6.2.3 Catecholamines (CAs)

Both epinephrine and norepinephrine display diurnal variations in blood and urine samples from unstressed humans and mice, with a peak in the beginning of the active phase (Linsell *et al.*, 1985). Daily rhythms of CA release from the adrenal medulla parallel diurnal changes in sympathetic tone, suggesting central regulation of sympathetic adrenomedullary system activity by the SCN. In line with this, SCN lesions in rats abolish circadian rhythms of heart rate and blood pressure, mainly controlled by the sympathetic system, without affecting activity and sleep–wake cycles (Janssen *et al.*, 1994).

6.2.4 Adrenal clocks

The above findings demonstrate that the SCN clock is critical for maintaining daily rhythmicity of adrenal hormones. However, several lines of evidence suggest that the adrenal gland itself harbors an intrinsic circadian oscillator. Firstly, clock gene expression in the adrenal of rodents and primates is highly rhythmic (Oster *et al.*, 2006a, 2006b). Interestingly, circadian rhythms in the expression of clock genes are different in different adrenal regions (Oster *et al.*, 2006b) (Fig. 6.2). Moreover, approximately 5% of the adrenal transcriptome is expressed in a circadian fashion (Oster *et al.*, 2006a), including genes involved in cholesterol uptake and transport, regulators of steroid biosynthesis, ACTH signaling, and CA metabolism (*Maoa, Nr4a2, Pnmt*). Circadian variations in expression of key transcripts involved in CA synthesis (*Th, Pnmt*) and reuptake (*Slc6a2*) were also found in an independent microarray study of monkey adrenals (Lemos *et al.*, 2006). Interestingly, it has been shown that StAR, a key rate-limiting cholesterol transporter, is also rhythmically expressed and under direct regulation by the clock machinery (Son *et al.*, 2008). In 1964, Andrews and Falk demonstrated that cultured hamster adrenal glands maintain circadian patterns of respiration and steroid secretion *ex vivo* (Andrews and Folk, 1964). Similarly, adrenocortical Y-1 cells display a circadian rhythm of GC synthesis *in vitro* (Son *et al.*, 2008) and transplanted wild-type adrenal grafts can maintain rhythmic clock gene expression and glucocorticoid production under entrained conditions in clock-deficient transgenic mice (Oster *et al.*, 2006b).

6.2.5 Local control of MC rhythms

Adrenalectomy severely affects circadian variations in blood pressure and heart rate in wild-type mice. Moreover, the components of the RAAS are also produced locally in the adrenal cortex in response to ACTH, regulating sensitivity of adrenocortical cells to Ang II. However, it is unclear whether the sensitivity to Ang II changes throughout the day. Okamura and colleagues have provided strong evidence for a role of the adrenal circadian clock in aldosterone-mediated regulation of blood pressure (Doi *et al.*, 2010; Chapter 9). *Cry1/2* double deficient mice lacking a functional circadian clock display abnormally high levels of plasma aldosterone. This effect is due to overexpression of *Hsd3b6* in *Cry* mutant adrenals, which encodes a steroidogenic enzyme that acts upstream of aldosterone synthesis. *Hsd3b6* is expressed exclusively in aldosterone-producing *zona glomerulosa* cells. When fed a high salt diet *Cry*-null mice become hypertensive. This elevation in blood pressure is aldosterone-dependent and can be reversed by

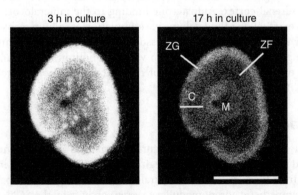

Fig. 6.2 The adrenal clock is sustained in culture. Luminescence imaging of *PER2::LUC* mouse adrenal slices. C: cortex; M: medulla; ZG: zona glomerulosa; ZF: zona fasciculata; scale bar is 1 mm.

treatment with the aldosterone blocker eplerenone. It remains to be shown whether the adrenocortical clock itself is sufficient to maintain aldosterone rhythmicity or whether it coordinates the sensitivity of the steroidogenic machinery to systemically driven rhythmic cues.

6.2.6 Local control of GC rhythms

In vitro data suggest that the adrenal clock is essential for gating the adrenal responsiveness to ACTH stimulation. In cultured clock-deficient (*Per2/Cry1* double mutant) adrenal slice cultures circadian variations in the corticoid response to ACTH stimulation is abolished (Oster *et al.*, 2006b) and the magnitude of this response is also highly compromised upon suppression of *Bmal1* (Son *et al.*, 2008). Two different approaches have been used so far to dissect a functional role of the adrenal clock *in vivo*. Our group performed adrenal transplantations between arrhythmic *Per2/Cry1* double mutant and wild-type mice (Oster *et al.*, 2006b). It was found that an intact adrenal clock is sufficient for maintaining GC rhythmicity in a *Clock*-deficient host under 12h:12h light–dark conditions, but rhythms are lost after removing the external *Zeitgeber*. Alternatively, Son and coworkers performed genetic ablation of the adrenal clock (Son *et al.*, 2008), knocking down *Bmal1* by overexpressing an antisense transcript under the control of the ACTH receptor gene (*Mc2r*) promoter. In these mice GC rhythms were strongly dampened in constant darkness, but not in light–dark conditions, suggesting that the adrenal clock is required for maintaining high amplitude GC oscillations.

Interestingly, under certain conditions the adrenal clock is also involved in the synchronization of clocks in other peripheral tissues. Fast traveling over several time zones results in misalignment of endogenous clocks. This is reflected in a range of symptoms affecting sleep timing, appetite and digestion, cognitive performance, and immune responses, covered under the term *jetlag*. During jetlag circadian clocks of different organs (including the liver) re-entrain at different speed, creating a transient state of internal desynchrony. Adrenal clocks coordinate global resetting via rhythmic regulation of GC levels. Pharmacologically shifting GC profiles prior to a jetlag can promote the re-entrainment process, at least in mice (Kiessling *et al.*, 2010).

Of note, GC production has two general modes of control. Besides circadian modulation of basal GC levels there is acute induction of GC synthesis by stressful stimuli—physical, psychological, inflammatory, or metabolic. Both modes can potentially influence each other. Circadian changes may define an activation threshold of the HPA axis to acute stressors and, vice versa, stress-induced GC surges may serve as resetting signals for other peripheral clocks. It is known that the intensity of stress-induced GC responses depends on the time of day, but the results to date are far from being conclusive. Some reports in rodents and humans show that HPA axis responses are more pronounced at the beginning of the activity phase (Buijs *et al.*, 1993), while other reports found an opposite pattern (Kalsbeek *et al.*, 2003) or failed to detect any diurnal changes. SCN lesion studies provide further evidence for a role of the central clock in maintaining daily stress sensitivity (Buijs *et al.*, 1993). Interestingly, the type of stress stimulus appears critical in this context. While novelty exposure in rats elicits maximal ACTH and corticosterone responses in the early morning, insulin-induced hypoglycemia stimulated GC release peaks in the early night (Kalsbeek *et al.*, 2003). These findings suggest the existence of at least two different clock-controlled stress pathways that can activate adrenal GC secretion.

6.3 Circadian control of liver function

The liver is (after the skin) the largest organ of the body. Its primary function is the metabolization of nutrients and the storage of glucose and, to a lesser extent, lipids as energy fuels for the body. It further shares an important role with the kidneys in detoxification and excretion processes. More recently, the liver has also been identified as an endocrine organ, secreting hormones such as insulin-like growth factor-1 (IGF-1), angiotensinogen, thrombopoeitin, and hepcidin. Structurally the mammalian liver consists of several large lobes (four in humans and rodents). Roughly 60% of the cells in the liver are made up of hepatocytes of parenchymal origin. Hepatocytes are also the largest cells of the liver, making up to 80% of the liver volume. Other cells include endothelial, macrophage-like Kupffer, and hepatic stellate cells (also known as Ito cells). Like many other growth factors, IGF-1 secretion follows a circadian rhythm with peak levels during the rest phase. Circadian rhythms of thrombopoietin, but not of hepcidin and angiotensinogen, have been described (Levi and Schibler, 2007). Diurnal variations of blood pressure seem to rather depend on rhythmic release of vasopressin from the hypothalamus and aldosterone from the adrenal (see above).

The functions of the liver in energy metabolism and detoxification are tightly linked to the diurnal variation of food intake. In fact, transcriptome studies in rodents suggest that food intake may be a stronger synchronizer of liver transcriptome rhythms than the circadian clock itself (Vollmers *et al.*, 2009). Together with nutrients, numerous substances are taken up that either need to be chemically modified to be useful to the body or, because of their toxicity, have to be removed again from the system. The liver prepares for these needs by regulating its transcriptional machinery to ready the enzymatic armory in times of need while saving energy during fasting times, for example, during the daily rest phase. Of note, feeding time is also a strong synchronizer of peripheral clocks and the liver clock can phase-reset in response to regularly timed food intake, an effect that becomes important during jetlag when adjusting mealtime can have dramatic effects on the re-entrainment process at the destination of travel (Angeles-Castellanos *et al.*, 2011).

6.3.1 Glucose metabolism

Glucose metabolism is probably the best described rhythmic process in the liver but its regulation is highly complex, influenced by both internal and external timing cues (Fig. 6.3). In the postprandial phase higher order carbohydrates are broken down to fructose and glucose and transported to the liver via the blood. Upon entry into hepatocytes glucose is quickly converted into glucose-6-phosphate – and by this taken out of the equilibrium – and either broken down to pyruvate for further conversion or stored as glycogen. Glycogen biosynthesis is high during the active (feeding) phase and glycogen breakdown becomes a major source of energy during the inactive (fasting) period of the day, that is, the night in humans or the day in nocturnal rodents (Kohsaka and Bass, 2007). The uptake into and release of glucose from liver storage is regulated by the insulin/glucagon endocrine system that responds to changes in blood glucose levels. Other hormones, such as cortisol and leptin/ghrelin, most of which are under the

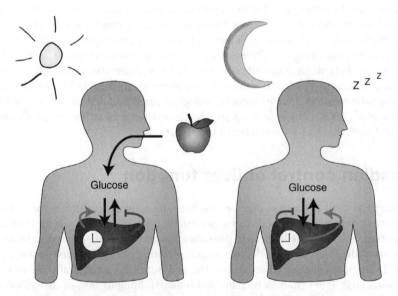

Fig. 6.3 Liver circadian clocks regulate blood glucose levels by the timing of glucose uptake and release.

control of the circadian clock, also play a role (Levi *et al.*, 2007). Cortisol induces gluconeogenesis, the *de novo* synthesis of glucose from pyruvate, and promotes the release of glucose into the blood. Leptin and ghrelin impinge on glucose metabolism primarily via indirect means, regulating appetite centers in the basal hypothalamus (Leproult and Van Cauter, 2010).

6.3.2 Lipid metabolism

Though circadian aspects of lipid metabolism have mostly been described for adipose tissues, similar to glucose, lipid metabolism in liver is tightly coupled to food intake. Lipids are transported in the blood in the form of lipoproteins. Upon food intake chylomicrons are assembled in the intestinal mucosa. Most chylomicrons are taken up from muscle and adipose tissues, but the so called *remnants* reach the liver where they can be used for conversion into lipid derivatives or for breakdown into acetyl-CoA. Acetyl-CoA is also the substrate for endogenous cholesterol. Cholesterol biosynthesis is robustly rhythmic with a peak during the late active phase (i.e., the evening in humans and the early morning in rats). Remnants become problematic when lipids are taken up excessively or at the wrong time of day, for example, under high fat (*Western*) diet conditions or in patients with night eating syndrome. Circadian disruption, which is also seen in night shift workers or during jetlag, has strong effects on liver lipid metabolism, promoting excessive lipogenesis and the development of nonalcoholic fatty liver disease (NAFLD)(Levi and Schibler, 2007).

6.3.3 Detoxification

The rhythmic regulation of biotransformation and detoxification processes in the liver has important implications for the clinics as a critical determinant of drug pharmacokinetics, -dynamics and the manifestation of side effects (Fig. 6.4). As just one example, the lethal toxicity of a fixed dose of the anesthetic halothane in mice can vary between 5 and 76%, depending on the time of day when the drug is given (Levi and Schibler, 2007). Similar effects are described for various anti-cancer agents and anti-biotics. Circadian variations in the efficacy of drugs have been documented for all relevant parameters, absorption, distribution, metabolism, and elimination (*ADME*), most of which are regulated by the liver (or, sometimes, the kidneys). This has giving rise to the field of *chronopharmacology* (Levi and

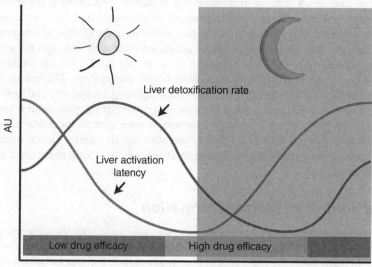

Fig. 6.4 The efficacy of many drugs dependents is determined by daily profiles of detoxification rate and activation latency in liver.

Schibler, 2007). It is worth considering that circadian rhythms differ between males and females and amongst individuals (of different *chronotypes*). Therefore, easy and efficient means of determining endogenous clock phase in patients are needed to better implement circadian knowledge into the clinical practice.

6.3.4 Hepatocyte clocks

Hepatocyte clocks have been excessively studied in rodents, while very little is known about clocks in other cells of the liver. The hepatocyte clockwork comprises the same set of clock genes described for the SCN pacemaker but clock phase is delayed by a couple of hours. In the hepatocyte, the clock components CLOCK and BMAL1 show highest activity around the day/night transition in both diurnal and nocturnal species, indicating that the interplay between liver clock function and metabolic regulation must differ between animals with different activity profiles. It is assumed that liver clocks are reset by the SCN in a similar way as has been proposed for the adrenal. Again, as for the adrenal, between 5 and 10% of the liver transcriptome follows a circadian expression rhythm. Interestingly, liver-specific genetic disruption of clock function abrogates most but not all of these rhythms, indicating that systemic cues exert a strong influence on liver physiology (Kornmann *et al.*, 2007). The communication pathways between the SCN and the liver clock are largely unknown. Of note, adrenal-derived hormones such as GCs and norepinephrine can also affect the liver clock, which offers the possibility of an indirect entrainment pathway. Light appears capable of directly modulating clock gene expression in the liver (Cailotto *et al.*, 2005). However, unlike what has been shown for the adrenal, the physiological implications of this process remain obscure.

6.3.5 Local control of energy metabolism

Insight on the effects of local liver clock function on metabolic processes comes mostly from studies on tissue-specific mouse mutants. Lamia and coworkers have shown that deleting the clock gene *Bmal1* in hepatocytes using the *Cre/loxP* gene targeting system affects glucose metabolism but has little overall effect on energy homeostasis (Lamia *et al.*, 2008). Liver-*Bmal1* mutant mice show hypoglycemia during the rest phase, exaggerated glucose clearance after insulin injection combined with a loss of the rhythmic expression of genes involved in glucose transport and the regulation of glucose utilization. The authors conclude that the liver clock may be important for buffering circulating glucose in a time-of-day dependent manner, thereby ensuring a constant supply of glucose as fuel for other organs such as the brain over the course of the day, while at the same time preventing the adverse effects of excessive blood glucose concentrations. Cho and colleagues have generated mice with liver specific mutations of two other clock components, *Rev-erbα* and *Rev-erbβ* (Cho *et al.*, 2012). Double mutants show clock dysfunction in hepatocytes together with deregulated lipid metabolism. Microarray analyses reveal enrichment for changes in transcripts involved in insulin signaling, amino acid and lipid metabolism in the livers of the double mutants, correlating with increased circulating glucose and triglyceride levels, and a reduction in the level of free fatty acids observed in mice with an inducible (global) deletion of *Rev-erbα/β*. Given that systemic and local (clock) controlled signals interact closely in the regulation of liver physiology more studies are needed to distinguish the function of local hepatocyte clocks from that of external regulatory factors.

6.3.6 Local control of biotransformation

The term *biotransformation* comprises metabolic processes associated with the conversion of biologically active substances (e.g., steroid hormones) and the modification and elimination of xenobiotics (such as drugs or toxins). In many cases the main goal of biotransformation is the polarization of lipophilic substances to increase their solubility and facilitate excretion via urine or bile. Detoxification can be divided into two major steps: modification and conjugation/excretion. Modification involves oxidatory reactions facilitated by the cytochrome P450 family of oxidases. Many P450 transcripts are controlled by the local clock machinery or by clock-controlled transcription factors, such as the PAR-domain basic leucine zipper transcription factors DBP, TEF, and HLF (Gachon *et al.*, 2006). P450 activity is high during the active phase. Conjugation involves esterification of metabolites with polar species such as glutathione, glycine, and sulfuric or glucuronic acid by broad specificity transferases. Hepatic glutathione-S-transferase and glutathione peroxidase activities are rhythmic in mice, indicating a role for the circadian clock in the regulation of transfer reactions. Transport of modified metabolites into the blood or bile, again, is regulated in a circadian way, but it remains to be shown to which extent local clocks are involved in these processes (Levi and Schibler, 2007).

6.4 Conclusion

In multicellular organisms, circadian timekeeping is organized in a complex hierarchical system with a central oscillator in the SCN and peripheral clocks in most tissues of the body. Adrenal and liver tissue clocks have been shown to impinge on the regulation of endocrine and physiological functions, including diurnal rhythms of glucocorticoid secretion and energy metabolism. While the SCN is entrained primarily by the light–dark cycle, peripheral clocks respond to different external stimuli such as food intake, emphasizing the tight interaction between peripheral clock function and metabolism and allowing for a high degree of plasticity in the entrainment of endogenous timers to the external environment. The good accessibility of peripheral clocks makes them prime targets for chronopharmacological approaches. On the other hand, assessment of peripheral clock phase may become an important tool for determining internal circadian phase and tailor medication in the clinical practice.

Acknowledgements

Henrik Oster is an Emmy Noether fellow of the German Research Foundation (DFG) and a Lichtenberg fellow of the Volkswagen Foundation.

References

Andrews, R.V., and Folk, G.E. Jr., (1964) Circadian metabolic patterns in cultured hamster adrenal glands. *Comparative Biochemistry and Physiology* **11**, 393–409.

Angeles-Castellanos, M., Amaya, J.M., Salgado-Delgado, R., *et al.* (2011) Scheduled food hastens re-entrainment more than melatonin does after a 6-h phase advance of the light-dark cycle in rats. *Journal of Biological Rhythms* **26**, 324–334.

Bader, M. (2010) Tissue renin-angiotensin-aldosterone systems: Targets for pharmacological therapy. *Annual Review of Pharmacology and Toxicology* **50**, 439–465.

Buijs, R.M., Kalsbeek, A., van der Woude, T.P., *et al.* (1993) Suprachiasmatic nucleus lesion increases corticosterone secretion. *American Journal of Physiology* **264**, R1186–1192.

Cailotto, C., La Fleur, S.E., Van Heijningen, C., *et al.* (2005) The suprachiasmatic nucleus controls the daily variation of plasma glucose via the autonomic output to the liver: are the clock genes involved? *The European Journal of Neuroscience* **22**, 2531–2540.

Cho, H., Zhao, X., Hatori, M., *et al.* (2012) Regulation of circadian behaviour and metabolism by REV-ERB-alpha and REV-ERB-beta. *Nature* **485**, 123–127.

Dallman, M.F., Engeland, W.C., Rose, J.C., *et al.* (1978) Nycthemeral rhythm in adrenal responsiveness to ACTH. *The American Journal of Physiology* **235**, R210–218.

Dibner, C., Schibler, U., and Albrecht, U. (2010) The mammalian circadian timing system: organization and coordination of central and peripheral clocks. *Annual Review of Physiology* **72**, 517–549.

Doi, M., Takahashi, Y., Komatsu, R., *et al.* (2010). Salt-sensitive hypertension in circadian clock-deficient Cry-null mice involves dysregulated adrenal Hsd3b6. *Nature Medicine* **16**, 67–74.

Gachon, F., Olela, F.F., Schaad, O., *et al.* (2006) The circadian PAR-domain basic leucine zipper transcription factors DBP, TEF, and HLF modulate basal and inducible xenobiotic detoxification. *Cell Metabolism* **4**, 25–36.

Guo, H., Brewer, J.M., Champhekar, A., *et al*. (2005) Differential control of peripheral circadian rhythms by suprachiasmatic-dependent neural signals. *Proceedings of the National Academy of Sciences of the USA* **102**, 3111–3116.

Havelock, J.C., Auchus, R.J., and Rainey, W.E. (2004) The rise in adrenal androgen biosynthesis: adrenarche. *Seminars in Reproductive Medicine* **22**, 337–347.

Ishida, A., Mutoh, T., Ueyama, T., *et al*. (2005) Light activates the adrenal gland: timing of gene expression and glucocorticoid release. *Cell Metabolism* **2**, 297–307.

Janssen, B.J., Tyssen, C.M., Duindam, H., and Rietveld, W.J. (1994) Suprachiasmatic lesions eliminate 24-h blood pressure variability in rats. *Physiology & Behavior* **55**, 307–311.

Kalsbeek, A., Ruiter, M., La Fleur, S.E., *et al*. (2003) The diurnal modulation of hormonal responses in the rat varies with different stimuli. *Journal of Neuroendocrinology* **15**, 1144–1155.

Kiessling, S., Eichele, G., and Oster, H. (2010) Adrenal glucocorticoids have a key role in circadian resynchronization in a mouse model of jet lag. *The Journal of Clinical Investigation* **120**, 2600–2609.

Ko, C.H. and Takahashi, J.S. (2006) Molecular components of the mammalian circadian clock. *Human Molecular Genetics* **15**(Suppl 2), R271–277.

Kohsaka, A. and Bass, J. (2007) A sense of time: how molecular clocks organize metabolism. *Trends in Endocrinology and Metabolism: TEM* **18**, 4–11.

Kornmann, B., Schaad, O., Bujard, H., *et al*. (2007) System-driven and oscillator-dependent circadian transcription in mice with a conditionally active liver clock. *PLoS Biology* **5**, e34.

Lamia, K.A., Storch, K.F., and Weitz, C.J. (2008) Physiological significance of a peripheral tissue circadian clock. *Proceedings of the National Academy of Sciences of the USA* **105**, 15172–15177.

Lemos, D.R., Downs, J.L., and Urbanski, H.F. (2006) Twenty-four-hour rhythmic gene expression in the rhesus macaque adrenal gland. *Molecular Endocrinology* **20**, 1164–1176.

Leproult, R. and Van Cauter, E. (2010) Role of sleep and sleep loss in hormonal release and metabolism. *Endocrine Development* **17**, 11–21.

Levi, F., and Schibler, U. (2007) Circadian rhythms: mechanisms and therapeutic implications. *Annual review of Pharmacology and Toxicology* **47**, 593–628.

Levi, F., Filipski, E., Iurisci, I., *et al*. (2007) Cross-talks between circadian timing system and cell division cycle determine cancer biology and therapeutics. *Cold Spring Harbor Symposia on Quantitative Biology* **72**, 465–475.

Linsell, C.R., Lightman, S.L., Mullen, P.E., *et al*. (1985) Circadian rhythms of epinephrine and norepinephrine in man. *The Journal of Clinical Endocrinology and Metabolism* **60**, 1210–1215.

Oster, H., Damerow, S., Hut, R.A., and Eichele, G. (2006a) Transcriptional profiling in the adrenal gland reveals circadian regulation of hormone biosynthesis genes and nucleosome assembly genes. *Journal of Biological Rhythms* **21**, 350–361.

Oster, H., Damerow, S., Kiessling, S., *et al*. (2006b) The circadian rhythm of glucocorticoids is regulated by a gating mechanism residing in the adrenal cortical clock. *Cell Metababolism* **4**, 163–173.

Son, G.H., Chung, S., Choe, H.K., *et al*. (2008) Adrenal peripheral clock controls the autonomous circadian rhythm of glucocorticoid by causing rhythmic steroid production. *Proceedings of the National Academy of Sciences of the USA* **105**, 20970–20975.

Stephan, F., and Zucker, H. (1972) Circadian rhythms in drinking behavior and locomotor activity of rats are eliminated by hypothalamic lesions. *Proceedings of the National Academy of Sciences of the USA* **69**, 1583–1586.

Ulrich-Lai, Y.M. and Herman, J.P. (2009) Neural regulation of endocrine and autonomic stress responses. *Nature Reviews Neuroscience* **10**, 397–409.

Vollmers, C., Gill, S., DiTacchio, L., *et al*. (2009) Time of feeding and the intrinsic circadian clock drive rhythms in hepatic gene expression. *Proceedings of the National Academy of Sciences of the USA* **106**, 21453–21458.

Waite, E.J., McKenna, M., Kershaw, Y., *et al*. (2012) Ultradian corticosterone secretion is maintained in the absence of circadian cues. *The European Journal of Neuroscience* **36**(8):3142–3150.

Yoo, S.H., Yamazaki, S., Lowrey, P.L., *et al*. (2004) PERIOD2::LUCIFERASE real-time reporting of circadian dynamics reveals persistent circadian oscillations in mouse peripheral tissues. *Proceedings of the National Academy of Sciences of the USA* **101**, 5339–5346.

Zhang, E.E., and Kay, S.A. (2010) Clocks not winding down: unravelling circadian networks. *Nature Reviews Molecular Cell Biology* **11**, 764–776.

Nutrition and Diet as Potent Regulators of the Liver Clock

7

Yu Tahara and Shigenobu Shibata

Department of Electrical Engineering and Bioscience, Waseda University, Tokyo, Japan

7.1 Introduction

This chapter centers on the new keyword "chrono-nutrition," which we define as the research field focused on understanding the relationship between circadian rhythm and nutrition/diet. Mammals have a master oscillator, the mammalian suprachiasmatic nucleus (SCN; Chapter 3), and another master oscillator, which we call the "food entrainable oscillator" (FEO). The FEO senses food timing and/or nutritional factors, and then organizes the circadian system independent of SCN regulation. Here, recent chrono-nutritional studies are discussed in order to understand the importance of the mutual interactions between circadian rhythms and nutrition/diet.

7.2 Food is a "zeitgeber": The FEO in the brain

7.2.1 Food entrainment and food anticipatory activity

Food can entrain peripheral circadian clocks in as strong or stronger manner than that of the light–dark (LD) cycle. Researchers have demonstrated food-induced phase-shifts of behavioral rhythms, independent of LD cycle-induced behavioral rhythms. In fact, feeding time restriction in mice (scheduled feeding, SF) of 3–6 hours in the daytime can change their behavior from nocturnal to diurnal (Fig. 7.1). Because mice have to eat food for their survival, food seeking behavior appears 2–3 hours before feeding time in this paradigm. We call this seeking behavior a "food anticipatory activity" (FAA) and believe that mice can recall feeding time using their own internal clock. In addition to the behavioral change, there are many physiological rhythms that can be changed by SF. Body temperature, blood hormone concentrations, blood glucose, and liver glycogen levels have classically been reported in this field to be entrained by SF (Shibata *et al.*, 2010). It is also possible to shift and even entrain clock gene expression patterns by SF in peripheral tissues such as those of liver, kidney, and adrenal gland (Chapter 6). Thus, the timing of food can have a major impact on the circadian system.

Circadian Medicine, First Edition. Edited by Christopher S. Colwell.
© 2015 John Wiley & Sons, Inc. Published 2015 by John Wiley & Sons, Inc.

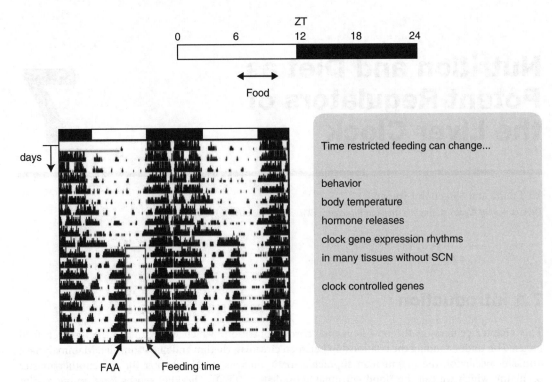

Fig. 7.1 Daytime scheduled feeding paradigm induces changes of many physiological factors. If feeding time is restricted to mice during several hours of the light phase, food anticipatory activity (FAA) will appear before their feeding time. In addition to the behavioral change, phases of expression of clock genes are entrained to the feeding time. Along with these changes, rhythms of other physiological factors, such as hormonal releases and body temperature, are also followed to the feeding time. ZT, zeitgeber time (ZT0, lights-on time)

7.2.2 Role of the SCN on the FEO

The SCN does not appear to participate in feeding cycle entrainment. Clock gene expression rhythms and neural firing rhythms in the SCN could not be entrained by daytime SF. In addition, a classic neurobehavioral study demonstrated that SCN-lesioned behaviorally arrhythmic mice were able to adapt to SF and show FAA prior to feeding time (Moore and Eichler, 1972). SCN-lesioned mice continue exhibit SF-induced rhythms of body temperature, corticosteroids, and clock gene expression in many tissues. As shown in Fig. 7.2, the SCN is strongly regulated by the LD cycle through the retinal–hypothalamic tract (RHT) (Chapter 3), but other brain sections and peripheral tissues are regulated by the restricted feeding paradigm. In fact, lesioning the central clock appears to enhance the levels of FAA, suggesting that the SCN normally inhibits food-induced FEO entrainment.

7.2.3 FEO formation and characteristics in the brain

Recently, many researchers have attempted to elucidate the location and mechanism of the FEO in the brain, as the discovery of the FEO is equivalent to the discovery of the second master oscillator in mammals. To locate the FEO, they have used FAA as an index of the activated FEO, studying abnormal mice that show no FAA despite SF conditioning, in order to determine the mechanism of the FEO. One possible approach is to locate the specific brain area(s) that control the FEO, like the SCN. Many brain regions have been examined by lesion studies, and lesion of the dorsomedial hypothalamus attenuated FAA formation in mice. However, a more recent study has shown that mice with combined destruction of the SCN and

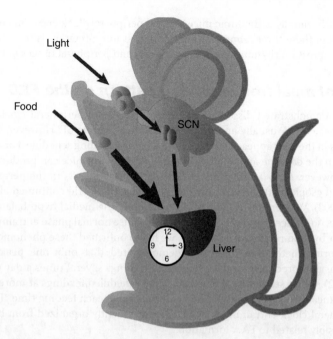

Fig. 7.2 Schematic cartoon of the liver clock entrained by light and food. The circadian system in the SCN is directly regulated by the light–dark cycle, and SCN regulates circadian clocks in a whole body. However, if food timing is restricted at the specific period in a day, the clock in the liver is strongly regulated by the food stimulus rather than by light.

the dorsomedial hypothalamus can still express normal FAA (Acosta-Galvan *et al.*, 2011). Thus, the current hypothesis is that neural networks among many parts of the brain organize the FEO for FAA.

Another strategy for locating the FEO was the use of genetic mutations in mice. Clock gene mutant mice showed no or small weak effects on FAA formation (Shibata *et al.*, 2010). Impairment of other genes such as *Rgs16* (regulator of G protein signaling) and *Melanocortin-3* showed reductions in FAA, but none showed a complete loss of FAA using mutant mice (Shibata *et al.*, 2010). Knockout of *Orexin*, an important neuropeptide for food intake behavior, was reported to reduce FAA in a mouse SF experiment. Therefore, not just the circadian clock systems but also food intake motivation may be involved in the formation of FAA. The FEO is governed by more complicated mechanisms than SCN oscillation, as it is an essential survival mechanism.

7.3 The FEO in peripheral tissues

7.3.1 Discovery of the FEO in peripheral tissues

In 2000, Damiola and coworkers demonstrated that the core clock genes in peripheral tissues were phase-shifted by daytime SF, but that the SCN clock was not (Damiola *et al.*, 2000). In this study, they also found that the entraining speed of *Dbp* gene expression rhythms by SF was faster in the liver than in the kidney, heart, or pancreas. In 2001, Stokkan and coworkers demonstrated that *Per1* gene expression rhythms in the liver were entrained by daytime SF within two days by using a *Per1-luc* transgenic rat, in which the luciferase gene was transfected under the control of the *Per1* promoter (Stokkan *et al.*, 2001). In addition, they showed that *Per1-luc* rhythm in the SCN was not entrained by SF. At the same time, our laboratory also demonstrated that *Per1* and *Per2* gene expression rhythms in the liver, cerebral cortex, and hippocampus were shifted by daytime SF in mice, but these same rhythms were not shifted in the SCN (Hara *et al.*, 2001). We also showed that a change in the LD cycle (a 7-h phase advance of the LD cycle) but no change in nighttime SF, could entrain SCN clocks to a new LD cycle, but not peripheral clocks. In addition, the SCN-lesioned behaviorally arrhythmic mice showed peripheral clock entrainment to SF. Taking into account the data from these three laboratories, the simplest interpretation is that the SF paradigm can entrain clock gene expression rhythms in many brain parts and peripheral tissues but not in the SCN.

7.3.2 Effect of meal frequency and pattern on the FEO

Some studies have demonstrated dissociations between FAA and peripheral clock gene entrainment under SF conditions, as FAA usually appears 3–4 days after starting SF. However, shifts in clock gene expression rhythms in the liver appear 1–2 days after starting a feeding schedule. For example, two meals per day (one meal in the daytime and another in the nighttime) for mice can produce FAA twice before each meal time; however, *Per1-luc* rhythms of *Per1-luc* transgenic rats in the peripheral tissues (liver, colon, stomach, and esophagus) showed only one peak phase and still continued along a 24-h rhythm (Davidson *et al.*, 2003). We demonstrated that destruction of the medial hypothalamus in mice did not cause the normal FAA (reduced amount of FAA) but did cause normal phase entrainment of PER2::LUC rhythms in the liver by food restriction. Recently, we have confirmed these phenomena using an *in vivo* PER2::LUC monitoring method in mice. We demonstrated that only one peak corresponding to PER2::LUC rhythms appeared in mice with scheduled feedings several times a day (2, 3, 4, or 6 meals) (Kuroda *et al.*, 2012). Other studies have elucidated that scheduled feedings at more than one meal per day (e.g., 2, 4, or 6 meals per day) can induce FAA formation at each feeding time. Thus, these findings suggest that peripheral clock entrainment by SF is independently organized from brain clock entrainment, which is possibly related to FAA formation.

7.3.3 Role of clock genes in FAA and FEO in the brain and FEO in peripheral tissues

Previous work using *Per2* mutant mice demonstrated a reduced amount of FAA but a normal shift in liver clock gene expression rhythms (e.g., *Bmal1*, *Rev-erba*, and *Dbp*) by daytime SF (Feillet *et al.*, 2006). In *Clock* mutant mice, their behavior in constant darkness (DD) is arrhythmic because of the weak clock function of the SCN, but they maintain normal FAA and normally entrained clock gene expression rhythms in peripheral tissues by SF, suggesting that *Clock* is not important for FAA and FEO formation (Shibata *et al.*, 2010). However, we showed that entrained liver clock gene expression rhythms were dampened earlier in *Clock* mutant mice than in wild-type mice during the fasting period after stopping SF. Therefore, as with the weak central clock in the SCN of *Clock* mutant mice in DD, FEO-induced peripheral rhythms also need *Clock* genes to maintain their rhythms when the feeding signal disappears.

7.4 What should we eat? What types of food can stimulate the peripheral clock?

7.4.1 Role of nutrients in the FEO

To understand the mechanism of the FEO, many types of food have been used for food-induced phase entrainment in the circadian system. Using many substituted foods, such as casein, gelatinized corn-starch, high amylose cornstarch, soybean oil, glucose, and sucrose, we demonstrated the differing roles of nutrients in the phase change of the liver clock (Hirao *et al*, 2010). When each nutrient was given alone (100% nutrient) to mice in the daytime for two days, an insignificant weak phase advance was found to be induced by cornstarch and soybean oil, and a large phase advance occurred with gelatinized corn-starch, but not with high amylose cornstarch. A combination of glucose and casein without oil, vitamin, or fiber caused a significant phase advance. Thus, glucose plus casein may be a good candidate nutrient for peripheral food entrainment.

Scheduled daytime access to chocolate in rodents was reported to induce FAA. Mendoza and coworkers demonstrated that the availability of a highly palatable meal (chocolate) during the daytime facilitated the entrainment of locomotor activity in free-fed rats (Mendoza *et al.*, 2005). This chocolate-induced FAA was smaller than food-induced FAA but was continuously maintained for at least four days after chocolate access deprivation, suggesting that FAA is driven by an intrinsic FEO. This experiment also suggests that a palatable meal-induced-related mechanism is important for the expression of FAA by the FEO. In terms of the use of glucose for entraining signals, glucose downregulates *Per1* and *Per2* expression *in vitro* and then synchronizes circadian clocks among cells, indicating that glucose is a "zeitgeber" in cultured cells. In addition, parenteral glucose administration during the 12 hours of daytime in rats affected liver clocks, as with time-restricted daytime feeding.

It was also shown that parenteral administration of amino acids could affect the liver clocks (Miki *et al.*, 2003). Parenteral nutrition can be directly administered in the blood; therefore, food entrainment in the peripheral clocks does not require intestinal digestion. Additionally, streptozotocin-induced type 1 diabetic mice, whose blood glucose level is high, showed phase-advanced peripheral clocks, which suggests that blood glucose concentration is an important factor for maintaining the peripheral clock phase (Lamia *et al.*, 2009). AMP kinase, an important energy-sensitive cell signaling regulator, has been reported to modify the speed of CRY protein degradation. In fact, low and high glucose concentrations cause longer and shorter periods of clock gene expression rhythms *in vitro*, respectively. CRY can inhibit glucocorticoid receptor-mediated transcription of *Pepck* to regulate glucose homeostasis. Taken together, glucose levels may play a role as a sensor of the FEO.

7.4.2 Foods beyond nutrients

Ex vivo tissue culture experiments have provided evidence that caffeine prolongs the period of the central SCN and peripheral circadian clocks (Oike *et al.*, 2011). Caffeine is an antagonist of adenosine receptors and also an inhibitor of phosphodiesterase, which increases cAMP concentrations. Although morning coffee clearly wakes us, drinking coffee often may cause a delay in our clocks. Dahl salt-sensitive rats, an animal model of hypertension, fed a high salt (4% NaCl) diet for six weeks showed significantly decreased levels of *Per2*, *Bmal1*, and *Dbp* in the heart and kidney compared with rats fed a normal salt diet. However, time-restricted drinking of saline in sodium-deprived rats had no effect on *Per2* rhythms in the limbic forebrain structures. A high fat diet lengthened free-running behavioral rhythms and attenuated circadian gene expression rhythms in fat cells (Kohsaka *et al.*, 2007). However, a high cholesterol diet did not affect the daily expression of *Per2*, *Bmal1*, *Dbp*, and *E4bp4* in the liver. Drinking alcohol alters *Period* gene expression rhythms in various brain regions, including the SCN.

7.4.3 Signal transduction in peripheral FEO

To clarify the mechanism of the FEO in peripheral clocks, several studies have investigated the direct entraining pathway of clock genes in peripheral tissues via food or nutrient stimulation. After overnight fasting in mice, daytime re-feeding rapidly caused an upregulation of *Per2* and *Dec1*, along with a downregulation of *Per1* and *Rev-erba* in the liver (Vollmers *et al.*, 2009; Tahara *et al.*, 2011). Decreased *Per1* mRNA was regulated by the transcriptional factor CREB, as livers in the re-fed mice showed a reduction in phosphorylated CREB, and the promoter region of the *Per1* gene possesses a CRE site. Increased *Per2* and decreased *Rev-erba* due to re-feeding were activated by food-induced insulin secretion, because streptozotocin-administered insulin-deficit mice failed to show these food-induced mRNA expression changes. In addition, insulin itself directly affected the phase of *Per2* gene expression rhythm in cultured fibroblasts through upregulation of *Per2* gene expression. Thus, food-induced insulin secretion is an important direct pathway for food entrainment in the liver circadian clock.

In Fig. 7.3, how clock gene expression rhythms are changed by food or insulin is illustrated. Food- or insulin-induced upregulation of *Per2* mRNA at the time of lower gene expression levels of *Per2* mRNA will cause peak mRNA levels, thus the peak time will be earlier than the normal peak phase. Conversely, food or insulin stimulation at the time of higher gene expression levels of *Per2* mRNA will cause peak expression again after the normal peak phase, and will then cause a delayed phase of gene expression rhythm. Yamajuku and coworkers have shown a phase-response curve by insulin-induced phase shifting

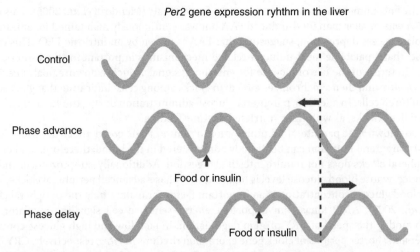

Fig. 7.3 Schematic graph of the phase shift of *Per2* gene expression rhythm by food or insulin stimulation in the liver. If the stimulus comes at the time when clock gene expression moves from trough to peak, food or insulin stimulation caused acute upregulation of expression of *Per2*, then the peak phase of *Per2* is phase-advanced compared to the intact condition. In contrast, if the stimulus comes at the time point from top to trough, the peak phase after stimulus will be phase-delayed. Therefore, there is usually time of day dependency in the phase-shift phenomena.

in *Per2-luc* transgenic rat hepatocytes (Yamajuku *et al*, 2012). This phase-response curve was very similar to that induced by light in SCN-driven circadian rhythms. However, streptozotocin-injected insulin-deficient mice showed normal FAA and food-induced phase-shift of clock gene expression rhythms in peripheral tissues after several days. Therefore, the insulin pathway is an adequate but not necessary signal for food entrainment. In other words, similar to the FEO in the brain, the FEO in the peripheral tissues intricately comprises many physiological mechanisms.

7.5 When should we eat? Application to human life science

The discussion now focuses on when we should eat in order to maintain our body clock at an appropriate time. To understand this question, several works are introduced that investigated how peripheral clocks respond to multiple feeding conditions. In the first experiment, we demonstrated that a one meal per day condition in mice can fix peripheral clocks at different times, dependent upon the feeding time of the single meal. This indicates that peripheral clocks can be determined by the time of feeding. In the next experiment, we examined the effect of two meals (one meal after 16 h of starvation and the other after 8 h of starvation) per day on peripheral clocks (Hirao *et al.*, 2010). The results demonstrated that food amount and starvation period clearly affected the phase of peripheral clocks. In fact, food after a long starvation (16 h) is more powerful in fixing the peripheral clock than food after a short starvation (8 h). In addition, if we give two meals per day to mice with identical intervals (12 h starvation for each meal), the food timing with a larger food amount has a stronger power to determine the phase. Finally, we have applied these findings to a three meals per day schedule (i.e., human eating habits) in mice (Kuroda *et al.*, 2012). Consistently, the phases of peripheral clocks (liver, kidney, and submandibular gland) were dependent on the intervals and amount of food.

In this study, we also examined the effect of a late night dinner on phase determination of the peripheral clock. Mice could take the meals at standard times (for humans), that is, breakfast at 8 a.m., lunch at 12 p.m., and dinner at 8 p.m. We then changed the dinner time from 8 p.m. to 10 p.m. or 11 p.m. When

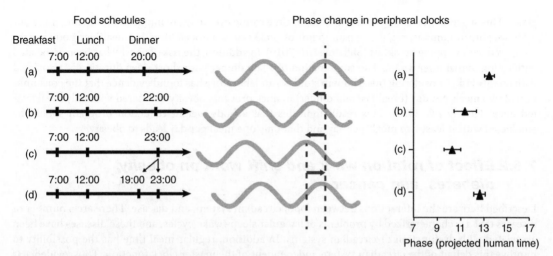

Fig. 7.4 Late night dinner caused irregular phase of peripheral clocks. In our recent paper (Kuroda *et al.*, 2012), we demonstrated that fasting duration was important to anticipate peripheral clock phase. Late night dinner will make longer fasting between lunch and dinner. As a result, late night dinner has strong resetting power for the peripheral clocks, and then the phase is shifted to the irregular phase. To reduce this effect, we divided the dinner foods into two meals (19:00 and 23:00); then, the phase was returned to the normal phase.

the dinner timing was shifted, mice peripheral clocks were also shifted depending on the dinner timing (Fig. 7.4). We next examined the effect of separation of dinner on the delayed dinner-induced phase shift of the peripheral clock. When mice ate food at 8 a.m. and 12 p.m., then took separate small meals at 7 p.m. and 11 p.m., the peripheral clock phase returned to the normal phase. Thus, we have shown that the peripheral clock phase is strongly determined by the timing of food intake, even under a three meals per day schedule.

Calorie restriction (e.g., 80% of food) has been reported to prolong life span in mice and many species. Calorie restriction can affect behavioral rhythms and, importantly, also affect SCN clocks. SCN clock and behavioral rhythms were phase-advanced during calorie restriction (Shibata *et al.*, 2010). We also demonstrated that a single day fast induced phase-advance of the liver clock. However, high fat diet-fed mice showed long free-running periods of behavioral rhythms. Taken together, it is assumed that the total amount of food is an important factor for determining the period of circadian rhythm in mammals.

7.6 Circadian rhythm and obesity and diabetes

7.6.1 Feeding frequency and patterns affect obesity and diabetes

Classically, it has been believed that late night eating causes obesity. Several reports have confirmed this in mice. Arble and coworkers showed that nocturnal mice fed a high fat diet only during the day gained more weight than mice fed only during the night (Arble *et al.*, 2009). Bray and coworkers divided the 12-h dark phase into three sections (breakfast, lunch, and dinner; each 4 h), then changed the meal type (normal or high fat diet) to determine the effects of time-of-day-dependent dietary fat consumption on cardio-metabolic syndrome parameters (Bray *et al.*, 2010). They demonstrated that a high fat meal during the dinner section led to increased weight gain, adiposity, glucose intolerance, hyperinsulinemia, hypertri-glyceridemia, and hyperleptinemia (Hatori *et al.*, 2012). Additionally, recent studies have demonstrated that time-restricted high fat feeding during either only daytime or nighttime in mice strongly reduced fat accumulation and body weight gain compared with freely fed mice. Additionally, time-restricted feeding improved CREB, mTOR, and AMPK pathway functions and oscillations of clock and clock-controlled genes. This suggests that eating habits with same-time eating everyday are important for maintaining our body weight. In humans, regular consumption of breakfast is associated with a healthier body weight compared with skipping breakfast (Shibata *et al.*, 2010). In addition, the risk of obesity has been associated with eating dinner after 8 p.m.. The combination of a late dinner with short sleep duration is associated with obesity risk. Considering these human studies, our laboratory has found evidence that the consumption of two meals per day (breakfast and dinner) in mice prevents obesity compared with only breakfast-fed mice (Fuse *et al.*, 2012). This result indicates that a body weight reduction program should be conducted with at least two meals per day and that only one meal per day leads to obesity.

7.6.2 Effect of rotation work and shift work on obesity, diabetes, and cancer

Described here are the interactions between food, circadian system, and disease. There are a number of diseases that are characterized by problems of irregular sleep–wake cycles, and these diseases have been associated with dysfunction of circadian systems. In addition, regular meal time has the possibility to improve this deficit of the circadian system, independent of the master clock function. Thus, evidence is presented of treatment of such diseases by regular food timing habits.

In 2007, WHO's International Agency for Research on Cancer demonstrated that shift work is a probable factor associated with cancer growth (Straif *et al.*, 2007; Chapters 12 and 13). In female shift workers, there was a 50% increased risk of breast cancer reported. Additionally, shift-work model mice, caused by changing their LD conditions (e.g., advanced 8-h phase-shift of the LD cycle every two days), showed an acceleration of implanted cancer development (Li *et al.*, 2010). Further, *Bmal1* knockout mice showed a high incidence of cancer. This is because the clock gene regulates important genes (*c-Myc* and *Wee1*), which regulate the cell cycle (Sahar and Sassone-Corsi, 2012). In rotating shift work conditions in humans or mice, the circadian clock does not function well. Therefore, researchers have attempted to reorganize the irregular clock in shift-work model mice and attempted to determine the recovery effect on their cancer development. They showed that implanted osteosarcoma development was inhibited by time-restricted feeding during either daytime or nighttime in mice, and that mice fed during the daytime could survive longer than free-fed mice with implanted osteosarcoma (Li *et al.*, 2010).

Rotating shift workers also suffer from obesity and type 2 diabetes (Chapter 13). *Clock* gene knockout mice are known to exhibit the same symptoms. There are many reasons why clock gene mutant mice show obesity. For example, they cannot produce insulin well due to irregular development of beta cells in the pancreas. Another reason is irregular clock-controlled metabolic gene expression in peripheral tissues due to irregular control of clock genes. To reorganize irregular clocks in shift-work model mice, time-restricted feeding helps their clocks independent of the irregular LD cycle. Salgado-Delgado and coworkers demonstrated that scheduled feeding during the nighttime can prevent obesity in shift-work model rats that were maintained on an eight-hour activity schedule in a rotating chamber during the daytime (Salgado-Delgado *et al.*, 2010). Disrupted or shifted blood glucose rhythms, triglycerides rhythms, corticosteroid rhythms, and body weight rhythms in shift work model rats were all corrected by restricted feeding during the nighttime.

7.6.3 Effect of calorie restriction on circadian rhythm and life span

Aging should be considered a factor of a weakened circadian system (Chapter 22). Low activity counts and flattened rhythmicity of behavior were reported in aged rodents. Neural firing in the SCN of aged mice was investigated using an *in vivo* multi-unit neural activity recording system, and reduction of the amplitude of the day–night difference was observed in neural firings. One older study from 1986 demonstrated that calorie restriction in either the daytime or nighttime could prolong life span in mice (Nelson and Halberg, 1986). The authors examined the effect of food timing with 25% calorie restriction on life span. (Please note here that calorie restriction itself has the power to extend the life span with increased activity of the sirtuin signaling pathway.) They prepared the following four groups: *ad libitum*, single meal at early light period, single meal at early dark period, and six smaller meals during the dark period with two-hour intervals. The results demonstrated that all three calorie-restricted groups showed similar life spans, which were longer than the *ad libitum* group. Therefore, they indicated that calorie restriction is a more important factor for aging than food timings. In the aged population, many neuro-degenerative disorders are related to abnormal sleep–wake cycles (Chapters 19–21). Huntington's disease model mice showed a disrupted sleep–wake cycle and abnormal expression of peripheral clock genes. However, daytime restricted feeding restored their abnormal behavioral rhythms and gene expression rhythms of the peripheral clock (Maywood, 2010). Therefore, organizing timing for eating might help fix the impaired circadian system in individuals with Huntington's disease.

7.6.4 Role of circadian rhythm in pharmacological and nutritional actions

Finally, we want to introduce the keyword "chrono-nutrition" (Fig. 7.5). In the most recent two decades, "chrono-pharmacology" has become a common word in medical research fields. Since many proteins or receptors have transcriptional or translational circadian rhythms, drug application time should be

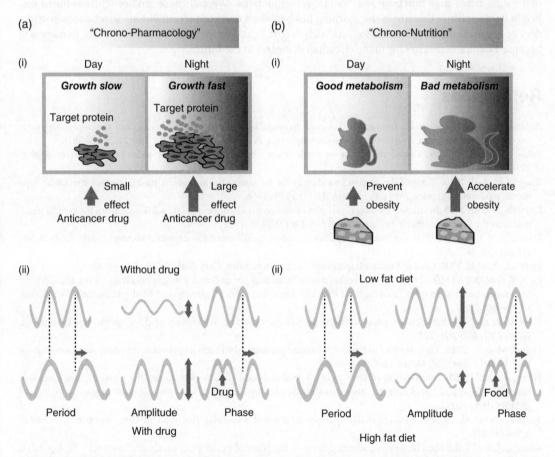

Fig. 7.5 Schematic illustration of "Chrono-Pharmacology" and "Chrono-Nutrition". (a) There are two aspects in chrono-pharmacology. One considers ADME (absorption, distribution, metabolism, excretion) and drug target to increase pharmacological effect and reduce side effect (i). The other considers the effect of drugs on controlling circadian clocks (ii). (b) Chrono-nutrition also has two aspects. One considers food timings or contents for keeping our health by understanding circadian clock-regulated metabolic pathways (i). The other considers the effect of food timing on controlling circadian clocks, because food has a power to entrain circadian clocks.

considered to produce the maximum effect of the drug and reduce side effects. For example, the antitumor effect of an angiogenesis inhibitor (VEGF inhibitor) was reported to cause a larger effect during daytime than during nighttime, due to increased VEGF protein in the daytime. In another view of chrono-pharmacology, many chemical compounds, such as CK1 inhibitors and GSK3B inhibitors, have been reported to affect the period of circadian rhythms. CK1 inhibitor prolongs the circadian period and the GSK3b inhibitor shortens it. Thus, there are at least two interactions between drug actions and circadian rhythms. We should consider the application time of drugs to obtain the optimal drug effect. We should also consider the application time of drugs to reset the circadian rhythms. Consequently, we call these studies "chrono-pharmacology."

Similar to "chrono-pharmacology," there are interactions between nutrient action and the circadian system. One is that we should consider food content and timing to maintain our health, as, for example, there are circadian variations of metabolic gene(s) expression throughout the day. As mentioned here, a late night dinner caused an increase in fat synthesis and a phase-shift of clock gene expression rhythms in peripheral clocks. The other is that food can become a "zeitgeber" to entrain the circadian system. We can organize our body clock time to an appropriate time by considering daily meal timings. The effect of food entrainment in humans is still unknown because of the lack of reports to date. However, we hope that eating times may function as a "zeitgeber" in humans. We call these studies "chrono-nutrition." Bright light exposure therapy in the morning has become a common treatment in circadian sleep disorders or seasonal affective depression. As with bright light therapy, we hope food timing therapy will become a common therapy for many circadian disorders in the future.

References

Acosta-Galvan, G. *et al.* 2011. Interaction between hypothalamic dorsomedial nucleus and the suprachiasmatic nucleus determines intensity of food anticipatory behavior. *Proc Natl Acad Sci USA* **108**(14):5813–5818.

Arble, D.M. *et al.* 2009. Circadian timing of food intake contributes to weight gain. *Obesity (Silver Spring)* **17**(11):2100–2102.

Bray, M.S. *et al.* 2010. Time-of-day-dependent dietary fat consumption influences multiple cardiometabolic syndrome parameters in mice. *Int J Obes (Lond)* **34**(11):1589–1598.

Damiola, F. *et al.* 2000. Restricted feeding uncouples circadian oscillators in peripheral tissues from the central pacemaker in the suprachiasmatic nucleus. *Genes Dev* **14**(23):2950–2961.

Davidson, A.J. *et al.* 2003. Is the food-entrainable circadian oscillator in the digestive system? *Genes Brain Behav* **2**(1):32–39.

Feillet, C.A. *et al.* 2006. Lack of food anticipation in Per2 mutant mice. *Curr Biol* **16**(20):2016–2022.

Fuse, Y. *et al.* 2012. Differential roles of breakfast only (one meal per day) and a bigger breakfast with a small dinner (two meals per day) in mice fed a high-fat diet with regard to induced obesity and lipid metabolism. *J Circadian Rhythms* **10**(1):4.

Hara, R. *et al.* 2001. Restricted feeding entrains liver clock without participation of the suprachiasmatic nucleus. *Genes Cells* **6**(3):269–278.

Hatori, M. *et al.* 2012. Time-restricted feeding without reducing caloric intake prevents metabolic diseases in mice fed a high-fat diet. *Cell Metab* **15**(6):848–860.

Hirao, A. *et al.* 2010. Combination of starvation interval and food volume determines the phase of liver circadian rhythm in Per2::Luc knock-in mice under two meals per day feeding. *CAm J Physiol Gastrointest Liver Physiol* **299**(5):G1045–1053.

Kohsaka, A. *et al.* 2007. High-fat diet disrupts behavioral and molecular circadian rhythms in mice. *Cell Metab* **6**(5):414–421.

Kuroda, H. *et al.* 2012. Meal frequency patterns determine the phase of mouse peripheral circadian clocks. *Sci Rep* **2**:711.

Lamia, K.A. *et al.* 2009. AMPK regulates the circadian clock by cryptochrome phosphorylation and degradation. *Science* **326**(5951):437–440.

Li, X-M. *et al.* 2010. Cancer inhibition through circadian reprogramming of tumor transcriptome with meal timing. *Cancer Res* **70**(8):3351–3360.

Maywood, E.S. *et al.* 2010. Disruption of peripheral circadian timekeeping in a mouse model of Huntington's disease and its restoration by temporally scheduled feeding. *J Neurosci* **30**(30):10199–10204.

Mendoza, J. *et al*. 2005. A daily palatable meal without food deprivation entrains the suprachiasmatic nucleus of rats. *Eur J Neurosci* **22**(11):2855–2862.

Miki, H. *et al*. 2003. Total parenteral nutrition entrains the central and peripheral circadian clocks. *Neuroreport* **14**(11):1457–1461.

Moore, R.Y. and Eichler, V.B. 1972. Loss of a circadian adrenal corticosterone rhythm following suprachiasmatic lesions in the rat. *Brain Res* **42**(1):201–206.

Nelson, W. and Halberg, F. 1986. Schedule-shifts, circadian rhythms and lifespan of freely-feeding and meal-fed mice. *Physiol Behav* **38**(6):781–788.

Oike, H. *et al*. 2011. Caffeine lengthens circadian rhythms in mice. *Biochem Biophys Res Commun* **410**(3):654–658.

Sahar, S. and Sessone-Corsi, P. 2012. Regulation of metabolism: the circadian clock dictates the time. *Trends Endocrinol Metab* **23**(1):1–8.

Salgado-Delgado, R. *et al*. 2010. Food intake during the normal activity phase prevents obesity and circadian desynchrony in a rat model of night work. *Endocrinology* **151**(3):1019–1029.

Shibata, S. *et al*. 2010. The adjustment and manipulation of biological rhythms by light, nutrition, and abused drugs. *Adv Drug Deliv Rev* **62**(9–10):918–927.

Stokkan, K-A. *et al*. 2001. Entrainment of the circadian clock in the liver by feeding. *Science* **291**(5503):490–493.

Straif, K., *et al*. 2007. Carcinogenicity of shift-work, painting, and fire-fighting. *Lancet Oncol* **8**:1065–1066.

Tahara, Y. *et al*. 2011. Refeeding after fasting elicits insulin-dependent regulation of Per2 and Rev-erbα with shifts in the liver clock. *J Biol Rhythms* **26**(3):230–240.

Vollmers, C. *et al*. 2009. Time of feeding and the intrinsic circadian clock drive rhythms in hepatic gene expression. *Proc Natl Acad Sci USA* **106**(50):21453–21458.

Yamajuku, D. *et al*. 2012. Real-time monitoring in three-dimensional hepatocytes reveals that insulin acts as a synchronizer for liver clock. *Sci Rep* **2**:439.

The Cardiovascular Clock

8

R. Daniel Rudic

Pharmacology and Toxicology, Georgia Regents University, Augusta, GA, USA

8.1 Introduction

The circadian clock is a signaling network that comprises the molecular basis of circadian rhythms. In the nervous system, the circadian clock is responsible for generating rhythmic behavior. The cardiovascular system of mammals also follows a circadian rhythm, exhibiting a functional oscillation of a 24-hour period. Blood pressure follows a 24-hour profile, rising in the daytime and falling at night. Heart rate, endothelial function, circulating levels of humoral signals, and myogenic tone also follow a circadian rhythm. This stems from the fact that the cardiovascular system is fully equipped with the same components of the circadian clock that are found in the suprachiasmatic nucleus (SCN) of the brain. The organs that control the function of the circulatory system (heart, blood vessels, and kidney) have an oscillating circadian clock. And each of these organs, comprised of a heterogeneous composition of cell types including endothelial cells, smooth muscle cells and fibroblasts, has its own circadian clock. In this chapter, the importance of the circadian clock and circadian rhythms is discussed with regard to their significance in cardiovascular cell signaling, blood pressure control, vascular function, and disease based on insights from human physiology and experimental animal models.

8.2 The vascular clock

Rhythmic oscillation of clock genes is responsible for rhythms in sleep and locomotor activity in the SCN of the brain (Chapters 3 and 4). The circadian clock is also present in the vasculature. The core molecular circadian clock (Chapters 1 and 2), which includes *Bmal1*, *Clock*, *Npas2*, *Per*, and *Cry*, is expressed and oscillating in vascular tissue (McNamara *et al.*, 2001; Rudic *et al.*, 2005a). The vascular tree is comprised of arteries, veins, and microvessels which all express the circadian clock. While the differences in the vascular tree are uniquely structured and functional, with arteries being elastic to propagate movement of blood, arterioles being abundant and contractile to control tissue delivery, and veins being pliable to amass fluid return, they all express a clock, but functionality and timing of the clock within the different blood vessel types is uniquely coordinated. Indeed, the timing of circadian oscillation in arteries is different than veins (as indexed by *Per2* oscillation), and these rhythms do persist *ex vivo* (Davidson *et al.*, 2005). The differences of circadian timing in blood vessels may be of an organic origin, or alternatively due to variations in blood flow and pressure across the vasculature. For example, the mechanical forces exerted by the pulsatile motion of blood vary by proximity to the heart and, as such, these forces may act as an entraining signal to the circadian clock, in a manner analogous

Circadian Medicine, First Edition. Edited by Christopher S. Colwell.
© 2015 John Wiley & Sons, Inc. Published 2015 by John Wiley & Sons, Inc.

to the light/dark (LD) cycle, which resets the central clock and food that entrains the liver clock (Chapters 6 and 7).

Evidence is emerging that numerous vasoactive signals also modulate circadian clock signaling in vascular cells. Indeed, circadian rhythms can be recapitulated *in vitro* (Balsalobre *et al.*, 2000). Though single cells in culture have an oscillating circadian clock, cultured cell populations *en masse* are arrhythmic due to asynchronous circadian clock oscillation among cells (Nagoshi *et al.*, 2004). Thus, a phase-aligning stimulus must be applied to cultured cells to elicit a uniform circadian rhythm (Welsh *et al.*, 2004). In cultured fibroblasts, exposure to a short duration, high concentration of horse serum or even glucose phase-aligns or synchronizes the circadian clock among cells, to then evoke a uniform oscillatory clock signal (i.e., *Bmal1*, *Per2* oscillation), while other signals alter the timing of the clock to phase advance or delay the rhythm (Balsalobre *et al.*, 1998; Hirota *et al.*, 2002). Recent studies have begun to identify these "vascular clock"-modifying signals. Surprisingly, signals with established roles in the control of vascular contractility, tone, and remodeling also impart a significant influence on the circadian clock. These include endothelin, prostanoids, angiotensin (AT), and even nitric oxide (NO).

8.3 Circadian clock regulation of the endothelial cell layer of blood vessels

Blood vessels comprise three layers: an inner endothelial cell layer that is in contact with circulating blood; an underlying layer comprised of smooth muscle cells; and an outer adventitial layer comprised of fibroblasts with each layer conferring a unique property (Fig. 8.1). The adventitia is an outer layer of connective tissue that provides a protective covering to the blood vessel. Smooth

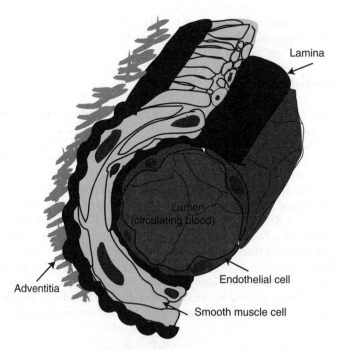

Fig. 8.1 The anatomy of the blood vessel. A blood vessel comprises three layers. An outer adventitial layer, a smooth muscle cell layer called the media, and an inner layer comprised of endothelial cells called the intima. Each layer is separated by a lamina (black line). *(See insert for color representation of the figure.)*

muscle cells of the media comprise the middle layer of contractile cells that allow the blood vessel to constrict and relax. The endothelial cells of the endothelium, being in direct contact with flowing blood, communicate mechanical forces caused by circulating blood into autocrine and paracrine biochemical signals to the smooth muscle and even adventitia. Indeed, with regard to the endothelium, the circadian clock plays an important role in the regulation of its function. The vasodilatory response to acetylcholine is reduced in *Per2* mutants, *Bmal1*-KO, and *Clock* mutant mice (Viswambharan *et al.*, 2007; Anea *et al.*, 2009). Acetylcholine relaxes blood vessels by activating endothelial muscarinic receptors to release intracellular calcium to activate the enzyme endothelial NO synthase (eNOS) to produce NO. NO, in turn, diffuses from endothelial cells to smooth muscle cells to cause relaxation. Despite this impairment in endothelial function, vascular smooth muscle cell function was normal in these mice. There is further evidence to suggest that these impairments are directly dependent on deterioration of circadian rhythms. *Clock* mutant mice have normal endothelial function in LD conditions but develop dysfunction only when placed in constant conditions (DD).

8.4 The circadian clock in vascular disease

Healthy endothelial function counterbalances pathological processes. Thus, it is not surprising that the endothelial function observed in circadian clock deficient mice manifests as gross abnormalities in the response to vascular injury. Thrombosis, which is the formation of blood clots, is accelerated during endothelial dysfunction and exhibits a circadian rhythm in a photochemically-induced thrombosis model in wild-type (WT) mice, but this rhythm is absent in *Clock* mutant mice (Westgate *et al.*, 2008). Surprisingly, *Clock* mutant mice seem to be protected from thrombosis, as evident by a delay in the duration of time taken to reach blood flow arrest after the laser injury. Mice with endothelial specific disruption of *Bmal1* also lose their rhythm in this time-of-day dependent thrombosis, but in contrast suffer blood flow arrest much faster due to thrombosis, a deleterious phenotype. Thus, the circadian clock conditions acute thrombotic events.

In addition to controlling the acute endothelium and circulating blood interactions that contribute to thrombosis, the genetic components of the circadian clock also exert a significant influence in the chronic adaptation of vascular wall through the restructuring process called vascular remodeling. Experimentally, adaptation of the vasculature can be induced by arterial ligation (Fig. 8.2a), which in normal animals causes the blood vessel to narrow and the blood vessel wall to thicken over a time span of several weeks. In mice with a dysfunctional circadian clock, arterial ligation of the common carotid artery leads to arterial wall thickening and proliferation of the inner lining surrounding the endothelium of the blood vessel in a process called intimal hyperplasia. Injury can also be induced by damaging the endothelium surgically by placing a small wire inside the lumen of the blood vessel (Fig. 8.2b). Again, in circadian clock mutant mice, this wire injury causes an exacerbated injury response, relative to WT mice (Anea *et al.*, 2009). Small blood vessel development is also impaired in circadian clock mutant mice. Small blood vessels sprout new vessels during conditions of metabolic stress. Ischemia in the hindlimb induced by ligation causes such angiogenesis, but the angiogenic response is reduced and results in susceptibility to limb loss in *Per2* mutant mice (Gao *et al.*, 2008).

Transplant arteriosclerosis is also worsened in circadian clock mutant mice. During organ transplants, blood vessels are connected to maintain blood circulation to the donor tissue. In an experimental model of blood vessel transplantation, blood vessels from circadian clock mutant mice (*Bmal1*-KO or *Period* KO mice) suffered increased vessel disease relative to normal WT donor blood vessels (Cheng *et al.*, 2011). These observations point to a significant role for the circadian clock in the progression of large artery and small vessel disease, which are common in human aging (Chapter 22). Indeed, one hallmark feature of an aging vasculature is the stiffening or hardening of the blood vessels. This process of stiffening is accelerated in circadian clock mutant mice (Anea *et al.*, 2010). *Bmal1* and *Per2* oscillations and expression are blunted in high passage (aged *in vitro*) human

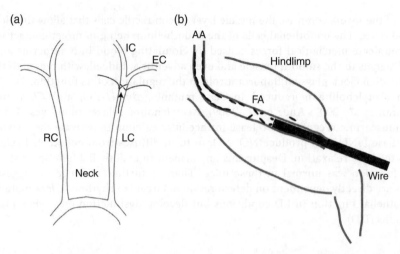

Fig. 8.2 Experimental models of vascular injury. (a) Ligation of the left common carotid artery (LC) by placement of a suture interrupts blood flow to the internal common carotid artery (IC) and external common carotid artery (EC). After two weeks of ligation, the LC narrows due to a process of vascular remodeling and is reduced in size relative to the contralateral right common carotid artery (RC). Some animals that have mutated genes, such as the circadian clock mutant mice, exhibit an abnormal response and instead of narrowing display a growth response. This model mimics the arterial blockages that can occur in human disease. (b) In the hind limb or leg of mice, the femoral artery (FA,) which branches from the abdominal aorta, (AA) can be surgically exposed and a wire placed inside the vessel to injure the endothelial layer. Again, circadian clock mutant mice exhibit a worsened response to the wire injury compared to normal mice. This model recapitulates the angioplasty approach that is used in medicine to treat arterial blockages.

aortic smooth muscle cells and *in vivo* in large arteries (aortae) from old WT mice, while endothelial cells and aortic tissue of *Per2* mutant mice have elevated markers of senescence (Gao *et al.*, 2008; Kunieda *et al.*, 2008).

8.5 The circadian clock and vascular cell signaling

Endothelial cells contain eNOS that releases NO to relax blood vessels via an enzymatic reaction that is dependent on cofactors to bind eNOS. Recent evidence has demonstrated that the circadian clock regulates eNOS signaling. The phosphorylated form of eNOS (P-eNOS) and its activating kinase Akt exhibit circadian oscillation in the vasculature of WT mice and comprise an important pathway that enhances NO production, protects cells from apoptosis, and modulates vascular function. *Bmal1*-KO mice exhibit decreased P-eNOS expression and, Akt, which phosphorylates eNOS, is also decreased. PDK-1, which phosphorylates Akt, is also misregulated in both *Bmal1*-KO and *Per2* mutant mice (Gao *et al.*, 2008; Anea *et al.*, 2009).

The relationship between NO and the circadian clock may be reciprocal. NO donors activate *Per1* transcriptional activity, and conversely increase *Bmal1* expression in endothelial cells. eNOS KO mice also exhibit a phase shift the circadian clock, while the NOS inhibitor L-NAME phase advances Per2 expression in smooth muscle cells. That L-NAME phase shifts *Per2* in cultured smooth muscle cells, suggests that the effect is eNOS-independent, since eNOS is only expressed in endothelial cells and that the neuronal NOS isoform (nNOS) is modulating the circadian clock in smooth muscle cells (Kunieda *et al.*, 2008). In contrast to the effect of NO in the vasculature, neither eNOS nor nNOS knockout mice have any aberration in behavioral circadian function, suggesting that endogenously produced NO may exert a vascular-specific role in control of the circadian clock (Kriegsfeld *et al.*,

1999, 2001). The phosphorylated, activated forms of Akt and eNOS are essential for vasodilatory responses in blood vessels and their levels are blunted in arteries from mice deficient in the circadian clock. Aging also plays a part in these signaling mechanisms (Luo *et al.*, 2000). Additional evidence suggests that elevation in presser mechanisms and, in particular, those mediated by Cyclooxygenase-1 (COX-1) may also play a part in the cardiovascular pathologies of aging. COX-1 protein expression is increased in aortae of *Per2* mutant mice, and the contractile response to indomethacin is exacerbated.

Understanding the signals that regulate the circadian clock in vascular cells may ultimately provide novel therapeutic tools to treat circadian dysfunction in the vasculature and the periphery. Glucocorticoids were shown to induce circadian gene oscillation in fibroblasts, liver cells, and vascular smooth muscle cells. In human vascular smooth muscle cells and murine aorta, retinoic acid was shown to phase shift the oscillation of circadian clock, evidence that humoral signals may act to influence the clock (McNamara *et al.*, 2001). ATII also entrains the circadian clock within vascular smooth muscle cells, an effect dependent on the ATII type 1 receptor, suggesting that circadian clock function may be perturbed during renin-dependent hypertension (Nonaka *et al.*, 2001). Though the presence of AT1 receptors in the SCN has been demonstrated, it may also be that AT and other vaso-active signals selectively act on the vascular clock, without impinging on central circadian rhythms (Thomas *et al.*, 2004). Catecholamines may also exert an influence on circadian timing, as norepinephrine and epinephrine can phase advance *Per2* expression in cultured human aortic smooth muscle cells, although, *in vivo*, peripheral circadian clock rhythms were preserved in dopamine beta-hydroxylase knockout mice (Reilly *et al.*, 2008).

Prostaglandins have also been shown to entrain the circadian clock. In cultured fibroblasts, PGE2 induced rhythmicity of *Per2*, while intraperitoneal injection in mice phase shifted *Per2* expression in heart, liver, and kidney, an effect that was also mimicked by the administration of an agonist to the EP1 receptor, a PGE2 receptor subtype important in the regulation of blood pressure (DeBruyne *et al.*, 2007; Sei *et al.*, 2008). In another study, a peptide and lipid library were used to screen for circadian activators in a rat fibroblast cell line stably expressing *Per2*-Luc. Endothelin, a potent vaso-constrictor and PGJ2, which has been linked to angiogenesis, and VEG-F signaling, were identified as inducers of circadian oscillation. In addition, PPARγ, which is activated by PGJ2, may also be an important circadian clock modifying signal (Baggs *et al.*, 2009). The PPARγ agonist rosiglitazone transactivated the *Bmal1* promoter in transformed endothelial and cancer cell lines, while in aortae of mice, endothelial and smooth muscle cell-specific deletion of PPARγ decreased *Bmal1* oscillation and expression. Future studies are needed to characterize additional agents that modify the circadian clock in vascular smooth muscle and endothelial cells and may yield important therapeutic agents in the control of vascular rhythms.

8.6 The circadian rhythm in blood pressure, nighttime hypertension, and cardiovascular disease in humans

While circadian rhythms in waking and sleeping are the most obvious, it is also well established that blood pressure exhibits circadian variation in humans and mice (Li *et al.*, 1999; Chapter 9). Elevated blood pressure or hypertension is a major risk factor for cardiovascular disease and death, causing impairments in the vasculature, including wall thickening, luminal narrowing, endothelial dysfunction, and wall stiffness, which as earlier described are influenced by the circadian clock. In healthy humans, there is a nighttime dip in blood pressure followed by a rise in the morning hours, while this rhythm is inverted in nocturnal animals such as mice. The circadian rhythm of blood pressure can be abnormal during hypertension, with blood pressure showing daily patterns, such as nondipping, extreme dipping, and reverse dipping (O'Brien *et al.*, 1988; Kario *et al.*, 1996, 2001). These disturbances in blood pressure rhythm cause increased cardiovascular disease and death (Timio *et al.*, 1995; Chobanian *et al.*, 2003). Thus, having high blood pressure at night, during resting or sleep can be even more harmful to health than daytime hypertension, which in part may reflect the difficulty in diagnosing the hypertension that would be potentially undetected in daytime office visits. Conversely, controlling nighttime hypertension is beneficial to health. Perhaps, this was exemplified in the Heart Outcomes Prevention Evaluation Study (HOPE trial). In this trial, the angiotensin converting enzyme (ACE) inhibitor ramipril had significant effects on the reduction in rates of death, myocardial infarction, and stroke (Yusuf *et al.*, 2000). While ramipril did not significantly lower blood pressure during office visits (daytime), a subsequent substudy revealed ramipril did lower blood pressure at night (Svensson *et al.*, 2001).

Aside from the rhythm in blood pressure, the time of day or night at which antihypertensive drugs are actually administered, called chronotherapy, also differentially influences blood pressure control (Lemmer, 1996, 2006). A calcium channel blocker (CCB), which reduces blood pressure by dilating blood vessels and reducing heart contractility, was shown to cause an improved blood pressure lowering effect on nighttime blood pressure when given at 8 p.m. compared to an 8 a.m. administration. Also, when given at nighttime, the CCB effect of lowering nighttime blood pressure restored the circadian rhythm in blood pressure (Portaluppi *et al.*, 1995). Similarly, an alpha adrenergic antagonist more successfully lowered blood pressure in hypertensive patients when given before bed compared to other times of day (Hermida *et al.*, 2004). Thus, the restoration of circadian variability in blood pressure appears to be an important factor in the control of cardiovascular disease.

Numerous control mechanisms are involved in the regulation of blood pressure (Chapter 9). The medulla of the brain controls blood pressure via sympathetic and parasympathetic drive of the heart, kidneys and vasculature. Catecholamines, the product of sympathetic drive are misregulated in experimental models where rhythms in blood pressure and activity are disrupted (Curtis *et al.*, 2007; Wang *et al.*, 2008a). In addition to autonomic drive, central clock-modifying signals may also play a role in blood pressure control. Vasoactive intestinal peptide (VIP) modulates central circadian clock function, impacts vascular function and is suppressed in hypertensive patients (Ignarro *et al.*, 1987; Goncharuk *et al.*, 2001). To provide another example, the rhythmically secreted hormone melatonin has also been implicated in blood pressure. In hypertensive patients with impaired circadian variation in blood pressure, melatonin supplementation can improve the lowering of nocturnal blood pressure (Scheer *et al.*, 2004). It remains unclear where these actions occur as melatonin receptors are found not just in the brain but are also expressed in the cardiovascular system (Dubocovich and Markowska, 2005).

Recent basic science studies have further implicated the circadian clock in the control of blood pressure. In mice, the genetic disruption of the core components of the circadian clock (*Bmal1*, *Clock*, *Npas2*, *Per*, and *Cry*) influence the circadian rhythm in baseline blood pressure. *Cry1/Cry2* deficient mice are hypertensive during their normal sleep time and lose the normal circadian variation in blood pressure (Masuki *et al.*, 2005). The ultimate effect is that *Cry* deficient mice have higher blood pressure during the rest period and exhibit fairly normal blood pressure in the activity period. *Bmal1*-KO mice also lose the circadian variation in blood pressure due to a decreased blood pressure during the activity period (Curtis *et al.*, 2007). The effect of *Bmal1* to regulate blood pressure seems to be independent of the endothelial layer of blood vessels, as the overall blood pressure rhythm remains intact in mice with endothelial-specific deletion of *Bmal1* (EC-Bmal1-KO) (Westgate *et al.*, 2008). These endothelial KO mice do exhibit a reduction in blood pressure at discrete times within the activity phase, but the effect is modest and not observed in the resting phase when it should be most pronounced. *Npas2* mutant mice retain the circadian variation in blood pressure but have a lower blood pressure overall. Similarly, mutation of *Clock* in mice also causes only subtle dampening of blood pressure variation in LD, which may reflect the influence of the LD cycle in these mice and the functional redundancy provided by the ability of BMAL1 to bind either CLOCK or NPAS2 (Curtis *et al.*, 2007; DeBruyne *et al.*, 2007; Sei *et al.*, 2008).

Other signals have been shown to interact with the circadian clock to modulate the circadian variation in blood pressure. Mice with targeted deletion of PPARγ in the endothelium are phenotypically similar to EC-Bmal1-KO mice with regard to blood pressure (Wang *et al.*, 2008b; Westgate *et al.*, 2008).

EC-PPARγ-KO mice have lower blood pressure at night, and normal blood pressure during the day. However, the daily blood pressure rhythm remains largely intact in contrast to the complete ablation of rhythm observed in *Bmal1*-KO mice. Smooth muscle cell disrupted PPARγ KO mice are phenotypically different from the endothelial knockouts. These KO mice have higher blood pressure in the daytime and trend to a lower blood pressure at night, while locomotor rhythms remain intact in both types of selective PPARγ KO mice (Wang *et al.*, 2008b). This is different from the core clock global KOs, which do exhibit impairments in locomotor function, but may suggest that circadian inputs into blood pressure regulation are not solely the result of central clock or activity rhythms. These same studies showed that PPARγ exhibits a direct interaction with BMAL1. Agonist-activation of PPARγ increases aortic *Bmal1* expression and correspondingly loss of PPARγ in the aorta of both EC and SMC-PPARγ-KO mice leads to reduced expression of the core circadian clock components.

EC-Bmal1-KO and EC-PPARγ-KO mice retain daily blood pressure rhythms, but this does not necessarily abrogate a role for the endothelial clock in the regulation of blood pressure rhythm. Circadian rhythms are robust and resistant to the perturbation of individual clock components, which may in part occur through redundancy, networking, and intercellular coupling of the circadian clock mechanism (Liu *et al.*, 2007; Baggs *et al.*, 2009). Many of the current studies extrapolated effects from the aorta or large arteries that do not control blood pressure. It is the small abundant arterioles that are most critical in controlling blood pressure through vasoconstriction and vasodilation, and studies in these peripheral resistance governing vessels are lacking.

8.7 Diabetes, obesity, and blood pressure

While obesity and metabolic dysfunction are major risk factors for the impaired control of blood pressure, recent evidence has also implicated the circadian clock (Chapter 11). In experimental rodent models of type II diabetes, blood pressure is increased (Carlson *et al.*, 2000; Osmond *et al.*, 2009). The elevation in blood pressure is also characterized by changes in the circadian variation of blood pressure (Su *et al.*, 2008; Goncalves *et al.*, 2009; Senador *et al.*, 2009). The daytime drop in blood pressure in mice is blunted (smaller drop) in animals with type II diabetes suggesting that the circadian clock and its management of blood pressure are impaired. This is also observed in humans with type II diabetes who have an increased frequency of nondipping blood pressure in up to 75% of patients (Czupryniak *et al.*, 2007). Again, the loss of nighttime blood pressure dipping is associated with increased cardiovascular mortality (Sturrok *et al.*, 2000; Izzedine *et al.*, 2006). In addition to type II diabetes, type I diabetes is also characterized by blunted circadian regulation of blood pressure, which seems to correlate with declining renal function (Lurbe *et al.*, 1993; Holl *et al.*, 1999).

In addition to the effects of diabetes to impair blood pressure rhythms, type II diabetes also affects the circadian regulation of heart rate and locomotor activity (Su *et al.*, 2008; Goncalves *et al.*, 2009). Other aspects of blood pressure control are also altered in animals with type II diabetes including renal function, circulating hormones, autonomic reflexes, vascular and sympathetic tone. These effects may be intricately related to the rhythms in locomotor activity, which is frequently used as a surrogate for the activity of the central clock, while lesion of the SCN also disrupts the rhythms of feeding, activity and blood pressure (Witte *et al.*, 1998). Indeed, mice with type II diabetes exhibit a gross reduction in locomotor activity that accompanies the impaired daily variations in blood pressure. Despite the gross reduction in locomotor activity, the circadian rhythm in activity remains intact. This may then be a consequence of the morbidly obese phenotype seen in diabetic mice, which may act as the primary constraint on activity rather than an alteration of the central clock. Consistent with the idea that these effects are central clock independent, expression of circadian clock genes is unaltered in the SCN of mice with type II diabetes (Kudo *et al.*, 2004). However, the oscillation of circadian genes in the periphery, isolated blood vessels and liver are impaired in diabetic mice (Kudo *et al.*, 2004; Su *et al.*, 2008). The link between type II diabetes and altered circadian timing is further complicated by the ability of the circadian clock itself to influence metabolism and ultimately obesity and diabetes (Chapter 11). These links support the concept that type II diabetes promotes asynchrony of peripheral and central circadian clocks and this asynchrony may contribute significantly to cardiovascular disease.

8.8 AT influences the circadian rhythm in experimental hypertension

Animal models of renin-angiotensin system(RAS)-induced hypertension reproduce an important manifestation of human hypertension. The renin-angiotensin-aldosterone system produces renin, which then cleaves angiotensinogen to angiotensin I(ATI); ATI is then converted to angiotensin II(ATII) by angiotensin-converting-enzyme(ACE). ATII exerts its biological effects to increase blood pressure by constricting blood vessels and by triggering the release of aldosterone, which increases blood volume by promoting sodium and water retention in the kidney.

There are different animal models with mutations in this pathway that exhibit hypertension and defects in blood pressure circadian rhythm. TGR(mREN2)27 rats are transgenic, hypertensive rats that possess an extra copy of the renin gene [TGR(mREN2)27]. TGR(mREN2)27 rats develop an inverse blood pressure rhythm (inverse/reverse dipper) six weeks after birth, transitioning from a blood pressure that peaks at night to a blood pressure that peaks in the day while circadian activity rhythms remain unperturbed (Witte and Lemmer, 1999). SHR rats exhibit a blood pressure rhythm with the peak blood pressure shifted further toward the resting period (Shimamura *et al.*, 1999). Activity rhythms are also impaired in SHRs as activity begins 1.5 hours earlier than in WKY control rats. The SHRs have a single nucleotide polymorphism in the essential circadian clock component *Bmal1*, suggesting an association between the hypertensive phenotype and the *Bmal1* mutation (Woon *et al.*, 2007). SHRs also exhibit enhanced expression of *Clock*, *Bmal1*, and *Per2* in heart tissue (Naito *et al.*, 2003). Furthermore, SHRs exhibit enhanced amplitudes in the oscillation of renin, angiotensinogen, ACE, and AT type 1a (AT1a) and type 2 (AT2) receptors in the heart (Naito *et al.*, 2002). Indeed, ATII does have significant effects on the circadian clock in vascular cells. In cultured vascular smooth muscle cells, ATII has potent effects on the circadian clock via synchronization of the circadian oscillations of *Per2* and *Bmal1* expression across the cell population (Nonaka *et al.*, 2001).

While there are genetic mutants in the RAS pathway, hypertension can additionally be induced by direct administration of ATII. Chronic ATII infusion by osmotic minipump in rats has more robust effects on circadian blood pressure compared to RAS-defective SHRs (Sampson *et al.*, 2008). Exogenous administration of ATII abolishes the circadian rhythm of arterial pressure in a gender-independent manner and further causes a modest reverse dipper phenotype in female rats, reminiscent of the response of TGR(mREN2)27 rats. With regard to effects on locomotor rhythms, although exogenous administration of ATII directly on SCN brain slices does stimulate neuronal depolarization, the behavioral rhythm remains intact in AngII infused mice despite profound effects on blood pressure rhythm (Brown *et al.*, 2008; Sampson *et al.*, 2008). These results suggest that blood pressure regulation is complex and cannot be explained solely by changes in activity.

Other mice with targeted genetic disruption to components of the RAS signaling pathway largely retain the baseline rhythm in blood pressure. However impairments do emerge during conditions of experimental hypertension. While ACE-KO mice maintain blood pressure rhythm, administration of a high salt diet enhances the amplitude of the rhythm in ACE heterozygote mice but blunts the rhythm in ACE KO mice(Carlson *et al.*, 2002). Similarly, in AT1a receptor–KO mice blood pressure rhythm is preserved but fructose feeding increases the difference in blood pressure between nighttime and daytime (Farah *et al.*, 2007). Again, in AT1a receptor-KO mice, five days of high salt diet abolishes the normal BP rhythm in AT1a-KO mice (Chen *et al.*, 2006). This may reflect altered AT2 receptor expression in kidney, blood vessels or brain. This is based on evidence showing that adenoviral transduction of the AT2 receptor in the ventral lateral medulla of rats abolished the circadian variation in blood pressure by blunting the night-time spike

(Gao *et al.*, 2008). Hypertensive disease may worsen clock function, which may feed forward to further impair the pressor response.

8.9 The circadian clock and fluid balance

The kidney is the major organ for long-term blood pressure regulation and is also under circadian regulation (Chapter 10). In nondipping human hypertensive patients, the normal circadian pattern of sodium excretion is blunted in concert with blood pressure (Dyer *et al.*, 1987). Sodium restriction can convert nondippers into dippers and, alternatively, sodium loading attenuates dipping suggesting a vital role for the kidney and fluid volume in this process. This may also reflect activation of the RAS pathway, as sodium restriction is a potent stimulus for AT, renin and aldosterone. Thiazide diuretics promote natriuresis (the excretion of sodium and water) and can also restore the nighttime reduction in blood pressure (Fujii *et al.*, 1999). Further evidence for a role of the kidney comes from studies showing that loss of renal function following nephrectomy correlates with impaired circadian variation in blood pressure (Goto *et al.*, 2005).

Recent studies have begun to uncover putative molecular targets of the circadian clock in the kidney that account for the rhythmic changes in blood pressure. The Na^+/H^+ exchanger (NHE3) appears to be a target of the circadian clock as its expression in the kidney oscillates with a circadian rhythm and its promoter contains functional E-boxes that are transactivated by *Bmal1* and *Clock* (Saifur *et al.*, 2005). However, the loss of NHE3 in mice does not appear to affect the circadian regulation of blood pressure (Noonan *et al.*, 2005). Similarly, loss of the Na-2Cl-K cotransporter does not affect blood pressure rhythm (Kim *et al.*, 2008a). Interestingly, deficiency of carbonic anhydrase II in mice, which is important in sodium and bicarbonate reabsorption in the kidney, alters the circadian period of locomotor rhythm (Kernek *et al.*, 2006).

Recent observations further describe a reciprocal relationship between a circadian clock component, the *Per1* gene, and sodium balance (Gumz *et al.*, 2009). Aldosterone, a steroid which has been shown to oscillate in plasma, regulates blood levels of potassium, sodium and water volume. Aldosterone increases sodium and water reabsorption, and hence blood pressure, by elevating expression of the epithelial sodium channel (ENaC) in the kidney. In these studies, aldosterone stimulated *Per1* expression in the kidney medulla *in vivo* and *in vitro*; this was further corroborated by reporter assay studies of transcriptional regulation of the *Per1* promoter. It was also shown that the alpha subunit of the renal epithelial sodium channel, αENaC, is an output of the circadian clock. *Per1* reduces the expression of αENaC leading to increased sodium and water excretion, decreasing blood pressure. The expression of αENaC is reduced in mice lacking functional *Period* genes and by *Per1* knockdown. These studies further demonstrated that urinary sodium excretion was increased in *Per*-deficient mice. Interestingly, these observations are consistent with observations in *Clock* mutant mice, which have decreased water intake (Sei *et al.*, 2008). These results suggest that the circadian clock may be important in the control of sodium balance.

8.10 The circadian clock and peripheral vascular resistance

The constriction of blood vessels leading to increased peripheral vascular resistance is a significant target of hypertension therapy. The vasoconstriction/vasodilation or vascular tone of blood vessels is known to exhibit a circadian variation (Panza *et al.*, 1991). Catecholamines clearly play a part in the circadian tone of blood vessels. Circadian clock deficient mice [*Bmal1*-KO and *Npas2* mutant] and EC-PPARγ-KO mice, which have reduced *Bmal1*, have reduced levels of norepinephrine and epinephrine in plasma in both the nighttime and daytime, consistent with the hypotensive phenotype of the mice (Curtis *et al.*, 2007; Wang *et al.*, 2008a). Mice with disruption of chromogranin A, which produces the catecholamine inhibitory fragment catestatin, have complete impairment in circadian blood pressure rhythm and reduction in adrenal catecholamine levels (Mahapatra *et al.*, 2005). While catecholamines stimulate beta adrenergic receptors to increase heart contractility and raise blood pressure by enhancing kidney renin release, β1/β2 adrenergic knockout mice exhibit a normal blood pressure rhythm (Kim *et al.*, 2008b). However, mice deficient in dopamine β-hydroxylase, the rate limiting enzyme in catecholamine production, do have an impaired blood pressure rhythm (Swoap *et al.*, 2004). Indeed, catecholamine release from nerve fibers localized on arterioles of the circulatory system stimulates alpha-1 adrenergic receptors to cause vasoconstriction, elevating blood pressure. Thus, it may be that catecholamines mediate circadian changes in blood pressure by controlling vascular resistance via alpha-1 adrenergic receptors as opposed to controlling blood pressure by increasing cardiac contractility via β-adrenergic receptors. This is supported by observations in *Cry*-deficient mice demonstrating alterations in the expression of α-adrenergic receptors and suppressed pressor response to a α1-adrenergic receptor agonist (Masuki *et al.*, 2005).

NO has also been implicated as a control mechanism for the circadian variation in blood pressure. There are three isoforms of NOS: neuronal (nNOS), inducible (iNOS) and endothelial (eNOS) that are responsible for the generation of NO in higher mammals. Indeed, recent data suggests that eNOS signaling and endothelial function is impaired in mice with dysfunctional circadian clocks (Rudic *et al.*, 2005b; Wang *et al.*, 2008b; Anea *et al.*, 2009). NO and the ability of the NOS inhibitor, L-NAME to increase blood pressure vary with time. L-NAME also decreases the diurnal variation in blood pressure and along with other NOS inhibitors can modulate the function of the SCN (Witte *et al.*, 1995; Kriegsfeld *et al.*, 1999). Additionally, the concentration of NO metabolites in the plasma also exhibits circadian variation (Mastronardi *et al.*, 2002). Posttranslational mechanisms regulating eNOS activity are compromised in mice with a targeted mutation of the circadian clock, consistent with observations demonstrating that eNOS activity exhibits circadian variation, which may be a consequence of its phosphorylation state (Tunctan *et al.*, 2002; Kunieda *et al.*, 2008, Wang *et al.*, 2008b; Anea *et al.*, 2009). Moreover, vascular disease is worsened in circadian clock mutant mice compared to WT mice when challenged by arterial ligation or vascular injury (Anea *et al.*, 2009). Despite this, the rhythm in blood pressure is retained in eNOS knockout mice suggesting that circadian rhythms in blood pressure are either not mediated by eNOS or are compensated for through other mechanisms (Van Vliet *et al.*, 2003; Lemmer *et al.*, 2004). Similarly, the function of the SCN is normal in nNOS knockout mice (Kriegsfeld *et al.*, 1999).

Another mechanism that might account for a reduction in nocturnal pressure is a loss of endothelial function in the arterioles in the circulatory system. That a circadian rhythm exists in the function of human blood vessels is long known (Kaneko *et al.*, 1968). Indeed, endothelial function varies according to time of day; this variation is altered in mice with mutated circadian clocks, while the downstream effector response to NO, through guanylyl cyclase, remains intact (Viswambharan *et al.*, 2007; Anea *et al.*, 2009). This is consistent with observations in humans demonstrating that the response to sodium nitroprusside does not vary according to time of day (Panza *et al.*, 1991). Small vessels or arterioles exhibit stiffening in *Bmal1*-KO and *Per*-KO mice, which may compromise vasodilatory processes important in blood pressure regulation (Anea *et al.*, 2010). In individuals with compromised endothelial function, which is often accompanied by vascular stiffening, the diurnal variation in blood vessel tone is blunted (Shaw *et al.*, 2001). Forearm blood flow is also compromised in nondipping versus dipping hypertensives (Higashi *et al.*, 2002). Moreover, hypertension is known to modify the circadian clock in the heart and vasculature. These findings raise important questions as to whether a loss of circadian rhythms causes endothelial dysfunction or if loss of endothelial function results in the disruption of circadian regulation or both. Indeed, hypertension is known to modify the circadian clock in the heart and vasculature (Young *et al.*, 2001; Mohri *et al.*, 2003; Naito *et al.*, 2003). Recent studies in fact show that endothelial dysfunction occurs in arteries from mice with genetic disruption of the circadian clock (Viswambharan *et al.*, 2007; Anea *et al.*, 2009).

Superoxide is a form of extremely reactive oxygen having a free electron, and its generation is a powerful antagonist to the vasculoprotective actions of NO and a frequent cause of endothelial dysfunction in cardiovascular disease states. Blood vessels from hypertensive animals overproduce superoxide and accompanying reactive oxygen species (ROS), which alter vascular tone and induce

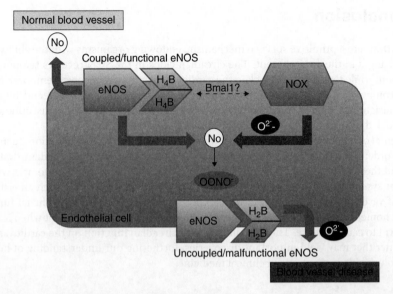

Fig. 8.3 Uncoupled endothelial NO synthase (eNOS). During normal conditions, the enzyme eNOS produces NO in part via interaction with tetrahydrobiopterin (H_4B), a cofactor that facilitates its NO-producing activity. Superoxide generated via NADPH oxidase enzymes (NOXes) can oxidize H_4B to H_2B to uncouple eNOS and produce superoxide (O^{2-}), impairing smooth muscle cell dilation and propagating vascular disease. The circadian clock component *Bmal1* has been shown to exert an important role in this pathway.

endothelial dysfunction (Rajagopalan *et al.*, 1996). Increased production of ROS occurs in kidneys and spleen from *Bmal1*-KO mice (Kondratov *et al.*, 2006). Moreover, the levels of superoxide production in brain and neutrophils have been shown to exhibit circadian variation (Muniain *et al.*, 1991). More recently, it was shown that superoxide production is increased in *Bmal1*-KO mice (Anea *et al.*, 2012). These data suggested that uncoupling of eNOS from its cofactor BH4 was a source of superoxide production (Fig. 8.3). Increased production of ROS can also disrupt the timing of the circadian clock, suggesting a potential mechanism for stimuli that induce ROS production, such as high blood pressure or diabetes, to disrupt the local circadian clock and promote vascular disease (Hardeland *et al.*, 2003; Zheng *et al.*, 2007).

It is evident that the regulation of the circadian clock influences multiple mechanisms involved in blood pressure regulation. The hands of the clock may directly touch upon the genes and proteins involved in blood pressure regulation through direct transcriptional control and posttranslational regulation. Perturbations to the circadian clock may occur in a behaviorally silent manner, perhaps influencing only peripheral clocks, as in nondipping hypertension, or through central behavioral aberrations, such as sleep apnea, sleep duration, and shift work (Fig. 8.1). One possibility is that the genetic components of the circadian clock act directly to modulate gene expression in tissues intrinsically important in blood pressure regulation. Alternatively, the molecular clock may exert influence on blood pressure regulation via tissues extrinsic to the pressor mechanism through the release of mediators such as hormones or circulating peptides.

Transcriptional activation by the positive limb of peripheral circadian clocks may transactivate genes important in vascular, cardiac, or renal function and these functions can be antagonized by proteins of the negative limb (Kita *et al.*, 2002; Storch *et al.*, 2002; Rudic *et al.*, 2005a). Future studies are needed to examine if there is an impact of ROS production in vascular function and blood pressure regulation in mice with a disrupted circadian clock as ROSs are established negative modulators of the molecular clock (Laursen *et al.*, 1997). Moreover, it will be important to identify the putative signals that act as intermediaries to blood pressure and circadian control.

8.11 Conclusion

Circadian rhythms are a primitive survival mechanism, endowing organisms with the ability to anticipate predictable changes in the environment. The circadian clock in the SCN receives temporal input from the environment while the circadian clock in the cardiovascular system receives temporal input from the internal environment of the body, from cells to organs, from circulating blood and humoral signals. While much insight has been gleaned from animals with genetically engineered disruption of the circadian clock, clock dysfunction also occurs in the absence of genetic mutation.

Environmental or behavioral aberrations that directly impact central clock function, such as shift work and sleep disorders, impinge on cardiovascular homeostasis. In addition, circadian dysfunction may extend beyond these centrally derived anomalies. Circadian clock function deteriorates with age in the cardiovascular system, impairing vascular cell signaling and function. Having such an elaborate role in the control of vascular cell signaling and in the control of daily cycles of endothelial function, blood pressure, and homeostasis, the impact of circadian clock dysfunction is significant when it malfunctions in the long term to cause disease. Thus, the influence of circadian function on the cardiovascular system is a new frontier that may yield important discoveries, furthering our understanding of human disease and leading to valuable innovations in clinical medicine.

References

Anea CB, Zhang M, Stepp DW, *et al.* 2009. Vascular disease in mice with a dysfunctional circadian clock. *Circulation* **119**:1510–1517.

Anea CB, Ali MI, Osmond JM, *et al.* 2010. Matrix metalloproteinase 2 and 9 dysfunction underlie vascular stiffness in circadian clock mutant mice. *Arterioscler Thromb Vasc Biol* **30**:2535–2543.

Anea CB, Cheng B, Sharma S, *et al.* 2012. Increased superoxide and endothelial no synthase uncoupling in blood vessels of bmal1-knockout mice. *Circ Res* **111**:1157–1165.

Baggs JE, Price TS, DiTacchio L, *et al.* 2009. Network features of the mammalian circadian clock. *PLoS Biol* **7**:e52.

Balsalobre A, Damiola F, Schibler U. 1998. A serum shock induces circadian gene expression in mammalian tissue culture cells. *Cell* **93**:929–937.

Balsalobre A, Brown SA, Marcacci L, *et al.* 2000. Resetting of circadian time in peripheral tissues by glucocorticoid signaling. *Science* **289**:2344–2347.

Brown TM, McLachlan E, Piggins HD. 2008. Angiotensin II regulates the activity of mouse suprachiasmatic nuclei neurons. *Neuroscience* **154**:839–847.

Carlson SH, Shelton J, White CR, Wyss JM. 2000. Elevated sympathetic activity contributes to hypertension and salt sensitivity in diabetic obese zucker rats. *Hypertension* **35**:403–408.

Chen Y, Oroszi TL, Morris M. 2006. Salt consumption increases blood pressure and abolishes the light/dark rhythm in angiotensin AT1a receptor deficient mice. *Physiol Behav* **88**:95–100.

Cheng B, Anea CB, Yao L, *et al.* 2011. Tissue-intrinsic dysfunction of circadian clock confers transplant arteriosclerosis. *Proc Natl Acad Sci USA* **108**:17147–17152.

Chobanian AV, Bakris GL, Black HR, *et al.* 2003. The seventh report of the joint national committee on prevention, detection, evaluation, and treatment of high blood pressure: The jnc 7 report. *JAMA* **289**:2560–2572.

Curtis AM, Cheng Y, Kapoor S, *et al.* 2007. Circadian variation of blood pressure and the vascular response to asynchronous stress. *Proc Natl Acad Sci USA* **104**:3450–3455.

Czupryniak L, Pawlowski M, Saryusz-Wolska M, Loba J. 2007. Circadian blood pressure variation and antihypertensive medication adjustment in normoalbuminuric type 2 diabetes patients. *Kidney Blood Press Res* **30**:182–186.

Davidson AJ, London B, Block GD, Menaker M. 2005. Cardiovascular tissues contain independent circadian clocks. *Clin Exp Hypertens* **27**:307–311.

DeBruyne JP, Weaver DR, Reppert SM. 2007. Clock and NPAS2 have overlapping roles in the suprachiasmatic circadian clock. *Nat Neurosci* **10**:543–545.

Dubocovich ML, Markowska M. 2005. Functional MT1 and MT2 melatonin receptors in mammals. *Endocrinolgy* **27**:101–110.

Dyer AR, Stamler R, Grimm R, *et al.* 1987. Do hypertensive patients have a different diurnal pattern of electrolyte excretion? *Hypertension* **10**:417–424.

Farah V, Elased KM, Morris M. 2007. Genetic and dietary interactions: Role of angiotensin AT1a receptors in response to a high-fructose diet. *Am J Physiol Heart Circ Physiol* **293**:H1083–H1089.

Fujii T, Uzu T, Nishimura M, *et al.* 1999. Circadian rhythm of natriuresis is disturbed in nondipper type of essential hypertension. *Am J Kidney Dis* **33**:29–35.

Gao L, Wang W, Wang W, *et al.* 2008. Effects of angiotensin type 2 receptor overexpression in the rostral ventrolateral medulla on blood pressure and urine excretion in normal rats. *Hypertension* **51**:521–527.

Goncalves AC, Tank J, Diedrich A, *et al.* 2009. Diabetic hypertensive leptin receptor-deficient db/db mice develop cardioregulatory autonomic dysfunction. *Hypertension* **53**:387–392.

Goncharuk VD, van Heerikhuize J, Dai JP, *et al.* 2001. Neuropeptide changes in the suprachiasmatic nucleus in primary hypertension indicate functional impairment of the biological clock. *J Comp Neurol* **431**:320–330.

Goto N, Uchida K, Morozumi K, *et al.* 2005. Circadian blood pressure rhythm is disturbed by nephrectomy. *Hypertens Res* **28**:301–306.

Gumz ML, Stow LR, Lynch IJ, *et al.* 2009. The circadian clock protein period 1 regulates expression of the renal epithelial sodium channel in mice. *The Journal of Clinical Investigation* **119**:2423–34.

Hardeland R, Coto-Montes A, Poeggeler B. 2003. Circadian rhythms, oxidative stress, and antioxidative defense mechanisms. *Chronobiol Int* **20**:921–962.

Hermida RC, Calvo C, Ayala DE, *et al.* 2004. Administration-time-dependent effects of doxazosin gits on ambulatory blood pressure of hypertensive subjects. *Chronobiol Int* **21**:277–296.

Higashi Y, Nakagawa K, Kimura M, *et al.* 2002. Circadian variation of blood pressure and endothelial function in patients with essential hypertension:A comparison of dippers and non-dippers. *J Am Coll Cardiol* **40**:2039–2043.

Hirota T, Okano T, Kokame K, *et al.* 2002. Glucose down-regulates per1 and per2 mrna levels and induces circadian gene expression in cultured rat-1 fibroblasts. *J Biol Chem* **277**:44244–44251.

Holl RW, Pavlovic M, Heinze E, Thon A. 1999. Circadian blood pressure during the early course of type 1 diabetes. Analysis of 1,011 ambulatory blood pressure recordings in 354 adolescents and young adults. *Diabetes Care* **22**:1151–1157.

Ignarro LJ, Byrns RE, Buga GM, Wood KS. 1987. Mechanisms of endothelium-dependent vascular smooth-muscle relaxation elicited by bradykinin and vip. *Am. J. Physiol* **253**:H1074–H1082.

Izzedine H, Launay-Vacher V, Deray G. 2006. Abnormal blood pressure circadian rhythm: A target organ damage? *Int J Cardiol* **107**:343–349.

Kaneko M, Zechman FW, Smith RE. 1968. Circadian variation in human peripheral blood flow levels and exercise responses. *J Appl Physiol* **25**:109–114.

Kario K, Matsuo T, Kobayashi H, *et al.* 1996. Nocturnal fall of blood pressure and silent cerebrovascular damage in elderly hypertensive patients. Advanced silent cerebrovascular damage in extreme dippers. *Hypertension* **27**:130–135.

Kario K, Pickering TG, Matsuo T, *et al.* 2001. Stroke prognosis and abnormal nocturnal blood pressure falls in older hypertensives. *Hypertension* **38**:852–857.

Kernek KL, Trofatter JA, Mayeda AR, *et al.* 2006. A single copy of carbonic anhydrase 2 restores wild-type circadian period to carbonic anhydrase II-deficient mice. *Behav Genet* **36**:301–308.

Kim SM, Eisner C, Faulhaber-Walter R, *et al.* 2008a. Salt sensitivity of blood pressure in NKCC1-deficient mice. *Am J Physiol Renal Physiol* **295**:F1230–F1238.

Kim SM, Huang Y, Qin Y, *et al.* 2008b. Persistence of circadian variation in arterial blood pressure in beta1/beta2-adrenergic receptor-deficient mice. *Am J Physiol Regul Integr Comp Physiol* **294**:R1427–R1434.

Kita Y, Shiozawa M, Jin W, *et al.* 2002. Implications of circadian gene expression in kidney, liver and the effects of fasting on pharmacogenomic studies. *Pharmacogenetics* **12**:55–65.

Kondratov RV, Kondratova AA, Gorbacheva VY, *et al.* 2006. Early aging and age-related pathologies in mice deficient in BMAL1, the core componentof the circadian clock. *Genes Dev* **20**:1868–1873.

Kriegsfeld LJ, Demas GE, Lee SE Jr., *et al.* 1999. Circadian locomotor analysis of male mice lacking the gene for neuronal nitric oxide synthase (nNOS-/-). *J Biol Rhythms* **14**:20–27.

Kriegsfeld LJ, Drazen DL, Nelson RJ. 2001. Circadian organization in male mice lacking the gene for endothelial nitric oxide synthase (eNOS-/-). *J Biol. Rhythms* **16**:142–148.

Kudo T, Akiyama M, Kuriyama K, *et al.* 2004. Night-time restricted feeding normalises clock genes and PAI-1 gene expression in the db/db mouse liver. *Diabetologia* **47**:1425–1436.

Kunieda T, Minamino T, Katsuno T, *et al.* 2008. Reduced nitric oxide causes age-associated impairment of circadian rhythmicity. *Circ Res* **102**:607–614.

Laursen JB, Rajagopalan S, Galis Z, *et al.* 1997. Role of superoxide in angiotensin II-induced but not catecholamine-induced hypertension. *Circulation* **95**:588–593.

Lemmer B. 1996. Chronopharmacology of hypertension. *Ann NY Acad Sci* **783**:242–253.

Lemmer B. 2006. The importance of circadian rhythms on drug response in hypertension and coronary heart disease--from mice and man. *Pharmacol Ther* **111**:629–651.

Lemmer B, Arraj M, Thomas M, Zuther P. 2004. Enos-knock-out mice display a disturbed 24-h rhythm in heart rate but not in blood pressure. *Am J Hypertens* **17**:S79–S79.

Li P, Sur SH, Mistlberger RE, Morris M. 1999. Circadian blood pressure and heart rate rhythms in mice. *Am J Physiol Regul Integr Comp Physiol* **276**:R500–R504.

Liu AC, Welsh DK, Ko CH, *et al.* 2007. Intercellular coupling confers robustness against mutations in the scn circadian clock network. *Cell* **129**:605–616.

Luo Z, Fujio Y, Kureishi Y, *et al.* 2000. Acute modulation of endothelial akt/pkb activity alters nitric oxide-dependent vasomotor activity in vivo. *J Clin Invest* **106**:493–499.

Lurbe A, Redon J, Pascual JM, *et al.* 1993. Altered blood pressure during sleep in normotensive subjects with type i diabetes. *Hypertension* **21**:227–235.

Mahapatra NR, O'Connor DT, Vaingankar SM, *et al.* 2005. Hypertension from targeted ablation of chromogranin a can be rescued by the human ortholog. *J Clin Invest* **115**:1942–1952.

Mastronardi CA, Yu WH, McCann SM. 2002. Resting and circadian release of nitric oxide is controlled by leptin in male rats. *Proc Nat Acad Sci USA* **99**:5721–5726.

Masuki S, Todo T, Nakano Y, *et al.* 2005. Reduced alpha-adrenoceptor responsiveness and enhanced baroreflex sensitivity in cry-deficient mice lacking a biological clock. *J Physiol* **566**:213–224.

McNamara P, Seo SP, Rudic RD, *et al.* 2001. Regulation of CLOCK and MOP4 by nuclear hormone receptors in the vasculature: A humoral mechanism to reset a peripheral clock. *Cell* **105**:877–889.

Mohri T, Emoto N, Nonaka H, *et al.* 2003. Alterations of circadian expressions of clock genes in dahl salt-sensitive rats fed a high-salt diet. *Hypertension* **42**:189–194.

Muniain MA, Rodríguez MD, Romero A, *et al.* 1991. Circadian variations in the superoxide production, enzyme release and neutrophil aggregation in patients with rheumatoid arthritis and controls. *Rheumatology* **30**:138–140.

Nagoshi E, Saini C, Bauer C, *et al.* 2004. Circadian gene expression in individual fibroblasts: Cell-autonomous and self-sustained oscillators pass time to daughter cells. *Cell* **119**:693–705.

Naito Y, Tsujino T, Fujioka Y, *et al.* 2002. Augmented diurnal variations of the cardiac renin-angiotensin system in hypertensive rats. *Hypertension* **40**:827–833.

Naito Y, Tsujino T, Kawasaki D, *et al.* 2003. Circadian gene expression of clock genes and plasminogen activator inhibitor-1 in heart and aorta of spontaneously hypertensive and wistar-kyoto rats. *J Hypertens* **21**:1107–1115.

Nonaka H, Emoto N, Ikeda K, *et al.* 2001. Angiotensin II induces circadian gene expression of clock genes in cultured vascular smooth muscle cells. *Circulation* **104**:1746–1748.

Noonan WT, Woo AL, Nieman ML, *et al.* 2005. Blood pressure maintenance in NHE3-deficient mice with transgenic expression of NHE3 in small intestine. *Am J Physiol Regul Integr Comp Physiol* **288**:R685–R691.

O'Brien E, Sheridan J, O'Malley K. 1988. Dippers and non-dippers. *Lancet* **2**:397.

Osmond JM, Mintz JD, Dalton B, Stepp DW. 2009. Obesity increases blood pressure, cerebral vascular remodeling, and severity of stroke in the zucker rat. *Hypertension* **53**:381–386.

Panza JA, Epstein SE, Quyyumi AA. 1991. Circadian variation in vascular tone and its relation to alpha-sympathetic vasoconstrictor activity. *N Engl J Med* **325**:986–990.

Portaluppi F, Vergnani L, Manfredini R, *et al.* 1995. Time-dependent effect of isradipine on the nocturnal hypertension in chronic renal failure. *Am J Hypertens* **8**:719–726.

Rajagopalan S, Kurz S, Munzel T, *et al.* 1996. Angiotensin II-mediated hypertension in the rat increases vascular superoxide production via membrane nadh/nadph oxidase activation. Contribution to alterations of vasomotor tone. *J Clin Invest* **97**:1916–1923.

Reilly DF, Curtis AM, Cheng Y, *et al.* 2008. Peripheral circadian clock rhythmicity is retained in the absence of adrenergic signaling. *Arterioscler Thromb Vasc Biol* **28**:121–126.

Rudic RD, Curtis AM, Cheng Y, FitzGerald G. 2005a. Peripheral clocks and the regulation of cardiovascular and metabolic function. *Methods Enzymol* **393**:524–539.

Rudic RD, McNamara P, Reilly D, *et al.* 2005b. Bioinformatic analysis of circadian gene oscillation in mouse aorta. *Circulation* **112**:2716–2724.

Saifur Rohman M, Emoto N, Nonaka H, *et al.* 2005. Circadian clock genes directly regulate expression of the na+// h+ exchanger NHE3 in the kidney. *Kidney Int* **67**:1410–1419.

Sampson AK, Widdop RE, Denton KM. 2008. Sex-differences in circadian blood pressure variations in response to chronic angiotensin II infusion in rats. *Clin Exp Pharmacol Physiol* **35**:391–395.

Scheer FA, Van Montfrans GA, van Someren EJ, *et al.* 2004. Daily nighttime melatonin reduces blood pressure in male patients with essential hypertension. *Hypertension* **43**:192–197.

Sei H, Oishi K, Chikahisa S, *et al.* 2008. Diurnal amplitudes of arterial pressure and heart rate are dampened in CLOCK mutant mice and adrenalectomized mice. *Endocrinology* **149**:3576–3580.

Senador D, Kanakamedala K, Irigoyen MC, *et al.* 2009. Cardiovascular and autonomic phenotype of db/db diabetic mice. *Exp Physiol* **94**:648–658.

Shaw JA, Chin-Dusting JPF, Kingwell BA, Dart AM. 2001. Diurnal variation in endothelium-dependent vasodilatation is not apparent in coronary artery disease. *Circulation* **103**:806–812.

Shimamura T, Nakajima M, Iwasaki T, *et al.* 1999. Analysis of circadian blood pressure rhythm and target-organ damage in stroke-prone spontaneously hypertensive rats. *J Hypertens* **17**:211–220.

Storch KF, Lipan O, Leykin I, *et al.* 2002. Extensive and divergent circadian gene expression in liver and heart. *Nature* **417**:78–83.

Sturrock ND, George E, Pound N, *et al.* 2000. Non-dipping circadian blood pressure and renal impairment are associated with increased mortality in diabetes mellitus. *Diabet Med* **17**:360–364.

Su W, Guo Z, Randall DC, *et al.* 2008. Hypertension and disrupted blood pressure circadian rhythm in type 2 diabetic db/db mice. *Am J Physiol Heart Circ Physiol* **295**:H1634–H1641.

Svensson P, de Faire U, Sleight P, *et al.* 2001. Comparative effects of ramipril on ambulatory and office blood pressures: A hope substudy. *Hypertension* **38**:E28–E32.

Swoap SJ, Weinshenker D, Palmiter RD, Garber G. 2004. Dbh(-/-) mice are hypotensive, have altered circadian rhythms, and have abnormal responses to dieting and stress. *Am J Physiol Regul Integr Comp Physiol* **286**:R108–R113.

Thomas MA, Fleissner G, Stohr M, *et al.* 2004. Localization of components of the renin-angiotensin system in the suprachiasmatic nucleus of normotensive sprague-dawley rats: Part b. Angiotensin II (AT1)-receptors, a light and electron microscopic study. *Brain Res* **1008**:224–235.

Timio M, Venanzi S, Lolli S, *et al.* 1995. "Non-dipper" hypertensive patients and progressive renal insufficiency: A 3-year longitudinal study. *Clin Nephrol* **43**:382–387.

Tunctan B, Weigl Y, Dotan A, *et al.* 2002. Circadian variation of nitric oxide synthase activity in mouse tissue. *Chronobiol Int* **19**(2):393–404.

Van Vliet BN, Chafe LL, Montani J-P. 2003. Characteristics of 24 h telemetered blood pressure in enos-knockout and c57bl/6j control mice. *J Physiol* **549**:313–325.

Viswambharan H, Carvas JM, Antic V, *et al.* 2007. Mutation of the circadian clock gene per2 alters vascular endothelial function. *Circulation* **115**:2188–2195.

Wang CY, Wen MS, Wang HW, *et al.* 2008a. Increased vascular senescence and impaired endothelial progenitor cell function mediated by mutation of circadian gene per2. *Circulation* **118**:2166–2173.

Wang N, Yang G, Jia Z, *et al.* 2008b. Vascular ppargamma controls circadian variation in blood pressure and heart rate through bmal1. *Cell Metab* **8**:482–491.

Welsh DK, Yoo SH, Liu AC, *et al.* 2004. Bioluminescence imaging of individual fibroblasts reveals persistent, independently phased circadian rhythms of clock gene expression. *Curr Biol* **14**:2289–2295.

Westgate EJ, Cheng Y, Reilly DF, *et al.* 2008. Genetic components of the circadian clock regulate thrombogenesis in vivo. *Circulation* **117**:2087–2095.

Witte K, Lemmer B. 1999. Development of inverse circadian blood pressure pattern in transgenic hypertensive TGR(mREN2)27 rats. *Chronobiol Int* **16**:293–303.

Witte K, Schnecko A, Zuther P, Lemmer B. 1995.Contribution of the nitric oxide-guanylyl cyclase system to circadian regulation of blood pressure in normotensive wistar-kyoto rats. *Cardiovasc Res* **30**:682–688.

Witte K, Schnecko A, Buijs RM, *et al.* 1998. Effects of SCN lesions on circadian blood pressure rhythm in normotensive and transgenic hypertensive rats. *Chronobiol Int* **15**:135–145.

Woon PY, Kaisaki PJ, Braganca J, *et al.* 2007. Aryl hydrocarbon receptor nuclear translocator-like (BMAL1) is associated with susceptibility to hypertension and type 2 diabetes. *Proc Natl Acad Sci USA* **104**:14412–14417.

Young ME, Razeghi P, Taegtmeyer H. 2001. Clock genes in the heart: Characterization and attenuation with hypertrophy. *Circ Res* **88**:1142–1150.

Yusuf S, Sleight P, Pogue J, *et al.* 2000. Effects of an angiotensin-converting-enzyme inhibitor, ramipril, on cardiovascular events in high-risk patients. The heart outcomes prevention evaluation study investigators. *N Engl J Med* **342**:145–153.

Zheng X, Yang Z, Yue Z, *et al.* 2007. Foxo and insulin signaling regulate sensitivity of the circadian clock to oxidative stress. *Proc Natl Acad Sci USA* **104**:15899–15904.

Hypertension Caused by Disruption of the Circadian System: Blood Pressure Regulation at Multiple Levels

9

Hitoshi Okamura, Miho Yasuda, Jean-Michel Fustin, and Masao Doi
Department of Systems Biology, Graduate School of Pharmaceutical Sciences, Kyoto University, Sakyo-ku, Kyoto, Japan

9.1 Introduction

In daily human life, blood pressure increases after getting up in the morning, peaks towards the end of the afternoon then decreases gradually until its nadir at around midnight. When the daily cycles of our routine life are disrupted by shift work or chronic extended wakefulness, blood pressure has been shown to increase (Suwazono *et al.*, 2008; Scheer *et al.*, 2009). This suggests that stable biological rhythms of activity are an important issue to maintain normal blood pressure. With the collaboration of Dr van der Horst in the Netherlands (van der Horst *et al.*, 1999), we addressed the lack of molecular clock oscillatory machinery in both central and peripheral organs of *Cry*-null (*Cry1⁻/⁻Cry2⁻/⁻*) mice (Okamura *et al.*, 1999; Yagita *et al.*, 2001). Comprehensive analysis of these mice to understand the role of biological rhythms in the maintenance of physiological blood pressure led to the discovery that *Cry*-null mice showed hyperaldosteronemia and developed salt-induced hypertension (Doi *et al.*, 2010). Surprisingly, however, *Cry*-null mice did not show hypertension under a normal diet despite aldosterone levels 5–10 times higher than normal. Here, the etiology of hyperaldosteronism in *Cry*-null mice is described and the mechanisms of blood pressure regulation in these mice further defined.

9.2 Effects of deleting *Cry* genes

Deletion of Cry genes causes complete loss of circadian rhythms and leads to hyperaldosteronism and salt-sensitive hypertension. The transcription/translation feedback loop is composed of clock genes regulating their own expression which generate circadian rhythms at the cellular level, accompanied by dynamic changes of cellular metabolism (Reppert and Weaver, 2000; Okamura, 2004; Eckel-Mahan and Sassone-Corsi, 2013). These cellular oscillations, which are generated by trillions

Circadian Medicine, First Edition. Edited by Christopher S. Colwell.
© 2015 John Wiley & Sons, Inc. Published 2015 by John Wiley & Sons, Inc.

of cells in the body, are all synchronized by one central clock in the hypothalamic suprachiasmatic nucleus (SCN) of the brain (Chapter 3). The SCN sends time signals to the surrounding subparaventricular zone (SPVZ), thalamic paraventricular nucleus and various other hypothalamic nuclei, including the dorsomedial hypothalamic nucleus, arcuate nucleus and paraventricular nucleus. These signals are finally sent out of the brain to the whole body via sympathetic and parasympathetic routes, synchronizing all peripheral cellular rhythms (Buijs RM, Kalsbeek, 2001; Ishida *et al.*, 2005). The SCN is indispensable for the generation of circadian rhythms at the systemic level, since lesion of this nucleus abolishes all physiologically relevant rhythms, including behavioral and hormonal rhythms. Therefore, the circadian system is composed of oscillating peripheral clocks orchestrated by the SCN.

What molecular mechanisms are involved in generating these rhythms? Clock genes control the daily expression of thousands of clock-controlled genes (ccg) in mammals (Chapters 1 and 2). Ccg rhythms are generated at the transcriptional level directly by clock genes (Reppert and Weaver, 2000) or indirectly via RNA processing (Koike *et al.*, 2012). Ccgs are important not only for universal cellular function, such as cell cycle (Matsuo *et al.*, 2003), and universal metabolism, such as nucleic acids (Fustin *et al.*, 2012), but also for cell-specific functions, such as production of neurotransmitter/hormone vasopressin (Jin *et al.*, 1999). Thus, the characterization of ccgs is important to unveil the pathogenic mechanisms of diseases originating from a malfunction of the circadian clock.

In *Cry*-null mice, circadian clocks are unable to oscillate in both the central SCN and peripheral organs (e.g., heart blood vessels, adrenal glands, kidneys) involved in blood pressure regulation. Although the mean arterial pressure (MAP) of these mice is within the normal range under a normal salt diet (Fig. 9.1a), placing these mice on a high salt diet (3.15% sodium) markedly elevated the MAP, leading to a nondipper type of salt-sensitive hypertension (Chapter 8). Screening *Cry*-null mice to identify possible mechanisms, it was found that the aldosterone plasma concentration was 5–10 times higher in *Cry*-null mice than normal (Doi *et al.*, 2010) (Fig. 9.1b). Because plasma renin activity was low, it was surmised that the increased aldosterone was not due to an activated renin–angiotensin system (RAS) but rather to an intrinsic mechanism within the adrenal.

DNA microarray analyses of adrenal glands transcriptome were conducted to compare *Cry*-null with wild-type (WT) mice. Among dozens of steroid synthetic enzymes, *Hsd3b6*, a new type of 3β-hydroxylsteroid dehydrogenase (3β-HSD), was markedly overexpressed in *Cry*-null mice (Doi *et al.*, 2010). This gene is specifically expressed in aldosterone-producing cells in the zona glomerulosa (ZG) and its expression is enhanced and suppressed by clock genes *Dbp* and *E4BP4*, respectively (Fig. 9.1c). Since *Dbp* is constantly high and *E4bp4* constantly low in the adrenal of *Cry*-null mice, levels of *Hsd3b6* transcription are elevated in *Cry*-null mice. *Hsd3b6* is, therefore, a ccg converting pregnenolone to progesterone in the steroidogenesis pathway (Fig. 9.1c). Administration of a 3β-HSD inhibitor (trilostane, 2α-cyano-4α,5α-epoxy-17β-ol-androstane-3-one) dose-dependently decreased the plasma aldosterone levels in *Cry*-null mice, revealing this step as rate limiting for aldosterone synthesis.

To translate this finding to humans, we searched for the homologue enzyme in humans and found that human *HSD3B1* gene is the functional counterpart to the mouse *Hsd3b6*: both genes are expressed mainly in aldosterone-producing cells in the adrenal zona glomerulosa (Doi *et al.*, 2010). Moreover, recent findings suggest a relationship between SNPs of HSD3B1 and essential hypertensive patients (Shimodaira *et al.*, 2010).

Aldosterone induces reabsorption of ions and water in the kidneys, thereby increasing blood volume, leading to higher blood pressure. An excess of aldosterone production in the adrenal gland is called primary aldosteronism (PA); it accounts for 10% of total hypertension cases (Funder, 2011). PA is caused either by aldosterone-producing adenoma (APA) and/or by bilateral hyperplasia causing idiopathic hyperaldosteronism (IHA) in PA patients. Since PA carries a higher risk of developing cardiovascular complications, accurate diagnosis and treatment of this disease are particularly important. So far, however, there have been no appropriate animal models of PA. *Cry*-null mice are proposed as a possible animal model for PA, and particularly for IHA, in which aldosterone synthesis increase is bilateral due to the overexpression of *HSD3B1/Hsd3b6* in the ZG.

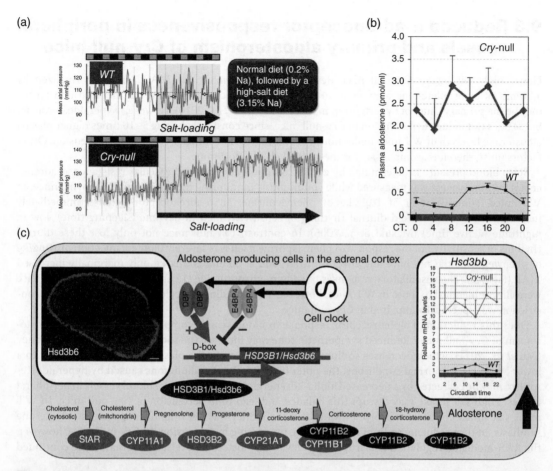

Fig. 9.1 Diagram of the mammalian circadian system and hypertension in *Cry*-null mice. (a) *Cry*-null mice exhibit salt-sensitive hypertension. Shown are representative recordings of temporal profiles of mean arterial pressure (MAP) of wild-type (*WT*) mice (8-day recording) and *Cry*-null mice (15-day recording). In both groups, animals were kept in constant darkness and fed a normal salt diet (0.2% sodium) for the first four days; the salt-loaded group was transferred to a high salt diet (3.15% sodium) on the fifth day. Gray and black boxes below the graphs represent the subjective day and subjective night, respectively. BP data were collected in 30-second bouts at 5-min intervals and plotted using a 1-h moving average. The 24-h means of each day are shown by open squares. Horizontal dotted lines indicate the mean value of the BP in days 1 through 4, on the normal salt diet. (b) Twenty-four–hour profiles of plasma aldosterone concentration (PAC) in *WT* and *Cry*-null mice in constant darkness (n=5–12 mice per time point). The values at CT0 are double plotted. Values are means±s.e.m. (c) Cellular clocks regulate steroidogenesis in the aldosterone-producing cells in the zona glomerulosa of the adrenal gland. *HSD3B1/Hsd3b6* is a clock controlled gene regulated via D-boxes in the promoter region by DBP and its antagonist E4BP4. In the *Cry*-null adrenal gland, however, constitutive activation of DBP shifts the balance towards overproduction of DBP-regulated *Hsd3b6* gene (bottom). HSD3B1/Hsd3b6 is a key enzyme for aldosterone production in *Cry*-null mice. Immunohistochemistry of Hsd3b6 protein in a *Cry*-null adrenal gland (upper left). (Some parts of this figure are adapted from Doi *et al.*, 2010.) *(See insert for color representation of the figure.)*

9.3 Reduced α-adrenoceptor responsiveness in peripheral vessels and primary aldosteronism of *Cry*-null mice

Under high salt intake *Cry*-null mice develop hypertension,but the MAP can be normalized by administration of eplerenone, a mineralocorticoid receptor blocker, suggesting that elevated aldosterone may be the primary cause of hypertension in these mice (Doi *et al.*, 2010). However, hyperaldosteronism *per se* does not induce hypertension in *Cry*-null mice, since constantly having 5–10 times higher plasma aldosterone levels than WT mice under normal conditions is not sufficient to cause hypertension. Other factors must, therefore, compensate for the high levels of aldosterone.

Since blood pressure is determined by cardiac output and peripheral vascular resistance, α-adrenoceptor responsiveness was measured while continuously monitoring the MAP in freely moving mice. In WT mice, administration of 10 µg/kg of phenylephrine, an α-adrenoceptor agonist, immediately increased MAP with marked diurnal rhythms of sensitivity: high in daytime (sleeping time), low in nighttime (active time) (Masuki et a., 2005). In contrast, *Cry*-null mice not only lost these diurnal rhythms of sensitivity but the response to phenylephrine itself was severely blunted: injection of 10 µg/kg of phenylephrine did not have any effect on MAP, and at 50 and 200 µg/kg only marginally increased MAP (Fig. 9.2). The vasodilatory responses to sodium nitroprusside (15 and 30 µg/kg) of *Cry*-null mice were almost identical to those in WT mice, however. These findings revealed that sympathetic vasoconstriction was specifically impaired in *Cry*-null mice.

Does this reduction of alpha receptor response in blood vessels compensate for the hyperaldosteronism of *Cry*-null mice? Reduced sympathetic tone may increase the sodium clearance in the kidney (Mu *et al.*, 2011), which decreases sodium ion concentration in the plasma, and lead ultimately to a lower MAP. Under normal conditions, the potential increase of sodium ions caused by hyperaldosteronism may be corrected by a decreased alpha-adrenergic responsiveness of blood vessels in peripheral tissues. High salt intake may disrupt this balance and lead to hypertension in *Cry*-null mice. In WT mice, salt intake induces reabsorption of salt in the kidney but RAS rapidly suppresses aldosterone synthesis, in turn reducing sodium reabsorption, preventing hypertension. In *Cry*-null mice, however, the RAS-mediated regulation is disrupted by elevated aldosterone levels, which may cause continued

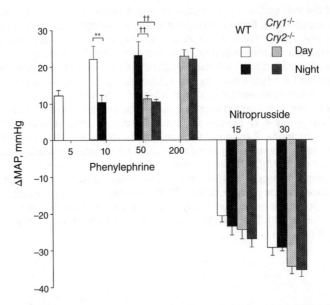

Fig. 9.2 MAP response to 5, 10, 50 and 200 µg kg⁻¹ of phenylephrine or 15 and 30 µg kg⁻¹ of sodium nitro-prusside. Columns show means ± S.E.M. for six wild-type (WT) and 5 *Cry1⁻ᐟ⁻Cry2⁻ᐟ⁻* mice. **Significant difference from *WT* mice in the day at P < 0.01. ††Significant differences from WT mice in the night at P < 0.01. (Adopted from Masuki *et al.*, 2005.)

reabsorption of sodium ions in the kidneys, leading to hypertension. These pathological conditions of *Cry*-null mice may play an important role in unraveling the pathophysiology of PA and salt-sensitive hypertension in humans.

Intriguingly, Miyajima *et al.* (1991) reported that muscle sympathetic nerve activity increased in essential hypertension and renovascular hypertension but decreased in PA. Although it is still unknown why sympathetic nervous system is suppressed in PA, the decrease of sympathetic nerve activity may compensate the persistent high levels of sodium reabsorption in the kidneys. Further pathological analyses in the kidneys, blood vessels, and central/peripheral nervous system in *Cry*-null mice will be useful to understand the pathophysiology of PA.

9.4 Rapid blood pressure control system: enhanced baroreflex in *Cry*-null mice

Examined next was the baroreflex regulation in *Cry*-null mice for the rapid regulation of blood pressure. Baroreceptors are extension receptors located in the aortic arch and carotid sinuses, their information transmitted to the nucleus of the tractus solitarius (NTS) of the medulla oblongata by the visceral sensory neurons (Fig. 9.3). NTS neurons transmit this visceral sensation to the cardiovascular center in

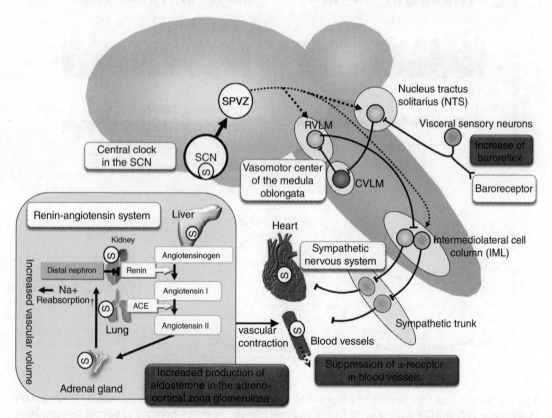

Fig. 9.3 Schematic representations of central/peripheral clocks, afferent/efferent pathways of the barore-flex, and renin–angiotensin system. Time signals generated in the SCN go to the SPVZ; these signals are then transmitted multisynaptically to the vasomotor centers of the medulla oblongata. Peripheral clocks exist in all organs consisted with the renin–angiotensin system. Pathophysiological findings observed in *Cry*-null mice are shown in white characters in gray-backed squares. Abbreviations: CVLM, caudal ventrolateral medulla; IML, intermediolateral cell column; RVLM, rostral ventrolateral medulla; NTS, nucleus of the tractus solitarius; SCN, suprachiasmatic nucleus; SPVZ, subparaventricular zone.

the rostral ventrolateral medulla (RVLM). RVLM cells send efferents to the intermediolateral cell column of the spinal cord, and these preganglionic neurons suppress cardiac output and dilate blood vessels. This baroreflex provides a negative feedback loop in which an elevated MAP reflexively reduces heart rate (HR), causing MAP to decrease; instead, decreased MAP activates heart rate, causing an immediate increase in MAP.

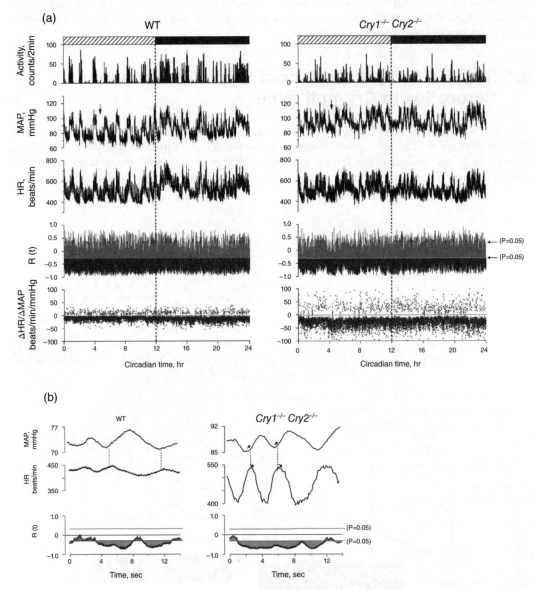

Fig. 9.4 Twenty-four hour profiles of activity, MAP, HR and spontaneous baroreflex sensitivity (ΔHR/ΔMAP) in wild-type (*WT*) and *Cry*-null mice. (a) Typical example of measurements, from top to bottom: activity, MAP, HR, cross-correlation function (R(t)) between MAP and HR, ΔHR/ΔMAP in a *WT* (left) and a *Cry*-null mice (right). R(t) above (red) and below (blue) the lines of P = 0.05 indicate significantly positive and negative correlations, respectively, which were used to determine positive (red) and negative (blue). (b) The areas indicated by arrows in A were enlarged to show dynamic change in MAP and HR. The HR response to a given change in MAP was greater in the *Cry*-null mouse than in the *WT* mouse. R(t) in blue indicates a significantly negative correlation at P < 0.05, used to determine ΔHR/ΔMAP. (Adopted from Masuki *et al.*, 2005.)

This baroreflex is very important for rapid regulation of blood pressure. In WT mice, the magnitude of the baroreflex (ΔHR/ΔMAP) showed a diurnal rhythm, with a nighttime magnitude twofold higher than during the day (Masuki et al., 2005). In Cry-null mice, however, this diurnal difference disappeared but the baroreflex magnitude was much larger than that in WT mice (Fig. 9.4a). Cry-null mice therefore dramatically change their heart rate in response to minute change of MAP, which suggests that their baroreflex is constantly hypersensitive (Fig. 9.4b). In WT mice, cardiac output and peripheral vascular resistance equally contribute to the sustained blood pressure at rest. In Cry-null mice, however, peripheral vascular resistance does not contribute to maintaining the blood pressure; blood pressure was maintained only by cardiac output: high baroreflex sensitivity may be necessary as a compensatory response. In humans, Munakata et al. (1995) measured the baroreflex sensitivity by analysing heart rate variability on electrocardiogram and reported that baroreflex sensitivity in patients with primary aldosteronism was significantly increased; baroreflex sensitivity returned to normal after removal of the adrenal adenoma.

9.5 Conclusion

The regulation of blood pressure is crucially important and, thus, is controlled by multilayered regulatory systems. Shift work and late working hours, which disturb the inherent biologic rhythms, increase the risk of hypertension and other lifestyle-related diseases. Clock genes regulate many physiologically relevant genes at the cellular level in all systems. In the case of aldosterone-producing cells in the adrenal, a new type of 3β-HSD enzyme, HSD3B1/Hsd3b6, is a clock-controlled gene. Investigations into how ccgs are regulated will contribute to the understanding of the molecular origin of hypertension and will provide potential new targets for its treatment.

Acknowledgments

The research from our laboratory reported in this chapter was supported by Grants-in-Aid from the Ministry of Education, Culture, Sports, Science and Technology of Japan, SRF, Takeda Foundation, and Health Labour Sciences Research.

References

Buijs, R.M. and Kalsbeek, A. (2001) Hypothalamic integration of central and peripheral clocks. Nat Rev Neurosci, 2(7):521–526.

Doi, M., Takahashi, Y., Komatsu, R., et al. (2010) Salt-sensitive hypertension in circadian clock-deficient mice involves dysregulated adrenal Hsd3b6. Nat Med, 16(1):67–74.

Eckel-Mahan, K. and Sassone-Corsi, P. (2013) Metabolism and the circadian clock converge. Physiol Rev, 93(1):107–135.

Funder, J.W. (2011) The genetics of primary aldosteronism. Science, 331(6018):685–686.

Fustin, J-M., Doi, M., Yamada, H., et al. (2012) Rhythmic nucleotide synthesis in the liver: Temporal segregation of metabolites. Cell Rep, 1:341–349.

Ishida, A., Mutoh, T., Ueyama, T., et al. (2005) Light activates the adrenal gland: Timing of gene expression and glucocorticoid release. Cell Metab, 2:297–307.

Jin, X., Shearman, L.P., Weaver, D.R., et al. (1999) A molecular mechanism regulating rhythmic output from the suprachiasmatic nucleus. Cell, 96:57–68.

Koike, N., Yoo, S.H., Huang, H.C., et al. (2012) Transcriptional architecture and chromatin landscape of the core circadian clock in mammals. Science, 338(6105):349–354.

Masuki, S., Todo, T., Nakano, Y., et al. (2005) Reduced alpha-adrenoceptor responsiveness and enhanced baroreflex sensitivity in Cry-deficient mice lacking biological clock. J Physiol, 566:213–224.

Matsuo, T., Yamaguchi, S., Mitsui, S., et al. (2003) Control mechanism of the circadian clock for timing of cell division. Science, 302:255–259.

Miyajima, E., Yamada, Y., Yoshida, Y., *et al.* (1991) Muscle sympathetic nerve activity in renovascular hypertension and primary aldosteronism. *Hypertension*, **17**(6 Pt 2):1057–1062.

Mu, S., Shimosawa, T., Ogura, S., *et al.* (2011) Epigenetic modulation of the renal β-adrenergic-WNK4 pathway in salt-sensitive hypertension. *Nat Med*, **17**(5):573–580.

Munakata, M., Aihara, A., Imai, Y., *et al.* (1995) Increased gain in baroreceptor-heart rate reflex in patients with primary aldosteronism. *J Hypertens*, **13**(12 Pt 2):1648–1653.

Okamura, H. (2004) Clock genes and cell clocks: Roles, actions and mysteries. *J Biol Rhythms*, **19**:388–399.

Okamura, H., Miyake, S., Sumi, Y., *et al.* (1999) Photic induction of mPer1 and mPer2 in cry deficient mice lacking a biological clock. *Science*, **286**:2531–2534.

Reppert, S.M. and Weaver, D.R. (2002) Coordination of circadian timing in mammals. *Nature*, **418**(6901):935–941.

Scheer, F.A., Hilton, M.F., Mantzoros, C.S., *et al.* (2009) Adverse metabolic and cardiovascular consequences of circadian misalignment. *Proc Natl Acad Sci USA*, **106**(11):4453–4458.

Shimodaira, M., Nakayama, T., Sato, N., *et al.* (2010) Association of HSD3B1 and HSD3B2 gene polymorphisms with essential hypertension, aldosterone level, and left ventricular structure. *Eur J Endocrinol*, **163**:671–680.

Suwazono, Y., Dochi, M., Sakata, K., *et al.* (2008) Shift work is a risk factor for increased blood pressure in Japanese men: a 14-year historical cohort study. *Hypertension*, **52**(3):581–586.

van der Horst, G.T., Muijtjens, M., Kobayashi, K., *et al.* (1999) Mammalian Cry1 and Cry2 are essential for maintenance of circadian rhythms. *Nature*, **398**(6728):627–630.

Yagita, K., Tamanini, F., van der Horst, G., and Okamura H. (2001) Molecular mechanisms of the biological clock in cultured fibroblasts. *Science*, **292**:278–281.

Chronobiology of Micturition

10

Akihiro Kanematsu[1] and Hiromitsu Negoro[2]

[1] Department of Urology, Hyogo College of Medicine, Nishinomiya, Hyogo, Japan
[2] Department of Urology, Graduate School of Medicine, Kyoto University, Sakyo, Kyoto, Japan

10.1 Introduction

The micturition frequency is determined by the amount of urine produced by the kidneys and the ability of the urinary bladder to hold urine without leakage (termed bladder capacity). The urine amount produced in the kidneys is determined by the amount of blood flow to the glomeruli and by the reabsorption of water in tubules. The former is determined by fluid intake and constriction/relaxation of afferent vessels regulated in part by the renin–angiotensin system and autonomic nervous system. The latter is determined by the hormonal system, including antidiuretic hormone (ADH, also called vasopressin) and aldosterone, working on ion transporters and channels. The function of the bladder to hold and expulse urine when desired is controlled by a complicated network of autonomous and parietal innervation. This network transmits the sensation of bladder fullness to spinal micturition center, which plays a pivotal role in generating micturition reflex. The central nervous system (CNS) controls this spinal center, so that micturition reflex takes place only when desired.

These basic processes show a daily rhythm in healthy humans such that kidneys produce more urine and the urinary bladder keeps more urine while awake than while asleep, resulting in a dramatically decreased micturition frequency during the sleep time. Unless a problem develops, we are generally unaware of this rhythm and take it for granted. One type of problem in the timing of urination is nocturnal enuresis, that is, involuntary loss of urine during sleep, experienced by 5–15% of school children. Loss of urine in the bed is harmful for children's self-esteem but, fortunately, nocturnal enuresis subsides in most children by adolescence. The other common timing problem is nocturia, that is, waking up for micturition during sleep. This is experienced by more than 60% of people over 60 years old. This nightly need for micturition interrupts sleep and is undoubtable part of the problem of fragmented sleep seen with the aging process (Chapter 22). These abnormal conditions illustrate the importance of the daily micturition cycle for healthy life.

It is not yet known how this micturition cycle is created and how to correct the problem when it is disturbed. The circadian clock exists in most peripheral tissues and organs (Chapters 6–14), including kidney and urinary bladder, which are critical for this daily rhythm. This chapter describes our current understanding of the science underlying the micturition cycle. It provides an overview of the field including behavioral phenomenology and, more recently, the beginnings of molecular insight.

Circadian Medicine, First Edition. Edited by Christopher S. Colwell.
© 2015 John Wiley & Sons, Inc. Published 2015 by John Wiley & Sons, Inc.

10.2 Human studies

10.2.1 Children and nocturnal enuresis

Control of day and nighttime micturition takes place during the toilet-training phase, typically occurring around 2–3 years of age. Generally, establishment of daytime micturition habit affords continence (dryness) during daytime before the establishment of continence during the night. Micturition in neonates involves reflex voiding, which gradually becomes regulated by the CNS along with postnatal development, accompanied by enlargement of bladder capacity, resulting in coordination between bladder contraction and sphincteric relaxation. The details of this developmental transition are not yet understood. Most likely it is a genetically controlled event, modified by postnatal habit and supportive education. In the majority of the cases, the nighttime continence is established by school age. However, at least 10% of school-aged children struggle with nocturnal continence (Neveus, 2009; Robson, 2009).

10.2.2 Aging and nocturia

Studies have shown that the established day-and-night micturition cycle is gradually disturbed in many elderly people, a condition known as nocturia (Nakamura *et al.*, 1996; Bosch and Weiss, 2010). Traditionally, nocturia used to be considered as one of the symptoms of benign prostatic hyperplasia (BPH). In BPH, a hypertrophied prostate gland compressing the urethra causes obstruction of urinary flow from the bladder, resulting in a poor urine stream, urinary urgency, or urinary frequency. BPH patients could be cured from these symptoms by either alpha-blocker medication, which relaxes the tonus of the prostate, or by transurethral resection of prostate (TUR-P), an endoscopic surgery to remove the hypertrophied inner portion of the prostate and create a wider channel for urinary flow. However, in a sharp contrast with the beneficial effect for other obstructing symptoms, the treatments for BPH provide only mild relief for nocturia. This suggests that nocturia is distinct from BPH and is a disorder with various correlates, such as age, hypertension, diabetes, cerebrovascular history (Yoshimura, 2012). When nocturia occurs two to three times per night, it has a major negative impact on the person's quality of life and is correlated with increased mortality (Nakagawa *et al.*, 2010).

10.2.3 Nocturnal polyuria

Nocturnal polyuria, that is, excessive production of urine during sleep time (nocturnal volume >20–33% of total 24-h volume), is documented as a major cause for both enuresis and nocturia. The amount of urine production is determined by oral intake of fluid and food, and one may well assume that eating and drinking behavior should be the major determinant of urine production rate. However, urine production is also controlled by altered reabsorption of water and ions in renal tubules. It is known that even when large amount of fluid or food is taken before going to bed, we do not necessarily wake up for micturition for the following several hours during sleep. This means that the water is retained in the body, reabsorbed into circulation via renal tubules after filtration by glomerulus. Furthermore, when humans are maintained under a constant routine, when food and drink are taken equally throughout the daily cycle in constant dim light, urine production keeps the same daily rhythm as people in a normal cycle. This indicates that there is an intrinsic circadian rhythm in urine production. This urine production rhythm has been known to be maintained, at least partly, by the diurnal rhythm of ADH produced in the pituitary gland.

Interestingly, enuretic children or elderly people with nocturia often show the loss or inversion of the normal rhythm in plasma ADH. Thus, reduction of urine production is a viable therapeutic method for these patients. Desmopressin, a synthesized antidiuretic hormone, is now a standard medication for enuretic children showing nocturnal polyuria. Similarly, in the elderly with refractory nocturia, the inversion of rhythm could be related to decreased natriuresis during daytime, which results in increased urine production during nighttime. Therefore, administration of diuretics during daytime is one treatment for nocturia.

10.2.4 Daily change in bladder capacity

It is also documented that functional bladder capacity shows temporal variation between daytime and nighttime in healthy subjects. Healthy adults urinate the largest volume of urine at the first voiding after they wake up, which has been stored during sleep in the bladder. The urinary bladder is composed of three layers: the innermost stratified epithelial layer called "urothelium" functioning as barrier against urine; the "suburothelial" layer consisting of connecting tissue and myofibrolasts; and the outermost smooth muscle layer, also called the "detrusor muscle". The bladder capacity is determined by sensation of fullness in the bladder and suppression of involuntary bladder contraction.

The mechanism generating the sensation of fullness in the bladder is not fully elucidated yet, but both the urothelium and detrusor layer have been shown to play important roles, in coordination with suburothelial peripheral nerves. Contraction of the detrusor muscle can occur in a dramatic manner, with a rapid and large contraction of the bladder wall to expel the urine. This contraction is mediated by cholinergic stimulus of the voiding reflex in response to sensation of urinary fullness in the bladder. Less well known, bladder muscle also shows spontaneous contraction as a localized, asynchronous event in normal bladders (Hashitani et al., 2004; Ikeda et al., 2007). Such spontaneous contractions evoke afferent nerve firing in mouse bladder (McCarthy et al., 2009) and are related to sensation of urinary fullness. In pathological conditions, increased spontaneous excitations within the smooth muscle cells in the bladder related to enhanced propagation of the signal is considered as a myogenic cause of bladder overactivity. However, it is unknown why the bladder radically changes its capacity between day and night.

Reduction in the nighttime functional of bladder capacity is a common feature in pathogenesis of refractory nocturnal enuresis (Yeung et al., 2002) and nocturia in the elderly (Weiss and Blaivas, 2002). Enuretic children and healthy children are capable of holding similar volumes of urine during daytime under a holding exercise, but early-morning voiding volume in enuretic children is smaller than that in healthy children (Van Hoeck et al., 2007a, 2007b). Early-morning voided volume reaches maximal volume voided per micturition in a day in 72% of healthy children but only in 28% of enuretic children. This fact indicates that pathogenesis of enuresis may not be related to the structural bladder size itself but to the regulatory mechanism of day/night change in functional bladder capacity instead. In parallel with this, the elderly have a significantly decreased capacity for normal desire to void during the night compared with middle-aged men (Satoh and Nakada, 1999); such a decrease in nighttime functional bladder capacity also characterizes nocturia (Weiss and Blaivas, 2002).

Day/night shift in bladder function is also recognized for the micturition stream, which is the other dynamic aspect of detrusor muscle contraction. The urine flow rate at voiding time can be measured by a device called "uroflowmeter", equipped in most urology clinic as a noninvasive tool to assess micturition. The flow rate of urine in normal subjects also shows day and night variation, decreased during night and increased during day. Taken together, the bladder contracts less during sleep, which may be associated with a less acute sensation of fullness during sleeping time.

10.2.5 Central control of the kidneys and the bladder

Kidneys and bladder are innervated by a complex network of autonomic and parietal nerves. Thus, regulation of the kidneys and the bladder is intricately associated with the sleep–awake cycle of the brain. The brain also controls production of ADH, thereby controlling urine production from kidneys. In a classical view of physiology, it has been supposed that the CNS regulation could be the only way by which peripheral organs function differently between day and night. However, in such a view, dissociation between the organ functions and arousal status seen in the pathological conditions could not be explained. Why do the kidneys produce an excessive amount of urine, disturbing sound sleep, in enuretic children or nocturic elderly? Why does the nocturnal bladder capacity remain small in both groups of patients? Why do these peripheral organs not follow CNS command in these cases? Before answering these questions, it should first be recognized that it is still not known why and how these daily rhythms are generated in humans and that it is necessary to turn to basic research to solve these problems.

10.3 Animal models

10.3.1 Rats

Rodents are nocturnal animals that are awake during the dark and sleep during the day. Early studies in rodents on the micturition cycle were performed using rats for technical reasons (Andersson et al., 2011). Studies showed that the bladder capacity of rats is increased during sleep and decreased during wake (Schmidt et al., 2001). Our group has replicated those experiments (Fig. 10.1) and found that the urine volume voided per micturition (UVVM), representing functional bladder capacity, shows a robust day/night difference (Negoro et al., 2011). The rats also urinate less frequently in the light than in the dark. Notably, such change was also recorded by cystometrogram, a simulation test of bladder filling and emptying using saline injected through an indwelled catheter connected to a recorder for monitoring the pressure inside the bladder, which is not affected by the urine production rate (Kiddoo et al., 2006). Although rats have been a valuable resource for studying micturition behavior, there are also limitations. As genetically modified mice have become readily available, research has shifted to the use of this species.

10.3.2 Mice

The same kind of day/night variation in micturition frequency seen in rats has also been recognized in mice by researchers, although accurate diachronic measurement of UVVM remains challenging. The UVVM in mice is so small, sometimes less than 50 μl, that it cannot be measured accurately using the electric balance system developed for rats. For studying mouse micturition, researchers have employed urine stain on filter paper as a surrogate of voided volume (Birder et al., 2002; Sugino et al., 2008). In this method, researchers left mice on the lattice, with a filter paper placed below to trap urine drops. The size on the stained filter paper is then converted into UVVM. In order to get information about time, an approach was devised that we call the automated voided stain on paper (aVSOP) method. A rolled laminated filter paper pre-treated to turn the edge of urine stains deep purple is used; this is moved at a constant speed below the mice cage. Using the aVSOP method, the micturition of free-moving mice over the course of several days can be recorded. This method clearly recorded the day and night rhythm of micturition in mice, consisting of daily changes in urine production and bladder capacity to avoid urination during sleep. Importantly, this rhythm was maintained even in constant dark conditions (DD, Fig. 10.2), suggesting that micturition is driven by a circadian clock. We speculate that avoiding micturition during sleep time may be beneficial for rodents as well as for humans.

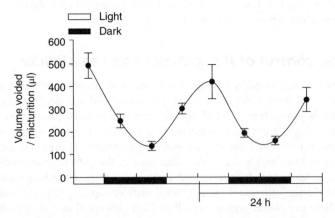

Fig. 10.1 Diurnal rhythm in the bladder capacity of rats, which shows that rats urinate less in light cycle and more in dark cycle (n = 15, 1,001 micturitions for 2 days).

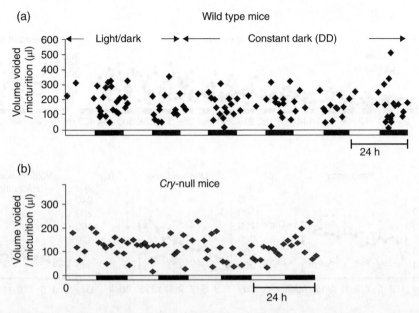

Fig. 10.2 (a) A representative chart showing that diurnal micturition rhythm of a normal mouse in LD cycle is maintained when the rat is kept in constant dark conditions (DD). (b) A representative chart showing that a *Cry*-null mouse lacks circadian micturition rhythm.

We have been investigating the development of micturition rhythms in mice. Newborn mice before weaning cannot urinate without the assistance of their mother, who licks their genitalia to evoke micturition reflex; without this maternal behavior, the newborn can actually die as a result of urinary retention. The weaning phase, when infant mice leave their mother and urinate independently, may correspond to the toilet-training period of humans. The aVSOP system could make an accurate diachronic recording of micturition even in the mice immediately after weaning. According to the recording of infant C57/BL6 mice, a micturition rhythm emerges with a urine production rhythm appearing at 3–4 weeks of age, followed by maturation of a diurnal change in bladder capacity occurring around five weeks of age (Negoro *et al.*, 2013) (Fig. 10.3). Thus, the diurnal micturition rhythm in mice is not yet established by the time of weaning. Thus, we suggest that the developing mouse can provide a model of the control of urination in humans.

10.4 The circadian clock and micturition

As the micturition cycle appears to be a circadian rhythm that continues in constant conditions, it is expected that mutations in the molecular circadian clock would impact the timing of urination (Stow *et al.*, 2012). Indeed, *Cry*-null mice, having a defective circadian clock, show arrhythmic pattern of micturition, urine production, and bladder capacity (Fig. 10.2). *Per1* and *Per2* double knockout (dKO) mice lose the diurnal rhythm of urine volume (Shiromani *et al.*, 2004). The question then arises whether the mutations are acting in the central clock in the SCN or in peripheral clocks found in the kidneys or bladder.

There are rapidly accumulating findings indicating the involvement of a kidney clock for diuresis rhythm. Circadian excretion and reabsorption of water and major electrolytes in urine have been shown physiologically (Roelfsema *et al.*, 1980; Minors and Waterhouse, 1982). The recent molecular chronobiology revealed the corresponding genetic circadian oscillation in transcription of the molecules related to such physiological findings (Zuber *et al.*, 2009). One group of these molecules is related to regulation

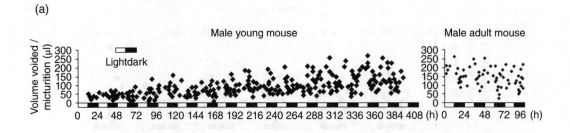

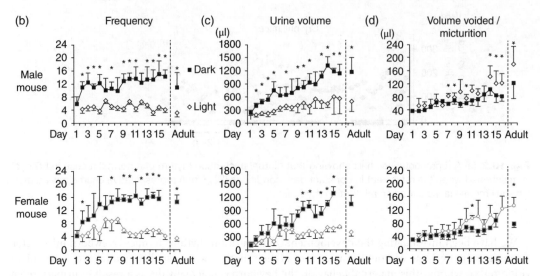

Fig. 10.3 (a) A representative chart illustrating the development of the micturition rhythm. Development of night-and-day changes in micturition parameters in infant mice immediately after weaning shown in (b) miturition frequency, (c) urine volume, and (d) volume voided per micturition, representing the bladder capacity (*: p<0.05).

of water reabsorption: aquaporin-2, 3 and 4, and type 2 vasopressin receptor. Another group is related to regulation of electrolytes movement: control of the sodium transport mediated by epithelial sodium channel (ENaC), the chloride movement across the epithelia, and the potassium excretion. The transcription of many of these genes appears to be rhythmic although the specific role played by each molecule needs further study.

10.5 The clock in the bladder

10.5.1 The bladder has rhythm: demonstration of the circadian clock in the bladder

Involvement of the circadian timing system in the bladder has been explored by our group (Negoro *et al.*, 2012). The existence of a functional peripheral clock in the mouse bladder was proven by three methods. Firstly, it was shown that the circadian expression of clock genes in the bladder collected from mice sacrificed at regular intervals throughout the day and night. The urinary bladder has a strong oscillation rhythm in core clock genes (Chapters 1 and 2), *Per2*, *Bmal1*, *Cry1/2* and *Clock*, and also in regulators, such as *Rev-erbα/β*. Such oscillations were lost in the *Cry*-null mice. Secondly, it was shown that circadian rhythms in bioluminescence could be recorded from the isolated bladder from PER2::LUC knock-in mice (Yoo *et al.*, 2004). This result demonstrates that the peripheral clock in the bladder can function without central cues. Thirdly, rhythms in clock gene expression were demonstrated in primary cultures of bladder smooth muscle cells, which were serum-shocked to synchronize their cellular oscillators (Balsalobre *et al.*, 1998).

With this data, the bladder joins the ranks of other organs, such as liver, kidney, or adrenal gland (Chapter 6), as organs in which a circadian clock has been identified. If these molecular rhythms are related to bladder physiology, one would reason that it should be related with regulation of bladder capacity or contraction, the most conspicuous example of bladder function showing day-to-night change. A microarray analysis of urinary bladder retrieved from C57BL/6 mice under DD conditions revealed that there are thousands of oscillating genes (deposited in Gene Expression Omnibus under accession code GSE35795; Negoro *et al.*, 2012). Most of major molecules related to bladder capacity, such as muscarinic acetylcholine receptors (Andersson, 2010) and transient receptor potential channels (Gevaert *et al.*, 2007), did not show clear oscillations. One key exception has been *Connexin43* (*Cx43*), which emerged as a major regulator of circadian rhythm of the bladder capacity.

10.5.2 Connexin43 (Cx43) is a clock-controlled gene in the bladder

Connexin43 (Cx43) is a gap junction protein in the urinary bladder. There are other types of connexin in the bladder but evidence accumulated thus far implicates only Cx43 as important for bladder capacity. Increases in Cx43 has been associated with bladder overactivity following bladder outlet obstruction. Specifically, the increase in Cx43 enhances intercellular electrical and chemical transmission and sensitizes the response of bladder muscles to cholinergic neural stimuli, thereby decreasing functional bladder capacity and increasing micturition frequency in rats (Imamura *et al.*, 2009). Based on these findings, we investigated the function of Cx43 by analyzing micturition behavior of the *Cx43* heterozygote mice (homozygotes mutants do not survive) and their WT littermates. The aVSOP system revealed that genetic ablation of *Cx43* increased bladder capacity and decreased micturition frequency.

The dynamic oscillation of *Cx43* mRNA in WT mice, demonstrated by microarray and confirmed by real-time reverse transcription polymerase chain reaction (RT-PCR), was also reflected in circadian change in Cx43 protein level, since Cx43 protein has a relatively rapid turnover time, ranging from two to six hours. The circadian oscillation of *Cx43* transcripts and protein was also recognized in cultured bladder smooth muscle cells *in vitro*, confirming that the *Cx43* rhythm is an internally controlled circadian rhythm. Since *Cx43* mRNA oscillates without systemic cues, it was readily hypothesized that a circadian clock regulated circadian oscillation of *Cx43* transcriptions.

Identification of the elements driving the rhythmic transcription of *Cn43* has become an interesting story. On the promoter region of the *Cx43* gene there was neither consensus E-box, D-box, nor canonical retinoic acid receptor-related orphan receptors response element (RORE) sequences recruiting the binding of clock proteins. Surprisingly, promoter–reporter assay of *Cx43* promoter revealed that Rev-erbα, the clock component molecule known to be transcriptional suppressor, enhanced transcription of *Cx43*. This finding was confirmed by downregulation of *Cx43* transcripts after reduction of Rev-erbα by RNA interference in cultured bladder smooth muscle cells (Fig. 10.4a).

These findings have lead us to suggest a novel paradigm for control of circadian gene expression: an oscillating circadian clock component (Rev-erbα) can modulate the activity of transcription factors coded by nonoscillating nonclock genes (*Sp1*) by functioning as transcriptional cofactors, and produce genetic oscillation of a target gene (*Cx43*). It is worth noting that genome-wide screening of putative clock-associated sequences has revealed that many genes showing circadian oscillation do not have binding sequences for clock proteins (Panda *et al.*, 2002; Ueda *et al.*, 2005). Thus, we propose the possibility that some of these genes could be regulated by the clock protein, Rev-erbα, acting as a cofactor.

Finally, is this oscillation of *Cx43* transcripts and protein physiologically or clinically relevant? It should be, since the rise of Cx43 protein corresponds to the waking time of mice and, also, bladder smooth muscle cells cultured *in vitro* shows temporal change in cell-to-cell diffusion of fluorescent dyes, which occurs in parallel with a shift in Cx43 protein level. In short, the bladder "wakes up" in the beginning of

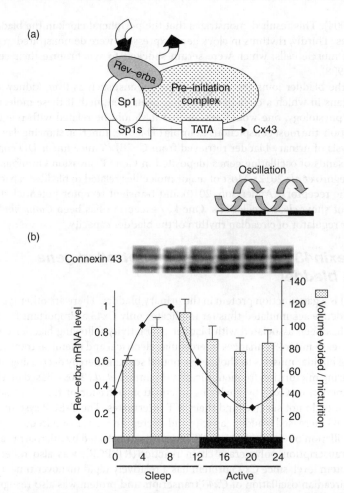

Fig. 10.4 (a) A mechanistic scheme of *Cx43* oscillation, controlled by the Rev-erbα and Sp1 complex binding to Sp1 sites of the *Cx43* promoter. (b) Circadian rhythms of *Rev-erbα* mRNA expression, Cx43 protein expression and volume voided per micturition. Note that the rhythm of Cx43 protein expression follows that of *Rev-erbα* mRNA expression and that when Cx43 expression is at the peak, volume voided per micturition is at the bottom, and vice versa.

the active phase with a rise in Cx43, allowing transmission of stimulus promoting micturition, and "falls asleep" at the end of the active phase with a decrease in Cx43, which shuts down the gate for the cells to intercommunicate (Fig. 10.4b). The daily increase in cell-to-cell communication should lead to increased spontaneous contraction in muscle layer, or facilitate sensation of urinary fullness to be propagated through afferent nerves.

10.6 Future directions

10.6.1 Basic research

What are the next steps in basic research into the mechanisms underlying the micturition rhythm? Comprehensive analyses like microarray have already presented a list of oscillating genes in the kidney and in the bladder. The function of these genes should be analyzed one by one. The amount of candidate genes could be limited by focusing on those with a high amplitude oscillation. This work would need to be undertaken by researchers with expertise in nephrological and the urological sciences. Ideally, the genetic mutations would be targeted to just kidneys or bladder to isolate the impact of the manipulation to a single structure. Therefore, though not feasible yet, generating and analyzing animals with kidney- or bladder-specific genetic modification would make fundamental progress for investigating the role of the candidate genes as well as the circadian clock in these organs. Such animals would become models of enuresis or nocturia, where rhythms of brain, kidneys, and bladder are dissociated or mismatched between each other.

In the bladder, the function of the circadian clocks in the three main cell populations, including the smooth muscle layer as well as the urothelium and suburothelial layers, will need to be explored. For example, the urothelium has recently been conceived as mechanosensor that detects fullness of urine in the bladder, acting as a starting end of afferent neural transmission (Birder and de Groat, 2007). In other regions, the sensory fibers are "gated" by the circadian system and this may turn out to be the case in urothelium. Another important area for future research is to discover the signals that synchronize or disturb the bladder clock. Although the signals from the central clock in the SCN should play a significant role via innervation to the bladder, the bladder clock is likely to be synchronized or tuned by bladder-specific mechanisms. These mechanisms and the impact of disease on this synchronization are not understood. Finally, more evidence is needed that the molecular clockwork impacts the daily rhythm in micturition and how this timing is altered by disease.

10.6.2 Clinical research

What could be done to advance this field into clinical practice and to determine the role of the circadian clock for micturition rhythm as well as a therapeutic target in treating enuresis and nocturia? One strategy is to focus on each target organ, the kidneys and the bladder. By altering the urine production rhythm in the kidneys, one could aim to develop novel drugs to suppress nighttime urine production, other than desmopressin, which is the only drug available on the market. For the bladder, one could consider a organ-specific gap-junction inhibitor for treating patients with enuresis and nocturia. Unfortunately, the currently available gap-junction inhibiting molecules are not specific for the bladder and cause a variety of adverse reactions. For example, our preliminary clinical trial of glytirrhetic acid, a gap junction inhibitory agent, for treating overactive bladder patients was performed but had to be suspended because of adverse effects, such as hypokalemia or hypertension, seen in the treated patients (unpublished data). However, history has shown with an alpha-blocker for prostate hypertrophy, and anticholinergics for overactive bladder, that revolutionary drugs can be created if the drugs whose action is specific to the bladder can be identified. We predict that a bladder-specific gap-junction inhibitor without systemic adverse effect would be a promising measure to treat the patients with lower urinary tract symptoms.

The other, much broader, strategy for treating enuresis or nocturia is to deal with circadian system itself. While not yet causally established, our data indicate that enuresis and nocturia may well be related to mistiming in the circadian system. If so, this opens up a new set of interventions that could be used. For example, melatonin and melatonin receptor agonists like ramelteon may well improve the synchronization of the circadian system and, through this mechanism, increase bladder capacity and reduce the bother of nocturia. Similarly, improvements in lifestyle are known to affect the symptoms of nocturia significantly (Soda *et al.*, 2010). Therefore, we can speculate that scheduled light exposure, exercise, and meals (Schroeder and Colwell, 2013) could be new candidates for treatment and prevention of enuresis and nocturia. In short, the recognition that the bladder and kidneys have peripheral circadian clocks has provided a new perspective for considering highly prevalent micturition problems like enuresis and nocturia.

References

Andersson KE. 2010. Antimuscarinic mechanisms and the overactive detrusor: an update. *Eur Urol* **59**:377–386.

Andersson KE, Soler R, Fullhase C. 2011. Rodent models for urodynamic investigation. *Neurourol Urodyn* **30**:636–646.

Balsalobre A, Damiola F, Schibler U. 1998. A serum shock induces circadian gene expression in mammalian tissue culture cells. *Cell* **93**:929–937.

Birder LA, Nakamura Y, Kiss S, *et al.* 2002. Altered urinary bladder function in mice lacking the vanilloid receptor TRPV1. *Nat Neurosci* **5**:856–860.

Birder LA, de Groat WC. 2007. Mechanisms of disease: involvement of the urothelium in bladder dysfunction. *Nat Clin Pract Urol* **4**:46–54.

Bosch JL, Weiss JP. 2010. The prevalence and causes of nocturia. *J Urol* **184**:440–446.

Gevaert T, Vriens J, Segal A, *et al.* 2007. Deletion of the transient receptor potential cation channel TRPV4 impairs murine bladder voiding. *J Clin Invest* **117**:3453–3462.

Hashitani H, Brading AF, Suzuki H. 2004. Correlation between spontaneous electrical, calcium and mechanical activity in detrusor smooth muscle of the guinea-pig bladder. *Br J Pharmacol* **141**:183–193.

Ikeda Y, Fry C, Hayashi F, *et al.* 2007. Role of gap junctions in spontaneous activity of the rat bladder. *Am J Physiol Renal Physiol* **293**:F1018–F1025.

Imamura M, Negoro H, Kanematsu A, *et al.* 2009. Basic fibroblast growth factor causes urinary bladder overactivity through gap junction generation in the smooth muscle. *Am J Physiol Renal Physiol* **297**:46–54.

Kiddoo DA, Valentino RJ, Zderic S, *et al.* 2006. Impact of state of arousal and stress neuropeptides on urodynamic function in freely moving rats. *Am J Physiol Regul Integr Comp Physiol* **290**:R1697–R1706.

McCarthy CJ, Zabbarova IV, Brumovsky PR, *et al.* 2009. Spontaneous contractions evoke afferent nerve firing in mouse bladders with detrusor overactivity. *J Urol* **181**:1459–1466.

Minors DS, Waterhouse JM. 1982. Circadian rhythms of urinary excretion: the relationship between the amount excreted and the circadian changes. *J Physiol* **327**:39–51.

Nakamura S, Kobayashi Y, Tozuka K, *et al.* 1996. Circadian changes in urine volume and frequency in elderly men. *J Urol* **156**:1275–1279.

Nakagawa H, Niu K, Hozawa A, *et al.* 2010 Impact of nocturia on bone fracture and mortality in older individuals: a Japanese longitudinal cohort study. *J Urol* **184**:1413–1418.

Negoro H, Kanematsu A, Imamura M, *et al.* 2011. Regulation of connexin 43 by basic fibroblast growth factor in the bladder: transcriptional and behavioral implications. *J Urol* **185**:2398–2404.

Negoro H, Kanematsu A, Doi M, *et al.* 2012. Involvement of urinary bladder Connexin43 and the circadian clock in coordination of diurnal micturition rhythm. *Nat Commun* **3**:809–.

Negoro H, Kanematsu A, Matsuo M, *et al.* 2013. Development of diurnal micturition pattern in mice after weaning. *J Urol* **189**(2):740–746.

Neveus T. 2009. Diagnosis and management of nocturnal enuresis. *Curr Opin Pediatr* **21**:199–202.

Panda S, Antoch MP, Miller BH, *et al.* 2002. Coordinated transcription of key pathways in the mouse by the circadian clock. *Cell* **109**:307–320.

Robson WL. 2009. Clinical practice. Evaluation and management of enuresis. *N Engl J Med* **360**:1429–1436.

Roelfsema F, van der Heide D, Smeenk D. 1980. Circadian rhythms of urinary electrolyte excretion in freely moving rats. *Life Sci* **27**:2303–2309.

Satoh W, Nakada T. 1999. Characteristics of circadian change in urinary frequency, bladder capacity and residual urine volume in elderly men with lower urinary tract symptoms. *Nurs Health Sci* **1**:125–129.

Schmidt F, Yoshimura Y, Ni RX, *et al.* 2001. Influence of gender on the diurnal variation of urine production and micturition characteristics of the rat. *Neurourol Urodyn* **20**:287–295.

Schroeder AM, Colwell CS. 2013. How to fix a broken clock. *Trends Pharmacol Sci* **34**:605–619.

Shiromani PJ, Xu M, Winston EM, *et al.* 2004. Sleep rhythmicity and homeostasis in mice with targeted disruption of mPeriod genes. *Am J Physiol Regul Integr Comp Physiol* **287**:R47–R57.

Soda T, Masui K, Okuno H, *et al.* 2010. Efficacy of nondrug lifestyle measures for the treatment of nocturia. *J Urol* **184**:1000–1004.

Stow LR, Richards J, Cheng KY, *et al.* 2012. The circadian protein period 1 contributes to blood pressure control and coordinately regulates renal sodium transport genes. *Hypertension* **59**:1151–1156.

Sugino Y, Kanematsu A, Hayashi Y, *et al.* 2008. Voided stain on paper method for analysis of mouse. *Neurourol Urodyn* **27**:548–552.

Ueda HR, Hayashi S, Chen W, *et al.* 2005. System-level identification of transcriptional circuits underlying mammalian circadian clocks. *Nat Genet* **37**:187–192.

Van Hoeck K, Bael A, Lax H, *et al.* 2007a. Urine output rate and maximum volume voided in school-age children with and without nocturnal enuresis. *J Pediatr* **151**:575–580.

Van Hoeck K, Bael A, Lax H, *et al.* 2007b. Circadian variation of voided volume in normal school-age children. *Eur J Pediatr* **166**:579–584.

Weiss JP, Blaivas JG. 2002. Nocturnal polyuria versus overactive bladder in nocturia. *Urology* **60**:28–32.

Yeung CK, Sit FK, To LK, *et al.* 2002. Reduction in nocturnal functional bladder capacity is a common factor in the pathogenesis of refractory nocturnal enuresis. *BJU Int* **90**:302–307.

Yoo SH, Yamazaki S, Lowrey PL, *et al.* 2004. PERIOD2::LUCIFERASE real-time reporting of circadian dynamics reveals persistent circadian oscillations in mouse peripheral tissues. *Proc Natl Acad Sci USA* **101**:5339–5346.

Yoshimura K. 2012. Correlates for nocturia: a review of epidemiological studies. *Int J Urol* **19**:317–329.

Zuber AM, Centeno G, Pradervand S, *et al.* 2009. Molecular clock is involved in predictive circadian adjustment of renal function. *Proc Natl Acad Sci USA* **106**:16523–16528.

Disruption of Circadian Rhythms and Development of Type 2 Diabetes Mellitus: Contributions to Insulin Resistance and Beta-cell Failure

11

Aleksey V. Matveyenko

Department of Physiology and Biomedical Engineering, Mayo Clinic, Rochester, MN, USA; Department of Medicine, University of California Los Angeles, Los Angeles, CA, USA

11.1 Introduction

The incidence of Type 2 diabetes mellitus (T2DM) has truly reached an epidemic proportion worldwide. Recent estimates show that nearly 360 million people globally have been diagnosed with T2DM, resulting in nearly five million yearly deaths attributed to this debilitating disease (Whiting *et al.*, 2011). Alarmingly, the incidence of T2DM worldwide is expected to continue to rise and projected to afflict nearly 600 million people within the next two decades. Since clinical manifestation of T2DM is still poorly defined and diabetes testing is rare, it has been estimated that most patients with T2DM are often diagnosed several years after the disease onset, suggesting that current diabetes prevalence figures often significantly underestimate the global impact of diabetes burden worldwide.

T2DM is associated with severe harmful health complications that afflict both the quality and the length of life and burden health care systems with direct global spending estimated at nearly US$500 billion per year (Whiting *et al.*, 2011). Macrovascular complications in diabetes increase risk of coronary heart disease, stroke and hypertension whereas microvascular complications commonly lead to blindness, kidney failure, peripheral neuropathy and increased risk of amputations (Stratton *et al.*, 2000). In addition, patients with T2DM are more likely to develop a variety of common cancers, as cancer increasingly becoming one of the leading causes of mortality and morbidity associated with T2DM (Braun *et al.*, 2011). Undoubtedly, there is an urgent need for the development of novel therapeutic and lifestyle altering strategies to combat the rise in T2DM prevalence worldwide. However, to meet this objective it is critical to thoroughly elucidate environmental, physiological and molecular mechanisms underlying pathogenesis of T2DM in the 21st century.

Circadian Medicine, First Edition. Edited by Christopher S. Colwell.

11.2 Mechanisms underlying pathophysiology of Type 2 diabetes mellitus: interaction between insulin resistance and beta-cell failure

T2DM diagnosis is defined by onset of fasting and postprandial hyperglycemia, commencement of which involves a complex interaction among polygenetic predispositions and numerous confounding environmental contributors. When induction of hyperglycemia in T2DM is examined longitudinally in humans, the transition from normoglycemia to hyperglycemia is characterized by (i) a prolonged (up to several years) period of slow linear increases in glucose concentrations (period termed pre-diabetes) followed by (ii) a rapid phase of glucose decompensation during which there is an exponential rise in fasting and postprandial glucose occurring within 1–3 years of clinical diagnosis (Mason *et al.*, 2007). The observation that the initial rise in glycemia in T2DM patients exhibits slow decade-long linear increases (which often remain asymptomatic and undetected), provides important insights into the complexities of diabetes diagnosis and implementation of preventative strategies.

Physiologically, the initiation of hyperglycemia in T2DM occurs as a result of the failure to maintain adequate pancreatic beta-cell insulin secretion (i.e., beta-cell failure) to compensate for a progressive decline in insulin action/sensitivity (insulin resistance) (Bergman *et al.*, 1981). Although the precise mechanisms and timelines by which insulin resistance and beta-cell failure interact to induce hyperglycemia still remain an active area of investigation and some controversy, both factors are prominent features of T2DM and imperative for full manifestation of the disease. The relationship between insulin secretion and insulin sensitivity in health and diabetes can be graphically illustrated as a hyperbolic curve (Fig. 11.1), as first described in classic experiments undertaken by Bergman and colleagues (DeFronzo, 1988). The x-axis of the hyperbolic curve represents a measure of insulin sensitivity whereas the y-axis represents a determinant of beta-cell insulin secretion. In nondiabetic individuals, the mathematical product of insulin secretion and insulin sensitivity (termed disposition index) falls "on" or "above" the hyperbolic curve, thus representing an adequate insulin release required to appropriately activate insulin signaling in insulin-sensitive tissues. On the other hand, in patients with T2DM, disposition index falls "below" the hyperbolic curve, thus indicating inappropriate or failed stimulation of insulin secretion in lieu of prevailing insulin sensitivity. The next question to be addressed is: What physiological and molecular mechanisms underlie declines in insulin sensitivity and insulin secretion in T2DM patients?

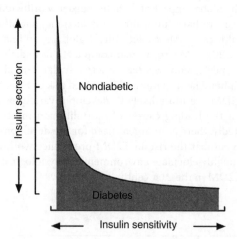

Fig. 11.1 Graphical relationships between insulin secretion and insulin sensitivity in health and T2DM in humans.

Insulin resistance is defined as a reduction in insulin's ability to activate cellular insulin signaling cascade and, consequently, stimulate insulin-mediated biological processes. Insulin resistance in T2DM primarily manifests in the liver and the skeletal muscle. However, newer studies suggest that abnormal insulin signaling in other cell types (e.g., hypothalamic neurons and adipocytes) may also contribute to hyperglycemia in T2DM (Defronzo, 2009). Specifically, in the liver, insulin resistance is associated with inappropriately elevated rates of hepatic glucose production at fasting, attributed in part to failed insulin-mediated suppression of gluconeogenesis. Hepatic insulin resistance is also associated with failure to suppress hepatic glucose production in the postprandial state, attributed to failed suppression of gluco-neogenesis, glycogenolysis and inappropriate hepatic glucose uptake (Rizza, 2010). In skeletal muscle, insulin resistance manifests due to diminished insulin-stimulated recruitment of GLUT-4 glucose trans-porter protein to the plasma membrane, decrease in glycogen storage and glucose oxidation resulting in inappropriate activation of skeletal muscle glucose clearance following a meal.

Although genetic susceptibility undoubtedly plays a contributory role in pathogenesis of insulin resis-tance, lifestyle factors, such as obesity and physical inactivity, are considered to be the primary determi-nants of insulin action in T2DM (Koivisto et al., 1986). Specifically, evidence suggests that induction of insulin resistance in T2DM at the molecular level is largely attributed to ectopic lipid accumulation in insulin–sensitive tissues (i.e., liver, skeletal muscle and adipose tissue) largely attributed to induction of obesity and related phenotype (Samuel and Shulman, 2012).

Over the years, a number of potential molecular mechanisms have been proposed to explain the ori-gins of obesity-induced insulin resistance in T2DM. In muscle and liver, ectopic lipid deposition due to obesity-induced intracellular accumulation and consequent trafficking of lipid signaling intermediates (i.e., ceramides and diacylglycerols) play a major role in development of impaired activation of cellular insulin signaling cascade (Samuel and Shulman, 2012). Specifically, intracellular accumulation of diacyl-glycerols and ceramides contributes to insulin resistance through deleterious effects of these lipid inter-mediates on activation of the insulin signaling molecules, such as insulin receptor substrate 1/2(IRS-1/2) and AKT2 mediated in part through activation of serione/threonine kinases such as Protein Kinase C θ. In addition, obesity in T2DM is also associated with impaired adipocytes metabolism resulting in (i) excessive lipolysis and consequent increase in plasma free fatty acid levels and (ii) excessive production and secretion of pro-inflammatory cytokines (i.e., TNF-α, Il-6 etc.) which are thought to originate from activated adipose tissue macrophages (Hotamisligil, 2006). Thus, aberrant adipose tissue metabolism in T2DM can directly contribute to insulin resistance in target tissues through increase in lipid accumulation or indirectly through cytokine-mediated disruption of the insulin signaling cascade in the liver and skeletal muscle as a result of activating cytokine-mediated pro-inflammatory pathways. Finally, it is also important to point out that once hyperglycemia develops, chronic elevations in prevailing glycemia (termed glucotoxicity) can further diminish activation skeletal muscle and hepatic insulin signaling, thus further exacerbating ongoing insulin resistance in T2DM (Defronzo, 2009).

Defective insulin secretion in T2DM is a characteristic metabolic abnormality and develops as a result of impaired pancreatic beta-cell secretory function (i.e., inappropriate release of insulin by pancreatic beta cells) and the deficit in beta-cell mass (i.e., reduction in total number of beta-cells in the pancreas) (Meier, 2005). Importantly, a near complete loss of glucose-stimulated insulin secretion is already evi-dent prior to clinical diagnosis of T2DM (i.e., during the pre-diabetes or impaired fasting glucose (IFG) stage) (Kahn, 2001). Furthermore, disturbances in glucose-stimulated insulin secretion can also be detected in normoglycemic first degree relatives of patients with T2DM, suggesting that the loss of insulin secretion in T2DM precedes induction of hyperglycemia and exhibits a strong genetic compo-nent (Kahn, 2001). In support of this, genome wide association studies have identified several T2DM-associaited gene variants purported to control beta-cell molecular pathways that mediate beta-cell secretory function, beta-cell development, proliferation and survival (Florez, 2008).

The quantitative contribution of beta-cell secretory dysfunction versus the loss of beta-cell mass to impaired insulin secretion in T2DM remains unknown. This problem is largely attributed to the inability to accurately predict or measure beta-cell mass *in vivo* in humans. However, some insights into beta-cell pathology can be gleaned from studies that utilized autopsy pancreata from patients diagnosed with IFG (pre-diabetes) and/or T2DM (Matveyenko and Butler, 2008). These studies report that there is already an approximately 50% deficit in beta-cell mass in people with IFG, and an approximately 65% decrease in beta-cell mass in those patients with T2DM (Butler *et al.*, 2003). This suggests that the quantitative loss of beta-cell numbers is a relatively "early" abnormality in T2DM, occurring prior to clinical diagnosis. Further evidence for the importance of beta-cell loss in the pathophysiology of IFG and T2DM comes from numerous animal models of reduced beta-cell mass (e.g., rodents, pigs, dogs and nonhuman primates), in which reduction of beta-cell mass to the extent reported in humans with IFG and T2DM (about 50–65%) results in induction of hyperglycemia (Matveyenko and Butler, 2008). Taken together, loss of beta-cell mass and secretory function is an "early" pathophysiological event in diabetes progression which underlies diminished glucose-stimulated insulin secretion and failed adaptation to insulin resistance. Next, an overview is provided on the molecular mechanisms responsible for the loss of beta-cell secretory function and mass in T2DM.

The maintenance of appropriate beta-cell mass relies on a sufficient early-life beta-cell formation as well as regulated turnover of beta-cell numbers during adulthood, a process driven by an intricate balance between beta-cell proliferation, neogenesis and apoptosis (Butler *et al.*, 2007). The early-life formation of beta-cell mass in humans occurs rapidly during the first years of life and plateaus by 5–10 years of age. Importantly, studies in humans indicate that early-life formation of beta-cell mass is influenced by multiple genetic as well as epigenetic factors, which can subsequently modulate susceptibility to T2DM in adulthood. For example, genome wide association studies report that variants in beta-cell genome controlling cell cycle regulation increase susceptibility to T2DM in humans, likely through regulation of fetal and postnatal beta-cell formation/programming (Florez, 2008). The deficit in beta-cell mass seen in patients with T2DM in adulthood has been also attributed to increased beta-cell loss as a consequence of increased beta-cell attrition (Butler *et al.*, 2003). Indeed pancreatic islets in T2DM patients display increased frequency of beta-cell apoptosis associated with induction of endoplasmic and oxidative stress. Although the exact etiology of increased beta-cell apoptosis in T2DM remains an area of investigation, a number of potential mechanisms have been proposed; these include interactions among the toxicity due to exposure to high glucose levels (*glucotoxicity*), toxicity due to exposure to high concentrations of free fatty acids (*lipotoxicity*) and toxicity due to intracellular formation of human islet amyloid polypeptide (h-IAPP) oligomers (*proteotoxicity*) (Haataja *et al.*, 2008).

The cause of defective beta-cell secretory function in T2DM also shows a strong genetic component given the fact that glucose-stimulated insulin secretion is already deficient in first degree-relatives of T2DM patients, presumably prior to any loss of beta-cell mass (Kahn, 2001). In addition, induction of gluco- and lipotoxicity associated with T2DM phenotype also profoundly disrupts beta-cell secretory function and, thus, constrains glucose-stimulated insulin secretion *in vivo*. The mechanisms likely include increased formation of mitochondrial reactive oxygen species leading to depletion of insulin stores due to decrease in genes regulating insulin production/secretion, that is, insulin and pancreatic duodenal homeobox 1 (PDX-1) (Poitout and Robertson, 2007). Furthermore, prolonged hyperglycemia/ hyperlipidemia also impairs beta-cell secretory function by altering expression of genes regulating beta-cell glucose sensing and glycolytic flux such GLUT2 and glucokinase (Laybutt *et al.*, 2002). Taken together, decline in beta-cell secretory function is an early event in the etiology of T2DM that exhibits strong genetic susceptibility. In addition, as diabetes evolves induction of hyperglycemia/hyperlipidemia further disrupts beta-cell function, which together with already deficient beta-cell mass results in accelerated beta-cell failure characterized by loss of fasting and postprandial insulin release.

In summary, Fig. 11.2 graphically illustrates the interactions between induction of insulin resistance and beta-cell failure during progression to T2DM in humans. In short, elevations in prevailing glycemia in T2DM develops as a result of interplay between impaired insulin sensitivity, primarily manifesting at the level of the liver and skeletal muscle, and an inadequate compensatory stimulation of insulin secretion, attributed to the decline in beta-cell mass and secretory function. The current view indicates that the decline in insulin sensitivity in T2DM is largely due to lifestyle factors, such as obesity and physical inactivity, resulting in consequent ectopic lipid accumulation in insulin sensitive cell types. On the other hand, decline in beta-cell secretory function and mass is primarily, but not exclusively, attributed to genetic and developmental factors that are exacerbated by induction of gluco- and lipotoxicity and consequent oxidative stress. Having overviewed pathophysiology of T2DM onset, the next question to be

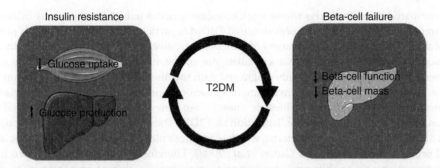

Fig. 11.2 Pathophysiology of Type 2 diabetes. Type 2 diabetes is a complex metabolic disease, the pathophysiology of which involves an interaction between genetic predisposition and environmental triggers. Hyperglycemia occurs as a result of pancreatic beta-cell failure in response to insulin resistance. Beta-cell failure in T2DM is associated with a deficit in beta-cell mass and beta-cell function. Insulin resistance in T2DM primarily manifests at the level of the liver and the skeletal muscle, characterized by impaired insulin-stimulated glucose disposal and failure to adequately suppress hepatic glucose production.

addressed is how does disruption of circadian rhythms contributes to growing global epidemic of T2DM and what mechanisms underlie this phenomenon.

11.2.1 Circadian disruption and predisposition to Type 2 diabetes mellitus: accumulating evidence from epidemiological, clinical and animal studies

As discussed in detail in preceding chapters, the mammalian circadian system is organized as a multi-level oscillator network. The main circadian oscillator is localized in the suprachiasmatic nucleus (SCN) (Chapter 3) and synchronized to the changes in the light/dark (LD) cycle through specialized retinal ganglion cells with light serving as the principal entrainment stimuli. The SCN, in turn, plays a pivotal role in synchronizing the rhythms of the peripheral circadian clocks to the 24-hour LD cycle. Subsequently, the SCN employs neuroendocrine, autonomic and hormonal cues to synchronize an organism's physiological and molecular circadian rhythms to anticipate diurnal behavioral changes such as sleep–wake and fast–feeding cycles. This complex multilevel circadian oscillator system undoubtedly provides an evolutionary advantage for human health and survival, however this system becomes disadvantageous when lifestyle factors impose time constrains that produce misalignment between internal circadian oscillators and their functions and the external environment (i.e., *circadian disruption*).

In the last few decades, global human population has become increasingly exposed to conditions associated with disruption of normal circadian rhythms resulting in numerous deleterious health consequences, which include increased predisposition to T2DM (Chapter 13). This trend can be attributed to numerous factors, some of which include, but are not limited to, (i) increased reliance on rotational shift work and extended work schedules, (ii) advent of new media technologies with 24-hour cycles of news and entertainment, and (iii) technological advances in lighting leading to light pollution (Wyse *et al.*, 2011). In the United States alone, more than 70% of adults report inadequate sleep quality and duration (Beihl *et al.*, 2009) and nearly 20 million people are exposed to daily shift work conditions (Basner *et al.*, 2007). Alarmingly, circadian disruption is particularly prevalent in adolescents, a group in which there has been a recent marked decline in sleep quality and duration associated with increased nocturnal light exposure due to extensive use of media technology (Kohyama, 2009). Importantly, this recent spike in circadian disruption in adolescence has coincided with a marked increase in the incidence of T2DM and metabolic syndrome in the same age group (Weigensberg and Goran, 2009).

Numerous epidemiological studies report an association between work conditions characterized by circadian disruption (i.e., shift/night work) and susceptibility to Type 2 diabetes (Chapter 13). For example, individuals assigned to work all three daily shifts have a three times higher prevalence of diabetes compared to counterparts whose work schedule is restricted to day shifts only (Mikuni *et al.*, 1983). A significant increment in the prevalence of T2DM is particularly seen in individuals performing rotational shift work, reported across variety of professional industries (Kivimaki *et al.*, 2011). In addition, epidemiological studies also show that circadian disruption negatively impacts the treatment and management of diabetes in those already diagnosed with the disease. However, it is important to point out that a number of confounding environmental, socioeconomic and health-related variables (i.e., socioeconomic status, health habits, lifestyle choices, etc.) may contribute to the observed positive association between shift work and predisposition to T2DM. For example, shift work is typically associated with disrupted/deficient sleep patterns, which is another independent factor closely associated with increased prevalence of T2DM (Van Cauter *et al.*, 2008). Therefore, some studies examined impact of circadian disruption akin to shift work conditions on regulation of glucose homeostasis in controlled laboratory settings in healthy human volunteers (Scheer *et al.*, 2009; Buxton *et al.*, 2012). In those studies, exposure to circadian misalignment during which individuals ate, slept and functioned 12 hours out of phase of their typical daily living schedules (shift work paradigm) raised prevailing glucose concentrations and induced glucose intolerance in as little as 10 days. Interestingly, Scheer and colleagues show that in a subset of individuals (about 40%) 10 days of circadian misalignment led to the level of glucose intolerance that can be classified as "pre-diabetic" according to American Diabetes Association diagnostic criteria. It is intriguing to hypothesize that, as with other known environmental triggers such as obesity, circadian misalignment may promote development of T2DM in the subset of the population with genetic predisposition.

Epidemiological and clinical studies in humans undoubtedly present an advantage of being more relevant to conditions of daily living and direct relevance to human health. However, interpretation of these studies may be hindered by confounding social, psychological and physiological variables associated with induction of circadian disruption. For this reason, investigators have turned to rodent models to examine the impact of circadian disruption on regulation of glucose homeostasis and predisposition to T2DM independent of potential confounding variables (Fonken *et al.*, 2010; Gale *et al.*, 2011; Husse *et al.*, 2012). Specifically, experimental disruption in the light/dark cycle produced by either prolonged exposure to constant light or frequent six-hour advances in the light cycle induce impaired glucose tolerance and accelerate development of T2DM in diabetes-prone rodents (Gale *et al.*, 2011). Similar results are obtained in rodent models where animals are kept awake and active during the "inactive" phase of the LD cycle and vice versa, thus designed to recapitulate conditions associated with human shift work (Husse *et al.*, 2012).

Additional support for the association between circadian disruption and T2DM comes from mice genetics experiments. Specifically, whole body genetic mutations in the core intracellular circadian clock components, such as *Clock, Bmal1, Per1* and *Per2*, are all associated with disrupted glucose homeostasis leading to glucose intolerance and prevailing hyperglycemia (Turek *et al.*, 2005; Lamia *et al.*, 2008). Furthermore, studies show that alterations in glucose homeostasis can also be observed in rodents with conditional mutations in circadian clock components in the liver (Lamia *et al.*, 2008), skeletal muscle (Andrews *et al.*, 2010) and the beta-cell (Marcheva *et al.*, 2010), tissues critical for maintenance of proper glucose control in health and T2DM.

11.3 Mechanisms underlying the association between circadian disruption and T2DM; potential role of obesity and insulin resistance

As previously overviewed, hyperglycemia in T2DM develops as a result of an interaction between insulin resistance (primarily manifested at the level of liver, skeletal muscle and adipose tissue) and pancreatic beta-cell failure (Fig. 11.2). We will first address potential mechanisms underlying the association between circadian disruption and insulin resistance, with particular emphasis on predisposition to obesity. Pathophysiology of insulin resistance in T2DM is largely attributed to ectopic lipid accumulation in insulin–sensitive tissues as a consequence of increased weight gain, visceral adiposity and consequent induction of obese phenotype (Samuel and Shulman, 2012). Epidemiological studies link circadian disruption to predisposition to obesity in humans. For example, rotational shift work displays strong association with increased body mass index (BMI), visceral fat accumulation and hypertriglyceridemia, partially attributed to increased preference for high energy foods and disrupted feeding patterns (Wyse et al., 2011). Moreover, shift work is also associated with ectopic lipid accumulation in insulin-sensitive organs such as the liver, a condition highly correlated to hepatic insulin resistance and predisposition to T2DM in humans (Lin and Chen, 2012). Notably, the association between shift work and obesity in humans appears to be independent from numerous lifestyle and occupation related, confounding variables supporting the postulate that circadian disruption associated with shift work is indeed is the primary inducer of the obesity-related phenotype (Suwazono et al., 2009).

In support of this premise, experiments in rodents also clearly show that circadian disruption is associated with increased weight gain, body adiposity and food intake. Accelerated weight gain due to increased adiposity in laboratory rodents has been observed following exposure to (i) repeated shifts in the LD cycle (Tsai et al., 2005), (ii) shortened LD cycle period (20 h) (Karatsoreos et al., 2011), as well as (iii) exposure to constant light (LL) (Fonken et al., 2010). Moreover, animal experiments also demonstrate a relationship between the endogenous circadian period (tau) and susceptibility to obesity. Specifically, an increase in susceptibility to obesity is observed in rodent strains in which an endogenous circadian period exhibits largest deviation from the environmental 24-hour period, whereas rodent strains characterized by robust high amplitude circadian rhythms of about 24 hours display reduced caloric consumption, increased life span and resistance to metabolic syndrome (Campuzano et al., 1999; Froy et al., 2006). These studies suggest that the deviation of genetically predetermined endogenous circadian period from 24 hours may also underlie increased susceptibility to obesity and metabolic syndrome in mammalian species. This postulate is supported by studies demonstrating an association between polymorphisms and/or genetic variants in key clock genes (Clock, Per2) and susceptibility to obesity in humans (Scott et al., 2008; Garaulet et al., 2010). Specifically, Per2 polymorphism in humans is associated with increased abdominal adiposity and, more interestingly, with modulation of the eating behavior resulting in the attrition to weight-loss treatment (Garaulet et al., 2010). In addition, whole body Clock and Bmal1 mutant mice display similar increased adiposity phenotype characterized by abnormal plasma lipid profile and fragmented feeding patterns (Turek et al., 2005; Lamia et al., 2008). These observations raise an important next question. What physiological and molecular mechanisms underlie increased susceptibility to adiposity in response to circadian disruption?

Alteration in the proper circadian timing of food consumption has been hypothesized to mediate deleterious effects of circadian disruption on the propensity to develop obesity. Circadian organization of food consumption is driven by the SCN and under normal LD cycle conditions is restricted to the activity phase (light cycle in humans and night cycle in rodents). In animal models, circadian disruption due to either (i) SCN ablation, (ii) exposure to light at night, (iii) forced wakefulness during the rest period or (iv) Clock gene mutation leads to shifting of the time of food intake from the activity to the rest period of daily circadian cycle. Importantly, this shift in the timing of the food consumption results in excessive weight gain and propensity to develop metabolic syndrome despite the fact that the cumulative caloric consumption remains unchanged (Arble et al., 2009; Hatori et al., 2012). A similar phenomenon is observed in humans undergoing shift/night work or individuals afflicted with "night eating syndrome" who consume nearly two thirds of their daily caloric intake outside of the circadian activity phase (Colles et al., 2007). Consistent with animal experiments (Chapter 7), these individuals display accelerated weight gain and predisposition to metabolic syndrome. Importantly, correcting the phase of circadian eating patterns by restricting food intake to typical activity phase prevents excessive weight gain and reverses metabolic abnormalities associated with obesity and metabolic syndrome (Hatori et al., 2012).

Mechanisms behind accelerated adiposity and metabolic dysregulation following misaligned feeding patterns remain an area of active investigation. It has been hypothesized that dysregulation in circadian feeding patterns leads to transcriptional reprogramming of tissues involved in regulation of lipid storage and disposal (i.e., the liver and adipose tissue; Chapter 6). For example, a significant transcriptional reprogramming of white adipose tissue has been observed after as little as five days of mimicking night shift schedule in mice (Husse *et al.*, 2012). Specifically, a majority of genes upregulated in response to night shift work conditions in mice that were involved in control of lipid biosynthesis (Acetyl-coenzyme A carboxylase and Diacylglycerol acyltransferase) and glycolytic pathways. This indicates that as little as five-day exposure to circadian disruption can effectively reprogram the adipose tissue transcriptional profile to favor lipid accumulation and storage, a transcriptional profile associated with propensity for increased adiposity and metabolic syndrome in humans. Thus, alteration in the proper circadian timing of food consumption has been shown to result in adipose tissue hypertrophy, increased immune infiltration and increased expression of pro-inflammatory cytokines (Hatori *et al.*, 2012). It is important to note, too, that circadian misaligned feeding patterns have also been shown to promote transcriptional reprogramming in the liver, leading to favor hepatic lipid biosynthesis and subsequent lipid accumulation (hepatic steatosis), a condition prerequisite for induction of hepatic insulin resistance in T2DM.

Altered clock gene expression in tissues mediating glucose homeostasis (i.e., liver and skeletal muscle) is another potential mechanism purported to mediate deleterious effects of circadian disruption on predisposition to insulin resistance and T2DM in humans. Circadian disruption results in marked attenuation in key clock gene diurnal expression, as well as altered phase and period of clock transcriptional oscillation in the liver (Barclay *et al.*, 2012). This results in a profound loss of diurnal rhythmicity in metabolic genes known to regulate carbohydrate metabolism in the liver. This includes key genes known to regulate insulin-mediated suppression of hepatic glucose production and uptake [e.g., Insulin receptor substrate 2 (IRS2) and Forkhead box 01 (FOXO1)]. Similar loss in diurnal rhythmicity and circadian regulation in hepatic glycolytic and gluconeogenic transcriptome was evident in liver-specific *Bmal1* knockout mice (Lamia *et al.*, 2008). Furthermore, study of functional protein interactions between the intracellular clock and various biological pathways revealed that at least 19 components of the insulin signaling pathway are under direct transcriptional control by the circadian clock (Zhang *et al.*, 2009).

In some parallels to the liver, alteration in the skeletal muscle clock gene expression also results in impaired skeletal muscle structural and functional abnormalities, which have been associated with induction of insulin resistance. Specifically, skeletal muscle *Clock* and *Bmal1* mutant mice exhibit profound loss in structural architecture and disrupted metabolism associated with reduction in mitochondrial function and volume (Andrews *et al.*, 2010). This is particularly important since reduction in mitochondrial volume and function in humans is strongly associated with development of insulin resistance and T2DM. Therefore, these accumulating observations lend further support to the notion that liver and skeletal muscle circadian clocks play an important role in the regulation of daily rhythms in metabolic and glucose fluxes, whereas either genetic or environmentally-induced alteration in tissue clock gene expression/function may lead to alterations in glucose homeostasis and predisposition to insulin resistance in T2DM.

11.4 Mechanisms underlying the association between circadian disruption and T2DM; potential role of impaired beta-cell secretory function and mass

The association between circadian disruption and T2DM has also been attributed in part to promotion of beta-cell failure associated with the loss of beta-cell insulin secretory function and/or loss of beta-cell mass (Butler *et al.*, 2007; Marcheva *et al.*, 2010; Gale *et al.*, 2011). Studies have long demonstrated that insulin secretion exhibits a robust circadian secretory pattern that becomes more pronounced with the rise in prevailing glucose concentrations (Boden *et al.*, 1996). It is important to point out that the circadian rhythm in insulin release has been shown to be independent of diurnal changes in feeding, an observation supported by presence of robust circadian rhythms in insulin secretion in isolated pancreatic islets *in vitro* (Peschke and Peschke, 1998). Specifically, in mammals, meal or glucose-stimulated insulin secretion is reported to be maximal at the onset of the activity phase and minimal during the rest phase of the circadian activity cycle, a relationship that is impaired upon exposure to circadian disruption (Kalsbeek and Strubbe, 1998). Importantly, disruption of circadian rhythms in humans as a result of three weeks of recurring 28-hour "days" leads to loss of circadian rhythmicity of insulin secretion and, more importantly, pronounced decrease in both fasting and postprandial insulin release despite an increase in prevailing glucose levels (Buxton *et al.*, 2012). Interestingly, deleterious effects of circadian disruption on insulin secretion were largely reversed after as little as nine days of circadian re-entrainment, suggesting that these effects were likely attributed to alteration in beta-cell secretory function rather than any changes in beta-cell mass. Taken together these data suggest that regulation of the beta-cell circadian clock may be an important determinant of insulin secretory function at fasting and in response to hyperglycemia in humans.

Indeed, as previously reported for various peripheral tissues, isolated pancreatic islets in culture exhibit robust circadian rhythms in clock gene and protein expression oscillating at a near 24-hour period (Fig. 11.3a). Interestingly, when examined individually, pancreatic islets display robust in-phase transcriptional oscillations in clock gene expression, whereas the amplitude of transcriptional oscillations tends to significantly vary among individual pancreatic islets (Fig. 11.3a). Importantly, genetic disruption of the key circadian clock components in pancreatic islets (*Clock* and *Bmal1*) results in the loss of diurnal insulin release and overall reduction in glucose-stimulated insulin secretion observed *in vivo* and *in vitro*. This leads to induction of glucose intolerance and hyperglycemia in beta-cell specific clock mutant mice (Marcheva *et al.*, 2010). Importantly, loss of beta-cell secretory function in clock mutant mice is also associated with the loss of secretory response to nonglucose secretagoges (e.g., Forskolin and KCl), suggesting that the impairment in insulin secretion is associated with disrupted insulin vesicular recruitment and/or exocytosis. In support of this premise, altered expression in genes regulating beta-cell insulin vesicular fusion and trafficking has been documented in beta-cells from *Clock* and *Bmal1* mutant mice.

In addition, further support for the role of the beta-cell circadian clock in regulation of beta-cell secretory function comes from rodents exposed to global circadian disruption due to prolonged exposure to light at night or frequent shifts in the light/dark cycle akin to jet lag (Gale *et al.*, 2011). In these studies investigators report that exposure to global circadian disruption significantly alters islet circadian clock function through impairment in the amplitude, phase and inter-islet synchrony of islet clock transcriptional oscillations (Fig. 11.3b). As a result, circadian disruption leads to accelerated development of hyperglycemia in diabetes-prone human islet amyloid transgenic (HIP) rats independent of the weight again and, importantly, associated with deterioration in glucose-stimulated insulin secretion (Fig. 11.3c, 11.3d).

Accumulating evidence also support a potential role for the beta-cell circadian clock in regulation of beta-cell mass and turnover through modulation of beta-cell growth, proliferation and survival molecular pathways. For example, microarray analysis shows that *Clock* mutant mice show altered expression of genes regulating islet growth, maturation and proliferation (e.g., CyclinD1, PDX-1 and NeuroD1), consistent with previous observation in the liver and skeletal muscle (Marcheva *et al.*, 2010). In support of these findings, *Clock* mutant mice also display diminished rate of islet cell proliferation and a reduction in the islet size. Furthermore, diminished rate of beta-cell proliferation has also been observed in primary beta-cells treated with siRNA for *Rev-erbα* (key component of the circadian molecular loop) (Vieira *et al.*, 2012). These data are consistent with an accumulating body of evidence suggesting that cell cycle and proliferation is under transcriptional control of the circadian clock (Chapter 12). It remains unexplored whether aberrant beta-cell clock gene expression contributes to beta-cell failure in T2DM by influencing beta-cell formation/proliferation. However, *Clock* mutation in fibroblast have been previously shown to inhibit cell growth, proliferation as well as response to regeneration in fibroblasts (Miller *et al.*, 2007). Clearly, additional work is needed to understand the role of the beta-cell circadian clock in regulation of beta-cell growth and proliferation and whether it plays a contributory role in beta-cell failure.

Collective evidence from different organisms suggests that regulation of cell survival is under transcriptional control of the circadian clock. Specifically, cellular response to oxidative stress has been reported to be under direct transcriptional control of the circadian clock (Kondrtov *et al.*, 2006; Lee *et al.*, 2013). This is significant because oxidative stress is a pathological feature of beta-cells in patients with T2DM (Sakuraba *et al.*, 2002). For instance, oxidative stress arises due to imbalance between production and clearance of reactive oxygen species (ROS), produced as byproducts of the mitochondrial respiratory chain reaction with potential to induce cellular protein, lipid and DNA damage (Balaban *et al.*, 2005). In beta-cells, accumulation of ROS is associated with an increase in beta-cell "workload" due to hyperglycemia and/or hyperlipidemia as well as accumulation of mis-folded proteins and contributes to beta-cell loss by decreasing mitochondrial ATP production (Maechler and Wollheim, 2001), inhibiting insulin and PDX-1 mRNA expression as well as contributing to DNA fragmentation.

In order to prevent a detrimental rise of intracellular ROS, cells developed a coordinated antioxidant enzymatic defense response to remove reactive superoxide anions. This response is orchestrated mainly, but not exclusively, by three antioxidant enzymes: superoxide dismutase (SOD), glutathione perioxidase (Gpx), and

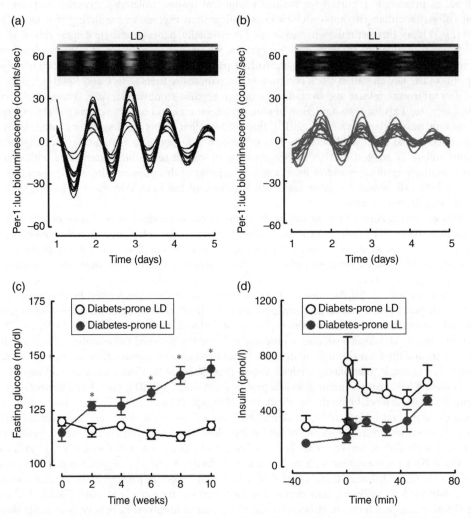

Fig. 11.3 Effects of circadian disruption of the beta-cell circadian clock and susceptibility to beta-cell failure and T2DM in rats. (A and B) Representative examples of *Per*-driven diurnal bioluminescence rhythms imaged by ICCD camera at the level of individual islets (n = 13) from *Per1:luc* rats exposed to either 10 weeks of typical light/dark cycle (LD) (a) or circadian disruption due to exposure to light at night (LL) (b). Each black or grey line represents a *Per*-driven bioluminescence signal from an individual islet. Note loss of the amplitude and synchrony in *Per1:luc* expression among individual islets in LL rats. (c) Effects of circadian disruption due to exposure to light at night (LL) on fasting glucose levels in diabetes-prone HIP rats (LD cycle (open circles) and LL cycle (grey circles)). (d) Glucose-stimulated insulin secretion during a hyperglycemic clamp (0–60 minutes) in diabetes-prone HIP rats exposed to either 10 weeks of typical LD (open circles) or disrupted LL cycle (grey circles). Note loss of glucose-stimulated insulin secretion in LL exposed rats. *(See insert for color representation of the figure.)*

catalase. Evidence suggests that cellular antioxidant defense response is under transcriptional control of the circadian clock. Firstly, diurnal rhythms in ROS production as well as antioxidant enzyme activity/expression has been described in several organisms as well as in different mammalian tissues (Hardeland *et al.*, 2003). Daily rhythms in antioxidant enzyme activity are particularly evident in cell types responsive to diurnal fluctuations in nutrient availability, such as the gut, the liver and the pancreas (Neuschwander-Tetri and Rozin, 1996). Secondly, clock gene mutants exhibit elevated ROS level, reduced expression and rhythmicity of antioxidant enzymes, and predisposition to oxidative stress associated with beta-cell failure, aging and neurodegeneration (Kondratov *et al.*, 2006; Krishnan *et al.*, 2012; Lee *et al.*, 2013). Additional studies are needed to address whether circadian disruption contributes to beta-cell loss as a consequence of compromised response to oxidative stress. However, in support of this premise, circadian disruption due to prolonged exposure to light at night in rats increased beta-cell vulnerability to apoptosis and beta-cell loss associated with overexpression of human islet amyloid polypeptide (a known inducer of oxidative stress in beta-cells) (Gale *et al.*, 2011).

11.5 Conclusion

The incidence of T2DM worldwide has reached an epidemic proportion and demonstrates an accelerated rise that threatens the health of the global population as well as economic stability. T2DM is a complex metabolic disease characterized by initiation of fasting and postprandial hyperglycemia as a result of pancreatic beta-cell failure in lieu of prevailing insulin resistance. Beta-cell failure in T2DM is largely attributed to genetic predispositions and manifests as a deficit in beta-cell mass and insulin secretory function. Insulin resistance in T2DM is largely attributed to ectopic lipid accumulation due to obesity and leads to impaired skeletal muscle and hepatic glucose disposal as well as inappropriately elevated hepatic glucose release.

Lifestyle choices and environmental conditions have long been known to modulate susceptibility to T2DM in humans. However, in recent years environmental conditions associated with disruption of

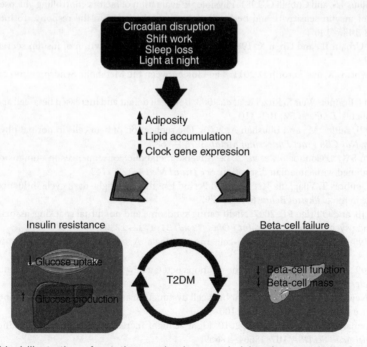

Fig. 11.4 Graphical illustration of putative mechanisms underlying the association between circadian disruption and induction of insulin resistance and beta-cell failure in T2DM.

circadian rhythms (e.g., shift work, light at night, sleep loss) have become increasingly prevalent in the modern societies and reported to significantly augment susceptibility to T2DM by promoting induction of both insulin resistance and beta-cell failure in humans (Fig. 11.4). The mechanisms underlying predisposition to circadian disruption-induced insulin resistance likely include (i) increased adiposity and consequent ectopic lipid accumulation in insulin-sensitive tissues as well as (ii) disrupted clock gene expression in tissues mediating glucose homeostasis. The mechanisms underlying predisposition to circadian disruption-induced beta-cell failure likely include disruption in beta-cell clock components resulting in (i) impaired beta-cell insulin secretory function, (ii) altered rate of beta-cell growth and proliferation as well as (iii) increased beta-cell attrition due to augmented susceptibility to oxidative stress. Understanding molecular and physiological mechanisms responsible for increased risk for T2DM in people experiencing daily disruptions in circadian rhythms will be important in development of novel therapeutic and lifestyle altering strategies to combat the global rise in diabetes prevalence in the 21st century.

References

Andrews JL, Zhang X, McCarthy JJ, *et al*. 2010. CLOCK and BMAL1 regulate MyoD and are necessary for maintenance of skeletal muscle phenotype and function. *Proc Natl Acad Sci USA* **107**: 19090–19095.

Arble DM, Bass J, Laposky AD, *et al*. 2009. Circadian timing of food intake contributes to weight gain. *Obesity (Silver Spring)* **17**: 2100–2102.

Balaban RS, Nemoto S, and Finkel T. 2005. Mitochondria, oxidants, and aging. *Cell* **120**: 483–495.

Barclay JL, Husse J, Bode B, *et al*. 2012. Circadian desynchrony promotes metabolic disruption in a mouse model of shiftwork. *PLoS One* **7**: e37150.

Basner M, Fomberstein KM, Razavi FM, *et al*. 2007. American time use survey: sleep time and its relationship to waking activities. *Sleep* **30**: 1085–1095.

Beihl DA, Liese AD, and Haffner SM. 2009. Sleep duration as a risk factor for incident type 2 diabetes in a multiethnic cohort. *Ann Epidemiol* **19**: 351–357.

Bergman RN, Phillips LS, and Cobelli C. 1981. Physiologic evaluation of factors controlling glucose tolerance in man: measurement of insulin sensitivity and beta-cell glucose sensitivity from the response to intravenous glucose. *J Clin Invest* **68**: 1456–1467.

Boden G, Ruiz J, Urbain JL, and Chen X. 1996. Evidence for a circadian rhythm of insulin secretion. *Am J Physiol* **271**: E246–252.

Braun S, Bitton-Worms K, and Leroith D. 2011. The Link between the Metabolic Syndrome and cancer. *Int J Biol Sci* **7**: 1003–1015.

Butler AE, Janson J, Bonner-Weir S, Ritzel R, *et al*. 2003. Beta-cell deficit and increased beta-cell apoptosis in humans with type 2 diabetes. *Diabetes* **52**: 102–110.

Butler PC, Meier JJ, Butler AE, and Bhushan A. 2007. The replication of beta cells in normal physiology, in disease and for therapy. *Nat Clin Pract Endocrinol Metab* **3**: 758–768.

Buxton OM, Cain SW, O'Connor SP, *et al*. 2012. Adverse metabolic consequences in humans of prolonged sleep restriction combined with circadian disruption. *Sci Transl Med* **4**: 129ra143.

Campuzano A, Cambras T, Vilaplana J, *et al*. 1999. Period length of the light-dark cycle influences the growth rate and food intake in mice. *Physiol Behav* **67**: 791–797.

Colles SL, Dixon JB, and O'Brien PE. 2007. Night eating syndrome and nocturnal snacking: association with obesity, binge eating and psychological distress. *Int J Obes (Lond)* **31**: 1722–1730.

DeFronzo RA. 1988. The triumvirate: beta-cell, muscle, liver. A collusion responsible for NIDDM. *Diabetes* **37**: 667–687.

Defronzo RA. 2009. From the triumvirate to the ominous octet: a new paradigm for the treatment of type 2 diabetes mellitus. *Diabetes* **58**: 773–795.

Florez JC. 2008. Newly identified loci highlight beta cell dysfunction as a key cause of type 2 diabetes: where are the insulin resistance genes? *Diabetologia* **51**: 1100–1110.

Fonken LK, Workman JL, Walton JC, *et al*. 2010. Light at night increases body mass by shifting the time of food intake. *Proc Natl Acad Sci USA* **107**: 18664–18669.

Froy O, Chapnik N, and Miskin R. 2006. Long-lived alphaMUPA transgenic mice exhibit pronounced circadian rhythms. *Am J Physiol Endocrinol Metab* **291**: E1017–1024.

Gale JE, Cox HI, Qian J, *et al.* 2011. Disruption of circadian rhythms accelerates development of diabetes through pancreatic beta-cell loss and dysfunction. *J Biol Rhythms* **26**: 423–433.

Garaulet M, Corbalan-Tutau MD, Madrid JA, *et al.* 2010. PERIOD2 variants are associated with abdominal obesity, psycho-behavioral factors, and attrition in the dietary treatment of obesity. *J Am Diet Assoc* **110**: 917–921.

Haataja L, Gurlo T, Huang CJ, and Butler PC. 2008. Islet amyloid in type 2 diabetes, and the toxic oligomer hypothesis. *Endocr Rev* **29**: 303–316.

Hardeland R, Coto-Montes A, and Poeggeler B. 2003. Circadian rhythms, oxidative stress, and antioxidative defense mechanisms. *Chronobiol Int* **20**: 921–962.

Hatori M, Vollmers C, Zarrinpar A, *et al.* 2012. Time-restricted feeding without reducing caloric intake prevents metabolic diseases in mice fed a high-fat diet. *Cell Metab* **15**: 848–860.

Hotamisligil GS. 2006. Inflammation and metabolic disorders. *Nature* **444**: 860–867.

Husse J, Hintze SC, Eichele G, *et al.* 2012. Circadian clock genes *per1* and *per2* regulate the response of metabolism-associated transcripts to sleep disruption. *PLoS One* **7**: e52983.

Kahn SE. 2001. The importance of beta-cell failure in the development and progression of type 2 diabetes. *J Clin Endocrinol Metab* **86**: 4047–4058.

Kalsbeek A and Strubbe JH. 1998. Circadian control of insulin secretion is independent of the temporal distribution of feeding. *Physiol Behav* **63**: 553–558.

Karatsoreos IN, Bhagat S, Bloss EB, *et al.* 2011. Disruption of circadian clocks has ramifications for metabolism, brain, and behavior. *Proc Natl Acad Sci USA* **108**: 1657–1662.

Kivimaki M, Batty GD, and Hublin C. 2011. Shift work as a risk factor for future type 2 diabetes: evidence, mechanisms, implications, and future research directions. *PLoS Med* **8**: e1001138.

Kohyama J. 2009. A newly proposed disease condition produced by light exposure during night: asynchronization. *Brain Dev* **31**: 255–273.

Koivisto VA, Yki-Jarvinen H, and DeFronzo RA. 1986. Physical training and insulin sensitivity. *Diabetes Metab Rev* **1**: 445–481.

Kondratov RV, Kondratova AA, Gorbacheva VY, *et al.* 2006. Early aging and age-related pathologies in mice deficient in BMAL1, the core componentof the circadian clock. *Genes Dev* **20**: 1868–1873.

Krishnan N, Rakshit K, Chow ES, *et al.* 2012. Loss of circadian clock accelerates aging in neurodegeneration-prone mutants. *Neurobiol Dis* **45**: 1129–1135.

Lamia KA, Storch KF, and Weitz CJ. 2008. Physiological significance of a peripheral tissue circadian clock. *Proc Natl Acad Sci USA* **105**: 15172–15177.

Lee J, Moulik M, Fang Z, *et al.* 2013. Bmal1 and beta-cell clock are required for adaptation to circadian disruption, and their loss of function leads to oxidative stress-induced beta-cell failure in mice. *Mol Cell Biol* **33**: 2327–2338.

Lin YC and Chen PC. 2012. Persistent rotating shift work exposure is a tough second hit contributing to abnormal liver function among on-site workers having sonographic fatty liver. *Asia Pac J Public Health*. Epub ahead of print.

Maechler P and Wollheim CB. 2001. Mitochondrial function in normal and diabetic beta-cells. *Nature* **414**: 807–812.

Marcheva B, Ramsey KM, Buhr ED, *et al.* 2010. Disruption of the clock components CLOCK and BMAL1 leads to hypoinsulinaemia and diabetes. *Nature* **466**: 627–631.

Mason CC, Hanson RL, and Knowler WC. 2007. Progression to type 2 diabetes characterized by moderate then rapid glucose increases. *Diabetes* **56**: 2054–2061.

Matveyenko AV and Butler PC. 2008. Relationship between beta-cell mass and diabetes onset. *Diabetes Obes Metab* **10**(Suppl 4): 23–31.

Meier JJ. 2005. Insulin secretion. In: *Endocrinology* (eds DeGroot LJ and Jameson JJ). Elsevier Saunders, Philadelphia, PA, pp. 961–973.

Mikuni E, Ohoshi T, Hayashi K, and Miyamura K. 1983. Glucose intolerance in an employed population. *Tohoku J Exp Med* **141**(Suppl): 251–256.

Miller BH, McDearmon EL, Panda S, *et al.* 2007. Circadian and CLOCK-controlled regulation of the mouse transcriptome and cell proliferation. *Proc Natl Acad Sci USA* **104**: 3342–3347.

Neuschwander-Tetri BA and Rozin T. 1996. Diurnal variability of cysteine and glutathione content in the pancreas and liver of the mouse. *Comp Biochem Physiol B Biochem Mol Biol* **114**: 91–95.

Peschke E and Peschke D. 1998. Evidence for a circadian rhythm of insulin release from perifused rat pancreatic islets. *Diabetologia* **41**: 1085–1092.

Poitout V and Robertson RP. 2007. Glucolipotoxicity: fuel excess and {beta}-cell dysfunction. *Endocr Rev* **29**(3):351–366.

Rizza RA. 2010. Pathogenesis of fasting and postprandial hyperglycemia in type 2 diabetes: implications for therapy. *Diabetes* **59**: 2697–2707.

Sakuraba H, Mizukami H, Yagihashi N, *et al.* 2002. Reduced beta-cell mass and expression of oxidative stress-related DNA damage in the islet of Japanese Type II diabetic patients. *Diabetologia* **45**: 85–96.

Samuel VT and Shulman GI. 2012. Mechanisms for insulin resistance: common threads and missing links. *Cell* **148**: 852–871.

Scheer FA, Hilton MF, Mantzoros CS, and Shea SA. 2009. Adverse metabolic and cardiovascular consequences of circadian misalignment. *Proc Natl Acad Sci USA* **106**: 4453–4458.

Scott EM, Carter AM, and Grant PJ. 2008. Association between polymorphisms in the Clock gene, obesity and the metabolic syndrome in man. *Int J Obes (Lond)* **32**: 658–662.

Stratton IM, Adler AI, Neil HA, *et al.* 2000. Association of glycaemia with macrovascular and microvascular complications of type 2 diabetes (UKPDS 35): prospective observational study. *BMJ* **321**: 405–412.

Suwazono Y, Dochi M, Oishi M, *et al.* 2009. Shiftwork and impaired glucose metabolism: a 14-year cohort study on 7104 male workers. *Chronobiol Int* **26**: 926–941.

Tsai LL, Tsai YC, Hwang K, *et al.* 2005. Repeated light-dark shifts speed up body weight gain in male F344 rats. *Am J Physiol Endocrinol Metab* **289**: E212–217.

Turek FW, Joshu C, Kohsaka A, *et al.* 2005. Obesity and metabolic syndrome in circadian Clock mutant mice. *Science* **308**: 1043–1045.

Van Cauter E, Spiegel K, Tasali E, and Leproult R. 2008. Metabolic consequences of sleep and sleep loss. *Sleep Med* **9**(Suppl 1): S23–28.

Vieira E, Marroqui L, Batista TM, *et al.* 2012. The clock gene Rev-erbalpha regulates pancreatic beta-cell function: modulation by leptin and high-fat diet. *Endocrinology* **153**: 592–601.

Weigensberg MJ and Goran MI. 2009. Type 2 diabetes in children and adolescents. *Lancet* **373**: 1743–1744.

Whiting DR, Guariguata L, Weil C, and Shaw J. 2011. IDF Diabetes Atlas: Global estimates of the prevalence of diabetes for 2011 and 2030. *Diabetes Res Clin Pract.* **103**(2): 137–149.

Wyse CA, Selman C, Page MM, *et al.* 2011. Circadian desynchrony and metabolic dysfunction; did light pollution make us fat? *Med Hypotheses* **77**: 1139–1144.

Zhang EE, Liu AC, Hirota T, *et al.* 2009. A genome-wide RNAi screen for modifiers of the circadian clock in human cells. *Cell* **139**: 199–210.

Circadian Clock Control of the Cell Cycle and Links to Cancer

12

T. Katherine Tamai and David Whitmore

Centre for Cell and Molecular Dynamics, Department of Cell and Developmental Biology, University College London, London, UK

12.1 Introduction

Human beings, as with most primates, are extremely diurnal. Most of us tend to sleep at night and, of course, are most active during the daylight hours, vampires and students being possible exemptions to this rule. Fundamentally, this daily rhythm in activity and sleep is regulated by our circadian clocks, which reside not only within the suprachiasmatic nucleus (SCN) within our hypothalamus but also within most of the cells that make up our bodies. These clocks are set or entrained by light, which, at least in the case of mammals, is detected by specialized cells within the retina (Hankins *et al.*, 2008). For most of us, and undoubtedly for our ancestors, this system has worked well. However, life is much more complicated nowadays in the "modern" world. Almost all of us travel, often internationally across time zones, and many individuals, especially those in the medical profession or in the travel/transportation industries, perform shift work. This "24/7" lifestyle impacts our biology and physiology in many ways, and one of the major consequences is that our biological timing system, including our sleep regulation, is often disrupted. This has clear and quite dramatic consequences on our health, which, of course, is one of the fundamental issues addressed in this book. Amongst the most significant effects of clock disruption is an apparent increased risk of cancer. In the remainder of this chapter, how this might occur is explored by addressing how the circadian clock could influence the cell cycle and cell division. Subsequently, potential ways of "using" the circadian system to improve our approaches to the treatment of cancer are discussed.

12.2 Epidemiology

Numerous work groups within our society are regularly exposed to circadian disruption, often through the requirement to perform night shifts. In particular, this includes members of the medical profession, such as doctors and nurses, individuals in the travel and transportation industries, as well as workers in large-scale industrial companies that work "around the clock." This provides the research community

Circadian Medicine, First Edition. Edited by Christopher S. Colwell.
© 2015 John Wiley & Sons, Inc. Published 2015 by John Wiley & Sons, Inc.

with highly defined groups of individuals for whom medical records and health reports can be explored for clear increased frequencies of any specific illnesses.

Medical professionals offer a very "appealing" study group, because of their inherent understanding and close involvement in health matters. Consequently, much of the cancer-clock correlative data and epidemiology has been collected from Nurse Health Study cohorts (Megdal *et al.*, 2005). The design and results from such studies are explored extensively in this book in the chapter written by Dr Schernhammer (Chapter 13). To avoid repetition, we will simply jump to the bottom line. Two large-scale nurse cohorts, in which the number of individuals was close to or exceeded 120,000, came to the same conclusion, that there was approximately a 36% increase in the risk of breast cancer, a 35% increase in colorectal cancer and a 43% increase in endometrial cancer as a consequence of extended periods of shift work (Megdal *et al.*, 2005; Innominato *et al.*, 2010). This phenomenon is not only restricted to women but also includes men, with a significant increase in prostate cancer emerging from two male cohort studies (Conlon *et al.*, 2007). Such findings have led the World Health Organization to conclude that shift work, and its resulting impact on clock function, does act as a clear carcinogen for people who undertake it (Straif *et al.*, 2007). There are obvious ethical and financial implications that result from this, as demonstrated by the decision by the Danish government to compensate women with breast cancer who have worked night shifts for over 20 years (http://www.ask.dk/en/English/News/News-archive/Night-shift-work-and-the-risk-of-breast-/Many-recognised-cases-of-breast-cancer-a.aspx). This perhaps represents the beginning of a much wider impact such results will have on government policy, as well as the economies of developed countries over the next few years.

12.3 Does circadian clock disruption have any relevance in a clinical setting?

This issue is relatively unexplored to date. However, the fact of being diagnosed with cancer itself is likely to have a negative impact, both psychologically and physiologically, on circadian clock synchrony and, certainly, on sleep consolidation. Furthermore, the hospital environment itself is not conducive to having normal circadian activity for the staff, or for the patients. Anyone who has spent even a small period of time in hospital can relate to the sensation of "jet lag" such environments can produce. So, does either environmentally-induced clock disruption or asynchrony as a consequence of the illness itself have a negative consequence on cancer progression?

Though there are few explicit studies in this area, it is clear that circadian perturbation in a patient correlates dramatically with poor prognosis and distinctly reduced survival rates compared to individuals with robust circadian function (Sephton *et al.*, 2000). Perhaps the most significant of these studies monitored individual patient's general activity levels, using wrist-worn activity monitors, which are not only easily available but also represent a noninvasive method of measuring a subject's circadian state (Innominato *et al.*, 2009). In this example, 322 patients with metastatic colorectal cancer had their clock "robustness" determined over a 72-hour period prior to the onset of chemotherapy. The results are quite remarkable, with approximately a 50% reduction in average survival rates occurring in patients with marked disrupted clock function. Simply put, individuals with poor clock function and cancer die quicker and in larger numbers than patients with robust daily rhythms (Fig. 12.1). Now, of course, the mechanistic basis of this is far from understood and is undoubtedly complex. However, the implications are significant. The idea of "improving" the circadian environment for cancer patients, in the hospital or even prior to their admittance, has barely been explored, but the outcome for these patients could be considerable. This could be achieved either by simple improvements in lighting, compared to the rather constant illumination of most hospitals, especially intensive care wards, or one could even conceive of intervening with the use of drug applications, such as melatonin treatments or other agents to improve circadian synchrony. This type of treatment is wide open for further development and exploitation.

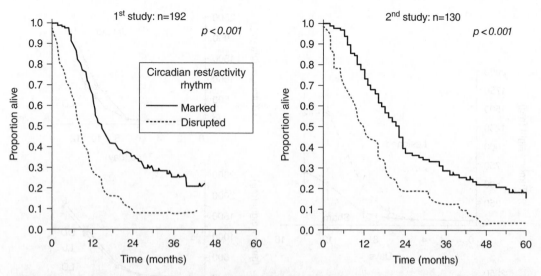

Fig. 12.1 A summary of the results from two studies showing that patients with cancer and disrupted circadian clock function tend to have shorter a life-span and reduced survival expectations compared to individuals that retain robust daily rhythmicity (Innominato *et al.*, 2009).

Animal studies shed light on and certainly support these human correlative data sets. Several fascinating studies, performed largely by the group of research oncologist Francis Levi in Paris, have clearly shown that clock disruption leads to an acceleration in the rate of tumor growth (Filipski *et al.*, 2006). It is not yet clear whether this is the causal event in humans that leads to accelerated death in those with poor clock function. In the mouse studies, individual animals were given bilateral subcutaneous injections of Glasgow osteosarcoma (GOS) or pancreatic adenocarcinoma cells. The circadian system in these animals was then subsequently disrupted, either by lesioning the clock center within the SCN, or by applying a desynchronizing "jet-lag" lighting regime to these animals (Filipski *et al.*, 2006). Controls either received sham SCN operations or were exposed to a normal 12:12 light–dark cycle.

The results are quite clear and are shown in Fig. 12.2. Tumors grow faster in the animals in which clock function has been disrupted, either surgically or through simple jet lag conditions. This means, of course, that either the proliferative rates of the cells within these tumors has been accelerated by the lack of daily rhythmicity, or inherent cell death is reduced. A rather fascinating addendum to these studies is that restricting the meal times of these mice to a four-hour window each day had a dramatic effect, not only on reducing their weight loss due to "illness" but also reducing the accelerated growth rate of their tumors (Filipski and Levi, 2009). Restricted or timed feeding is known to act effectively as a zeitgeber to set or entrain peripheral body clocks, even in the absence of "higher order" entraining signals, such as light or signals from the SCN (Stephan, 2002). This raises the interesting possibility that tightly regulating the meal times of patients in a clinical setting might also act positively to improve their peripheral tissue circadian synchrony, and subsequently improve their prognosis following chemotherapy, or related cancer treatments.

12.4 Circadian clock control of the cell cycle in healthy tissues

The clinical aspects of the circadian clock and cancer progression will be returned to later in the chapter. However, all of the above findings are based on the idea that the endogenous circadian clock can regulate cell cycle timing and the rate of cell cycle progression. So what is the evidence for this and what is the potential mechanism behind this process?

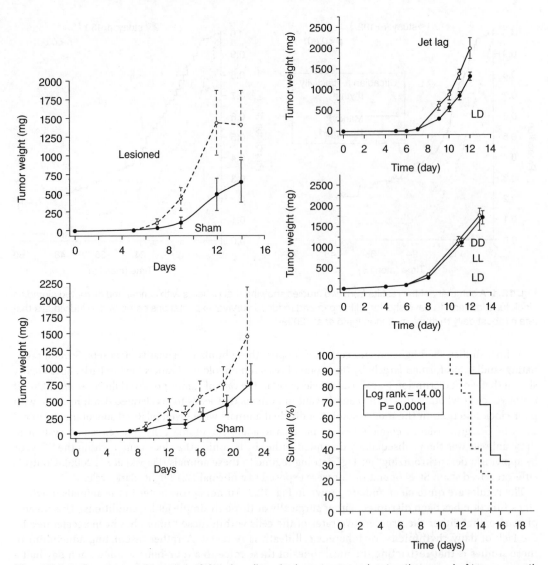

Fig. 12.2 In the mouse, disruption of the circadian clock system accelerates the speed of tumor growth and reduces subsequent life-span. In the left-hand graphs, mice had their "master" clock in the SCN surgically ablated. Transplanted osteosarcoma (GOS) or pancreatic adenocarcinoma cells were then transplanted into the animals subcutaneously. Compared to sham operated animals, tumors grew faster in the behaviorally arrhythmic population. Similar results were seen in animals that were systematically "jet lagged" versus controls on a normal light–dark cycle, or under free-running conditions (right-hand graphs). Jet-lagged animals with such tumors die faster than control animals with normal clock function (Filipski et al., 2006).

Many cells types in different tissues continue to divide or proliferate in the adult animal. This phenomenon has been described for many decades but has only relatively recently been "re-packaged" under the concept of adult stem cells. The tissues where this is most common is quite apparent and includes: hematopoietic stem cells (HSCs) that reside within the bone marrow and generate a number of blood cell types; adult mesenchymal stem cells (MSCs), falling under the "fibroblast" label; skin and oral mucosa stem cell populations; intestinal stem cells, critical for renewal of cells in the gut lining; stem cells in the cornea of the eye; and even adult neural stem cells, which appear to be restricted to specific regions of the mature brain. A loss of cell cycle regulation within these specific cell populations is, of course, thought to be a critical step in the formation of tumors within these areas of the body.

It has been known since at least the 1950s, if not even earlier, that the circadian clock influences the timing of these cell cycle events *in vivo*. The majority of data was collected, of course, using mouse models, but the observation is directly transferable to humans. Examination of the mitotic index (percentage of cells in mitosis) was shown to be strongly rhythmic in liver parenchyma by Franz Halberg in the late 1950s and was summarized at the first "circadian" meeting at Cold Spring Harbor in 1960 (Halberg, 1960). Subsequent studies, exploring the levels of DNA synthesis or S-phase of the cell cycle, expanded such rhythmic observations to the oral mucosa, tongue epithelium, five regions of the gut, bone marrow and corneal epithelium (Scheving *et al.*, 1978; Bjarnason *et al.*, 2001). More recent studies have extended this even further to describe rhythms in the stem cells of the skin, as well as daily oscillations of neurogenesis within regions of the adult brain, such as the hippocampus and within oligodendrocyte precursor cells (Janich *et al.*, 2011; Matsumoto *et al.*, 2011). Fundamentally, the clock controls the timing of the cell cycle within adult tissues, such that specific stages of the cell cycle are restricted to certain times of day. This phenomenon is not restricted to mammals but can also be found in a variety of species, ranging from unicellular organisms, through to developmental stages in zebrafish, and even within cells isolated in culture (Mori and Johnson 2000; Dekens *et al.*, 2003; Tamai *et al.*, 2012).

Our view of how this clock-cell cycle regulation might occur has changed dramatically over the last few years. The classical view of circadian organization is one of a highly centralized circadian timing system, based within the SCN of mammals, and the retina and pineal gland of lower vertebrates. This central clock was then thought to "drive" downstream rhythms within the body, presumably through either endocrine or neural pathways. Work in the late 1990s, initially both in zebrafish and mammalian cell culture, demonstrated that a functional circadian clock resided within all tissues and many cells in culture (Balsalobre *et al.*, 1998; Whitmore *et al.*, 1998, 2000). The circadian system in zebrafish was shown to be even further decentralized with the demonstration that individual cells and tissues were themselves directly light responsive (Whitmore *et al.*, 2000). Similar observations regarding the presence of a cellular circadian oscillator were extended later to adult mammalian tissues and were shown using transgenic mice containing luminescent gene reporter constructs (Yoo *et al.*, 2004). Tissues then dissected and placed into culture showed robust circadian gene expression rhythms for many days and even weeks.

The existence of peripheral clocks in mammals, coordinated by signals from the SCN in the hypothalamus, makes it highly likely that the circadian clock within each cell regulates the timing of the cell cycle directly and in a cell autonomous manner. This certainly appears to be the case for clock-cell cycle interactions examined in zebrafish cells in culture (Tamai *et al.*, 2012). It is also very likely to be true for mammalian cells as well, although there is considerably more debate regarding this issue. Furthermore, this idea of cell autonomous regulation of the cell cycle does not mean that added levels of complexity and regulation do not exist. On the contrary, cell–cell interactions within a tissue are also likely to play a role in cell cycle regulation, though this needs further experimental examination; and within the context of the whole body, of course, many factors, including endocrine, metabolic changes and so on, will add levels of complexity to this process of time-regulated cell division.

12.5 How might the cellular circadian clock regulate cell cycle timing?

Determining the mechanistic link between the cellular circadian oscillator and the cell cycle mechanism will undoubtedly require and benefit from studies using a wide range of model systems. This research will be greatly aided by the fact that the fundamental components of the cell cycle, and for that matter the circadian clock as well, are highly conserved across a wide range of species. Zebrafish offer a number of key advantages for such studies, especially in cell culture. Zebrafish cell lines are themselves directly light responsive. This means that, effectively, all of the "key ingredients" of a complete clock system are contained within a single cell. Consequently, it is possible to synchronize the cell cycle within these cultures simply by adjusting appropriately the lighting conditions of the incubator. This interesting piece of biology is a great aid in studying downstream, clock output processes, as no pharmacological intervention is required to synchronize clock function within the cell population. Studies to date in zebrafish have shown that both the timing of mitosis and S-phase/DNA replication occur at specific circadian times in both zebrafish cell lines, as well as developing embryos (Dekens et al., 2003; Tamai et al., 2012). A wide range of cell cycle genes and regulators are clock controlled, but this is especially true for the timing of *Cyclin B1* expression. Rhythms in expression of this central cell cycle gene correlate perfectly with the peak timing of mitosis and, presumably, in part at least, control the daily phasing of this cellular event, such that it occurs in the late night/early morning (Fig. 12.3). Further studies are now exploring how S-phase is regulated in cell culture and developing embryos.

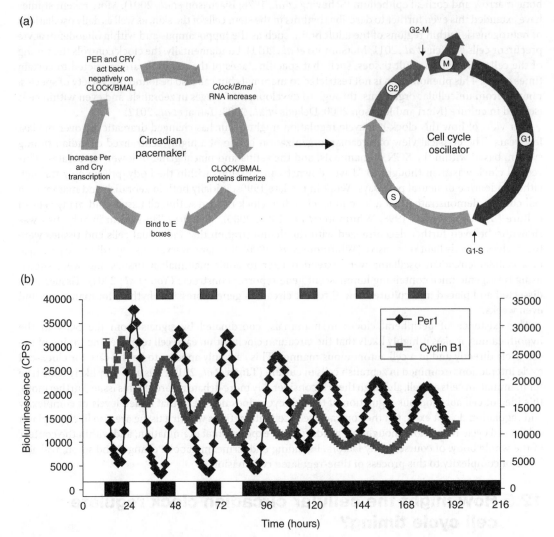

Fig. 12.3 The circadian clock directly regulates the timing of the cell cycle in many biological systems and cells, including human proliferative tissues. Typically, the clock seems to regulate entry into mitosis, at the G2 to M transition, and DNA replication or S-phase, at the G1-S transition. To date, much of this regulation appears to be transcriptional. Panel B shows the precision of this transcriptional rhythm in living zebrafish cell lines. Luminescent reporters for the clock gene *Period 1* and the cell cycle gene, *Cyclin B1*, show how the clock regulates peak *Cyclin B1* expression to occur in the late night – corresponding to the peak timing of mitosis (pink squares) in culture (Tamai et al., 2012). *(See insert for color representation of the figure.)*

One study that has shed considerable light on the clock-cell cycle interaction comes from work performed by Matsuo and colleagues using partial hepatectomy in mouse (Matsuo *et al.*, 2003). If a mouse liver is surgically reduced by about two-thirds, it will rapidly enter a proliferative state and regenerate back to the original starting size. Interestingly, if such surgery is performed at two different times of day, dawn and eight hours later, there is a distinct difference in the lag or timing of mitosis. The differential timing of this response suggests that a circadian clock is underlying the entry of these cells into mitosis but not into S-phase. An extensive analysis of rhythmic cell cycle-related genes by DNA microarray was performed and then confirmed by Northern blot analysis. Of 68 cell cycle genes analyzed, three in particular showed altered timing in peak expression that matched the differences seen in timed hepatectomy. As shown above for mitotic regulation in zebrafish cell lines, *Cyclin B1* transcript levels were strongly rhythmic, as well as expression of *Cdc2*, which codes for the protein partner of *Cyclin B1*. The third gene that showed significant clock regulation was *Wee1*, a tyrosine kinase and well described mitotic cell cycle regulator. The circadian oscillation in *Wee1* expression appears to be under direct control by the circadian clock, as E-box regulatory elements (CACGTG) within the *Wee1* promoter are important for the generation of this rhythm. This DNA sequence within the regulatory or promoter region of a gene is well established as a critical binding site for the two core clock proteins, CLOCK and BMAL. The CLOCK-BMAL protein dimer is known to bind to these key sequences and activate downstream transcription. So in this particular situation, as also seen in the case of zebrafish, the clock appears to be regulating critical cell cycle components at the transcriptional level.

Taken together, these results have led to a proposed model for how the circadian clock might regulate cell cycle timing within a regenerating liver (Fig. 12.4). A strong circadian rhythm in *Wee1* expression is produced by the core clock proteins CLOCK and BMAL positively activating transcription of *Wee1* in dividing hepatocytes at a point in the cycle when their protein levels peak. Inhibition of this positive transcriptional drive by core clock repressors, in particular Cryptochromes, at the opposite time in the cycle leads to an inhibition of CLOCK and BMAL and a subsequent drop in *Wee1* expression. A matching oscillation in the WEE1 kinase then leads to direct phosphorylation and inhibition of the CDC2-Cyclin B1 (also called CDK1-Cyclin B1) protein complex. These components of the cell cycle are essential for cells to enter mitosis, and phosphorylation of this complex blocks the G2/M transition. Consequently, a high level of WEE1 protein leads to high levels of CDC2-Cyclin B1 phosphorylation and an inhibition of entry into mitosis. Low levels of WEE1, conversely, facilitate or promote the timed entry of cells into mitosis. Significantly, alteration of key

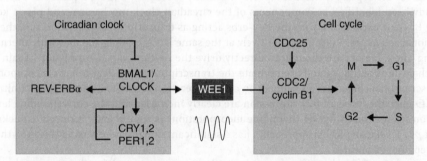

Fig. 12.4 Proposed mechanism for cell cycle control in the regenerating mouse liver. The exact molecular details of how the clock regulates cell cycle timing might vary slightly from one system to the other. However, certain key control points have been identified. In regenerating mouse liver, the circadian clock appears to regulate directly the expression of *Wee1* kinase through E-box elements in its promoter. This protein then phosphorylates the CDC2/Cyclin B1 stopping cells from entering mitosis, holding them in the G2 phase of the cell cycle. In this way, the rhythm in *wee1* expression is thought to produce a "gate" or "window" when cells can enter the mitotic stage of the cell cycle at a specific time of day (adapted from Matsuo *et al.*, 2003).

core clock gene expression has a predictable impact on *Wee1* expression. This is especially apparent in *Cryptochrome*-deficient mice (*Cry1/Cry2* double mutants), where the critical inhibition of CLOCK and BMAL function is reduced. Under such circumstances, the levels of *Wee1* expression are predictably increased. The opposite is true in cases where the levels of functional CLOCK protein are reduced, as in the *clock* mutant mouse. These data confirm a direct regulation of *Wee1* by core clock proteins, with a resulting impact on cell cycle progression. Though these data are very compelling, it must be stressed that this finding is based on one study in regenerating liver. The situation is undoubtedly much more complex and these results only represent "the tip of the iceberg" in terms of cellular mechanism. More work is clearly required in this important area of circadian biology.

This added complexity is alluded to by data from a series of microarray studies in different tissues and model systems, which have identified a wide range of rhythmic cell cycle regulators. In addition to *Cyclin B1* and *Wee1* described above, other *Cyclins*, including *D*, *E* and *A*, have been shown to oscillate, as well as other cell cycle factors, such as *c-Myc* and *Mdm2* (Fu *et al.*, 2002; Borgs *et al.*, 2009). Furthermore, a number of critical regulators of cell proliferation and apoptosis, including p53, are basally regulated by clock genes, even if they themselves do not show oscillatory expression. Aspects of circadian *p53* regulation may be tissue specific. So, for example, in *Clock* mutant mouse, the levels of *p53* expression are significantly reduced (Miller *et al.*, 2007). Microarray and RNA sequencing approaches are excellent at identifying rhythmic targets but, of course, provide little data as to how these factors are actually regulated or how they might influence cell cycle timing.

However, in the case of the cyclin-dependent kinase inhibitor gene *p21*, considerably more is known about its circadian clock regulation and control of cell proliferation (Grechez-Cassiau *et al.*, 2008). As its name suggests, p21 inhibits the activity of cyclin-dependent kinase CDK2-Cyclin E and, consequently, acts as a check point protein preventing cells entering S phase from G1. The *p21* gene is also an important downstream target of p53, which is typically activated by DNA damage, a fact that critically stops cells from progressing through the cell cycle with such damage. It is very apparent that *p21* gene expression is under clock control in a number of peripheral mouse tissues, including liver, heart and skeletal muscle, where peak expression occurs around dawn (Grechez-Cassiau *et al.*, 2008). These rhythms are again disrupted in clock mutant animals, in this particular case, in the *Bmal1* mutant mouse. A detailed analysis of the *p21* promoter has revealed a number of critical "circadian" DNA binding sites that actively regulate the rhythmic expression of this gene. Specifically, the *p21* promoter contains Rev-Erb/ROR response elements (RREs) ([A/T]A[A/T]NT[A/G]GGTCA), which are target binding sites for the orphan nuclear receptors, the family of Rev-erb and ROR proteins. These proteins have already been identified as components of the circadian clock mechanism and play a key role in regulating BMAL1 expression, with the Rev-erbs acting as transcriptional repressors and the RORs as transcriptional activators. Acting competitively at the same DNA binding site, but with alternate circadian timing, these factors are thought to directly drive the rhythm in *p21* expression. Again, the core clock mechanism is acting directly to regulate the transcription of critical cell cycle components. Do these transcriptional changes really impact on cell proliferation rates? The answer is a definitive yes, as in *Bmal* KO mice the levels of *p21* expression are clearly increased and the corresponding level of cell proliferation (as measured by 3H-thymidine incorporation) is significantly reduced. Knocking down this raised *p21* level using RNAi approaches has a significant impact on reversing this growth defect in primary hepatocyte cultures.

What is apparent from the above examples is that in normal, proliferative tissues, the circadian clock can and does regulate the timing of the cell cycle and rate of cell proliferation. The majority of studies support a direct transcriptional regulatory connection between these two cellular processes, but it is certain that over the next few years the level of mechanistic interaction between these two fundamental cellular processes will only increase, as posttranscriptional and translational events are taken into account. This idea begs the obvious question: Is the core clock disrupted in specific forms of cancer?

12.6 Clock disruption and cancer

The epidemiological data mentioned above support the idea that general "whole body" circadian clock disruption leads to an increased propensity towards developing cancer, but obviously, cancer can also be caused by many other factors. So within a developing tumor, what happens to circadian clock function? An examination of clock gene expression in numerous tumor types, especially breast, colorectal and prostate, have shown distinct "clock disruption" in these malignancies, compared to neighboring healthy tissue (Innominato *et al.*, 2010; Lahti *et al.*, 2012). It should be noted that much of this kind of data is based on single time point sampling and comparison, rather than a detailed analysis of clock gene rhythms. The reason for this limitation is rather self-evident when one considers that one is dealing with quite ill patients and the problem of surgically obtaining tissue biopsies from them.

The large-scale cancer gene expression databases, such as Oncomine (www.oncomine.org), are invaluable tools for directly comparing clock gene expression between tumors and nonmalignant tissues. An analysis of approximately 50 data sets, performed by Francis Levi and colleagues, showed that the *Period* genes were frequently downregulated in at least six types of human tumors (Innominato *et al.*, 2010). This is particularly true for *Per1* and *Per2*, which encode well known transcriptional repressors within the core clock mechanism. However, this was also true for *Per3*, which has been more strongly implicated in aspects of sleep regulation. Rather curiously, in this particular analysis, several of the core clock genes did not seem to show altered expression, including *Bmal1*, *Clock*, *Npas2* and the *Cryptochromes*. In some ways, this is rather unexpected, as these genes form an oscillatory transcription–translation negative feedback loop (Chapters 1 and 2), so it might be expected that disruption of one core clock component would influence expression of many others. Without a full rhythmic analysis of clock function, it is hard to say exactly what might be happening with the molecular clock; it also raises the likely possibility that clock genes may have independent noncircadian (core clock) consequences on downstream gene expression. This is very likely, as in essence the central clock mechanism is composed of numerous fundamental transcriptional activators and repressors.

In fact, *Per2* is often described as a tumor suppressor gene, which is supported by numerous studies in mouse. Early studies performed by Lee and colleagues using *Per2* mutant mice showed a dramatic increase in the probability and rate of tumor development in gamma-irradiated individuals compared to wild-type (WT) controls (Fu *et al.*, 2002). These clock defective animals have a shortened circadian period, with a tendency towards rapid clock damping under constant dark conditions. Approximately seven months following irradiation, all *Per2* mutant mice showed signs of teratoma compared to none in the WT controls, as well as other signs of "aging," including hair loss and greying (one sympathizes!). By 16 months, 71% of the *Per2* mutant animals had malignant lymphoma and showed a dramatically reduced life span compared to normal individuals. A number of key cell cycle genes are disrupted in these clock mutant animals, as would be expected, but perhaps one of the most significant is *c-Myc*. The levels of *c-Myc* are significantly increased in *Per2* mutant mice, as measured in the liver. One likely outcome of this deregulation of *c-Myc* is that cells will tend to remain proliferative, that is, stay within the cell cycle and undergo less apoptosis, a result clearly seen in the *Per2* mutants. The result of this, of course, will be increased cell proliferation, tumor growth rates, and enhanced sensitivity to DNA damaging treatments. Counter-experiments, where *Per2* was overexpressed in several mouse cancer cell lines, showed reduced *c-Myc* expression levels, amongst others and an increase in *p53* gene expression (Hua *et al.*, 2006). These overexpressing cells showed decreased cell proliferation and enhanced levels of apoptosis. It is very apparent that *Per2* levels can have a dramatic impact on cell division, either acting as a core clock component, or independently as a transcriptional regulator of other, downstream genes.

The *Period* genes are not the only clock components that are disrupted in tumors. Additional studies, particularly in breast and prostate cancers, have shown alterations in the expression of *Bmal1*, *Clock*, *Cry1*, *Cry2*, *Casein kinase 1 epsilon*, and *Npas2* (Lahti *et al.*, 2012). Whether these changes correlate with specific types of cancer will be addressed by "mining" these ever expanding human tumor databases over the next few years.

It is very clear that clock gene expression is disrupted in numerous types of human tumors, though only in a relatively few studies has such data been collected across the whole of a circadian cycle, as opposed to a single time point in the day. Such results could be interpreted in several ways. One possibility is that the circadian clocks within these tumors are "broken," there is no longer a molecular oscillation and the resulting steady state expression of these transcription factors disrupts the cell cycle. However, another explanation is that the clocks continue to oscillate within each cell in the tumor, but that a large degree of synchrony has been lost between cells, either because they are no longer responding to systemic entraining signals or there is a loss of coupling between malignant cells. Of course, the reality is likely to be a mix of these events and, in fact, clock function might well change as a tumor develops. In addition, it is very likely that clock function across a solid tumor is not uniform or equal, as changes in pH and hypoxic conditions in the center of the mass are likely to alter timing events. Though not well understood at this time, the difference between rhythmicity and nonrhythmicity within a tumor could have a significant impact on new ways of treating cancer progression. Regardless, the global outcome of these changes appears to be alterations in clock function, which are very likely to add to the general deregulation of cell cycle control.

12.7 Does alteration in clock gene expression in human tumors correlate with the survival of patients?

From a relatively limited number of high quality studies, this certainly appears to be the case. In colorectal cancer, *Per2* appears to be the most commonly mutated central clock gene (Sjöblom *et al.*, 2006). In a study of 133 patients with colorectal cancer, again performed by Levi and colleagues, an analysis of the number of cells staining positively for the PER2 protein in primary tumors strongly correlated with the outcome of chemotherapy, in this case, treatment with oxaliplatin, 5-FU and folinic acid (Iacobelli *et al.*, 2008). For 67 patients with more than 60% cells in the tumor having high PER2 expression, there was a 42% decrease in early death and extended lifespan compared to 66 patients with less than 10% of cells expressing PER2. Low PER2 levels correlate with a poorer prognosis in patients. It would be interesting to expand this analysis to other human tumors and determine how widely PER2 levels reflect the general outcome of cancer treatment in patients, as well as the speed at which the disease progresses. On a more speculative note, it might also be interesting to explore treatments that act to increase PER2 expression levels in these patients and determine if this, in combination with standard chemotherapeutic approaches, enhances shrinkage of the tumor, and the overall success rate of the treatment. Similar correlative data has been presented for studies on breast cancer, where levels of *Npas2* expression, rather than *Per2*, appear to be an indicator of survival rates and tumor progression within the selected cohort of patients (Zhu *et al.*, 2008).

12.8 Circadian-based chemotherapy (Chronotherapy): timing cancer treatment to improve survival

As described throughout this book, human physiology is extremely rhythmic, both at the whole body and cellular levels. Drugs taken orally may and will be absorbed differently at different times of day. Drug metabolism, plasma concentration and breakdown will also be rhythmic. The tumor itself resides within a rhythmic environment, being exposed to daily changes in cortisol, insulin, numerous growth factors, cytokines and many more. In addition, the tumor itself may retain some clock function, even if this is desynchronized between cells, such that the basic cell biology of the malignant cell, its metabolic state, receptor expression, and, obviously, cell cycle condition are changing with the time of day.

The majority of chemotherapeutic drug treatments, especially in a hospital environment, are given only during the working hours of the institution. This raises an obvious question: Can specifically targeting the delivery of an anti-cancer drug to a particular time of day improve the outcome of that treatment, when compared to either random or continuous application? The simple answer is, of course, yes. However, there are numerous caveats to this statement, relating to the specifics of the drug, the nature of its daily application, and even the gender of the patient. So the situation is a little more complex than might be immediately apparent. The aim of any chemotherapeutic treatment is to "kill" the largest number of malignant cells possible, while at the same time doing minimal damage to any surrounding, healthy tissue. If the clinician concerned is applying a drug that, for example, inhibits DNA replication or S-phase, it may be optimal to use that compound at a time of day when DNA replication is at its lowest level in healthy cells. Clearly, knowing the circadian phase of the cell cycle for the healthy tissue versus that for the tumor in a given individual is invaluable information for deciding the best time to administer that drug. In addition, knowing if there are timing or phase differences in the cell cycle between the tumor and neighboring tissue would strongly influence the timing of drug application. There are then additional considerations relating to drug toxicity/side effects, which are also likely to be time-of-day dependent. Furthermore, in the context of a study, should the drug be administered as a single, once a day bolus, or infused at varying concentrations across the day? Analyzing the data for continuous infusion itself can be complex, because even with constant exposure, due to rhythmic drug processing and metabolism, the levels of active compound in the bloodstream are very likely to be rhythmic. This phenomenon has been clearly demonstrated in the context of 5-fluorouracil (5-FU) use, where continuous infusion leads to higher concentrations in the plasma at night, depending on the amount of drug used and the rhythmic regulation of its breakdown by the enzyme, dihydropyrimidine dehydrogenase (Milano and Chamorey, 2002). Of course, rhythmic detoxification is a property of all drugs used in chemotherapy, not only 5-FU, and has been shown for a variety of compounds, including seliciclib, irinotecan and docetaxel. Simplistically put, the control by the circadian clock of enzymes involved in drug metabolism and detoxification in the liver is a critical component for the circadian treatment of cancer. A full understanding of the daily pharmacokinetics of a drug, the clock regulation of its metabolism, will greatly aid in its efficient use as an anti-cancer agent.

So two key factors come into play with chronotherapy, one is the rhythmic tolerance to the drug (chronotolerance), which is reflected in the maximum doses that can be applied to the patients, and the lowest number or level of side effects that are produced. And the second is the chronoefficacy of the drug, relating to how effective the compound is at "killing" cells when it reaches the tumor (Levi *et al.*, 2010). Empirically it would seem that these two tend to temporally coincide. This is a key concept, and perhaps counterintuitive, in that applying the drug when it is best tolerated, or least toxic, seems to correspond to the time when it is also most effective at treating the cancer. If this idea holds true as more and more studies are performed, then the consequences for the patient are clearly beneficial and quite dramatic. The development of advanced drug delivery technologies, that is, programmable pumps, also allows for these compounds to be delivered to the patient efficiently at hours that are not convenient for the hospital or clinician. Currently, over 95% of all cancer drug treatments occur between 9 a.m. and 5 p.m. The establishment of "user friendly" technology means that adoption of this chronotherapeutic approach in a medical setting is only going to increase.

It is impossible to go through all of the results from clinical trials for chronotherapeutic treatments (Levi *et al.*, 2010). However, the results are generally clear and very positive. In studies of patients with metastatic colorectal cancer, the specifically timed application of 5-FU-leucovorin-oxaliplatin versus constant infusion had a dramatic impact on the level of side effects experienced by the patient. The level of ulceration of the digestive tract (mucositis) was reduced by up to fivefold and sensory neuropathies were halved. The number of patients needing to attend the hospital due to drug toxicity problems was also greatly reduced, possibly by as much as threefold. An alteration in the specific timing of the daily drug application caused a shift in the level of severe toxic response from 16% in an optimal setting to 80% in a reversed schedule. Under such circumstances not only do patients obviously feel better but they are much more likely to stick with the prescribed chemotherapeutic regime.

In randomized trials, a comparison of constant infusion of the above drugs versus temporally-controlled application improved tumor regression (reduction by more than 50%) in 51% of patients with timed application versus 29% in constant-rate infusion. Curiously, in the total cohort, overall survival was not significantly improved. This rather unexpected result appears to be due to the gender of the patient. In men, the response to timed drug application was clearly beneficial, with approximately 25% of male patients showing improved survival. However, for female patients, this response was reversed, with 38% showing reduced life-span on the chrono-modulated schedule (Giacchetti *et al.*, 2006). Clearly, gender effects are dramatic in terms of not only analyzing the results of such clinical trials, but also in terms of determining the optimal treatment regimes. The underlying biological basis for this gender difference is being actively explored, but it may imply that different circadian schedules for drug application simply vary between men and women, and that a much higher level of personalization of medical intervention is required. New clinical trials are underway with the aim of addressing exactly such issues.

12.9 Conclusion

In this chapter, we have discussed how the circadian clock can strongly influence and regulate the timing of the cell cycle in a variety of animals and tissues, a fact that is also true for humans. Our knowledge of the molecular mechanisms that link the clock and the cell cycle is improving and many key candidates have been described. Yet this area of research is still in its early days, and a full understanding of the molecular interactions between the clock and cell division has not yet been achieved. Disruption of the circadian clock, by a variety of means, causes alterations in the regulation of the cell cycle, with a corresponding increase in cancer risk. In fact, many tumors appear to have disrupted clock gene expression. Again, much more work is needed to determine at what level this clock dysfunction occurs; it may well vary from tumor to tumor. An understanding of this biology is critical in a clinical setting. The timed, circadian application of drugs, chronotherapy, has already been shown to have clear benefits, especially regarding drug tolerance and toxicity. In many studies, the survival benefits to the patients are also clear, but this situation may be more complex than initially hoped. However, we are only at the beginning of this process. The clinicians and researchers of the future need to optimize these treatments in a temporal way, by understanding more about the kinetics of drug action as well as detailed consideration of each patient's circadian condition. Pharmaceutical companies also need to take temporal changes of the body into consideration when designing new drugs for cancer treatment. The future is bright, but there is still much work to do.

References

Balsalobre, A., Damiola, F., Schibler, U. 1998. A serum shock induces circadian gene expression in mammalian tissue culture cells. *Cell* **93**:929–37.

Bjarnason, G.A., Jordan, R.C., Wood, P.A., *et al.* 2001. Circadian expression of clock genes in human oral mucosa and skin: association with specific cell-cycle phases. *Am J Pathol* **158**:1793–801.

Borgs, L, Beukelaers, P., Vandenbosch, R., *et al.* 2009. Cell "circadian" cycle: new role for mammalian core clock genes. *Cell Cycle* **8**:832–7.

Conlon, M., Lightfoot, N., Kreiger, N. 2007. Rotating shift work and risk of prostate cancer. *Epidemiology* **18**:182–3.

Dekens, M.P., Santoriello, C., Vallone, D., *et al.* 2003. Light regulates the cell cycle in zebrafish. *Curr Biol* **13**:2051–7.

Filipski, E., Levi, F. 2009. Circadian disruption in experimental cancer processes. *Integr Cancer Ther* **8**:298–302.

Filipski, E., Li, X.M., Levi, F. 2006. Disruption of circadian coordination and malignant growth. *Cancer Causes Control* **17**:509–14.

Fu, L., Pelicano, H., Liu, J., *et al.* 2002. The circadian gene Period2 plays an important role in tumor suppression and DNA damage response *in vivo*. *Cell* **111**:41–50.

Giachetti, S., Bjarnason, G., Garufi, C., *et al.* 2006. Phase III trial comparing 4-day chronomodulated therapy versus 2-day conventional delivery of fluorouracil, leuovorin, and oxaliplatin at first-line chemotherapy of metastatic colorectal cancer: the European Organization for Research and Treatment of Cancer Chronotherapy Group. *J Clin Oncol.* **24**:3562–69.

Grechez-Cassiau, A., Rayet, B., Guillaumond, F., *et al.* 2008. The circadian clock component BMAL1 is a critical regulator of p21WAF1/CIP1 expression and hepatocyte proliferation. *J Biol Chem* **283**:4535–42.

Halberg, F. 1960. Temporal coordination of physiologic function. *Cold Spring Harb Symp Quant Biol* **25**:289–310.

Hankins, M.W., Peirson, S.N., Foster, R.G. 2008. Melanopsin: an exciting photopigment. *Trend Neurosci* **31**:27–36.

Hua, H., Wang, Y., Wan, C., *et al.* 2006. Circadian gene mPer2 overexpression induces cancer cell apoptosis. *Cancer Sci* **97**:589–96.

Iacobelli, S., Innominato, P., Piantelli, M., *et al.* 2008. Tumor clock protein PER2 as a determinant of survival in patients (pts) receiving oxaliplatin-5-FU-leucovorin as first-line chemotherapy for metastatic colorectal cancer (MCC). *J Clin Oncol* **26**(15S, May 20 suppl): abstract 11032.

Innominato, P.F., Focan, C., Gorlia, T., *et al.* 2009. Circadian rhythm in rest and activity: a biological correlate of quality of life and a predictor of survival in patients with metastatic colorectal cancer. *Cancer Res* **69**:4700–7.

Innominato, P.F., Levi, F.A., Bjarnason, G.A. 2010. Chronotherapy and the molecular clock: Clinical implications in oncology. *Adv Drug Deliv Rev* **62**:979–1001.

Janich, P., Pascual, G., Merlos-Suarez, A., *et al.* 2011. The circadian molecular clock creates epidermal stem cell heterogeneity. *Nature* **480**:209–14.

Lahti, T., Merikanto, I., Partonen, T. 2012. Circadian clock disruptions and the risk of cancer. *Ann Med* **44**:847–53.

Levi, F., Okyar, A., Dulong, S., *et al.* 2010. Circadian timing in cancer treatments. *Annu Rev Pharmacol Toxicol* **50**:377–421.

Matsumoto, Y., Tsunekawa, Y., Nomura, T., *et al.* 2011. Differential proliferation rhythm of neural progenitor and oligodendrocyte precursor cells in the young adult hippocampus. *PLoS One* **6**:e27628.

Matsuo, T., Yamaguchi, S., Mitsui, S., *et al.* 2003. Control mechanism of the circadian clock for timing of cell division *in vivo*. *Science* **302**:255–9.

Megdal, S.P., Kroenke, C.H., Laden, F., *et al.* 2005. Night work and breast cancer risk: a systematic review and meta-analysis. *Eur J Cancer* **41**:2023–32.

Milano, G., Chamorey, A.L. 2002. Clinical pharmacokinetics of 5-fluorouracil with consideration of chronopharmacokinetics. *Chronobiol Int* **19**:177–89.

Miller, B.H., McDearmon, E.L., Panda, S., *et al.* 2007. Circadian and CLOCK-controlled regulation of the mouse transcriptome and cell proliferation. *Proc Natl Acad Sci USA* **104**:3342–7.

Mori, T., Johnson, C.H. 2000. Circadian control of cell division in unicellular organisms. *Prog Cell Cycle Res* **4**:185–92.

Scheving, L.D., Burns, E.R., Pauly, J.E., Tsai, T.H. 1978. Circadian variation in cell division of the mouse alimentary tract, bone marrow and corneal epithelium. *Anat Rec* **191**:479–86.

Sephton, S.E., Sapolsky, R.M., Kraemer, H.C., Spiegel D. 2000. Diurnal cortisol rhythm as a predictor of breast cancer survival. *J Natl Cancer Inst* **92**:994–1000.

Sjöblom, T., Jones, S., Wood, L.D., *et al.* 2006. The consensus coding sequences of human breast and colorectal cancers. *Science* **314**:266–74.

Stephan, F.K. 2002. The "other" circadian system: food as a Zeitgeber. *J Biol Rhythms* **17**:284–92.

Straif, K., Baan, R., Grosse, Y., *et al.* 2007. Carcinogenicity of shift-work, painting, and fire-fighting. *Lancet Oncol* **8**:1065–6.

Tamai, T.K., Young, L.C., Cox, C.A., Whitmore, D. 2012. Light acts on the zebrafish circadian clock to suppress rhythmic mitosis and cell proliferation. *J Biol Rhythms* **27**:226–36.

Whitmore, D., Foulkes, N.S., Strahle, U., Sassone-Corsi, P. 1998. Zebrafish Clock rhythmic expression reveals independent peripheral circadian oscillators. *Nat Neurosci* **1**:701–7.

Whitmore, D., Foulkes, N.S., Sassone-Corsi, P. 2000. Lights acts directly on organs and cells in culture to set the vertebrate circadian clock. *Nature* **404**:87–91.

Yoo, S.H., Yamazaki, S., Lowrey, P.L., *et al.* 2004. PERIOD2::LUCIFERASE real-time reporting of circadian dynamics reveals persistent circadian oscillations in mouse peripheral tissues. *Proc Natl Acad Sci USA* **101**:5339–46.

Zhu, Y., Stevens, R.G., Leaderer, D., *et al.* 2008. Non-synonymous polymorphisms in the circadian gene NPAS2 and breast cancer risk. *Breast Cancer Res Treat* **107**:421–5.

How Shift Work and a Destabilized Circadian System may Increase Risk for Development of Cancer and Type 2 Diabetes

13

An Pan[1], Elizabeth Devore[2], and Eva S. Schernhammer[3,4]

[1] School of Public Health, Tongji Medical College, Huazhong University of Science and Technology, Wuhan, Hubei Province, China
[2] Channing Division of Network Medicine, Department of Medicine, Brigham and Women's Hospital and Harvard Medical School, Boston, MA, USA
[3] Department of Epidemiology, Harvard School of Public Health, Boston, MA, United States
[4] Department of Epidemiology, Centre of Public Health, Medical University of Vienna, Austria

13.1 Introduction

People spend much of their lives at work and occupational exposures can affect workers' health in many aspects. The potential association of occupational exposures with cancer and metabolic disorders, such as type 2 diabetes, has recently attracted considerable attention, with shift work appearing to have significant health implications. Shift work is common and is becoming increasingly prevalent in the so-called "24/7" society. According to the International Agency for Research on Cancer (WHO, 2010), about 15–30% of the working population in Europe and the United States is engaged in shift work (defined by the International Labor Organization as "a method of organization of working time in which workers succeed one another at the workplace so that the establishment can operate longer than the hours of work of individual workers").

In the scientific literature and for the general public, the term "shift work" has been widely used and usually includes any arrangement of daily working hours outside of regular daytime hours (7/8 a.m. to 5/6 p.m.). Therefore, shift workers include all individuals working evening shift, night shift, rotating shifts, split shifts, or irregular or on-call schedules – both during the week and on weekends. Obviously, people who work on shift schedules may be subject to desynchronized circadian rhythm, particularly those working in the night and on a rotating pattern. Emerging scientific evidence suggests that daily cycles of sleep–wake, regulation of hormones, and many physiological processes are often misaligned with behavioral patterns during shift work, especially rotating night shift work, leading to an increased risk of developing cancer and metabolic disorders, including obesity, metabolic syndrome, and type 2 diabetes.

Circadian Medicine, First Edition. Edited by Christopher S. Colwell.
© 2015 John Wiley & Sons, Inc. Published 2015 by John Wiley & Sons, Inc.

In 2007, the International Agency for Research on Cancer classified shift work as a possible carcinogen, based on what they called "convincing experimental evidence and suggestive epidemiologic data" to this effect (Straif *et al.*, 2007). Indeed, experimental data on the association between shift work and cancer has consistently demonstrated that simulated shift work can lead to a higher incidence of cancer in animal models. Shift work disrupts the normal light entrainment of the biological clock, as the suprachiasmatic nuclei (SCN) receives environmental light–dark information directly from the retina. This mechanism, which is also regulated by genes (Fu and Lee, 2003; Konopka and Benzer, 2011; Chapters 1 and 2), appears to have evolved to detect changes in day length/season (for functions like migration and hibernation).

Melatonin is a hormone and marker of circadian rhythmicity intimately linked to the circadian system that demonstrates cancer-protective properties (Vijayalaxmi *et al.*, 2002). Melatonin diffuses from the pineal gland into the cerebrospinal fluid and capillary blood, freely crossing the blood–brain barrier (Le Bars *et al.*, 1991). The effects of melatonin in the periphery can be roughly divided into direct effects, such as scavenging of free radicals, and receptor mediated effects (via its two receptors, MT_1 and MT_2) (Dubocovich, 2007). Relevant functions of melatonin related to cancer risk have been discussed elsewhere in greater detail (Vijayalaxmi *et al.*, 2002). Most prominent mechanisms that are currently being studied are melatonin's effect on estradiol (Brzezinski, 1997; Mediavilla *et al.*, 1999); its activity as an indirect antioxidant and free radical scavenger; its action on the immune system through activation of the cytokine system, thereby inhibiting growth over tumor cells; melatonin's suppression of fatty acid uptake and metabolism; its ability to increase the degradation of calmoduline, which is a key player in cell proliferation; and by inducing apoptosis and possibly acting as a natural antiangiogenetic molecule (Lissoni *et al.*, 2001; Blask *et al.*, 2002; Vijayalaxmi *et al.*, 2002; Sainz *et al.*, 2003).

In humans, epidemiologic data on an association between night shift work and cancer risk continue to accumulate, with the majority of studies indicating that a history of shift work is related to a modest increase in the risk of breast cancer. Initial studies have identified links between shift work and other cancers as well, although this evidence is very limited. A recent systematic review and meta-analysis, published in 2013 (Kamdar *et al.*, 2013), found a 21% increased risk of breast cancer (95% CI(confidence interval) 1.00 – 1.47, p = 0.056) among women who ever worked rotating night shifts.

Importantly, increasing evidence suggests that shift workers are more often obese compared to non-shift workers, which might be attributable to the metabolic and behavioral effects of circadian disruption – a common phenomenon among shift workers. In particular, individuals with circadian disruptions tend to have lower levels of leptin (an enzyme that signals satiation) and less healthy eating habits (e.g., consuming more food at night). Therefore, these mechanisms might explain the association between shift work and obesity, which is described in greater detail later (see also Table 13.3). In addition, obesity is a strong risk factor for many cancers, including breast cancer, colon cancer, and endometrial cancer, to name a few (Hursting and Dunlap, 2012). As a result, obesity is a potential mediator of the observed association between shift work and cancer risk and, in addition, may link shift work to other diseases that are strongly linked to obesity, such as type 2 diabetes (Gale *et al.*, 2011; Sherwin and Jastreboff, 2012). It is important to evaluate whether previous analyses support this hypothesis. In this chapter, epidemiologic studies of shift work and cancer risk are reviewed firstly, followed by a review existing of literature on shift work and type 2 diabetes, with an emphasis on the role of obesity in modifying these associations. The chapter concludes with a summary and suggested implications of this research.

13.2 Shift work and cancer

13.2.1 Epidemiologic studies of shift work and breast cancer risk

To date, 16 epidemiologic studies have examined the association of shift work and breast cancer (summarized in Table 13.1), Twelve of these studies have been conducted using a retrospective study design (i.e., the exposure – in our case, occupational exposure to night shift work – was measured *after* the outcome occurred), while four studies have been performed prospectively (i.e., the exposure

Table 13.1 Epidemiologic studies relating shift work with breast cancer risk among women.

Study author and date	Study design	Setting	Exposure	Outcome	Results
Tynes, 1996	Retrospective, nested case-control study	Cohort of all 2619 female radio and telegraph operators in Norway 1920–1980	Individual employment histories obtained from Norweigian seamen registries	50 cases occurring between 1961–1991, identified through the Norway Cancer Registry; 4–7:1 age-matched controls	Positive association
Schernhammer, 2001	Prospective cohort study	78,562 women participating in the Nurses' Health Study	Self-reported history of rotating night shift work	2441 cases occurring 1988–1998, identified by self-report and verified by medical records	Positive association
Davis, 2001	Retrospective case-control study	Women, aged 20–74 years, who lived in the Seattle metropolitan area during 1992–1995	Self-reported lifetime occupational history	813 cases occurring 1992–1995, identified by the Cancer Surveillance System of the Fred Hutchinson Cancer Center (Seattle); frequency-matched controls (5-year age strata), identified by random-digit dialing	Positive association
Hansen, 2001	Retrospective case-control study	Women, aged 30–54 years, with a work history in Denmark and born during 1935–59	Employment histories were reconstructed from national employment records, then combined with survey information about jobs that involving primarily night work	7035 cases having occurred by 1989, identified by the Danish Cancer Registry; 1:1 age-matched controls, identified from the Central Population Registry	Positive association
Schernhammer, 2006	Prospective cohort study	115,022 women participating in the Nurses' Health Study II	Self-reported history of rotating night shift work	1352 cases occurring 1989–2001, identified by self-report and verified by medical records	Positive association
Lie, 2006	Retrospective, nested case-control study	Cohort of 44,835 nurses educated 1914–1980 in Norway	Individual employment histories obtained from the Norwegian nurse registry, combined with census data in 1960, 1970, and 1980	537 cases occurring 1960–1982, identified by the Norway Cancer Registry; controls were matched 4:1 using incidence density sampling within the Norwegian nurse registry	Positive association

(Continued)

Table 13.1 (*continued*)

Study author and date	Study design	Setting	Exposure	Outcome	Results
O'Leary, 2006	Retrospective case-control study	Women, aged <75years, who had lived on Long Island at least 15 years in 1996–1997	Self-reported employment histories obtained by interview	576 cases occurring 1996–1997, identified by rapid ascertainment from local hospitals; frequency-matched controls (in 5-year age strata), identified by random-digit dialing and government records	No association
Schwartzbaum, 2007	Retrospective cohort study	1,148,661 female employees working at least half-time in 1970 in Sweden	Census information about employment histories, combined with survey information about jobs that involving primarily night work	70 cases occurring 1971–1989 among shift workers, identified by the Swedish Cancer Register; comparison group was all other women in the study base	No association
Pukkala, 2009	Prospective cohort study	7,454,847 women, aged 30–64 years, in the 1960–1990 censuses in Denmark, Finland, Iceland, Norway, and Sweden	Occupations reported on censuses between 1960–1990	7682 cases occurring through 2005 in nurses, identified by national cancer registries; comparison group was all other women in the study	Positive association
Pronk, 2010	Prospective cohort study	73,049 women, aged 40-70 years, cancer free, living in Shanghai (China), and having been employed outside of the home in 1996–2000	Self-reported employment histories obtained by interview	717 cases occurring 1996/2000–2007, identified by biennial interviews and the Shanghai Cancer Registry, and verified by home visits and medical records	No association
Pesch, 2010	Retrospective case-control study	Women, aged ≤80years, living in Bonn, Germany during 2000–2004	Self-reported occupational histories obtained by interview	1143 cases occurring within 6 months of study enrollment, identified from major hospitals in the region; frequency-matched controls (in 5-year age strata) from population registries	No association

Villeneuve, 2011	Retrospective case-control study	Women, aged 25–75 years, living in two specific areas of France	Self-reported occupational histories obtained by interview	1230 cases occurring 2005–2007, identified from major cancer hospitals; frequency-matched controls (5-year age strata), identified randomly by telephone directory	Positive association
Lie, 2011	Retrospective, nested case-control study	Cohort of 49,402 Norwegian nurses	Lifetime occupational history obtained by interview	699 cases occurring 1990–2007, identified by the Cancer Registry of Norway; 2:1 frequency-matched controls (in 5-year age strata)	Positive association
Hansen, 2012	Retrospective, nested case-control study	Cohort of 91,140 female members of the Danish Nurses Association	Lifetime occupational history obtained by interview	267 cases occurring 2001–2003, identified by the Danish Cancer Registry; age-matched controls (1 year), identified by incidence density sampling	Positive association
Hansen, 2012	Retrospective, nested case-control study	Cohort of 18,551 women who served in the Danish military 1964–1999	Self-reported occupational history	132 cases occurring 1990–2003, identified by the Danish Cancer Registry; age-matched controls were selected by incidence density sampling	Positive association
Menegaux, 2013	Retrospective case-control study	Women, aged 25–75 years, living in two specific areas of France	Lifetime occupational history obtained by interview	1232 cases occurring 2005–2007, identified from major cancer hospitals; frequency-matched controls (in 10-year age strata), identified randomly by telephone directory	Positive association

was measured *before* the outcome occurred). Overall, most studies have found some evidence in favor of an association between exposure to shift work and an increased risk of breast cancer, although a few studies have reported no such association.

13.2.1.1 Retrospective studies showing increased risk of breast cancer among shift workers

Nine retrospective studies have indicated that shift work might be associated with higher risk of breast cancer, including: three studies in Norway, three studies in Denmark, two studies in France, and one study in the United States.

As one of the earliest studies providing such evidence, Tynes *et al.* conducted a study of 2619 female Norwegian radio and telegraph operators certified between 1920 and 1980; over 30 years of follow-up (1961–1991), they documented 50 incident breast cancer cases (Tynes *et al.*, 1996). Night work was defined as "work at night with exposure to artificial light". The authors observed a significantly increased standardized incidence ratio for breast cancer among women working in this occupation compared to women in the general Norwegian population (standardized incidence ratio adjusted for duration of employment = 1.5, 95% CI 1.1–2.0). Moreover, in a subset of this cohort with detailed work histories, cumulative exposure to shift work was suggestively (albeit with very limited power) related to breast cancer risk in women aged <50 years (p-trend = 0.31; odds ratio (OR) 1.9, 95% CI 0.5–7.0 comparing high levels of shift work versus no shift work) or women aged ≥50 years (p-trend = 0.13; OR 4.3, 95% CI 0.7–26.0). Certainly, a limitation of this study was the small number of breast cancer cases (n = 50) included in the case-control study, which led to wide confidence intervals and thus limited interpretation of these data particularly in the stratified analyses.

In the first of three Danish studies, a population-based case-control analysis with 7035 breast cancer cases was utilized to evaluate breast cancer risk among women in "night-work trades" versus "nonnight-work trades"(Hansen, 2001). This study found that those in "night-work trades" had a 50% higher risk of breast cancer (OR 1.5, 95% CI 1.3–1.7) compared to those in "nonnight-work trades". "Night-work trades" were defined as occupations in which ≥60% of employees worked at night, based on a national employment survey; "nonnight-work trades" were defined as those with <40% of employees working at night. Of note, in this study night shift work was defined based on thresholds derived from national-level data; in other words, specific information on each participant's night work exposure was not collected. This approach probably led to considerable exposure misclassification, and therefore the reported association was likely to be underestimated.

Two further studies from Denmark focused specifically on shift worker populations, in which detailed employment histories were obtained from individual participants. One study was a case-control analysis with 267 breast cancer cases, nested within a large cohort of female members of the Danish Nurses Association. In this study, women with a history of rotating night shift work – after midnight – had an 80% increased risk of breast cancer compared to women with a history of permanent day work (OR 1.8, 95% CI 1.2–2.8), and the risk of breast cancer was even higher among women with a history of both rotating shift work and permanent night work (OR 2.9, 95% CI 1.1–8.0) (Hansen and Stevens, 2012). A second case-control study in Denmark (n = 132 breast cancer cases), nested within a cohort of female military employees, reported that long-term night shift work was related to a higher risk of breast cancer (e.g., p-trend = 0.03, OR 2.1, 95% CI 1.0–4.5 for ≥15 years of night shift work versus none) (Hansen and Lassen, 2012). Although these two studies of shift worker populations had much smaller case numbers, and therefore lower power, compared to the initial population-based study in Denmark, the greater accuracy of their exposure measurements based on individual employment histories may have enabled the detection of significant associations between night shift work and breast cancer risk.

Two additional studies evaluated associations between shift work and breast cancer within a cohort of >40,000 nurses in Norway. One of these studies reported that longer duration of night work was associated with an increased risk of breast cancer (n = 537 cases; p-trend = 0.01, OR 2.21, 95% CI 1.10–4.45 comparing nurses with ≥30 years of night work versus none) (Lie *et al.*, 2006). Although this finding was significant, the study determined participants' exposure status based on assumptions about which clinical positions tended to involve night work, and resulting exposure misclassification may have limited the ability to detect stronger associations in this study. A second study in this cohort found that women working ≥5 years, with schedules involving ≥5 consecutive night shifts, had a higher breast cancer risk compared to those who never worked night shifts (OR 1.6, 95% CI 1.0–2.4) (Lie et al., 2011). Unlike the first Norwegian study, this study involved an extensive telephone interview to ascertain each individual's employment history, which is likely to have provided much more accurate exposure classification regarding night work.

Two additional analyses were based in a French case-control study, comprising approximately 2500 women with extensive employment histories, including 1200 breast cancer cases. One study reported that working as a nurse for ≥10 years might be associated with a higher risk of breast cancer compared to working in other occupations (OR 1.4, 95% CI 0.9–2.1), although this association did not reach statistical significance (Villeneuve et al., 2011). However, in a second analysis using this study population, women with any history of night work had an elevated breast cancer risk when they were compared to women who never worked at night (OR 1.35, 95% CI 1.01–1.80) (Menegaux et al., 2013). Importantly, additional exposure metrics related to frequency and duration of night work indicated that longer-term exposure was related to an increased risk of breast cancer as well (e.g., OR 1.40, 95% CI 1.01–1.92 for women with ≥4.5 years of night work experience versus none). As noted previously for other studies, the availability of detailed information on employment history from each participant was an important strength of this study design, which enabled better detection of the associations of interest.

Finally, extensive employment histories among individuals were also used to identify relations between night shift work and breast cancer in a case-control study based in Seattle, Washington (Davis et al., 2001). In particular, women with a history of overnight shift work had greater odds of breast cancer than women who had never worked such shifts (n = 813 cases; OR 1.6, 95% CI 1.0–2.5), and there was evidence of a linear trend toward greater risk of breast cancer with increasing time spent on overnight shifts (p-trend = 0.04, OR 2.3, 95% CI 1.0–5.3 comparing women with ≥5.7 hours per week versus none).

13.2.1.2 Retrospective studies showing no association between shift work and breast cancer risk

Three studies with retrospective designs, to date, identified no association between shift work and breast cancer risk.

A case-control study, nested within the Long Island Cohort, found no association between evening or overnight shift work with risk of breast cancer (e.g., n = 576 cases; standardized incidence ratio = 1.04, 95% CI 0.79–1.38), although the authors limited exposure recall to the past 15 years of work experience (O'Leary et al., 2006). Thus, one possible explanation for their null finding is that shift work prior to this time period is etiologically relevant for breast cancer risk, and not accounting for earlier shift work exposure might have contributed to this null result. Furthermore, the unusually high incidence of breast cancer in the Long Island area might have masked any effects of shift work on breast cancer, and therefore these results may not provide insight into this association for the general population.

Another nested case-control study, conducted in Germany, found that women with a history of shift work had a similar breast cancer risk compared to women with no history of shift work (n = 1143 cases; OR 0.96, 95% CI 0.67–1.38), the same result was evident when women with prior involvement in night shift work specifically were compared to those with no shift work experience (OR 0.91, 95% CI 0.55–1.49)(O'Leary et al., 2006). Other shift work metrics, including greater cumulative number of lifetime night shifts and greater duration of night shift work, were associated with nonsignificantly elevated risks of breast cancer (e.g., OR 1.73, 95% CI 0.71–4.22 comparing women with ≥807 cumulative lifetime nights shifts versus none, and OR 2.48, 95% CI 0.62–9.99 comparing women with ≥20 years of night shift work versus none). However, these comparisons were based on a small number of breast cancer cases, as the prevalence of shift work was low (13%) in this population; as a result, wide confidence intervals made interpretation difficult.

Finally, a retrospective cohort study among >1 million female employees in Sweden found that shift work (defined as occupations that have ≥40% of employees in shift work) was not associated with breast cancer incidence compared to other types of work (defined as occupations with <30% of employees in shift work) (standardized incidence ratio = 0.94, 95% CI 0.74–1.18)(Schwartzbaum et al., 2007). As previously noted, the use of national-level data to establish thresholds defining exposure status is likely to cause considerable misclassification, and thus underestimation, of the association of interest.

13.2.1.3 Prospective studies of shift work and breast cancer risk

Three of four currently published prospective studies have provided evidence in favor of an association between shift work and breast cancer.

In the two Nurses' Health Studies, Schernhammer *et al.* (2001, 2006) described that women reporting the most extensive histories of rotating shift work had a modestly increased risk of breast cancer compared to those reporting no rotating shift work. Specifically, in premenopausal women, those with ≥20 years of shift work experience had a 79% higher risk (95% CI 1.06–3.01) than their counterparts; in postmenopausal women, breast cancer risk was elevated by 36% (95% CI 1.04–1.78) among those with ≥30 years versus no history of rotating shift work. One limitation of these studies is that women were asked to report durations of "rotating night work" defined as at least three nights per month in addition to days or evenings in that month; however, participants were not specifically asked about permanent night shift work, and therefore women with such work histories may have provided the same response as women without any shift work history. To the extent this occurred, women with permanent night shift experience were included in the reference group with nonshift workers, which may have biased the observed associations toward the null because permanent night workers are hypothesized to have intermediate circadian disruptions (and, therefore, possibly intermediate breast cancer risk) compared to nonshift workers and rotating night shift workers. Other limitations include the small case numbers in strata with longer durations of shift work and the potentially limited generalizability of these findings to other occupational groups.

Another prospective cohort study, conducted among 7.5 million women in five Nordic countries during 1961–2005, identified those in the nursing occupation as being at moderately greater risk of breast cancer compared to women working in other occupations (crude standardized incidence ratio = 1.18, 95% CI 1.15–1.20), although the possibility remains that other occupational exposures might explain this association (Pukkala *et al.*, 2009).

Finally, in a prospective cohort study in Shanghai, a history of working night shifts was not associated with breast cancer (HR = 1.0, 95% CI 0.9–1.2 comparing women with any night shift work versus none); additional shift work metrics that incorporated frequency, duration, and cumulative exposure were not related to breast cancer risk either (Pronk *et al.*, 2010). Limitations of this study, however, were the lack of information to distinguish fixed versus rotating shift work and low prevalence of extreme durations of shift work (e.g., ≥20 years). Either or both of these issues has the potential to have contributed to null findings, and thus could explain why shift work was not associated with breast cancer risk in this study. Nonetheless, findings from this study do not support an association between shift work and breast cancer, which contrasts with the other three prospective studies that have reported modest relations between shift work or the nursing profession and increased risk of breast cancer.

13.2.2 Epidemiologic studies of shift work and prostate cancer

Three observational studies – one retrospective study and two prospective studies – have examined the association between shift work and prostate cancer risk (Table 13.2).

The retrospective study, a case-control design based on 760 prostate cancer cases and 1632 frequency-matched controls, found that men who normally worked full-time rotating shifts had higher odds of prostate cancer compared to men who did not normally work such shifts (OR 1.19, 95% CI 1.00–1.42). However, this result should be interpreted with caution, as it is modest in magnitude and only borderline significant (Conlon *et al.*, 2007). There was also a suggestion that men with the longest duration of rotating shifts might have greater odds of prostate cancer compared to those who did not work rotating shifts (OR 1.30, 95% CI 0.97–1.74), although no dose-response relation was observed across five categories of shift work duration (p-trend = 0.4), and other shift work metrics were not related to prostate cancer risk. One limitation of this research was the crude exposure assessment, which asked participants to report their "usual" work time as day, evening/night, or rotating. Thus, exposure misclassification may have caused some underestimation of the associations of interest, as men who engaged in rotating shift work occasionally, but not predominantly, would not have contributed to risk in the rotating shift work group.

A prospective cohort study in Japan reported that men who worked rotating shifts had a significantly higher risk of prostate cancer compared to those working daytime shifts (risk ratio(RR) 3.0, 95% CI

Table 13.2 Epidemiologic studies relating shift work with prostate and other cancers.

Study author and date	Cancer type	Study design	Setting	Exposure	Outcome	Results
Schernhammer, 2003	Colorectal	Prospective cohort study	78,586 women in the Nurses' Health Study	Self-reported history of rotating night shift work	602 cases occurring 1988–1998, identified by self-report and verified by medical records	Positive association
Kubo, 2006	Prostate	Prospective cohort study	14,052 working men, aged 40–65 years, in Japan	Self-reported work schedule via questionnaire	31 cases, identified by area cancer registries	Positive association
Conlon, 2007	Prostate	Retrospective case-control study	2392 men, aged 45–84 years, living in northeastern Ontario	Self-reported lifetime employment history via questionnaire	760 prostate cancer cases, occurring 1995–1998	Positive association
Viswanathan, 2007	Endometrial	Prospective cohort study	53,487 women participating in Nurses' Health Study	Self-reported history of rotating night shift work	515 cases occurring 1988–2004, identified by self-report and verified by medical records	Positive association
Lahti, 2008	Non-Hodgkin lymphoma	Prospective cohort study	1,669,272 men and women, aged 25–64 years, working in Finland	Census information about employment histories, combined with survey information about jobs that involving primarily night work	6307 cases, occurring 1971–1995, and identified by the Finnish Cancer Registry	Positive association in men only
Kubo, 2011a	Prostate	Prospective cohort study	4995 men, aged 49–65 years, working in a Japanese manufacturing corporation	Long-term work schedule obtained from corporation records	17 cases, identified from health insurance records	No association
Poole, 2011	Ovarian	Prospective cohort study	181,548 women participating in the Nurses' Health Study and Nurses' Health Study II	Self-reported history of rotating night shift work	718 cases, occurring 1988–2007 in Nurses' Health Study and 1989–2008 in Nurses' Health Study II, and identified by self-report and verified by medical records	No association

(Continued)

Table 13.2 (*continued*)

Study author and date	Cancer type	Study design	Setting	Exposure	Outcome	Results
Schernhammer, 2011	Skin	Prospective cohort study	68,336 women participating in the Nurses' Health Study	Self-reported history of rotating night shift work	10,799 cases, occurring 1988–2006, and identified by self-report and verified by medical records	Negative association
Parent, 2012	Cancer of 11 different anatomic sites	Population-based case-controls study of men	Quebec, Canada; 3137 men with cancer and 512 population controls	Self-reported job histories including work hours	3137 men with cancer occurring 1979–1985, and 512 population controls	Positive association for cancers of the lung, colon, bladder, prostate, rectum, pancreatic, and non-Hodgkin lymphoma; Negative association for cancer of the stomach, kidney, esophagus, melanoma

1.2–7.7), and men working fixed night shifts had a nonsignificantly increased risk (RR 2.3, 95% CI 0.6–9.2) (Kubo *et al.*, 2006). Due to the small number of cases (n = 31), these estimates have wide confidence intervals and, therefore, should be interpreted with caution. However, this study also had a crude exposure measurement based on a single report of a participant's most common work schedule, which would have contributed to exposure misclassification and possible underestimation of associations, as described for the previous study.

An additional study, also prospectively conducted in Japan, found an increased risk of prostate cancer related to the performance of shift work compared to daytime work (OR 1.79, 95% CI 0.57–5.68), although the association was not significant due to an even smaller number of prostate cancer cases (n = 17) in this cohort (Kubo *et al.*, 2011a).

Thus, overall, evidence for a relation between shift work and prostate cancer is very limited, both by the small number of studies and major limitations involved in those studies that have been conducted.

13.2.3 Epidemiologic studies of shift work and risk of other cancers

Several prospective studies have examined associations between shift work and other cancers as well (Table 13.2). In the Nurses' Health Study, women with the longest durations of rotating shift work had modestly increased risks of colorectal cancer (n = 602 cases; RR 1.35, 95% CI 1.03–1.77 for ≥15 years versus none) (Schernhammer *et al.*, 2003) and endometrial cancer (n = 515 cases; RR 1.47, 95% CI 1.03–2.10 for ≥20 years versus none)(Viswanathan *et al.*, 2007); there was no association between rotating shift work and ovarian cancer in an analysis of 181,548 women participating in the Nurses' Health Study and Nurses' Health Study II (n = 718 cases; RR 0.80, 95% CI 0.51–1.23 comparing women with ≥20 versus no years of shift work)(Poole *et al.*, 2011). In addition, women with longer durations of shift work had a decreased risk of skin cancer in the Nurses' Health Study cohort (n = 10,799 cases; RR 0.86, 95% CI 0.81-0.92 for ≥10 years versus none), although this association was modified by hair color and, therefore, might be explained by genetic factors that determine hair color and increase genetic susceptibility to skin cancer risk (Schernhammer *et al.*, 2011).

Another study, involving a cohort of >1.6 million Finnish employees, found a slightly higher risk of non-Hodgkin lymphoma among men with exposure to night shift work (n = 3813 cases; RR 1.10, 95% CI 1.03–1.19), although the association was not apparent for women (n = 2494 cases; RR 1.02, 95% CI 0.94–1.12)(Lahti *et al.*, 2008). One possibility is that estrogen-related mechanisms might explain this sex difference, although the very modest association observed among men could also be simply due to chance.

In the most recent, a population-based case-control study among men only, Parent *et al.* (2012) examined the risk of 11 anatomically distinct cancer sites in relation to shift work. In their analyses, the authors found the risk of several cancers, specifically the risk of lung cancer (OR 1.76; 95% CI 1.25–2.47), colon cancer (OR 2.03; 95% CI 1.43–2.89), bladder cancer (OR 1.74; 95% CI 1.22–2.49), prostate cancer (OR 2.77; 95% CI 1.96–3.92), rectal cancer (OR 2.09; 95% CI 1.40–3.14), pancreatic cancer (OR 2.27; 95% CI 1.24–4.15); and non-Hodgkin lymphoma (OR 2.31; 95% CI 1.48–3.61), to be higher among men who reported ever having worked night shifts. However, there was no association between night shift work and the risk of cancers of the stomach, kidney, and esophagus, or melanoma. Moreover, that the observed risks did not increase with increasing number of years of shift work casts some doubt on the findings from this retrospective study.

13.2.4 Summary of evidence for an association between shift work and cancer

Taken together, and as supported by several recent meta-analyses (Jia *et al.*, 2013; Kamdar *et al.*, 2013), the growing evidence of studies on night shift work and breast cancer risk supports, even after considering limitations inherent to the various study designs and methods, the risk of breast cancer to be elevated in night shift workers; this appears to primarily apply for women with longer durations of night shift work (Bonde *et al.*, 2012). In contrast, while evidence for an association between night shift work and the risk of prostate cancer is beginning to accumulate, for all other cancers (other than breast cancer), too few studies have yet been published to reach a meaningful conclusion as far as their association between night shift work is concerned.

13.2.5 Consideration of obesity in epidemiologic studies of night shift work and cancer risk

Most, but not all, studies of shift work and cancer risk considered body mass index (BMI) as a possible confounding factor by adjusting for this covariate in statistical models. However, none of the studies that reported adjusting for BMI indicated a substantial change in effect estimates as a result. Given the potential for obesity to be an effect modifier of associations between shift work and cancer risk, three studies also conducted stratified analyses based on obesity status. Two of these studies focused on shift work and breast cancer, and found that obesity did not modify observed associations; a third study of shift work and endometrial cancer found some indication of an interaction. Specifically, rotating shift work was primarily related to endometrial cancer among obese women (RR 2.09, 95% CI 1.24–3.52), but not among nonobese women (RR 1.07, 95% CI 0.60–1.92), in the Nurses' Health Study. Clearly, additional studies are needed to explore the hypothesis that obesity might modulate the association between shift work and cancer risk, and especially for endometrial cancer risk, which is heavily influenced by obesity.

13.3 Shift work and obesity, metabolic syndrome, and type 2 diabetes

Diabetes affected 366 million people worldwide in 2011 and this number will continue to increase to approximately 552 million by 2030 globally, with two-thirds of all diabetes cases occurring in low- to middle-income countries (International Diabetes Federation). The increasing prevalence of diabetes and related health complications has become a global public health crisis that threatens the economies of all nations. Diabetes is characterized by raised fasting glucose or postprandial glucose levels in serum, which are caused by insufficient insulin production from the pancreas, or insulin resistance that causes cells not to respond to circulating insulin. Diabetes is a multifactorial disease and the underlying etiological factors include environment and genetic factors and their interactions on glucose homeostasis. Type 2 diabetes makes up more than 90% of all diabetes cases and mainly results from insulin resistance together with relatively reduced insulin secretion. Because type 1 diabetes usually occurs early in life and has a strong genetic predisposition, the focus in this chapter is on type 2 diabetes (also see Chapter 11).

It has been a well-known fact that night shift work causes circadian disruption and sleep disturbance, which could increase fasting glucose and insulin levels after shift work (Theorell *et al.*, 1976). An early observation reported a higher prevalence of diabetes among rotating night shift workers in a male Japanese population (Mikuni *et al.*, 1983). The available epidemiological studies that have linked shift work with obesity and metabolic syndrome (conditions that are highly correlated to type 2 diabetes) and type 2 diabetes are summarized in Table 13.3.

13.3.1 Epidemiological studies of shift work and obesity and metabolic syndrome

As clearly demonstrated in Table 13.3 (cross-sectional studies, case-control studies, and cohort studies with a minimum sample size of 100), the majority of cross-sectional studies reported a high prevalence of obesity and metabolic syndrome among shift workers compared to regular day workers. This has been repeated in different countries and different occupations. However, cross-sectional studies may be subject to selection bias. Two important sources of selection bias should be considered when investigating shift work-related health effects. One is the primary selection of people selecting shift work. People are less likely to apply for a shift work job if they think they might not adapt to the shift work schedule. The primary

Table 13.3 Epidemiological studies relating shift work with metabolic syndrome, obesity, and type 2 diabetes.

Study author and date	Study design	Setting	Exposure	Outcomes	Results
Karlsson, 2001	Cross-sectional study	Västerbotten intervention Program, Sweden, 27,485 men and women	Shift work	MetS	The relative risks for shift working versus day working women with one, two, and three metabolic variables were 1.06, 1.20, and 1.71, respectively. The corresponding relative risks for men were 0.99, 1.30, and 1.63, respectively
Nagaya, 2002	Cross-sectional study	Male blue-collar workers, Japan; 2824 day and 826 shift workers	Shift work	Insulin resistance syndrome	Shift work was associated with insulin resistance markers (hyperglycemia, hypertension, hypertriglyceridemia, and greater numbers of these markers) in workers younger than 50 years, but not in people who were older than 50 years
Sookoian, 2007	Cross-sectional study	Male workers, Argentina; 877 day workers, and 474 rotating shift workers	Rotating shift work	MetS	The OR for MetS in rotating shift workers when compared with day workers was 1.51 (95% CI 1.01–2.25); rotating shift workers had elevated BMI, waist-hip ratio, and HOMA-IR
Esquirol, 2009	Cross-sectional study	Workers in petrochemical plant, France; 98 male strictly rotating shift workers, and 100 male regular day workers	Rotating shift work	MetS	The OR was 2.33 (95% CI 1.04–5.23) compared rotating shift work with day work
Kawada, 2010	Cross-sectional study	Workers in a car manufacturing company, Japan; 3007 men (1700 day and 1307 shift workers)	Shift work	MetS	Two-shift work was associated with lower risk of MetS (OR 0.77; 95% CI 0.61–0.98) compared to day workers, the association was not significant for three-shift workers (OR 1.39; 95% CI 0.92–2.09)
Mohebbi, 2012	Cross-sectional study	Drivers, Iran; 3039 shift work drivers and matched nonshift workers	Shift work	MetS	The metabolic syndrome was more common among the shift workers (OR 1.495; 95% CI 1.349–1.657) compared to day workers

(Continued)

Table 13.3 (continued)

Study author and date	Study design	Setting	Exposure	Outcomes	Results
Puttonen, 2012	Cross-sectional study	Employees of a large airline company, Finland; 297 day workers, 341 former shift workers, 418 2-shift workers, 283 night shift workers, and 472 in-flight workers	Former shift work, current 2-shift work, current night shift work, and current in-flight work	MetS	Compared to male day workers, the OR (95% CI) was 2.00 (1.26–3.19) for male former shift workers, 1.48 (0.93–2.24) for male 2-shift workers, 1.37 (0.84–2.22) for male night shift workers; no significant differences were found among females
Tucker, 2012	Cross-sectional study	No specific occupation, France; 1757 participants, 989 being current or former shift workers	Current or former shift workers	MetS	Compared with day workers, the OR was 1.78 (95% CI 1.03–3.08) in current or former shift workers, and the OR was 1.30 and 1.83 for workers with 1–10 years and >10 years of shift work experience
De Bacquer, 2009	Prospective cohort study with median 6.6 years of follow-up	BELSTRESS Study, Belgium; 1529 men	Rotating shift work	MetS	Rotating shift workers were at high risk of developing MetS (OR 1.56; 95% CI 1.15–2.11), and hyperglycemia (including T2D; OR 1.56; 95% CI 1.18–2.05) compared to day workers
Lin, 2009a	Retrospective cohort study with 5 years of follow-up	Female workers in electronic manufacturing Company, Taiwan; 387 women	Persistent rotating shift work	MetS	The OR was 3.5 (95% CI 1.3–9.0) for persistent rotating shift work compared with persistent day job
Lin, 2009b	Retrospective cohort study with 5 years of follow-up	Male workers in electronic manufacturing Company, Taiwan; 996 men	Persistent rotating shift work	MetS	Male workers with baseline elevated ALT plus persistent rotating shift work had a 2.7-fold (95% CI: 1.4–5.3) greater risk of developing MetS compared with those having neither initial elevated ALT nor shift work exposure
Pietroiusti, 2010	Prospective cohort study with 4 years of follow-up	Male and female nurses free from any component of MetS at baseline, Italy; 402 night shift workers, and 336 daytime workers	Night shift work	MetS	The cumulative incidence of MS was 9.0% (36/402) among night shift workers, and 1.8% (6/336) among daytime workers (HR 5.10; 95% CI 2.15–12.11)
Li, 2011	Nested case-control study with 4 years of follow-up	Subcohort of the Saku Cancer Etiology Surveillance Study, Japan; 6712 men and women	Shift work	MetS	Compared with the day workers, shift workers had a significantly higher risk of MetS (OR 1.87; 95% CI 1.13–3.08)

van Amelsvoort, 1999	Cross-sectional study	Workers in a waste incinerator plant, and nurses in hospitals, The Netherlands; 181 men and 196 women	Shift work	BMI and waist-hip ratio	The linear regression coefficients were 0.12 for BMI ($P<0.05$) per year in shift work and 0.0016 work for WHR ($P<0.05$) per year in shift work;
Karlsson, 2001	Cross-sectional study	Västerbotten intervention Program, Sweden; 27,485 men and women	Shift work	Obesity	The OR for obesity was 1.39 (95% CI 1.25–1.55) in women, and 1.44 (95% CI 1.27–1.64) in men compared shift work with day work
Parkes, 2002	Cross-sectional study	Male offshore workers on oil and gas installations, UK; 787 male day workers and 787 male day-night shift workers	Night shift work	BMI	No significant association with BMI was found comparing day-night shift workers with day workers, but among day-night shift workers, years of shift work was significantly associated with BMI
Di Lorenzo, 2003	Cross-sectional study	Glucose tolerant workers in a chemical industry, Italy; 134 male day workers and 185 shift workers	Shift work	Obesity	Obesity was more prevalent in shift workers (20.0%) than in day workers (9.7%)
Karlsson, 2003	Cross-sectional study	Subpopulation in the WOLF study, Sweden; 665 day workers and 659 three-shift workers	Shift work	Central obesity	The crude OR for abdominal obesity among shift workers was 1.34 (95% CI 1.07–1.69), while the OR decreased to 1.19 (95% CI 0.92–1.56) after controlling for other covariates
Ishizaki, 2004	Cross-sectional study	Male workers in a metal product factory, Japan; 3658 day workers and 585 night shift workers	Night shift work	BMI and waist-hip ratio	The standardized estimate β was 0.506 for BMI and 0.011 for waist-hip ratio (both $P<0.001$) associated with shift work
Ha, 2005	Cross-sectional study	Female nurses, Korea; 226 women	Rotating shift work	Overweight and waist circumference	Waist-hip ratio, but not BMI. was significantly associated with duration of shift work in female nurses who were 30 years old or more
Di Milia, 2009	Cross-sectional study	Workers in a coal industry and a regional university, Australia; 208 shift workers and 138 day workers	Shift work	BMI	Mean BMI was significantly higher in shift workers (28.1±5.4) than in day workers (26.2±4.4)
Bushnell, 2010	Cross-sectional study	A multinational chemical and coatings manufacturer; 26,442 workers	Night shift work, rotating shift work	Obesity	Compared to day workers, night shift workers had a higher prevalence of obesity, but not rotating shift workers

(Continued)

Table 13.3 (continued)

Study author and date	Study design	Setting	Exposure	Outcomes	Results
Chen, 2010	Cross-sectional study	Female workers in a semiconductor manufacturing factory, Taiwan; 1838 women	Fixed 12-h night shift work	Obesity	Women working in the clean room on fixed 12 h night shifts had significantly elevated odds ratios for obesity (OR 2.7; 95% CI 1.6–4.5) and central obesity (OR 2.9; 95% CI 1.7–5.1) compared to female office workers
Thomas, 2010	Cross-sectional study	Subjects from the 1958 British birth cohort, UK; 7839 men and women aged 45 years old	Night/morning shift work, evening/weekend shift work	BMI and waist circumference	Men regularly performing night/morning work had significantly higher BMI, WC and CRP compared with men who did not regularly do the shift work. The association was not found for evening/weekend work after adjustment, neither in women
Zhao, 2011	Cross-sectional study	Female nurses and midwives, Australia; 2494 participants (1259 day and 1235 shift workers)	Shift work	Overweight and obesity	Shift workers were 1.15 times more likely to be overweight/obese than day workers (95% CI 1.03–1.28 and 1.02–1.30, respectively)
Macagnan, 2012	Cross-sectional study	Workers in a poultry processing plant, Brazil; 800 night shift workers and 406 day workers	Night shift work	Overweight and central obesity	The prevalence ratios for overweight and abdominal obesity were 1.27 (95% CI 1.00–1.61) and 1.45 (95% CI 1.10–1.92), respectively, for the nightshift workers compared to the dayshift workers
Smith, 2013	Cross-sectional study	Female and male nurses, Canada; 9291 nurses	Night shift, evening shift, and mixed shift	BMI	Night shift schedule were significantly associated with higher BMI scores among female nurses (β estimate 0.60; P < 0.05), but not statistically significant in male nurses (β estimate 1.19; P = 0.28); no significant association was found for evening and mixed shift schedules
Jermendy, 2012	Cross-sectional study	Workers in the light industry or in public services, Hungary; 234 shift workers and 247 daytime workers	Shift work	BMI	Female shift workers had significant higher BMI levels compared to daytime workers, but the association was not found in males

Reference	Study design	Population	Exposure	Outcome	Results
Morikawa, 2007	Prospective cohort study with 10 years of follow-up	Male workers in a sash and zipper factory, Japan; 1529 men	Day-day, day-shift, shift-day, and shift-shift work	Weight gain	The mean increase in BMI for the day-shift and shift-shift workers was significantly larger than that of the day-day workers
Biggi, 2008	Retrospective cohort study with maximum 30 years of follow-up	Male workers in a large municipal enterprise, Italy; 488 men	Permanent night work	BMI increase	Both the inter-individual comparison and the intra-individual comparison between day and night workers among the workers showed a significant increase in BMI, total cholesterol, and tryglicerides associated with night work.
Suwazono, 2008	Prospective cohort study with 14 years of follow-up	A steel company, Japan; 4328 day workers and 2926 rotating shift workers	Rotating shift work	Weight gain	The OR for 5% increase in BMI was 1.14 (95% CI 1.06–1.23) comparing rotating shift workers with regular day workers
Oberlinner, 2009	Retrospective cohort study with 10 years of follow-up	Workers in the global chemical company BASF SE, Germany; 14,128 male rotating shift and 17,218 male day workers	Rotating shift work	Obesity	Rotating shift work was associated with a higher risk of obesity (HR 1.39; 95% CI 1.26–1.53)
Thomas, 2010	Retrospective cohort study with 3 years of follow-up	1958 British birth cohort, UK; 6775 men and women aged 42 years old	Any shift work	BMI	For men, there was a significant positive linear trend between number of shift-work types and increases in BMI over 3 years: 0.027 (95% CI 0.003, 0.051); the association was stronger for night/early morning shift work type: 0.060 (95% CI 0.015, 0.105); no significant associations were found in women
Itani, 2011	Retrospective cohort study with 7 years of follow-up	Workers of a local government organization, Japan; 11,424 men and 899 women	Shift work	Overweight	The OR of overweight comparing shift work with day work was 1.06 (95% CI 0.97–1.17) in men and 1.55 (95% CI 0.80–3.00) in women
Kubo, 2011b	Retrospective cohort study with 27.5 years of follow-up	Male workers in manufacturing Corporation, Japan; 8892 male daytime workers and 920 male shift workers	Rotating three-shift work	Overweight	Shift work was associated with an increased risk of overweight (RR 1.14, 95% CI 1.01–1.28)
Pan, 2011	Prospective cohort study with 18 years of follow-up	Nurses' Health Study II, USA; 107,663 female nurses	Rotating night shift work	Weight gain	Each 5-year increase in rotating night shift work was associated with an increase of 0.17 units in BMI (95% CI 0.14–0.19) and an increase of 0.45 kg in weight gain (95% CI 0.38–0.53)

(Continued)

Table 13.3 (*continued*)

Study author and date	Study design	Setting	Exposure	Outcomes	Results
Zhao, 2012	Prospective cohort study with 2 years of follow-up	Female nurses and midwives, Australia; 2078 participants	Day work maintainers, shift work maintainers, day to shift changers, and shift to day changers	BMI change	The shift to day changers had decreased in BMI over the 2-year follow-up period, in contrast, the shift work maintainers and the day to shift changers had increased in BMI over follow-up period
Mikuni, 1983	Cross-sectional study	Male factory workers, Japan; 2176 men	Shift work	T2D	The prevalence of T2D among three-shift workers was 2.1%, compared to 0.9% among day workers
Karlsson, 2005	Prospective cohort study with, maximum 50 years of follow-up	Male workers from two pulp and paper manufacturing plants, Sweden; 3088 male day workers and 2354 male shift workers	Shift work	Diabetes death	The standardized relative rate for mortality due to diabetes associated with shift work was 1.24 (95% CI 0.91–1.70). The risk of death due to diabetes increased as the number of shift years increased, particularly after restriction for length of follow-up to end at a maximum of 68 years of age
Morikawa, 2005	Prospective cohort study with 8 years of follow-up	Male workers in a sash and zipper factory, Japan; 2860 men	Shift work	T2D	Compared to fixed daytime blue collar workers, two-shift workers (HR 1.73; 95% CI 0.85–3.52) and three-shift workers (HR 1.33; 95% CI 0.74–2.36) were at nonsignificant high risk; the risk was higher if using white collar workers as the reference group
Suwazono, 2006	Prospective cohort study with 10 years of follow-up	A steel company, Japan; 3203 day workers and 2426 rotating shift workers	Rotating shift workers	T2D	The OR for T2D was 1.35 (95% CI 1.05–1.75) comparing rotating shift workers with regular day workers
Oberlinner, 2009	Retrospective cohort study with 10 years of follow-up	Workers in the global chemical company BASF SE, Germany; 14,128 male rotating shift and 17,218 male day workers	Rotating shift work	T2D, obesity	Rotating shift work was associated with a higher risk of incident diabetes (HR 1.33; 95% CI 1.14–1.55) and obesity (HR 1.39; 95% CI 1.26–1.53)

First author, year	Study design	Study population	Shift work exposure	Outcome	Results
Suwazono, 2009	Prospective cohort study with 14 years of follow-up	A steel company, Japan; 4219 day workers and 2885 rotating shift workers	Rotating shift workers	≥10% HbA1c increase	The OR for ≥10% HbA1c increase was 1.35 (95% CI 1.26–1.44) comparing rotating shift workers with regular day workers
Pan, 2011	Prospective cohort study with 18–20 years of follow-up	Nurses' Health Study I and II, USA; 177,184 female nurses	Rotating night shift work	T2D	Compared to day workers, the HR (95% CI) was 1.03 (0.98–1.08) for 1–2 years, 1.06 (1.00–1.11) for 3–9 years, 1.10 (1.02–1.18) for 10–19 years, and 1.24 (1.13–1.37) for ≥20 years among rotating night shift workers
Oyama, 2012	Retrospective cohort study with 10 years of follow-up	Japan; 6413 male employees	3-shift work and 2-shift work	HbA1c≥5.9%	The risk of developing elevated glycemia was significantly increased among both 3-shift workers (HR 1.78; 95% CI 1.49–2.14] and 2-shift workers (HR 2.62; 95% CI 2.17–3.17) compared with day workers
Vimalananda, 2015	Prospective cohort study with 8 years of follow-up	USA, 28,041 participants of the Black Women's Health Study (BWHS)	Night-shift work	T2D	Compared to never having worked the night shift, HRs (95% CI) for diabetes were 1.17 (1.04–1.31) for 1–2 years of night-shift work, 1.23 (1.06–1.41) for 3–9 years and 1.42 (1.19–1.70) for ≥10 years

Abbreviations: ALT, alanine aminotransferase; BMI, body mass index; CI, confidence interval; HR, hazard ratio; MetS, metabolic syndrome; OR, odds ratio; RR, relative risk; T2D, type 2 diabetes.

selection might be influenced by socioeconomic status given that shift workers are generally paid more compared to their counterparts who work in the regular daytime. Some studies also have shown that behavioral factors, like smoking status, body weight, and sleep pattern, might predict whether individuals choose to participate in shift work (van Amelsvoort *et al.*, 2004; Nabe-Nielsen *et al.*, 2008). The second selection bias occurs when shift workers move out of their jobs because of health reasons. In both selections, the "healthy worker effect" may exist: people who start shift work and/or stay in it for a longer times may be healthier and/or they have a higher tolerance for factors affecting health. Other factors may also play a role in the selection bias, like age, education level, personality, self-efficacy, job availability, and family conflicts, but these analyses of these factors have yielded inconsistent results. These two sources of selection bias have been widely recognized as methodological obstacle in shift work research.

Compared to cross-sectional studies, the cohort study design may overcome some of the methodological pitfalls imposed by selection bias. One nested case-control study, two prospective cohort studies, and two retrospective cohort studies have been conducted and all have reported a consistent positive association between shift work and risk of metabolic syndrome. The relative risks ranged from 1.56 to 5.00 (all $P < 0.05$), and one study observed a significant interaction with baseline elevated alanine aminotransferase (ALT) levels in male shift workers (Lin *et al.*, 2009b), suggesting that shift work aggravates metabolic syndrome development among middle-aged males with elevated ALT. With regard to body weight and obesity, four prospective cohort studies and five retrospective cohort studies all indicated an increased risk of overweight/obesity or weight gain among shift workers compared to daytime workers. One study with two years of follow-up in Australian nurses and midwives found that the shift to day changers had decrease in BMI, in contrast, the shift work maintainers and the day to shift changers had increase in BMI over the two-year follow-up period compared with the day work maintainers (Zhao *et al.*, 2012). Another prospective cohort study with 18 years of follow-up in over 100,000 American young nurses demonstrated a positive dose-response between duration of rotating night shift work and weight gain (Pan *et al.*, 2011); for example, each five-year increase of rotating night shift work was associated with 0.45 kg in weight gain (95% CI 0.38–0.53).

13.3.2 Epidemiological studies of shift work and type 2 diabetes

Six prospective cohort studies and two retrospective cohort studies have investigated associations between shift work and incident type 2 diabetes, with follow-up years ranging from 8 to 50 years. Four studies were conducted in Japanese workers, one study in Sweden, one study in Germany, and two studies in USA. Four studies were performed only in men, two exclusively in women and two studies with mixed genders. Despite heterogeneities in study design, population characteristics, and varying definitions of shift work, all of the studies have observed a positive association between shift work and risk of elevated glycemia, greater increase of hemoglobin A1c, new-onset type 2 diabetes, and death due to diabetes, although some of the associations were not statistically significant probably due to the limited power. The publication by Pan *et al.* (2011) provides compelling evidence of the link between shift work and type 2 diabetes in women, with the effect partly, but not exclusively, mediated through body weight. The large-scale study utilized the comprehensive data from two ongoing large prospective cohorts in American nurses and is the first to reveal a graded association between duration of working rotating night shifts and risk of incident type 2 diabetes. There are several strengths of the study, including its prospective design, the large sample size and detailed information on a wide range of potential confounders, and long-term and repeated measures during the follow-up. Although the generalizability of the results to other populations may be limited, the homogeneity of the study participants of health professionals minimized the confounding by socioeconomic status and enhanced the response rate and the quality of the questionnaire data. Moreover, a recently published prospective cohort study of black women (Vimalananda *et al.*, 2015), looking at associations between night-shift work and incident diabetes among their 28,041 African-American participants, also reported a dose-response relation between night-shift work and incident type 2 diabetes, which are very similar to those of Pan *et al.* (2011) among their predominantly Caucasian women. The consistent results from the two studies further strengthen the causal relation, but studies in men and other populations are still needed.

When interpreting the epidemiological evidence, in addition to the above mentioned selection bias, the heterogeneity of the definition of shift work is another important methodological consideration. The broad definition of shift work includes evening shift, night shift, rotating shifts, split shifts, or irregular or on-call schedules both during the week and on weekends. However, some of these shift work types may be less detrimental to circadian rhythms and health outcomes (e.g., evening shift or weekend shift), while some may be more (e.g., rotating night shift work). Many studies have used self-reported data on shift work and the definitions varied substantially, which increase the possibility of misclassification. Furthermore, flexible and temporary employment has grown increasingly in our rapidly-changing world. Thus, it becomes difficult to assess the accurate exposure data (e.g., duration and intensity) related to shift work and to maintain a large population for sufficiently long periods of follow-up, which are important factors when evaluating risk of chronic diseases.

Taken together, the current evidence from extensive epidemiological studies reveals a positive association between shift work and type 2 diabetes. Therefore, exploration of the potential mechanisms is crucial for the causal inference and future intervention strategies to reduce the inherent risk among shift workers.

13.3.3 Pathways linking shift work to type 2 diabetes

Shift work can increase the risk of type 2 diabetes by several independent but interrelated physiological, behavioral, and psychosocial mechanisms. The physiological mechanisms are related to the desynchronized circadian rhythms, activation of the autonomic nervous system, inflammation, changed lipid and glucose metabolism, endothelial function, digestive disturbance, appetite control, and several other risk factors related to type 2 diabetes (Chapter 11). The potential behavioral changes include reduced quantity and quality of sleep, weight gain, shift meal times and unhealthy diet, and increased smoking. The psychosocial pathways relate to the disturbed socio-temporal patterns caused by performing regular shift work; for example, decreased work–life balance, increased stress levels, working hours and work demand, job insecurity, low decision latitude, and poor recovery following work. The potential mechanisms have been summarized in Fig. 13.1; some of the evidence is compelling (e.g., the biological alterations by the disruption of circadian system), while other pathways remain controversial.

The human body has the tendency to maintain the equilibrium of blood glucose levels through various biochemical and physical processes, or so-called glucose homeostasis. It has been now widely

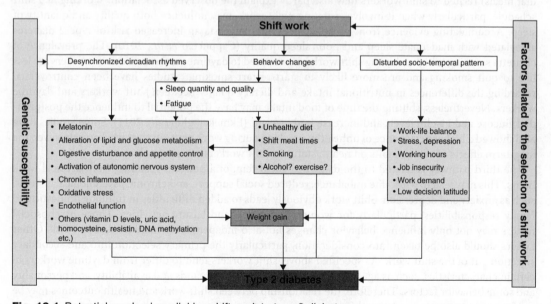

Fig. 13.1 Potential mechanisms linking shift work to type 2 diabetes.

acknowledged that the circadian rhythm regulates a wide range of biological processes, including wake–sleep cycle, body temperature, energy homeostasis, thermogenesis, hungry and feeding, cell cycle, hormone secretion, glucose and lipids metabolism. The principal endogenous circadian clock is located in the suprachiasmatic nuclei (SCN) of the anterior hypothalamus that responds to the environmental light–dark cycle. Circadian clocks have been identified within almost all mammalian organs and cells, such as the liver, intestine, adipose tissue, cardiomyocytes, vascular smooth muscle cells, endothelial cells and also pancreatic islets, to regulate cellular and physiological functions. The peripheral circadian clocks are influenced by the central clock and also the basis of feeding time and other environmental clues. As depicted in Chapter 11 in great detail, circadian rhythm is one important factor that influences the blood glucose and insulin levels, and the destabilized circadian system could lead to alterations of insulin secretion and disruption of glucose homeostasis.

Animal experiments have shown that the disruptions of both central and peripheral circadian clocks (by deletion of *Clock* and *Bmal1* genes) contribute directly to the insulin resistance and glucose homeostasis (Rudic *et al.*, 2004; Marcheva *et al.*, 2010). Human studies also show that circadian misalignment results in adverse metabolic and cardiovascular consequences, including a decrease in leptin, an increase in glucose and insulin, and an increase in arterial blood pressure (Scheer *et al.*, 2009).

Melatonin is a circulating hormone predominantly secreted from the pineal gland and has primarily been implicated in the regulation of circadian rhythms; the circulating levels of melatonin are high during the night and drop during daytime. Emerging evidence suggests that melatonin also has a role in the modulation of insulin secretion through the membrane receptors MT1 and MT2 in pancreatic islets (Peschke and Muhlbauer, 2010). Several genome-wide association studies have consistently revealed a close link between specific single nucleotide polymorphisms of the melatonin MT2-receptor (*MTNR1b*) locus and an increased risk of type 2 diabetes.

Shift work is generally associated with chronic destabilized circadian rhythms, which may increase risk of type 2 diabetes. Many other physiological pathways have also been affected, and studies have reported an increased risks of hypertension and dyslipidemia (Puttonen *et al.*, 2010), a higher levels of resistin (Burgueno *et al.*, 2010), systematic inflammation (Sookoian *et al.*, 2007; Puttonen *et al.*, 2011), oxidative stress (Sharifian *et al.*, 2005), impaired endothelial function (Suessenbacher *et al.*, 2011), elevated uric acid (Uetani *et al.*, 2006) but low vitamin D levels (Ward *et al.*, 2011) among shift workers, particularly when the shift work involves nighttime work, compared to daytime workers.

The unfavorable changes in health behaviors (such as sleep deprivation, increased smoking and irregular meals) related to shift workers may also partly explain the observed association. Working in a shift schedule, particularly when it involves rotating night work, may influence both quality and quantity of sleep. Accumulating evidence from prospective studies suggests an increased risk of type 2 diabetes associated with inadequate sleep and poor sleep quality (Cappuccio *et al.*, 2010). The prevalence of cigarette smoking is higher among shift workers compared to daytime workers, and shift workers are less like to quit smoking and are more likely to start/restart smoking. Studies have been controversial regarding the differences in nutritional intake and dietary quality between shift workers and daytime workers. Nevertheless, shifting the time of food intake may have the potential to influence the postprandial glucose and insulin levels and increase body weight (Ekmekcioglu *et al.*, 2011). Some studies have also showed a higher occurrence of unhealthy snacking during work hours in shift workers. However, the long-term effects of eating habits on health status in shift workers remain unclear.

The third pathway is related to the disturbed socio-temporal patterns resulting from atypical work hours. This may lead to work–life imbalance, reduced social support, and chronic psychological distress, such as anxiety and depression. Shift work obviously leads to added difficulties in fulfilling domestic and family responsibilities, particularly for women, and social and leisure activities. Those psychosocial factors may not only influence behavior changes but also independently increase diabetes risk. Other factors should also be taken into consideration, particularly the primary selection into and secondary selection out of the shift work. As specified above, shift workers tend to differ from daytime workers in certain characteristics, such as age, socioeconomic status, job demands and availability, and personality and some behavior factors. Therefore, the relationship between shift work and health outcomes may be confounded by those pre-existing differences.

13.4 Conclusions and perspective of future studies

Based on the literature that has been outlined in the previous sections, there is compelling evidence from animal experiments, cross-sectional comparison, and long-term prospective studies that shift work increases the risk of cancer, particularly breast and prostate cancer, and for developing type 2 diabetes. However, modern society has evolved to rely increasingly on 24-hour operations in many diverse settings, and shift work has become an occupational exposure that occurs virtually in all industries and is unavoidable. Thus, preventive strategies will ultimately be needed to reduce health risks among shift workers (Knauth and Hornberger, 2003).

Such preventive strategies could include regular health screening among shift workers, particularly targeted at identifying individuals at a high risk of cancer and type 2 diabetes. Secondly, there is a need to identify shift schedules (i.e., shift duration, direction of rotation, recovery times, and work/rest sequences) with the least detrimental effect on health. Improving eating as well as other lifestyle habits of employees who work night shifts (e.g., providing healthy foods, introducing incentives for exercise and smoking cessation, education in sleep hygiene) in an effort to lower shift work induced health disparities represents another important strategy. For example, a weight loss program among male overweight shift workers based on the Social Cognitive Theory has been shown to be effective in reducing body weight and waist circumference, improving blood pressure, increasing physical activity and decreasing sugary beverage intakes (Morgan *et al.*, 2011). However, no study has been done to investigate the long-term impact of those interventions. Future studies should continue to examine relations between shift work and specific aspects of chronic disease, including cancers and diabetes, and additionally test the effectiveness of specific interventions for ameliorating the adverse health consequences of shift work.

References

Biggi N, Consonni D, Galluzzo V, *et al.* 2008. Metabolic syndrome in permanent night workers. *Chronobiol Int* **25**(2):443–54.

Blask DE, Sauer LA, Dauchy RT. 2002. Melatonin as a chronobiotic/anticancer agent: cellular, biochemical, and molecular mechanisms of action and their implications for circadian-based cancer therapy. *Curr Trop Med Chem* **2**(2):113–32.

Bonde JP, Hansen J, Kolstad HA, *et al.* 2012. Work at night and breast cancer – report on evidence-based options for preventive actions. *Scand J Work Environ Health* **38**(4):380–90.

Brzezinski A. 1997. Melatonin in humans. *N Engl J Med* **336**(3):186–95.

Burgueno A, Gemma C, Gianotti TF, *et al.* 2010. Increased levels of resistin in rotating shift workers: a potential mediator of cardiovascular risk associated with circadian misalignment. *Atherosclerosis* **210**(2):625–9.

Bushnell PT, Colombi A, Caruso CC, *et al.* 2010. Work schedules and health behavior outcomes at a large manufacturer. *Ind Health* **48**(4):395–405.

Cappuccio FP, D'Elia L, Strazzullo P, *et al.* 2010. Quantity and quality of sleep and incidence of type 2 diabetes: a systematic review and meta-analysis. *Diabetes Care* **33**(2):414–20.

Chen JD, Lin YC, Hsiao ST. 2010. Obesity and high blood pressure of 12-hour night shift female clean-room workers. *Chronobiol Int* **27**(2):334–44.

Conlon M, Lightfoot N, Kreiger N. 2007. Rotating shift work and risk of prostate cancer. *Epidemiology* **18**(1):182–3.

Davis S, Mirick DK, Stevens RG. 2001. Night shift work, light at night, and risk of breast cancer. *J Natl Cancer Inst* **93**(20):1557–62.

De Bacquer D, Van Risseghem M, Clays E, *et al.* 2009. Rotating shift work and the metabolic syndrome: a prospective study. *Int J Epidemiol* **38**(3):848–54.

Di Lorenzo L, De Pergola G, Zocchetti C, *et al.* 2003. Effect of shift work on body mass index: results of a study performed in 319 glucose-tolerant men working in a Southern Italian industry. *Int J Obes Relat Metab Disord* **27**(11):1353–8.

Di Milia L, Mummery K. 2009. The association between job related factors, short sleep and obesity. *Ind Health* **47**(4):363–8.

Dubocovich ML. 2007. Melatonin receptors: role on sleep and circadian rhythm regulation. *Sleep Med* 8 Suppl 3:34–42.

Ekmekcioglu C, Touitou Y. 2011. Chronobiological aspects of food intake and metabolism and their relevance on energy balance and weight regulation. *Obes Rev* 12(1):14–25.

Esquirol Y, Bongard V, Mabile L, *et al*. 2009. Shift work and metabolic syndrome: respective impacts of job strain, physical activity, and dietary rhythms. *Chronobiol Int* 26(3):544–59.

Fu L, Lee CC. 2003. The circadian clock: pacemaker and tumour suppressor. *Nat Rev Cancer* 3(5):350–61.

Gale JE, Cox HI, Qian J, *et al*. 2011. Disruption of circadian rhythms accelerates development of diabetes through pancreatic beta-cell loss and dysfunction. *J Biol Rhythms* 26(5):423–33.

Ha M, Park J. 2005. Shiftwork and metabolic risk factors of cardiovascular disease. *J Occup Health* 47(2):89–95.

Hansen J. 2001. Increased breast cancer risk among women who work predominantly at night. *Epidemiology* 12(1):74–7.

Hansen J, Lassen CF. 2012. Nested case-control study of night shift work and breast cancer risk among women in the Danish military. *Occup Environ Med* 69(8):551–6.

Hansen J, Stevens RG. 2012. Case-control study of shift-work and breast cancer risk in Danish nurses: impact of shift systems. *Eur J Cancer* 48(11):1722–9.

Hursting SD, Dunlap SM. 2012. Obesity, metabolic dysregulation, and cancer: a growing concern and an inflammatory (and microenvironmental) issue. *Ann NY Acad Sci* 1271:82–7.

International Diabetes Fedaration. IDF Diabetes Atlas. http://www.idf.org/diabetesatlas/5e/diabetes (last accessed November 22, 2014).

Ishizaki M, Morikawa Y, Nakagawa H, *et al*. 2004. The influence of work characteristics on body mass index and waist to hip ratio in Japanese employees. *Ind Health* 42(1):41–9.

Itani O, Kaneita Y, Murata A, *et al*. 2011. Association of onset of obesity with sleep duration and shift work among Japanese adults. *Sleep Med* 12(4):341–5.

Jermendy G, Nadas J, Hegyi I, *et al*. 2012. Assessment of cardiometabolic risk among shift workers in Hungary. *Health Qual Life Outcomes* 10:18.

Jia Y, Lu Y, Wu K, *et al*. 2013. Does night work increase the risk of breast cancer? A systematic review and meta-analysis of epidemiological studies. *Cancer Epidemiol* 37(3):197–206.

Jones CR, Campbell SS, Zone SE, *et al*. 1999. Familial advanced sleep-phase syndrome: A short-period circadian rhythm variant in humans. *Nat Med* 5(9):1062–5.

Kamdar BB, Tergas AI, Mateen FJ, *et al*. 2013. Night-shift work and risk of breast cancer: a systematic review and meta-analysis. *Breast Cancer Res Treat* 38(1):291–301.

Karlsson B, Knutsson A, Lindahl B. 2001. Is there an association between shift work and having a metabolic syndrome? Results from a population based study of 27,485 people. *Occup Environ Med* 58(11):747–52.

Karlsson BH, Knutsson AK, Lindahl BO, *et al*. 2003. Metabolic disturbances in male workers with rotating three-shift work. Results of the WOLF study. *Int Arch Occup Environ Health* 76(6):424–30.

Karlsson B, Alfredsson L, Knutsson A, *et al*. 2005. Total mortality and cause-specific mortality of Swedish shift- and dayworkers in the pulp and paper industry in 1952-2001. *Scand J Work Environ Health* 31(1):30–5.

Kawada T, Otsuka T, Inagaki H, *et al*. 2010. A cross-sectional study on the shift work and metabolic syndrome in Japanese male workers. *Aging Male* 13(3):174–8.

Knauth P, Hornberger S. 2003. Preventive and compensatory measures for shift workers. *Occup Med (Lond)* 53(2):109–16.

Konopka RJ, Benzer S. 1971. Clock mutants of Drosophila melanogaster. *Proc Natl Acad Sci USA* 68(9):2112–6.

Kubo T, Ozasa K, Mikami K, *et al*. 2006. Prospective cohort study of the risk of prostate cancer among rotating-shift workers: findings from the Japan collaborative cohort study. *Am J Epidemiol* 164(6):549–55.

Kubo T, Oyama I, Nakamura T, *et al*. 2011a. Industry-based retrospective cohort study of the risk of prostate cancer among rotating-shift workers. *Int J Urol* 18(3):206–11.

Kubo T, Oyama I, Nakamura T, *et al*. 2011b. Retrospective cohort study of the risk of obesity among shift workers: findings from the industry-based shift worker's health study, Japan. *Occup Environ Med* 68(5):327–31.

Lahti TA, Partonen T, Kyyronen P, *et al*. 2008. Night-time work predisposes to non-Hodgkin lymphoma. *Int J Cancer* 123(9):2148–51.

Le Bars D, Thivolle P, Vitte PA, *et al*. 1991. PET and plasma pharmacokinetic studies after bolus intravenous administration of [11C]melatonin in humans. *Int J Rad Appl Instrum B* 18(3):357–62.

Li Y, Sato Y, Yamaguchi N. 2011. Shift work and the risk of metabolic syndrome: a nested case-control study. *Int J Occup Environ Health* 17(2):154–60.

Lie JA, Roessink J, Kjaerheim K. 2006. Breast cancer and night work among Norwegian nurses. *Cancer Causes Control* 17(1):39–44.

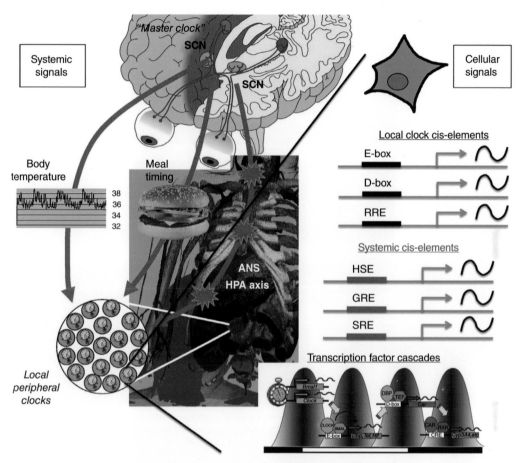

Fig. 2.1 Control of peripheral clocks. One set of signals controlling circadian physiology are systemic signals originating from the SCN or behaviors that it controls. These include meal timing, body temperature fluctuations, and activity of the autonomic nervous system (ANS) and hypothalamic–pituitary–adrenal (HPA) axis. These signals probably act upon clock- and clock-controlled gene expression via systemic cis-elements such as HSEs, GREs, and SREs. A second set of signals arises through local cell-autonomous circadian clocks and controls transcription through clock cis-elements such as E-boxes, D-boxes, and RRE elements. Other signals controlling circadian physiology, and in particular xenobiotic metabolism, arise via transcription factors cascades of PAR-bZIP family members.

Circadian Medicine, First Edition. Edited by Christopher S. Colwell.
© 2015 John Wiley & Sons, Inc. Published 2015 by John Wiley & Sons, Inc.

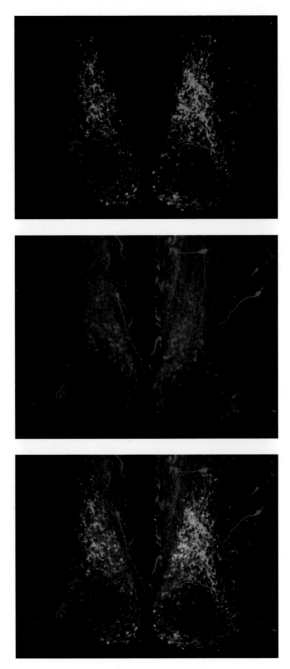

Fig. 3.1 The SCN is the master circadian clock in mammals. Neural cell populations within the SCN are defined by the expression of neuropeptides. The top panel shows expression of the peptide vasoactive intestinal peptide (VIP, green). The cell bodies of these neurons are located close to the optic chiasm. These neurons then project to the more dorsal cell populations and outward toward the subparaventrical zone (sPVZ) and other targets. The middle panel shows expression of the peptide arginine vasopressin (AVP, red). The bottom panel shows the merged image with yellow indicating the area of co-expression. The data are collected from adult male C57 mice using the technique of immunohistochemistry. The data are courtesy of Dr T. Kudo.

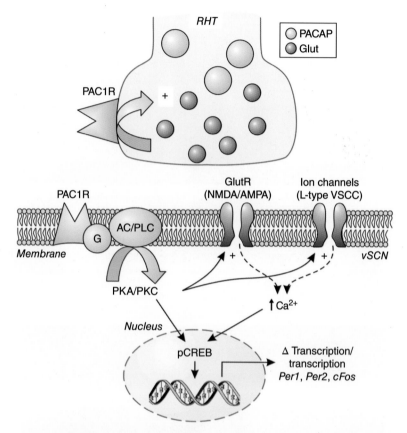

Fig. 3.4 Schematic of RHT/SCN synaptic connection illustrating the signaling events between the release of neurotransmitters and the transcriptional/translational regulation of *Per1*. The intrinsically photosensitive melanopsin-expressing retinal ganglion cells (ipRGC) encode ambient lighting and generate action potentials that travel down the RHT and innervate the SCN. The RHT terminals release glutamate and, under certain conditions, the neuropeptide pituitary adenylate cyclase activating peptide (PACAP). The glutamate release is detected by both AMPA and NMDA glutamate receptors (GluR). GluR induced membrane depolarization can be amplified by intrinsic voltage gated ion channels like the L-type calcium (Ca^{2+}) channel. The net result of RHT stimulation is an increase in firing rate and Ca^{2+} increase in SCN neurons. A number of signaling pathways are then activated and apparently converge to alter transcriptional and/or translational regulators, including CREB. Phosphorylated CREB is translocated into the nucleus where it can bind to CREs that in the promoter regions of *Per1* and *Per2* and drives transcription of these genes over the course of hours.

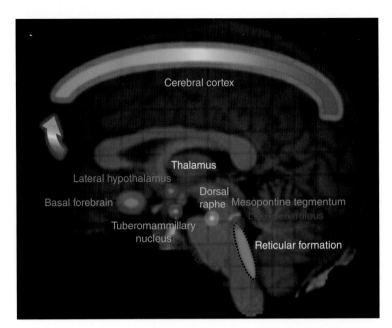

Fig. 5.2 The major structures of the arousal system. Cells in the reticular formation and other caudal regions, including noradrenergic neurons of the locus coeruleus, serotonergic raphe neurons, and dopaminergic neurons in the periaqueductal grey in the mesopontine tegmentum, project to more rostral areas via two pathways. A dorsal pathway via thalamus provides input to cerebral cortex. A ventral pathway provides input to the cerebral cortex via interconnected nuclei including orexigenic neurons in the lateral hypothalamus, histaminergic neurons in the tuberomammillary nucleus and cholinergic neurons in the basal forebrain. (View of the midline sagittal section of human brain from Allen Brain Atlas Resources [Internet]. Seattle (WA): Allen Institute for Brain Science ©2009. Available from: http://www.brain-map.org.)

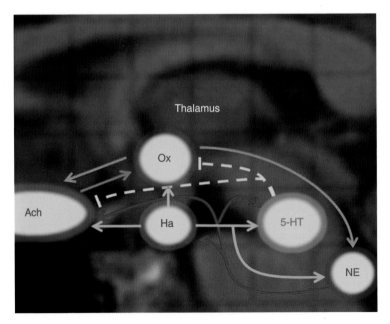

Fig. 5.3 Interactions of the main neuromodulatory systems that regulate wake within the arousal pathway. Cells in the basal forebrain producing acetylcholine (Ach) shown in green receive input from multiple regions. Excitatory projections from cells in the lateral hypothalamus expressing orexin (Ox) are shown in blue, projections from histamine (Ha)-producing cells in the tuberomammillary nucleus are shown in orange, projections from norepinephrine (NE)-containing cells in the locus coeruleus are shown in red. Inhibitory projections from cells in raphe nuclei expressing serotonin (5-HT) are shown by dashed lines. (Adapted from Brown *et al.*, 2012.)

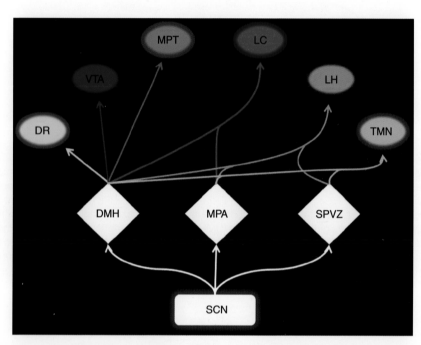

Fig. 5.4 Circadian signaling routes to govern regulation of sleep–wake and arousal pathways. Circadian pacemaker signals from the SCN project to three major relay nuclei, the dorsomedial nuclei of the hypothalamus (DMH), the medial preoptic area (MPA), and the subparaventricular zone (SPVZ). These areas then relay circadian information to areas within the arousal network including the dorsal raphe (DR), the ventral tegmental area (VTA), the mesopontine tegmentum (MPT), the locus coeruleus (LC), the lateral hypothalamus (LH) and the tuberomammillary nuclei (TMN).

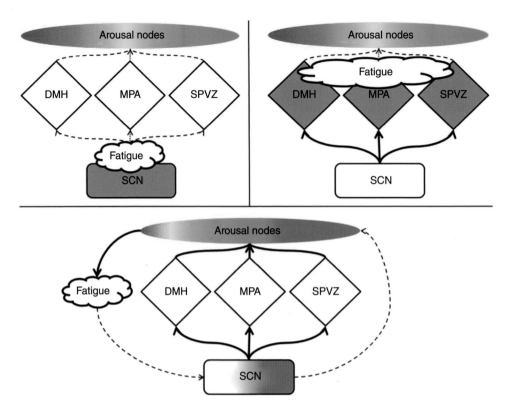

Fig. 5.5 Illustration highlighting the key areas impacted by disorders of arousal pathways and points where SCN regulation may either benefit or cause initial disorder. Top left: the induction of fatigue directly affects circadian regulation at the level of the SCN, resulting in impaired circadian output via the three major relay nuclei, the dorsomedial nuclei of the hypothalamus (DMH), the medial preoptic area (MPA), and the subparaventricular zone (SPVZ). Top right: the SCN is able to effectively signal circadian output to the three relay nodes; however, this signal is disrupted prior to innervation of the arousal network. Bottom: one or more nodes of the arousal network are directly affected by inducers of fatigue, reducing input to the circadian system and leading to subsequent declines in circadian output.

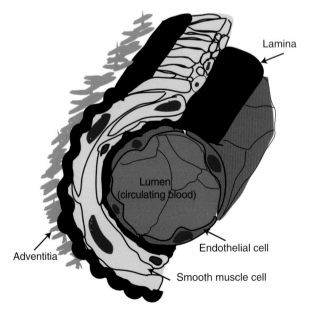

Fig. 8.1 The anatomy of the blood vessel. A blood vessel comprises three layers. An outer adventitial layer, a smooth muscle cell layer called the media, and an inner layer comprised of endothelial cells called the intima. Each layer is separated by a lamina (black line).

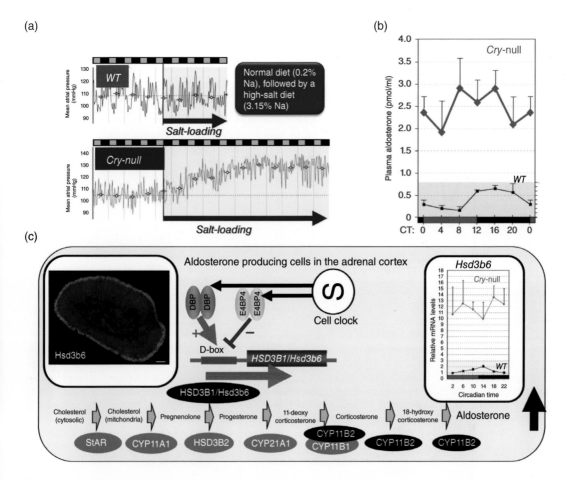

Fig. 9.1 Diagram of the mammalian circadian system and hypertension in *Cry*-null mice. (a) *Cry*-null mice exhibit salt-sensitive hypertension. Shown are representative recordings of temporal profiles of mean arterial pressure (MAP) of wild-type (*WT*) mice (8-day recording) and *Cry*-null mice (15-day recording). In both groups, animals were kept in constant darkness and fed a normal salt diet (0.2% sodium) for the first four days; the salt-loaded group was transferred to a high salt diet (3.15% sodium) on the fifth day. Gray and black boxes below the graphs represent the subjective day and subjective night, respectively. BP data were collected in 30-second bouts at 5-min intervals and plotted using a 1-h moving average. The 24-h means of each day are shown by open squares. Horizontal dotted lines indicate the mean value of the BP in days 1 through 4, on the normal salt diet. (b) Twenty-four–hour profiles of plasma aldosterone concentration (PAC) in *WT* and *Cry*-null mice in constant darkness (n=5–12 mice per time point). The values at CT0 are double plotted. Values are means±s.e.m. (c) Cellular clocks regulate steroidogenesis in the aldosterone-producing cells in the zona glomerulosa of the adrenal gland. *HSD3B1/Hsd3b6* is a clock controlled gene regulated via D-boxes in the promoter region by DBP and its antagonist E4BP4. In the *Cry*-null adrenal gland, however, constitutive activation of DBP shifts the balance towards overproduction of DBP-regulated *Hsd3b6* gene (bottom). HSD3B1/Hsd3b6 is a key enzyme for aldosterone production in *Cry*-null mice. Immunohistochemistry of Hsd3b6 protein in a *Cry*-null adrenal gland (upper left). (Some parts of this figure are adapted from Doi *et al.*, 2010.)

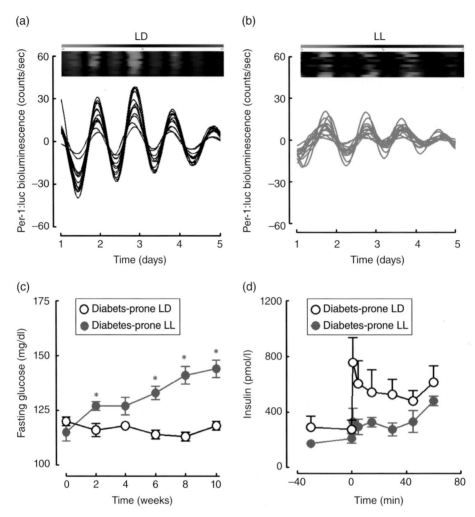

Fig. 11.3 Effects of circadian disruption of the beta-cell circadian clock and susceptibility to beta-cell failure and T2DM in rats. (a and b) Representative examples of *Per*-driven diurnal bioluminescence rhythms imaged by ICCD camera at the level of individual islets (n = 13) from *Per1:luc* rats exposed to either 10 weeks of typical light/dark cycle (LD) (a) or circadian disruption due to exposure to light at night (LL) (b). Each black or grey line represents a *Per*-driven bioluminescence signal from an individual islet. Note loss of the amplitude and synchrony in *Per1:luc* expression among individual islets in LL rats. (c) Effects of circadian disruption due to exposure to light at night (LL) on fasting glucose levels in diabetes-prone HIP rats (LD cycle (open circles) and LL cycle (grey circles)). (d) Glucose-stimulated insulin secretion during a hyperglycemic clamp (0–60 minutes) in diabetes-prone HIP rats exposed to either 10 weeks of typical LD (open circles) or disrupted LL cycle (grey circles). Note loss of glucose-stimulated insulin secretion in LL exposed rats.

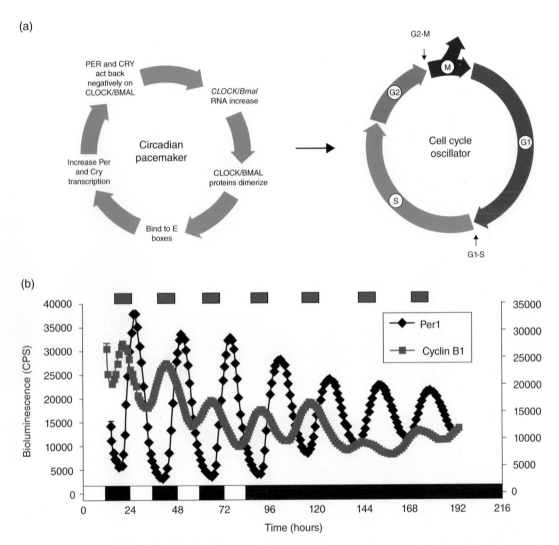

Fig. 12.3 The circadian clock directly regulates the timing of the cell cycle in many biological systems and cells, including human proliferative tissues. Typically, the clock seems to regulate entry into mitosis, at the G2 to M transition, and DNA replication or S-phase, at the G1-S transition. To date, much of this regulation appears to be transcriptional. Panel B shows the precision of this transcriptional rhythm in living zebra fish cell lines. Luminescent reporters for the clock gene *Period 1* and the cell cycle gene, *Cyclin B1*, show how the clock regulates peak *Cyclin B1* expression to occur in the late night – corresponding to the peak timing of mitosis (pink squares) in culture (Tamai *et al.*, 2012).

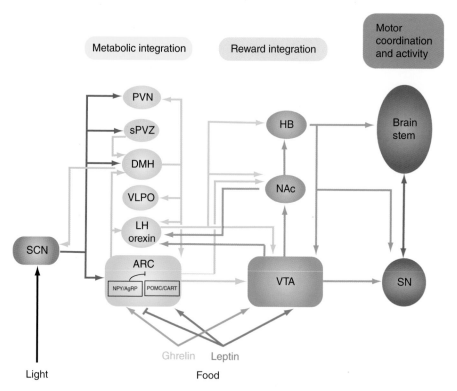

Fig. 15.2 Major neural pathways integrating light and feeding signals in mammals. Light signals are directly transmitted to the SCN. Light information is indirectly transmitted from the SCN (red arrows). The SCN projects to areas important for metabolic integration, including the PVN, sPVZ, DMH and ARC. Feeding signals (leptin and ghrelin) primarily affect two entities in the brain (green arrows): (i) the ARC, which is important for the metabolic integration of feeding signals (yellow), and (ii) the VTA, which is important for the integration of reward (blue). The structures important for metabolic integration (yellow) and reward integration (blue) exchange information with each other (yellow and blue arrows) and can affect the SCN timing center (red). Light and feeding signals combine and contribute to motor coordination and activity (purple). ARC, arcuate nucleus; DMH, dorsomedial hypothalamus; HB, habenula; ipRGC, intrinsically photosensitive retinal ganglion cell; LH, lateral hypothalamus; NAc, nucleus accumbens; Pin, pineal gland; PVN, paraventricular nucleus; SCN, suprachiasmatic nuclei; SN, substantia nigra; sPVZ, subparaventricular zone; VLPO, ventrolateral preoptic nucleus; VTA, ventral tegmental area.

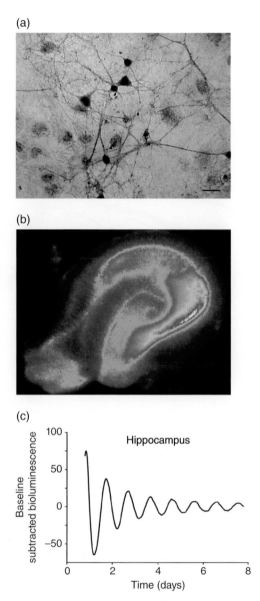

Fig. 16.1 The hippocampus is an "extra-SCN" circadian oscillator. (a) Expression of PER2 measured with immunohistochemical techniques in cultured hippocampal neurons. (b) Bioluminescence recorded from an organotypic hippocampal slice made from a PER2::LUC mouse. (c) The circadian rhythm in bioluminescence recorded from the hippocampal slice. Rhythmicity of bioluminescence damped over a period of several days (Modified from Wang *et al.*, 2009.)

Circadian regulation of monoamine circuitry

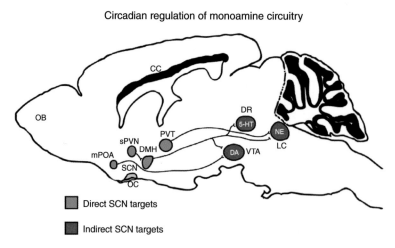

Fig. 17.2 The circadian system regulates multiple monoaminergic brain regions that control mood, anxiety and motivated behaviors, through local expression of clock genes as well as indirect connections originating from the master pacemaker in the suprachiasmatic nucleus (SCN). The SCN projects monosynaptically to multiple hypothalamic nuclei (in blue), which subsequently communicate with regions (in red) that synthesize dopamine (DA), serotonin (5-HT) and norepinephrine (NE). As a result, serotonin, norepinephrine and dopamine all have a circadian rhythm in their levels, release, and synthesis-related enzymes. Abbreviations: medial preoptic area (mPOA), subparaventricular nucleus of the hypothalamus (sPVN), dorsomedial hypothalamus (DMH), paraventricular nucleus of the thalamus (PVT), dorsal raphe (DR), ventral tegmental area (VTA), locus coeruleus (LC), optic chiasm (OC), corpus callosum (CC), olfactory bulb (OB).

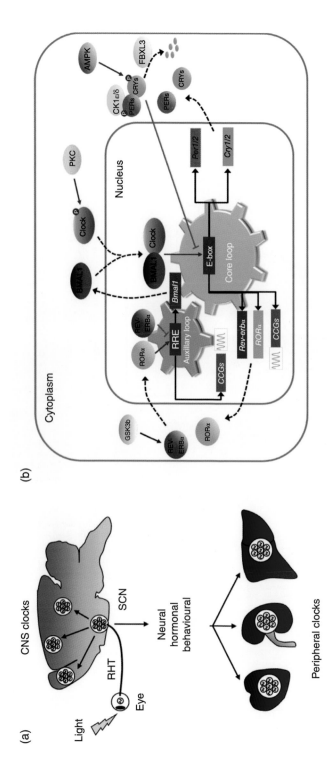

Fig. 18.1 The mammalian circadian system and the molecular clock. (a) The mammalian circadian system consists of intracellular oscillators found in both central nervous system and peripheral tissues throughout the body. These clocks are synchronized via neural, hormonal and behavioral time cues. The central circadian pacemaker is located in the suprachiasmatic nuclei (SCN) in the hypothalamus, which is entrained to the external light–dark cycle via light detected by retinal photoreceptors and conveyed via the retinohypothalamic tract (RHT). These peripheral clocks provide temporal regulation of local physiology. (b) Intracellular circadian oscillations are the product of a transcriptional-translational feedback loop (TTFL) comprised of core clock genes. This involves two interloping feedback loops – a core loop consisting of *Clock, Bmal1, Per1-2* and *Cry1-2* and auxiliary loop consisting of *Rev-erbα* and *Rorα* driving *Bmal1* expression. Various posttranslational modifications regulate the rate of the TTFL. Disruption of the components making up the TTFL may result in a change in circadian period (*tau*) or even complete arrhythmia. (TTFL figure based on that of Son *et al.*, 2011).

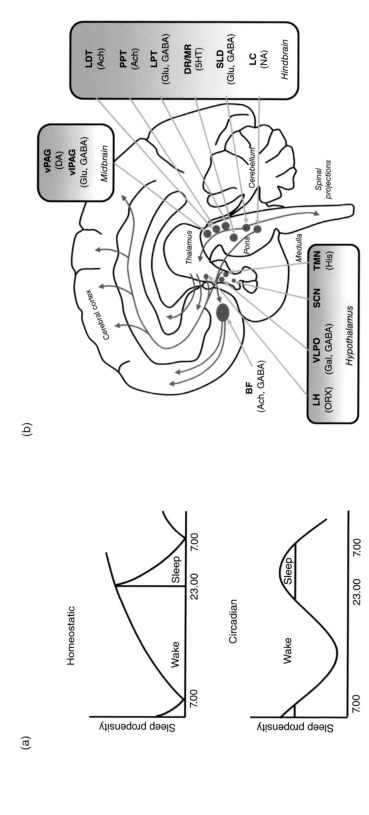

Fig. 18.2 Mechanisms involved in the regulation of sleep. (a) The homeostatic drive for sleep increases sleep propensity with prolonged wakefulness. Sleep pressure declines following sleep but increases again at waking. The circadian regulation of sleep creates a drive for wakefulness during the day, which declines at night. As such, sleep propensity is low during the day, but increases at night. (Figure based on that of Borbely, 1982.) (b) Sleep is the product of multiple brain regions and neurotransmitters. Abbreviations for brain regions: BF = Basal forebrain; DR/MR = Dorsal/medial raphe nucleus; LC = Locus coeruleus; LDT = Laterodorsal tegmental nuclei; LH = Lateral hypothalamus; LPT = Lateral pontine tegmentum; PPT = Pedunculopontine tegmental nuclei; SCN = Suprachiasmatic nuclei; SLD = Sublaterodorsal nucleus; TMN = Tuberomammillary nucleus; VLPO = Ventrolateral preoptic nuclei; vPAG = Ventral periaqueductal grey; vlPAG = Ventrolateral periaqueductal grey. Abbreviations for neurotransmitters: 5HT = Serotonin; Ach = Acetylcholine; DA = Dopamine; GABA = γ-Aminobutyric acid; Gal = Galanin; Glu = Glutamate; His = Histamine; NA = Noradrenaline; ORX = Orexin. (Figure based on that of Lockley and Foster, 2012).

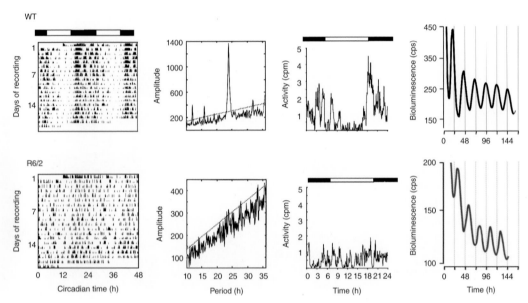

Fig. 21.3 R6/2 mutation disrupts activity–rest cycles in mPer1:Luciferase reporter mice used to analyze molecular time keeping in SCN *in vitro*. Representative actograms of WT (top) and R6/2 (bottom) mice held under 12 h light/dark cycle from 12 weeks of age onwards show a progressive deterioration of activity profile in R6/2 mice. Periodogram analyses of mice with circadian behavior show a highly significant peak in the WT but not in R6/2 mice. Mean daily activity profile of mice indicates more daytime and less nocturnal activity. Circadian bioluminescence recordings from SCN explants were obtained from two mice (one R6/2, one WT), whose activity is depicted in the actograms. The SCN from both R6/2 and WT mice showed functional molecular time keeping, as revealed by *in vitro* by bioluminescence gene expression. (Adapted from Pallier *et al.*, 2007.)

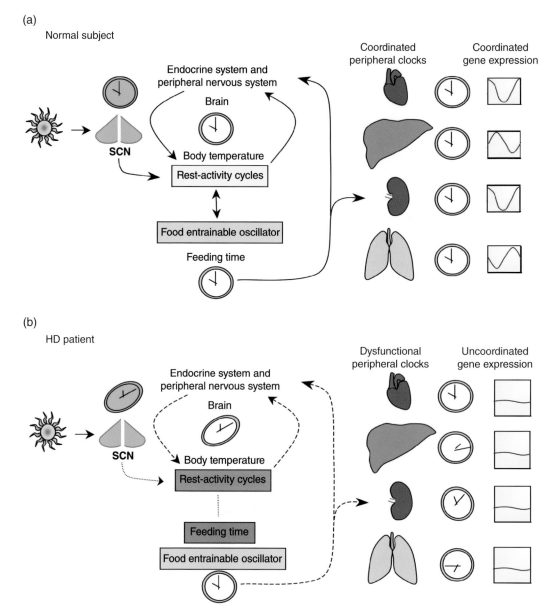

Fig. 21.5 Circadian control in HD subjects may be disturbed at multiple levels. In normal subjects, there is a sophisticated balance of feedback loops that regulates daily physiological function. Multiple aspects of this control system may be disturbed in HD patients, with the overall effect being either symptoms (such as abnormal daily activity) or hidden deficits (such as poorly coordinated metabolism).

Lie JA, Kjuus H, Zienolddiny S, *et al.* 2011. Night work and breast cancer risk among Norwegian nurses: assessment by different exposure metrics. *Am J Epidemiol* **173**(11):1272–9.

Lin YC, Hsiao TJ, Chen PC. 2009a. Persistent rotating shift-work exposure accelerates development of metabolic syndrome among middle-aged female employees: a five-year follow-up. *Chronobiol Int* **26**(4):740–55.

Lin YC, Hsiao TJ, Chen PC. 2009b. Shift work aggravates metabolic syndrome development among early-middle-aged males with elevated ALT. *World J Gastroenterol* **15**(45):5654–61.

Lissoni P, Rovelli F, Malugani F, *et al.* 2001. Anti-angiogenic activity of melatonin in advanced cancer patients. *Neuro Endocrinol Lett* **22**(1):45–47.

Macagnan J, Pattussi MP, Canuto R, *et al.* 2012. Impact of nightshift work on overweight and abdominal obesity among workers of a poultry processing plant in southern Brazil. *Chronobiol Int* **29**(3):336–43.

Marcheva B, Ramsey KM, Buhr ED, *et al.* 2010. Disruption of the clock components CLOCK and BMAL1 leads to hypoinsulinaemia and diabetes. *Nature* **466**(7306):627–31.

Mediavilla MD, Cos S, Sanchez-Barcelo EJ. 1999. Melatonin increases p53 and p21WAF1 expression in MCF-7 human breast cancer cells *in vitro*. *Life Sci* **65**(4):415–20.

Menegaux F, Truong T, Anger A, *et al.* 2013. Night work and breast cancer: a population-based case-control study in France (the CECILE study). *Int J Cancer* **132**(4):924–31.

Mikuni E, Ohoshi T, Hayashi K, *et al.* 1983. Glucose intolerance in an employed population. *Tohoku J Exp Med* **141**(Suppl):251–6.

Morgan PJ, Collins CE, Plotnikoff RC, *et al.* 2011. Efficacy of a workplace-based weight loss program for overweight male shift workers: the Workplace POWER (Preventing Obesity Without Eating like a Rabbit) randomized controlled trial. *Prev Med* **52**(5):317–25.

Morikawa Y, Nakagawa H, Miura K, *et al.* 2005. Shift work and the risk of diabetes mellitus among Japanese male factory workers. *Scand J Work Environ Health* **31**(3):179–83.

Morikawa Y, Nakagawa H, Miura K, *et al.* 2007. Effect of shift work on body mass index and metabolic parameters. *Scand J Work Environ Health* **33**(1):45–50.

Mohebbi I, Saadat S, Aghassi M, *et al.* 2012. Prevalence of metabolic syndrome in Iranian professional drivers: results from a population based study of 12,138 men. *PLoS One* **7**(2):e31790.

Nabe-Nielsen K, Garde AH, Tuchsen F, *et al.* 2008. Cardiovascular risk factors and primary selection into shift work. *Scand J Work Environ Health* **34**(3):206–12.

Nagaya T, Yoshida H, Takahashi H, *et al.* 2002. Markers of insulin resistance in day and shift workers aged 30–59 years. *Int Arch Occup Environ Health* **75**(8):562–8.

Oberlinner C, Ott MG, Nasterlack M, *et al.* 2009. Medical program for shift workers--impacts on chronic disease and mortality outcomes. *Scand J Work Environ Health* **35**(4):309–18.

O'Leary ES, Schoenfeld ER, Stevens RG, *et al.* 2006. Shift work, light at night, and breast cancer on Long Island, New York. *Am J Epidemiol* **164**(4):358–66.

Oyama I, Kubo T, Fujino Y, *et al.* 2012. Retrospective cohort study of the risk of impaired glucose tolerance among shift workers. *Scand J Work Environ Health* **38**(4):337–42.

Pan A, Schernhammer ES, Sun Q, *et al.* 2011. Rotating night shift work and risk of type 2 diabetes: two prospective cohort studies in women. *PLoS Med* **8**(12):e1001141.

Parent ME, El-Zein M, Rousseau MC, *et al.* 2012. Night work and the risk of cancer among men. *Am J Epidemiol* **176**(9):751–9.

Parkes KR. 2002. Shift work and age as interactive predictors of body mass index among offshore workers. *Scand J Work Environ Health* **28**(1):64–71.

Pesch B, Harth V, Rabstein S, *et al.* 2010. Night work and breast cancer – results from the German GENICA study. *Scand J Work Environ Health* **36**(2):134–41.

Peschke E, Muhlbauer E. 2010. New evidence for a role of melatonin in glucose regulation. *Best Pract Res Clin Endocrinol Metab* **24**(5):829–41.

Pietroiusti A, Neri A, Somma G, *et al.* 2010. Incidence of metabolic syndrome among night-shift healthcare workers. *Occup Environ Med* **67**(1):54–7.

Poole EM, Schernhammer ES, Tworoger SS. 2011. Rotating night shift work and risk of ovarian cancer. *Cancer Epidemiol Biomarkers Prev* **20**(5):934–8.

Pronk A, Ji BT, Shu XO, *et al.* 2010. Night-shift work and breast cancer risk in a cohort of Chinese women. *Am J Epidemiol* **171**(9):953–9.

Pukkala E, Martinsen JI, Lynge E, *et al.* 2009. Occupation and cancer – follow-up of 15 million people in five Nordic countries. *Acta Oncol* **48**(5):646–790.

Puttonen S, Harma M, Hublin C. 2010. Shift work and cardiovascular disease - pathways from circadian stress to morbidity. *Scand J Work Environ Health* **36**(2):96–108.

Puttonen S, Viitasalo K, Harma M. 2011. Effect of shiftwork on systemic markers of inflammation. *Chronobiol Int* **28**(6):528–35.

Puttonen S, Viitasalo K, Harma M. 2012. The relationship between current and former shift work and the metabolic syndrome. *Scand J Work Environ Health* **38**(4):343–8.

Rudic RD, McNamara P, Curtis AM, *et al*. 2004. BMAL1 and CLOCK, two essential components of the circadian clock, are involved in glucose homeostasis. *PLoS Biol* **2**(11):e377.

Sainz RM, Mayo JC, Rodriguez C, *et al*. 2003. Melatonin and cell death: differential actions on apoptosis in normal and cancer cells. *Cell Mol Life Sci* **60**(7):1407–26.

Scheer FA, Hilton MF, Mantzoros CS, *et al*. 2009. Adverse metabolic and cardiovascular consequences of circadian misalignment. *Proc Natl Acad Sci USA* **106**(11):4453–8.

Schernhammer ES, Laden F, Speizer FE, *et al*. 2001. Rotating night shifts and risk of breast cancer in women participating in the nurses' health study. *J Natl Cancer Inst* **93**(20):1563–8.

Schernhammer ES, Laden F, Speizer FE, *et al*. 2003. Night-shift work and risk of colorectal cancer in the nurses' health study. *J Natl Cancer Inst* **95**(11):825–8.

Schernhammer ES, Kroenke CH, Laden F, *et al*. 2006. Night work and risk of breast cancer. *Epidemiology* **17**(1):108–11.

Schernhammer ES, Razavi P, Li TY, *et al*. 2011. Rotating night shifts and risk of skin cancer in the nurses' health study. *J Natl Cancer Inst* **103**(7):602–6.

Schwartzbaum J, Ahlbom A, Feychting M. 2007. Cohort study of cancer risk among male and female shift workers. *Scand J Work Environ Health* **33**(5):336–43.

Sharifian A, Farahani S, Pasalar P, *et al*. 2005. Shift work as an oxidative stressor. *J Circadian Rhythms* **3**:15.

Sherwin R, Jastreboff AM. 2012. Year in diabetes 2012: The diabetes tsunami. *J Clin Endocrinol Metab* **97**(12):4293–301.

Smith P, Fritschi L, Reid A, *et al*. 2013. The relationship between shift work and body mass index among Canadian nurses. *Appl Nurs Res* **26**(1):24–31.

Sookoian S, Gemma C, Fernandez Gianotti T, *et al*. 2007. Effects of rotating shift work on biomarkers of metabolic syndrome and inflammation. *J Intern Med* **261**(3):285–92.

Straif K, Baan R, Grosse Y, *et al*. 2007. Carcinogenicity of shift-work, painting, and fire-fighting. *Lancet Oncol* **8**(12):1065–6.

Suessenbacher A, Potocnik M, Dorler J, *et al*. 2011. Comparison of peripheral endothelial function in shift versus nonshift workers. *Am J Cardiol* **107**(6):945–8.

Suwazono Y, Sakata K, Okubo Y, *et al*. 2006. Long-term longitudinal study on the relationship between alternating shift work and the onset of diabetes mellitus in male Japanese workers. *J Occup Environ Med* **48**(5):455–61.

Suwazono Y, Dochi M, Sakata K, *et al*. 2008. A longitudinal study on the effect of shift work on weight gain in male Japanese workers. *Obesity* **16**(8):1887–93.

Suwazono Y, Dochi M, Oishi M, *et al*. 2009. Shiftwork and impaired glucose metabolism: a 14-year cohort study on 7104 male workers. *Chronobiol Int* **26**(5):926–41.

Theorell T, Akerstedt T. 1976. Day and night work: changes in cholesterol, uric acid, glucose and potassium in serum and in circadian patterns of urinary catecholamine excretion. A longitudinal cross-over study of railway workers. *Acta Med Scand* **200**(1–2):47–53.

Thomas C, Power C. 2010. Shift work and risk factors for cardiovascular disease: a study at age 45 years in the 1958 British birth cohort. *Eur J Epidemiol* **25**(5):305–14.

Tucker P, Marquie JC, Folkard S, *et al*. 2012. Shiftwork and metabolic dysfunction. *Chronobiol Int* **29**(5):549–55.

Tynes T, Hannevik M, Andersen A, *et al*. 1996. Incidence of breast cancer in Norwegian female radio and telegraph operators. *Cancer Causes Control* **7**(2):197–204.

Uetani M, Suwazono Y, Kobayashi E, *et al*. 2006. A longitudinal study of the influence of shift work on serum uric acid levels in workers at a telecommunications company. *Occup Med (Lond)* **56**(2):83–8.

van Amelsvoort LG, Schouten EG, Kok FJ. 1999. Duration of shiftwork related to body mass index and waist to hip ratio. *Int J Obes Relat Metab Disord* **23**(9):973–8.

van Amelsvoort LG, Schouten EG, Kok FJ. 2004. Impact of one year of shift work on cardiovascular disease risk factors. *J Occup Environ Med* **46**(7):699–706.

Vijayalaxmi, Thomas CR, Jr., Reiter RJ, *et al*. 2002, Melatonin: from basic research to cancer treatment clinics. *J Clin Oncol* **20**(10):2575–601.

Villeneuve S, Fevotte J, Anger A, *et al*. 2011. Breast cancer risk by occupation and industry: analysis of the CECILE study, a population-based case-control study in France. *Am J Ind Med* **54**(7):499–509.

Vimalananda VG, Palmer JR, Gerlovin H, *et al*. 2015. Night-shift work and incident diabetes among African-American women. *Diabetologia*. Epub ahead of print. doi: 10.1007/s00125-014-3480-9.

Viswanathan AN, Hankinson SE, Schernhammer ES. 2007. Night shift work and the risk of endometrial cancer. *Cancer Res* **67**(21):10618–22.

Ward M, Berry DJ, Power C, *et al.* 2011. Working patterns and vitamin D status in mid-life: a cross-sectional study of the 1958 British birth cohort. *Occup Environ Med* **68**(12):902–7.

WHO (World Health Organization). 2010. IARC Monographs on the Evaluation of Carcinogenic Risks to Humans: Painting, Firefighting, and Shiftwork, Vol. 98. http://monographs.iarc.fr/ENG/Monographs/vol98/index.php (last accessed November 22, 2014).

Zhao I, Bogossian F, Song S, *et al.* 2011. The association between shift work and unhealthy weight: a cross-sectional analysis from the Nurses and Midwives' e-cohort Study. *J Occup Environ Med* **53**(2):153–8.

Zhao I, Bogossian F, Turner C. 2012. Does maintaining or changing shift types affect BMI? A longitudinal study. *J Occup Environ Med* **54**(5):525–31.

Circadian Rhythms in Immune Function

14

Kandis Adams, Oscar Castanon-Cervantes, and Alec J. Davidson

Department of Neurobiology and Neuroscience Institute, Morehouse School of Medicine, Atlanta, GA, USA

14.1 Introduction

Through surveillance and active defense mechanisms against a vast variety of antigens, the primary function of the immune system is to recognize self from non-self. As much as it is important to recognize and respond to an antigen, it is equally important to control and modulate the immune response, therefore preventing self-damage caused by an excessive reaction. The immune system has two main components: innate and adaptive. The innate immune system is the first line of defense and is characterized by nonspecific and rapid responses that occur within minutes to hours. The adaptive immune system is highly specific and requires more time to respond. The immune system not only protects from external pathogens, but also from internal pathological challenges that arise in cells and tissues that could lead to disease.

For decades the immune system was thought to rely on a simple mechanism by recognizing antigens with defensive responses intended to eliminate foreign material and then return to a standby or surveillance mode. A more modern view characterizes the immune system as a dynamic major player in the control of the homeostatic network. Such a role requires constant and precise communication with another major player of the homeostatic network, the *circadian system*: a sophisticated timing control mechanism based on the daily oscillations of well characterized clock genes that anticipates and adapts to daily changes in environmental and physiological variables. It is clear that the immune and the circadian system communicate with one another in a bidirectional fashion.

Components of the immune system at the tissue and cellular level receive circadian information by means of neural and endocrine signals. Most, if not all, immune cells contain molecular clock components. These cellular clocks mediate immune responses in natural killer cell activity, macrophage cell phagocytosis, and inflammation. Additionally, evidence from animal models has begun to clarify the potential mechanisms linking alterations in biological rhythms with pathological changes in the immune response. Therefore, in this chapter how the circadian regulation of the immune system contributes to the maintenance of an adequate and robust immune response is explored.

Circadian Medicine, First Edition. Edited by Christopher S. Colwell.

© 2015 John Wiley & Sons, Inc. Published 2015 by John Wiley & Sons, Inc.

14.2 Daily variations in health and disease

The most important role of the circadian system is to maintain precise temporal control among multiple physiological functions. The circadian system achieves this task by generating self-sustained molecular oscillations once about every 24 hours (Chapters 1 and 2). These circadian rhythms are organized at the systems level through both humoral and neural signals generated by a master circadian oscillator located in mammals in the hypothalamic suprachiasmatic nucleus (SCN) (Chapter 3). The SCN is a bilateral retino-recipient network of tightly coupled neuronal pacemakers that synchronize to the external lighting environment and act as an orchestra conductor by communicating timing information to targets throughout the brain and body.

The precise temporal control of physiological functions exerted by the clock, including the immune response, guarantees that biological processes are organized to be maximal at the time when a maximal response is needed (and appropriately minimal at other times). Thus, this temporal structure is thought to be an essential feature of a healthy homeostatic system. Therefore, alterations in the circadian system required to maintain temporal order of physiological responses may have severe health consequences. Pathological conditions that perturb sleep–wake patterns are likely to have consequences for the organization of temporal physiology by the circadian clock. Even in the absence of overt disease, behaviors or environments that chronically perturb circadian physiology, such as shift work schedules, frequent jet lag, and nighttime exposure to bright light or drug abuse, may disrupt the communication between physiological systems required to mount an appropriate response to a potential challenge. Although insufficient sleep is typically thought to be a major cause for dysregulation of immune function, circadian disruption that often coexists with loss of sleep may instead provide a mechanism for altered immune responses.

Prevalence of disease, particularly pathologies associated with chronic inflammation, is higher in people chronically exposed to circadian disruption. Described in the following sections are examples where significant changes in the immune response and modulation of these changes by circadian disruption occur with or without sleep loss, stressing the importance of the circadian system in the temporal control of physiology both in health, and disease.

14.3 Early evidence of circadian regulation on immunity

In 1960, Franz Halberg reported a diurnal rhythm of sensitivity to lethal doses of the bacterial endotoxin lipopolysaccharide (LPS). When the same dose of LPS was injected in the peritoneum of groups of mice, he noted that the mortality rate changed dramatically based on the time of day the injection was given (Fig.14.1). When the injection occurred during the last hours of the light cycle (right before the beginning of the activity period for nocturnal rodents), mortality rate was higher, and if the same injection was given in the middle of the dark period, mortality was lower (Halberg et al., 1960). This pattern revealed tight regulation of the inflammatory response and innate immunity by the circadian system.

A similar pattern was observed in response to tumor necrosis factor alpha (TNF-α) (Fig.14.1), a pro-inflammatory cytokine (Hrushesky et al., 1994). TNF-α is a mediator of the acute phase reaction, endotoxic shock and cell mediated host defense against bacteria and tumor cells. In addition to these experimental observations, there is evidence of modulation of immune responses by the circadian system in humans. Hospital deaths, many of them associated with sepsis, do not occur throughout the day randomly but most commonly between 2 a.m. and 6 a.m. (Smolensky et al., 1972). This time of day (right before the beginning of the activity period for a diurnal primate) corresponds to the time in the circadian cycle when LPS and TNF-α are each most often lethal in nocturnal rodents. The peak toxicity for TNF-α and LPS both occur at the time of day that is close to the usual daily cortisol peak. This is important because cortisol and glucocorticoids are essential in mediating the response to acute infectious and endotoxic challenges. Findings of this nature support the concept that the immune system is regulated by the circadian clock.

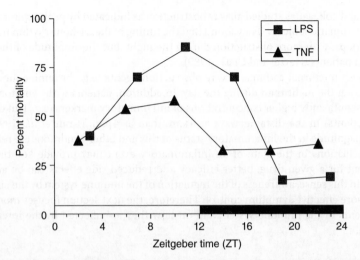

Fig. 14.1 24-hour changes in susceptibility to both lipopolysaccharide (LPS, a bacterial endotoxin) and tumor necrosis factor alpha (TNF-α, a pro-inflammatory cytokine). (Figure reprinted from Leone *et al.* (2007) with permission. The original data are from Halberg *et al.* (1960) (LPS) and Hrushesky *et al.* (1994) (TNF-a)).

Resolution of inflammatory and infectious challenges ultimately relies not only on innate but also on adaptive immunity. In this complementary aspect of the immune response, circadian control is also present. There are time-of-day differences associated with the effects of immunization and the peak concentrations for three major classes of immunoglobins undergo circadian changes (Haus and Smolensky, 1999). Rhythms in plasmatic levels of pro-inflammatory cytokines, as well peptide hormones produced and secreted by immune cells, have also been reported. Interleukin- 1β, 6, 10, and 12, TNF-α and interferon gamma (IFN-γ) exhibit high levels during the night and early morning in humans (Petrovsky and Harrison, 1997). This increase in cytokine plasma levels primes readiness for a robust immune response at the time of day when antigen presentation is most likely to occur. This anticipation, and the preparedness of an optimal physiological setting to produce an energy efficient response, is a core function of the circadian system in its regulation of nearly every physiological process in the time domain.

14.4 Clinical relevance of circadian regulation of the immune system

Besides the evidence for daily variations in immune responses provided by the aforementioned experiments, there are clinical data that reveal a strong correlation between time of day and manifestation of illnesses. For instance, rheumatoid arthritis symptoms such as joint pain, stiffness and functional disability occur in early morning hours (Cutolo and Straub, 2008). Key pro-inflammatory cytokines, TNF-α and IL-6, are under circadian regulation and play vital roles in the expression of rheumatoid arthritis symptoms. As previously mentioned, these cytokines have greatest expression during the early morning, prior to onset of activity. Interestingly, rheumatoid patients with elevated disease activity showed a markedly reduced circadian cortisol rhythm (Neeck *et al.*, 1990).

Asthma symptoms are also rhythmic; most asthma attacks occur at night (Litinski *et al.*, 2009). In fact, patients that have profound nocturnal asthma show increased morbidity and mortality compared to those that do not display such strong rhythmicity. There are three major components of asthma: chronic inflammation, airway hyperresponsiveness and reversible airway obstruction (Masoli *et al.*, 2005). Each of these components displays daily fluctuations with 4 a.m. being worse when compared to 4 p.m. For example, Hetzel and colleagues studied airway obstruction as indicated by peak expiratory flow (PEF) in 221 healthy and asthmatic subjects. They found that the timing of the 24-hour rhythm in PEF was similar between both groups, with more obstruction during the night, but the amplitude of the oscillation was greater in asthma patients (Hetzel and Clark, 1980).

For patients with nocturnal asthma, airway obstruction agents (e.g., histamine, house dust) have a greater effect during the night than during the day. In addition, patients with symptoms of "nocturnal asthma" exhibit significantly higher concentrations of inflammatory markers (e.g., leukocyte, neutrophil and eosinophil counts) in the distal airways at 4 a.m. than at 4 p.m. (Kraft *et al.*, 1996). Time of day changes of this magnitude in the inflammatory status of this and other conditions are relevant to clinical intervention. Oscillations in the state of an inflammatory event may provide key time windows for efficient treatment for a given drug; better efficacy and reduced side effects can be achieved without increasing dose. In this sense, awareness of the regulation of the immune system by the circadian network may be key for more effective symptom control. Therefore, the next section focuses more specifically on various components of the immune system and on how they are affected by the interaction with the circadian system.

14.5 The circadian system communicates time of day information to immune cells and tissues

The immune system is modulated by the circadian system by systemic signals and molecular clocks within immune cells. The central circadian pacemaker in the SCN of the anterior hypothalamus contains specialized neurons that receive photic input through the retinohypothalamic tract (RHT) and nonphotic cues by disparate neural inputs (Chapter 3). The convergence of these inputs in the SCN integrates both environmental and physiological signals in order to coordinate downstream brain areas and organ systems via neural and endocrine outputs (Guo *et al.*, 2006). Two important areas for regulating stress and immune responses are the paraventricular nuclei (PVN) and arcuate nuclei (ARC) (Saeb-Parsy *et al.*, 2000; Kalsbeek and Buijs, 2002). Although it is likely other pathways exist, the SCN conveys circadian information to the immune system by mediating activity of autonomic and endocrine neurons of the PVN. The neuroimmune axis is then comprised of the SCN, PVN and sympathetic nervous system, providing the basic framework that regulates the timing of immune cell function. Oscillatory expression of both immune-effector cell numbers, as well as physiological functions elicited by these cells (e.g., rhythmic phagocytosis) is synchronized so that proper homeostatic responses occur at the most suitable time of day.

14.6 Immune effector cells under circadian regulation

14.6.1 Natural killer cells

Natural killer (NK) cells participate in the immune response against infection and cancer. The cytotoxic activity of NK cells varies depending on the time of day (Arjona *et al.*, 2004); this rhythm is associated with the circadian variation in tumor clearance (Shakhar *et al.*, 2001). The expression of canonical clock genes, cytolytic factors and cytokines are all related to a rhythmic noradrenergic input to the spleen acting as a molecular time signal to NK cells and perhaps other spleen cells (Logan *et al.*, 2011; Logan and Sarkar, 2012). The expression of cytolytic factors, that is, granzyme B and perforin, in rat NK cells is high at the mRNA level during the light period and high at the protein level during the dark period (Arjona and Sarkar, 2005). Similar results are found for cytokines IFN-γ and TNF-α (Arjona and Sarkar, 2005, 2006). These oscillations persist in constant darkness, revealing the true circadian nature of the oscillatory function.

Perforin and granzymes have been largely recognized as fundamental components of the granule-mediated cytolytic activity. IFN-γ and TNF-α produced by NK cells act as self-activating molecules that promote NK cell-mediated killing. Interestingly, a cell line derived from the NK cell lineage in the rat (RNK16) exhibited a significant decrease of both perforin and granzyme B after functional mutation of *Per2* expression by siRNA.

14.6.2 Macrophages

Macrophages play an important role in the innate immune response. In mouse peritoneal macrophages, phagocytic function, and chemokine and cytokine expression of several proteins all display a circadian rhythm regulated by the molecular clock (Hayashi *et al.*, 2007; Keller *et al.*, 2009). Phagocytosis exhibits a circadian variation that peaks during the light period and is low during the dark period in rodents (Hayashi *et al.*, 2007). The strength of pro-inflammatory cytokine production from macrophages in response to bacterial endotoxin is determined by the circadian phase of the macrophage clock rather than by systemic circadian modulators such as rhythmic cortisol levels (Krieger, 1975). In peritoneal macrophages, for example, about 8% of transcripts are rhythmically expressed (Keller *et al.*, 2009). Hayashi and colleagues also demonstrated that clock gene expression of *Bmal1* in peritoneal macrophages exhibited daily oscillations and that the expression of the inflammatory factor monocyte chemo-attractant protein-1 (MCP-1/JE) is positively regulated by *Bmal1*. When *Bmal1* expression was suppressed by siRNA, nuclear factor kappa B (NF-κB) activity was decreased; this was followed by a downregulation in MCP-1/JE mRNA expression in macrophage cells (Hayashi *et al.*, 2007). Evolutionary adaptation to time of day-dependent pathogen pressure or activity correlated infection risk is a viable interpretation of these phenomena. Because macrophages are critical elements of the first line of defense against bacterial infections, anticipation of daily variation of infection risk is probably of great advantage. On the other hand, excessive responsiveness of these cells may be detrimental for the organism, and thus a tight regulation of its timing is likely to be beneficial.

14.6.3 T cells

T lymphocytes are essential in the adaptive response to infection. In the lymph nodes these cells encounter and recognize self from non-self. Fortier and colleagues showed that T cell function both *in vitro* and *in vivo* has daily variation (Fortier *et al.*, 2011). T cells exhibited a circadian rhythm of proliferation, and therefore mice immunized during the day showed a stronger T cell response than those mice immunized during the night. In humans, the maximal T cell proliferation in blood is during the night (Bollinger *et al.*, 2011). Absolute numbers of T cells in circulation are stably high from late evening throughout the early morning hours. Since mice are nocturnal and humans are diurnal, the highest T cell reactivity during daytime in mice is consistent with findings in humans who have highest T cell reactivity at night; in both species peak activity is during rest. T cell reactivity and proliferation is critical to secondary immune responses, and thus these rhythms have clinical relevance. Immunization timing for maximal T cell proliferation, rational timing of immunomodulatory drug intake, and blood sampling for immunological diagnostics are all potential therapeutic areas where rhythms are key. For example, T cell numbers are considerably more stable from the morning through the late afternoon in humans, which indicates that results from blood samples taken during routine clinical hours should not be subject to excessive intra-individual variability. However, nonroutine emergency situations during the night may yield higher cell counts and are, therefore, not comparable to similar samples obtained during regular clinic hours.

14.6.4 B cells

B cells are vital to memory and antibody production; they have the ability to differentiate into plasma cells (antibody producing cells) and memory cells. It has been shown that in splenic B cells, canonical clock genes such as *Bmal1* are expressed in a circadian pattern under normal lighting and constant darkness conditions (Silver *et al.*, 2012). *Bmal1* is vital to the development of B-cells (Sun *et al.*, 2006). In this study, a significant decrease of B cells in peripheral blood is reported on *Bmal1* deficient mice. It appears that the effect of *Bmal1* acts upon differentiation from pre-B cells to mature B cells.

In all, it has become apparent, that at the cellular level, the body does not randomly function but is temporally programmed to respond for optimal performance at specific times of day. The same is true for the immune system, which is paramount to the overall health of an organism.

In this section it has been shown that key immune cells, each performers of highly specialized functions in the immune system, are regulated by the circadian system. However, to better understand how the immune–circadian interaction works, it is necessary to examine how various human activities that counteract our normal circadian function influence health. The next section focuses on the effects of circadian disturbance on health and disease.

14.7 Circadian disruption role in immune pathology and disease

A major reason for understanding circadian rhythms is that they play a vital role in disease. Both epidemiological studies in humans and experimental animal research have shown that environmental desynchronization by external stressors (e.g., shift work and transmeridian travel) or by internal factors (e.g., genetic disorders) may lead to increased risks for the onset and progression of a variety of pathologies associated with chronic inflammation (Fig.14.2).

Various studies have established associations between disruptions in circadian clocks and disease development and progression. Nearly 20% of the working population in the United States engages in some sort of shift work, freely defined to include, static night shifts, flexible shifts, extended shifts, and rotating shifts (Bureau of Labor, 2005; Wright *et al.*, 2013). Exposure to nontraditional work schedules have been linked to increased risk of cancer (Schernhammer *et al.*, 2006; Bhatti *et al.*, 2013), gastric ulcers (Segawa *et al.*, 1987), diabetes (Morikawa *et al.*, 2005), and various cardiovascular diseases (Tuchsen *et al.*, 2006; Haupt *et al.*, 2008). Disturbances in the circadian system caused by the nontraditional work life style may lead to dysregulation of the immune system, which influences the exacerbation or development of various immune related diseases. Although the underlying mechanisms associated with shift work and disease are not yet clear, it is becoming more apparent that alterations in common circadian and immune pathways may potentially promote disease development.

A chronic schedule of environmental circadian disruption (ECD) in rodents, a lighting schedule that mimics some aspects of rotating human shift work, elicits dysregulated inflammatory responses to LPS both *in vivo* and *in vitro* (Castanon-Cervantes *et al.*, 2010; Adams *et al.*, 2013; Brager *et al.*, 2013). Mice on these schedules exhibit uncontrolled responses of the immune system, typified by increased cytokine secretion from peritoneal macrophages and whole blood, and endotoxemia and death at LPS doses that appear to have very mild consequences in control mice.

Similar chronic light-cycle perturbation has been shown to lead to the elevation of splenic and intestinal T-helper cells that protect against bacterial and fungal infections at mucosal surfaces. These mice were more prone to the development of dextran sulfate sodium (DSS)-induced colitis (Yu *et al.*, 2013). Since the circadian clock appears altered in immune cells after such light cycles

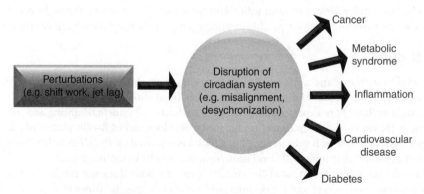

Fig. 14.2 Circadian disruption and disease.

(Castanon-Cervantes *et al.*, 2010; Yu *et al.*, 2013), it is reasonable to conclude that chronic disruption of the circadian system leads to pathological inflammatory responses.

14.8 The effects of clock gene alterations on immune functions

Disturbance of clock function through genetic manipulation also elicits changes in the regulation of the immune system. Among other pathologies associated with accelerated aging, *Bmal1* knockout mice develop progressive corneal inflammation and exhibit decreased numbers of lymphocytes (Kondratov *et al.*, 2006). Additionally, mice lacking both clock genes *Cry1* and *Cry2* exhibit exacerbated cytokine production and joint swelling after arthritic induction (Hashiramoto *et al.*, 2010).

    Clock-mutant mice showed phase-delayed circadian patterns in lymphocyte numbers and a bimodal pattern of plasma neutrophils compared with wild-type mice (Oishi *et al.*, 2006). *Per2* mutant mice did not show a circadian rhythm in IFN-γ mRNA expression that characterized wild-type control mice (Arjona and Sarkar, 2005). Furthermore, *Per2* deficient mice showed aberrations in cytokine production in response to LPS challenge, most significant of which was dramatically reduced levels of IFN-γ and IL-10 (Liu *et al.*, 2006). *Per2* mutant mice also demonstrate loss of a circadian pattern of resistance to LPS challenge that was well defined in the wild type, and the Per2 deficient mice were more resistant to LPS-induced death (Liu *et al.*, 2006). In addition, circadian disruption of rhythmic sympathetic input to the spleen alters circadian rhythms of cytokines and cytolytic factors in immune cells by disrupting the core components of the molecular clock (Logan *et al.*, 2011; Logan and Sarkar, 2012), supporting the view that circadian disruption desynchronizes central and peripheral immune clocks.

14.9 Conclusions

Human society has rapidly transformed into a 24 hour, 365 day/year active entity. We must understand how these altered routines and schedules change our biological functions and, in turn, influence our health. This chapter has covered how key cellular effectors of both the innate and adaptive arms of the immune system are under tight circadian regulation (Fig.14.3), thus affecting a wide variety of

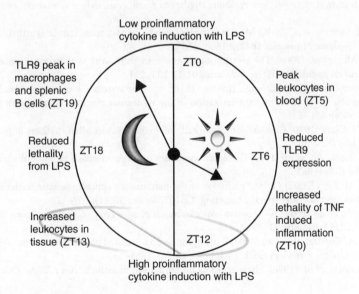

Fig. 14.3 Rhythms in immune cell function.

physiological functions. We have explained how alterations in clock gene function influence cellular behavior, development, and activation status. We have also shown how changes in the way human society organizes its activities beyond standard working hours typical of the pre-industrial revolution era has had severe health consequences that we have only just begun to appreciate. These challenges to our way of life are here to stay and the resulting disturbances to the circadian system will ultimately affect disease prevalence and outcome. Thus, a better understanding of the interactions between the circadian and the immune system including the mechanisms regulating these changes is needed.

References

Adams, K.L., O. Castanon-Cervantes, *et al.* (2013) Environmental circadian disruption elevates the IL-6 response to lipopolysaccharide in blood. *J Biol Rhythms* **28**(4): 272–277.

Arjona, A.and D.K. Sarkar (2005) Circadian oscillations of clock genes, cytolytic factors, and cytokines in rat NK cells. *J Immunol* **174**: 7618–7624.

Arjona, A.and D.K. Sarkar (2006) Evidence supporting a circadian control of natural killer cell function. *Brain Behav Immun* **20**(5): 469–476.

Arjona, A., N. Boyadjieva, *et al.* (2004) Circadian rhythms of granzyme B, perforin, ifn-γ, and NK cell cytolytic activity in the spleen: effects of chronic ethanol. *J Immunol* **172**: 2811–2817.

Bhatti, P., K.L. Cushing-Haugen, *et al.* (2013) Nightshift work and risk of ovarian cancer. *Occup Environ Med* **70**(4): 231–237.

Bollinger, T., A. Leutz, *et al.* (2011) Circadian clocks in mouse and human CD4+ T cells. *PLoS One* **6**(12): e29801.

Brager, A.J., J.C. Ehlen, *et al.* (2013) Sleep loss and the inflammatory response in mice under chronic environmental circadian disruption. *PLoS One* **8**(5): e63752.

Bureau of Labor Statistics (2005) Workers on flexible and shift schedules in May 2004. US Department of Labor, Washington, DC.

Castanon-Cervantes, O., M. Wu, *et al.* (2010) Dysregulation of inflammatory responses by chronic circadian disruption. *J Immunol* **185**(10): 5796–5805.

Cutolo, M.and R.H. Straub (2008) Circadian rhythms in arthritis:hormonal effects on the immune/inflammatory reaction. *Autoimmun Rev* **7**(3): 223–228.

Fortier, E.E., J. Rooney, *et al.* (2011) Circadian variation of the response of T cells to antigen. *J Immunol* **187**(12): 6291–6300.

Guo, H., J.M. Brewer, *et al.* (2006) Suprachiasmatic regulation of circadian rhythms of gene expression in hamster peripheral organs: effects of transplanting the pacemaker. *J Neurosci* **26**: 6406–6412.

Halberg, F., E.A. Johnson, *et al.* (1960) Susceptibility rhythm to E. coli endotoxin and bioassay. *Proc Soc Exp Biol Med* **103**: 142–144.

Hashiramoto, A., T. Yamane, *et al.* (2010) Mammalian clock gene Cryptochrome regulates arthritis via proinflammatory cytokine TNF-alpha. *J Immunol* **184**(3): 1560–1565.

Haupt, C. M., D. Alte, *et al.* (2008) The relation of exposure to shift work with atherosclerosis and myocardial infarction in a general population. *Atherosclerosis* **201**(1): 205–211.

Haus, E.and M.H. Smolensky (1999) Biologic rhythms in the immune system. *Chronobiol Int* **16**: 581–622.

Hayashi, M., S. Shimba, *et al.* (2007) Characterization of the molecular clock in mouse peritoneal macrophages. *Biol Pharm Bull* **30**(4): 621–626.

Hetzel, M.R.and T.J. Clark (1980) Comparison of normal and asthmatic circadian rhythms in peak expiratory flow rate. *Thorax* **35**(10): 732–738.

Hrushesky, W.J., T. Langevin, *et al.* (1994) Circadian dynamics of tumor necrosis factor alpha (cachectin) lethality. *J Exp Med* **180**(3): 1059–1065.

Kalsbeek, A.and R.M. Buijs (2002) Output pathways of the mammalian suprachiasmatic nucleus: coding circadian time by transmitter selection and specific targeting. *Cell Tissue Res* **309**(1): 109–118.

Keller, M., J. Mazuch, *et al.* (2009) A circadian clock in macrophages controls inflammatory immune responses. *Proc Natl Acad Sci USA* **106**(50): 21407–21412.

Kondratov, R.V., A.A. Kondratova, *et al.* (2006) Early aging and age-related pathologies in mice deficient in BMAL1, the core componentof the circadian clock. *Genes Dev* **20**(14): 1868–1873.

Kraft, M., R. Djukanovic, *et al.* (1996) Alveolar tissue inflammation in asthma. *Am J Respir Crit Care Med* **154**(5): 1505–1510.

Krieger, D.T. (1975). Rhythms of ACTH and corticosteroid secretion in health and disease, and their experimental modification. *J Steroid Biochem* **6**(5): 785–791.

Leone, M.J., J.J. Chiesa, *et al.* (2007) A time to kill, and a time to heal. Pathophysiological interactions between the circadian and the immune systems. *Physiological Mini Reviews* **2**(10): 60–69.

Litinski, M., F.A. Scheer, *et al.* (2009) Influence of the Circadian System on Disease Severity. *Sleep Med Clin* **4**(2): 143–163.

Liu, J., G. Malkani, *et al.* (2006) The circadian clock Period 2 gene regulates gamma interferon production of NK cells in host response to lipopolysaccharide-induced endotoxic shock. *Infect Immun* **74**(8): 4750–4756.

Logan, R.W.and D.K. Sarkar (2012). Circadian nature of immune function. *Mol Cell Endocrinol* **349**(1): 82–90.

Logan, R.W., A. Arjona, *et al.* (2011) Role of sympathetic nervous system in the entrainment of circadian natural-killer cell function. *Brain Behav Immun* **25**(1): 101–109.

Masoli, M., M. Weatherall, *et al.* (2005) The 24 h duration of bronchodilator action of the salmeterol/fluticasone combination inhaler. *Respir Med* **99**(5): 545–552.

Morikawa, Y., H. Nakagawa, *et al.* (2005) Shift work and the risk of diabetes mellitus among Japanese male factory workers. *Scand J Work Environ Health* **31**(3): 179–183.

Neeck, G., K. Federlin, *et al.* (1990) Adrenal secretion of cortisol in patients with rheumatoid arthritis. *J Rheumatol* **17**(1): 24–29.

Oishi, K., N. Ohkura, *et al.* (2006) Clock mutation affects circadian regulation of circulating blood cells. *J Circadian Rhythms* **4**: 13.

Petrovsky, N.and L.C. Harrison (1997) Diurnal rhythmicity of human cytokine production: a dynamic disequilibrium in T helper cell type 1/T helper cell type 2 balance? *J Immunol* **158**(11): 5163–5168.

Saeb-Parsy, K., S. Lombardelli, *et al.* (2000) Neural connections of hypothalamic neuroendocrine nuclei in the rat. *J Neuroendocrinol* **12**(7): 635–648.

Schernhammer, E.S., C.H. Kroenke, *et al.* (2006). Night Work and Risk of Breast Cancer. *Epidemiology* **17**(1): 108–111.

Segawa, K., S. Nakazawa, *et al.* (1987) Peptic ulcer is prevalent among shift workers. *Dig Dis Sci* **32**(5): 449–453.

Shakhar, G., I. Bar-Ziv, *et al.* (2001) Diurnal changes in lung tumor clearance and their relation to NK cell cytotoxicity in the blood and spleen. *Int J Cancer* **94**(3): 401–406.

Silver, A.C., A. Arjona, *et al.* (2012) Circadian expression of clock genes in mouse macrophages, dendritic cells, and B cells. *Brain Behav Immun* **26**(3): 407–413.

Smolensky, M.H., F. Halberg, *et al.* (1972). *Chronobiology of the Life Sequence.* Igaku Shoin, Tokyo.

Sun, Y., Z. Yang, *et al.* (2006) MOP3, a component of the molecular clock, regulates the development of B cells. *Immunology* **119**(4): 451–460.

Tuchsen, F., H. Hannerz, *et al.* (2006) A 12 year prospective study of circulatory disease among Danish shift workers. *Occup Environ Med* **63**(7): 451–455.

Wright, K.P., Jr, R. K. Bogan, *et al.* (2013) Shift work and the assessment and management of shift work disorder (SWD). *Sleep Med Rev* **17**(1): 41–54.

Yu, X., D. Rollins, *et al.* (2013) TH17 cell differentiation is regulated by the circadian clock. *Science* **342**(6159): 727–730.

Clocks in the Central Nervous System

Circadian Clock, Reward and Addictive Behavior

15

Urs Albrecht

Dept of Biology, Unit of Biochemistry, University of Fribourg, Fribourg, Switzerland

15.1 Introduction

The aim of this chapter is to highlight relationships between the circadian clock and reward that may influence addictive behavior. To begin, some of the key terms used in this chapter are defined.

The *circadian clock* is a biochemical mechanism that oscillates with a period of about 24 hours and can be coordinated with the day–night cycle. It consists of three major components: (i) a central oscillator with a period of 24 hours that is made up of several clock genes that regulate themselves in an autoregulatory manner allowing them to keep time (Chapters 1 and 2); (ii) a series of input pathways to the central oscillator to allow entrainment of the clock; and (iii) a series of output pathways tied to distinct phases of the oscillator allowing regulation of overt rhythms in biochemistry, physiology and behavior. If biochemical and physiological rhythms are described under the natural light–dark cycle of the environment (in contrast to constant conditions) these rhythms are defined as diurnal and not circadian.

Reward is a stimulus (positive or negative) that increases the intensity and occurrence of an associated behavior when presented more than once. This process is called reinforcement. Primary rewards are those necessary for survival, such as food, water, and sex. Secondary rewards derive their value from the primary rewards and include pleasant touch, music, and money (of which the latter two are probably for humans only). Rewards can be positive or negative. Positive rewards, such as drugs of abuse (e.g., alcohol, cocaine, nicotine), influence the reward system by improving subjective well-being and encourage repetitive drug use that eventually leads to addiction. In contrast, negative rewards, such as hunger or pain, induce searching behavior or avoidance of particular circumstances.

Addiction is the continued use or exposure to mood altering substances or cues despite adverse dependency consequences. This leads to chronic change of the reward system, motivation, memory and related circuitries in the brain, which is reflected in an individual by pursuing reward and/or relief by substance use and other behaviors.

15.2 Evidence for a time of day basis of addictive behavior

Many of the observations described in this section compare day to night and are best considered diurnal rhythms. There is evidence that time of day and addictive behaviors are linked. Drug addicts display disrupted sleep–wake and activity cycles as well as abnormal eating patterns, body temperature and

---

Circadian Medicine, First Edition. Edited by Christopher S. Colwell.

© 2015 John Wiley & Sons, Inc. Published 2015 by John Wiley & Sons, Inc.

hormone rhythms, and abnormal blood pressure (Wasielewski and Holloway, 2001; Jones *et al.*, 2003). These disruptions persist long after drug use and may contribute to relapse (Jones *et al.*, 2003) and it seems that drugs can affect diurnal rhythms. Similarly, it appears that the sensitivity to drugs of abuse is dependent on the time of day. Individuals experiencing a drug overdose are mostly admitted to emergency rooms between 6 and 7 p.m. (Raymond *et al.*, 1992), and cocaine sensitization displays a diurnal rhythm in rodents (Baird and Gauvin, 2000; Abarca *et al.*, 2002; Akhisaroglu *et al.*, 2004). These observations suggest a diurnal component in the body's response to drugs (also described in Chapter 17). A recent study in adult Finnish twins supports this view, because late type individuals (those with a slower clock) are more likely to become nicotine dependent than early type individuals (Broms *et al.*, 2011). Furthermore, people with genetic sleep disorders are more prone to addiction (Shibley *et al.*, 2008) and a rat strain with abnormal circadian rhythms shows increased ethanol preference (Rosenwasser *et al.*, 2005a).

15.3 Drugs, circadian clock genes and addictive behavior

There are various types of rewarding drugs; these can be subdivided into three main classes (Lüscher, 2007): (i) drugs that bind to transporters of biogenic amines; (ii) drugs that bind to ionotropic receptors and ion channels; and (iii) drugs that activate G protein-coupled receptors. Drugs that belong to the family of biogenic amines are cocaine and methamphetamine. Drugs that bind to ionotropic receptors and ion channels are alcohol and nicotine. Drugs that activate G protein-coupled receptors include opioids and cannabinoids. How these drugs affect the circadian clock and how the clock may be involved in the processing of the signals triggered by these drugs is discussed in the following sections.

15.3.1 Cocaine

Evidence for involvement of the circadian clock in the response to drugs of abuse came from studies performed in *Drosophila* (Andretic *et al.*, 1999). This study showed that flies mutant in various clock genes, including *Period* (*Per*), were lacking sensitization to repeated cocaine exposure and tyrosine decarboxylase was not induced as normally seen after cocaine exposure. This indicated that clock genes in the fly may directly or indirectly regulate tyrosine decarboxylase. In mice, similar observations were made. Cocaine modulates pathways for photic and nonphotic entrainment of the mammalian SCN circadian clock (Glass *et al.*, 2012). Mice lacking the *Per1* or the *Per2* gene displayed abnormal locomotor sensitization and conditioned place preference in response to cocaine (Abarca *et al.*, 2002). Expression of these genes was induced by cocaine in the dorsal striatum and the nucleus accumbens (NAc) (Yuferov *et al.*, 2003), brain regions important for cocaine mediated behavioral effects (Fig. 15.1). Interestingly, cocaine differentially affected clock gene expression in various brain regions depending on the treatment schedule (acute or chronic (Uz *et al.*, 2005). Cocaine and other drugs of abuse such as methamphetamine (see below) regulate the reward system via modulation of dopaminergic neurotransmission in the mesolimbic dopaminergic reward circuit, which includes the ventral tegmental area (VTA) and NAc of the striatum (Nestler and Carlezon 2006) (Fig. 15.1).

Interactions between the circadian clock and dopamine have been reported. In the retina, dopamine neurons regulate adaptation to light (Witkovsky, 2004) and mice lacking the dopamine D2 receptor display impaired light masking (Doi *et al.*, 2006). Signaling via the dopamine D2 receptor potentiates circadian transcriptional regulation in the retina (Yujnovsky *et al.*, 2006). Interestingly, retinal dopamine mediates multiple dimensions of light-adapted vision (Jackson *et al.*, 2012), which may indirectly affect the circadian system. This is supported by imaging analysis in *Drosophila* of clock neurons, which revealed that light buffers the wake-promoting effect of dopamine (Shang *et al.*, 2011). Dopamine in turn seems to act through *Cryptochrome* (*Cry*) to promote acute arousal in *Drosophila* (Kumar *et al.*, 2012). In rats, global depletion of dopamine disrupted normal circadian wheel-running patterns accompanied by altered *Per2* expression in the forebrain (Gravotta *et al.*, 2011). The effects of dopamine on PER2 protein in the rat striatum appeared to involve the daily activation of dopamine D2 receptors (Hood *et al.*, 2010). Together, these findings indicate that dopamine influences locomotor activity involving clock genes.

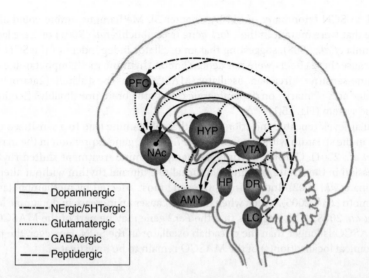

Fig. 15.1 Neural circuitry of addiction and mood. Several brain regions are implicated in the regulation of addiction. Besides the hippocampus (HP) and the prefrontal cortex (PFC), several subcortical structures are involved in reward, fear, and motivation. These include the nucleus accumbens (NAc), amygdala (AMY), and hypothalamus (HYP). The figure shows only a subset of the many known interconnections between these various brain regions. The ventral tegmental area (VTA) provides dopaminergic input to the NAc, AMY, and PFC. DR, Dorsal raphe nuclei; GABA, gamma-aminobutyric acid; LC, locus coeruleus; NE, norepinephrine; 5HT, serotonin.

The relationship between the circadian clock and dopamine signaling is further illustrated by analysis of mice mutant in clock genes. Animals with a point mutation in the gene *Clock* displayed increased excitability of dopamine neurons, and cocaine reward (McClung *et al.*, 2005; Chapter 17). In line with these findings is the observation that the animals showed mania-like behavior that is comparable to that observed in patients with bipolar disorder (Roybal *et al.*, 2007). Furthermore, it appeared that a mutation in *Clock* leads to altered dopamine receptor function (Spencer *et al.*, 2012). Especially, the ratio of D1:D2 receptors seemed to be significantly shifted towards the D2 receptor, which may affect proper synchronization between neurons. However, the mechanism by which *Clock* regulates the dopaminergic system is not understood but may involve systemic hormones, such as insulin, leptin and ghrelin, that are known to link feeding behavior and the reward system (see below). There appears to be a molecular link between the circadian clock mechanism and dopamine metabolism involving the clock proteins BMAL1, NPAS2 and PER2 (Hampp *et al.*, 2008). In mice, these proteins regulated expression levels and activity of monoamine oxidase A (MaoA), an enzyme important in dopamine degradation. PER2 acted as a coactivator of the BMAL1/NPAS2 heterodimer and, thereby, modulated dopamine levels in the mesolimbic dopaminergic system. As a consequence, mood-related behavior was altered, leading to the conclusion that the clock may influence mood. This conclusion is supported by the observation that seasonal affective disorder (SAD) in humans correlated with the frequency of specific single-nucleotide polymorphisms in *BMAL1*, *NPAS2* and *PER2* (Partonen *et al.*, 2007). A study also identified repeat variation in the human *PER2* gene as a genetic marker associated with cocaine addiction and brain dopamine D2 receptor availability (Shumay *et al.*, 2012).

15.3.2 Methamphetamine

Methamphetamine ((2*S*)-*N*-methyl-1-phenylpropane-2-amine) was one of the first drugs to be tested on circadian behavior in rats (Honma *et al.*, 1986). It affected the amount of locomotor activity and the period length of the activity rhythm. These effects persisted in constant darkness but disappeared after withdrawal of methamphetamine. Interestingly, methamphetamine could induce robust activity rhythms in rats that had no SCN (Honma *et al.*, 1987; Chapter 3). Methamphetamine could also induce such rhythms in mice that were mutant in the *Clock* gene (Masubuchi *et al.*, 2001) or were lacking the *Cry1/Cry2* genes (Honma *et al.*, 2008), suggesting that an oscillator independent of the SCN and these clock genes exists. Because these effects were not dependent on rhythmic methamphetamine consumption, a methamphetamine-sensitive circadian oscillator (MASCO) was postulated (Tataroglu *et al.*, 2006). Methamphetamine acts primarily on dopaminergic cells in the brain presumably affecting the mesolimbic dopaminergic system (Fig. 15.1).

At the molecular level, repeated injections of methamphetamine lead to a sensitized increase in *Per1* gene expression in the striatum without affecting *Per1* or *Per2* gene expression in the master clock of the SCN (Nikaido *et al.*, 2001). Chronic daytime methamphetamine treatment shifted rhythmic *Per1* and *Per2* gene expression in the striatum from a nocturnal to a diurnal rhythm without altering the rhythm in the SCN (Iijima *et al.*, 2002). Interestingly, the gene most affected by methamphetamine treatment was *Per2* (Yamamoto *et al.*, 2005), which when mutated causes an increase in dopamine levels in the striatum (Hampp *et al.*, 2008). This suggests that the *Per2* gene may be part of the MASCO, although the period of the MASCO is longer than the circadian oscillator in the SCN. However, the molecular make up and the anatomical localization(s) of the MASCO remain to be investigated.

15.3.3 Alcohol

Chronic alcohol intake in humans is associated with sleep disturbance and alterations in various daily physiological rhythms such as hormone secretion and EEG topography (Imatoh *et al.*, 1986; Fonzi *et al.*, 1994; Brower, 2001). Similarly, in rats chronic ethanol uptake is associated with alterations of clock parameters, such as free-running period and light response (Rosenwasser *et al.*, 2005b), suggesting that the chronobiological disruptions seen in human alcoholics are at least partially caused by ethanol-induced disruption of the circadian system. In support of this notion is the observation that ethanol administration in rats alters the circadian expression patterns of pro-opiomelanocortin (POMC) as well as *Per1* and *Per2* expression in the arcuate nucleus and in the SCN (Chen *et al.*, 2004). Furthermore, a reduced expression of circadian clock genes in male alcoholic patients has been observed (Huang *et al.*, 2010).

Alcohol not only affects clock gene expression but mutations in clock genes alter the response to alcohol. Mice with a mutation in the *Per2* gene displayed an increased ethanol intake (Spanagel *et al.*, 2005). This was associated with a decreased expression of a glutamate-aspartate transporter (*Glast* aka *Eaat1*) on astrocytes, which leads to a reduced efficiency of glutamate clearance from the synaptic cleft. As a consequence, glutamate levels in the striatum were increased (Spanagel *et al.*, 2005), most likely causing the excessive alcohol consumption (Tsai and Coyle, 1998). It has been suggested that the drug acamprosate acts on a hyper-glutamatergic state (Dahchour and De Witte, 2000) and blocks the increase in extracellular dopamine levels in the NAc (Cano-Cebrian *et al.*, 2003), which has also been observed in *Per2* mutant mice (Hampp *et al.*, 2008). Treatment of *Per2* mutant mice with acamprosate normalized their alcohol intake (Spanagel *et al.*, 2005). Acamprosate-responsive brain sites include the major reward (VTA, PPT and NAc) and circadian clock (IGL and SCN) areas of the brain (Brager *et al.*, 2011). However, it is still unclear how acamprosate mechanistically leads to this normalization. One study suggests the involvement of the *Per2* gene in the regulation of beta-endorphin neuronal responses to ethanol (Agapito *et al.*, 2010). Interestingly, *Per1* and *Per3* appear to play a role in stress-induced alcohol drinking. Mice lacking the *Per1* gene showed enhanced alcohol consumption in response to social defeat stress and an association with the frequency of heavy drinking in adolescents; a single nucleotide polymorphism in the human *Per1* gene was found (Dong *et al.*, 2011). In mice a polymorphism in the promoter of the *Per3* gene was associated with alcohol and stress responses (Wang *et al.*, 2012).

15.3.4 Nicotine

The effects of nicotine on the circadian system are not well studied. In rats, nicotine did not suppress the daily physiological rhythms but induced perturbations in daily rhythms of heart rate, body temperature, and locomotor activity (Pelissier *et al.*, 1998). In humans transdermal nicotine affected rhythms in blood pressure and was associated with the impairment of endothelium-dependent vasodilation (Yugar-Toledo *et al.*, 2005). It also appeared that chronotype, which is an attribute of human beings reflecting at what time of the day an individual's physical functions are active, was associated with smoking (Wittmann *et al.*, 2006). Decreased psychological well-being in late chronotypes appeared to be mediated by smoking and alcohol consumption (Wittmann *et al.*, 2010), with ethanol enhancing the effects of nicotine on timing and temporal memory (Meck, 2007). This indicates that social jet lag, that is, the discrepancy between social and biological timing, is probably one reason for smoking. This suggests that misalignment of the circadian clock with the environment encourages nicotine consumption. However, molecular evidence for such a potential mechanism is lacking and warrants further investigation.

15.3.5 Opioids

Opioids are used to treat acute pain after operations and are invaluable in the treatment of chronic pain. Therefore, it is of interest to study their temporal effects on the organism to optimize timing and dose of treatment (Junker and Wirz, 2010; Plante and VanItallie, 2010). Opioids bind to opioid receptors, which are coupled to G proteins, to activate an intracellular signaling cascade. These receptors are principally found in the central nervous system and the gastrointestinal tract.

Opioid receptor activation in rats affected the clock in the hypothalamus, which generates pulsatile growth hormone secretion, shortening the duration of the growth hormone burst (Willoughby and Medvedev, 1996). Daily injections of opiate drugs, such as fentanyl, have been reported to entrain increased locomotor activity around the time of the daily injection in rats (Gillman *et al.*, 2009) and the photic responsiveness of the circadian pacemaker in the hamster was modified, probably by influencing *Per* gene expression and electrical activity in the SCN (Vansteensel *et al.*, 2005). Withdrawal from opiates, a state characterized by profound physiological and motivational deficits, was associated with disturbances in circadian activity, sleep and hormone rhythms (Howe *et al.*, 1980; Stinus *et al.*, 1998; Shi *et al.*, 2007). Furthermore, opiate withdrawal affected transcriptional rhythms of clock genes *Per1* and *Per2* in the rat brain (Li *et al.*, 2009, 2010). Especially, *Per2* expression appeared to be altered in the limbic forebrain of rats after daily morphine injection and withdrawal (Hood *et al.*, 2011). Consistent with this is the observation that mice mutant in the *Per2* gene developed less tolerance and showed attenuated withdrawal signs after morphine treatment, indicating that *Per2* is involved in morphine induced tolerance and withdrawal (Perreau-Lenz *et al.*, 2010). Inhibition of *Per1* affected the response of mice to morphine, but already formed dependence was not affected (Liu *et al.*, 2005). It appeared that morphine-induced reward that affected *Per1* expression involved the ERK signaling pathway (Liu *et al.*, 2007). This signaling pathway also plays a major role in the photic response of the circadian clock (Motzkus *et al.*, 2000; Akashi *et al.*, 2008) indicating that photic signaling and opioid signaling pathways converge on the circadian clock by ERK signaling.

15.3.6 Cannabinoids

Data on the influence of cannabinoids on the circadian system are scarce. In the clinic, delta9-tetrahydrocannabinol (THC) is used to reduce nocturnal motor activity and agitation in severely demented patients (Walther *et al.*, 2006). This indicates that THC may influence the circadian clock. In line with this view is the finding that the cannabinoid type 1 receptor (CB1) was detected in the SCN of the hamster (Sanford *et al.*, 2008). This same study also showed that the period of circadian activity was not altered by application of a CB1 agonist. However, light-induced phase shifts were inhibited, which were reversed upon CB1 antagonist application. These findings were confirmed in mice and extended by showing that cannabinoids were excitatory within the SCN by a mechanism based on presynaptic CB1 attenuation of axonal GABA release (Acuna-Goycolea *et al.*, 2010). Taken together, these studies indicate that the endocannabinoid system may modulate the circadian system, which may explain the experience of time dissociation described by cannabinoid users.

15.4 Links between feeding, addictive behavior and the clock

Evidence has accumulated fostering the view that the consumption of both food and drugs of abuse converge on a shared pathway (Fig. 15.2) that mediates motivated behaviors (Simerly, 2006). Scheduled food or chocolate access entrained daily oscillations of the clock gene *Per1* in structures involved in metabolic homeostasis and reward in the limbic system (Angeles-Castellanos *et al.*, 2008) and this was accompanied by food-anticipatory activity (FAA). The persistence of these oscillations after interruption of the feeding schedule indicated an association of these oscillations with reward, suggesting that this oscillatory process may be part of temporal addictive behavior. Interestingly, FAA persisted in SCN-lesioned animals, demonstrating the existence of an SCN-independent food-entrainable oscillator (FEO) (Stephan *et al.*, 1979). The anatomical substrate of the FEO is still unknown but lesions in areas of the hypothalamus or limbic system have failed to identify a principal site (Mistlberger, 1992; Davidson *et al.*, 2000). This supports the possibility that the anatomical substrate

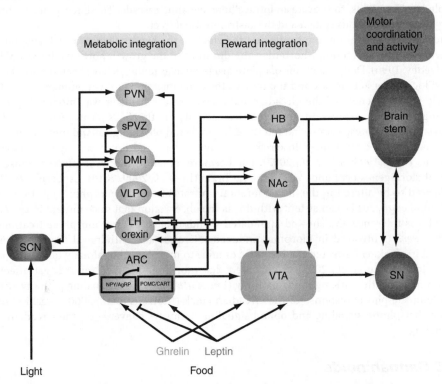

Fig. 15.2 Major neural pathways integrating light and feeding signals in mammals. Light signals are directly transmitted to the SCN. Light information is indirectly transmitted from the SCN (red arrows). The SCN projects to areas important for metabolic integration, including the PVN, sPVZ, DMH and ARC. Feeding signals (leptin and ghrelin) primarily affect two entities in the brain (green arrows): (i) the ARC, which is important for the metabolic integration of feeding signals (yellow), and (ii) the VTA, which is important for the integration of reward (blue). The structures important for metabolic integration (yellow) and reward integration (blue) exchange information with each other (yellow and blue arrows) and can affect the SCN timing center (red). Light and feeding signals combine and contribute to motor coordination and activity (purple). ARC, arcuate nucleus; DMH, dorsomedial hypothalamus; HB, habenula; ipRGC, intrinsically photosensitive retinal ganglion cell; LH, lateral hypothalamus; NAc, nucleus accumbens; Pin, pineal gland; PVN, paraventricular nucleus; SCN, suprachiasmatic nuclei; SN, substantia nigra; sPVZ, subparaventricular zone; VLPO, ventrolateral preoptic nucleus; VTA, ventral tegmental area. *(See insert for color representation of the figure.)*

of the FEO is dispersed in various brain regions or located in peripheral tissues (LeSauter *et al.*, 2009). Interestingly, deletion of various clock genes affected but did not abolish FAA (Dibner *et al.*, 2010), with the exception of a mutation in the *Per2* gene (Feillet *et al.*, 2006; Mendoza *et al.*, 2010). These findings are reminiscent of the results obtained with methamphetamine in search for the MASCO (see above), indicating that the FEO and the MASCO may share common properties, including a role of the *Per2* gene.

Food and drug-seeking behavior appear to be linked via hormones, which regulate not only feeding but also neuronal activity in the mesolimbic dopaminergic pathway. In particular, leptin appeared to reduce the firing rates of dopaminergic neurons (Hommel *et al.*, 2006), indicating that leptin acts on dopamine neurons via leptin receptors in the VTA (Fulton *et al.*, 2006). Leptin-deficient mice showed reduced levels of dopamine in the NAc, and leptin treatment increased the synthesis and activity of tyrosine hydroxylase (Fulton *et al.*, 2006). Interestingly, the amounts of hormones that regulate appetite and circulate in the bloodstream, such as leptin, ghrelin and orexin, are altered in *Clock* mutant mice (Turek *et al.*, 2005). These animals show metabolic syndrome (Turek *et al.*, 2005), altered dopaminergic transmission and cocaine reward (McClung *et al.*, 2005) with mania-like behavior (Roybal *et al.*, 2007). Because feeding regulates the production and/or secretion of these peptide hormones, feeding appears to play a role in the activity state of the reward system.

Several amino acids, including tryptophane, tyrosine, and glutamate, are precursors of neurotransmitters (such as catecholamines) or act as neurotransmitters. In fact, metabolic disturbance of amino acid metabolism leads in most cases to neurological pathologies. Interestingly, amino acids were found to be present in human saliva in a circadian fashion (Dallmann *et al.*, 2012), indicating that synthesis and degradation of amino acids is time-of-day dependent. Degradation of amino acids leads to the production of urea regulated by a process called nitrogen homeostasis. Recent observations indicated circadian clock regulation of nitrogen homeostasis (Jeyaraj *et al.*, 2012). In particular, Klf15, a transcription factor that is involved in the production of key enzymes of the urea cycle, was regulated by circadian clock components. The deletion of *Klf15* leads to altered nitrogen homeostasis and cognitive dysfunction. Hence, amino acid metabolism is at least partially linked via the circadian clock to brain function and, as a consequence, may affect the reward system.

15.5 Treatment of addiction changing the circadian clock

In the previous paragraphs how the circadian clock can affect addictive behavior via various pathways has been discussed. The question arises whether addiction could be, at least partially, treated using agents acting on clock components. Recently, several chemical agents have been identified that can modulate the activity of clock components (Albrecht, 2013). These molecules act mainly on nuclear receptors and kinases involved in the clock mechanism (Fig. 15.3).

A selective inhibitor of casein kinase 1 epsilon (CK1 epsilon) (PF-4800567) minimally affected the period length (Walton *et al.*, 2009) but modulated the sensitivity of mice to psychostimulants and opioids (Bryant *et al.*, 2012). The CK1delta inhibitor PF-670462 lengthened the circadian period accompanied by nuclear retention of the clock protein PER2 (Meng *et al.*, 2010). Injection of this CK1delta inhibitor prevented relapse-like alcohol drinking in mice (Perreau-Lenz *et al.*, 2012). These experiments suggest that CK1 inhibitors may be candidates for the development of drugs to treat addictive behaviors. The kinase GSK3beta may be another entry point to modulate the circadian clock and its effects on addiction. This kinase has been shown to be critical in the NAc core for methamphetamine-induced behavioral sensitization (Xu *et al.*, 2011). PER2 and REV-ERBalpha are both targets of GSK3beta (Iitaka *et al.*, 2005; Yin *et al.*, 2006). Lithium affects GSK3beta and produces strong phase delays in circadian rhythms (Johnsson *et al.*, 1983; Klemfuss, 1992) and impacts on amplitude and period of the molecular circadian clockwork (Li *et al.*, 2012). However, how the clockwork is linked to the drug sensitization mechanism is not understood, although both mechanisms involve GSK3beta.

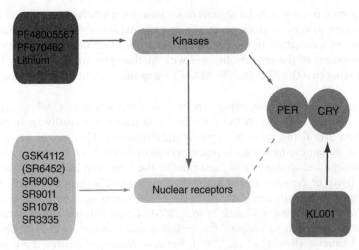

Fig. 15.3 Drugs that affect kinases (center top), nuclear receptors (center bottom), and clock components (right). The dashed line indicates protein interactions between nuclear receptors with PER or CRY proteins, respectively (Schmutz *et al.*, 2010; Lamia *et al.*, 2011).

Nuclear receptors such as those from the families of ROR (NR1F) and REV-ERB (NR1D) have been targets for the search of molecules modulating their action. Heme has been identified as a ligand that may influence the transcriptional potential of REV-ERBs (Yin *et al.*, 2007) and the synthetic agonist GSK4112 (SR6452) competed with heme for binding to REV-ERBs (Grant *et al.*, 2010). These molecules were identified as effective modulators of adipogenesis and indicated an important role of REV-ERBs in metabolic disease (Kumar *et al.*, 2010). Because GSK4112 exhibited poor plasma exposure, novel agonists binding to REV-ERBs with good plasma exposure were identified and tested (Solt *et al.*, 2012). Administration of these two agents (SR9011 and 9009) altered circadian behavior and clock gene expression in the hypothalamus as well as in the liver, skeletal muscle, and adipose tissue of mice. This resulted in a reduction of fat mass in diet-induced obese mice, improving dyslipidemia and hyperglycemia (Solt *et al.*, 2012). For the ROR family of nuclear receptors SR1078 as an agonist (Wang *et al.*, 2012) and SR3335 as an inverse agonist (Kumar *et al.*, 2011) have been identified. Future experiments will show how useful these molecules will be in the treatment of addiction and related behaviors.

A carbazole derivative (KL001) that binds to the clock proteins of the CRY family has been shown to prevent ubiquitin-dependent degradation of CRYs (Hirota *et al.*, 2012). As a consequence CRY was stabilized in the nucleus and glucagon-dependent induction of *Pck1* and *G6pc* genes was repressed, which led to inhibition of glucagon-mediated activation of glucose production. Since CRY proteins are involved in arousal and may affect addictive behavior (see above), KL001 may also be useful in the development of novel drugs for treatment of addiction.

Taken together, it is possible that drugs targeting components of the circadian clock mechanism or modifiers of it may be used to develop novel strategies to treat addictive behaviors. Because the circadian clock can be shifted by light, an additional strategy could be to use light pulses to modulate addictive behavior. However, this possibility has not yet been applied to treat addiction, but appeared to be beneficial to treat certain forms of depression (Chapter 17).

Acknowledgments

I would like to thank Dr J. Ripperger for critically reading the manuscript. Support by the Swiss National Science Foundation, the Velux Foundation, and the State of Fribourg is gratefully acknowledged.

References

Abarca, C., U. Albrecht, *et al.* (2002) Cocaine sensitization and reward are under the influence of circadian genes and rhythm. *Proc Natl Acad Sci USA* **99**(13): 9026–30.

Acuna-Goycolea, C., K. Obrietan, *et al.* (2010) Cannabinoids excite circadian clock neurons. *J Neurosci* **30**(30): 10061–6.

Agapito, M., N. Mian, *et al.* (2010) Period 2 gene deletion abolishes beta-endorphin neuronal response to ethanol. *Alcohol Clin Exp Res* **34**(9): 1613–8.

Akashi, M., Hayasaka, N., *et al.* (2008) Mitogen-activated protein kinase is a functional component of the autonomous circadian system in the suprachiasmatic nucleus. *J Neurosci* **28**(18): 4619–23.

Akhisaroglu, M., R. Ahmed, *et al.* (2004) Diurnal rhythms in cocaine sensitization and in Period1 levels are common across rodent species. *Pharmacol Biochem Behav* **79**(1): 37–42.

Albrecht, U. (2013) Circadian clocks and mood-related behaviors. In: *Circadian Clocks* (eds A. Kramer and M. Merrow), Handbook of Experimental Pharmacology, Vol. **217**. Springer, pp.227–39.

Andretic, R., S. Chaney, *et al.* (1999) Requirement of circadian genes for cocaine sensitization in Drosophila. *Science* **285**(5430): 1066–8.

Angeles-Castellanos, M., R. Salgado-Delgado, *et al.* (2008) Expectancy for food or expectancy for chocolate reveals timing systems for metabolism and reward. *Neuroscience* **155**(1): 297–307.

Baird, T.J. and D. Gauvin (2000) Characterization of cocaine self-administration and pharmacokinetics as a function of time of day in the rat. *Pharmacol Biochem Behav* **65**(2): 289–99.

Brager, A., R.A. Prosser, *et al.* (2011) Acamprosate-responsive brain sites for suppression of ethanol intake and preference. *Am J Physiol Regul Integr Comp Physiol* **301**(4): R1032–43.

Broms, U., J. Kaprio, *et al.* (2011) Evening types are more often current smokers and nicotine-dependent-a study of Finnish adult twins. *Addiction* **106**(1): 170–7.

Brower, K.J. (2001) Alcohol's effects on sleep in alcoholics. *Alcohol Res Health* **25**(2): 110–25.

Bryant, C.D., C.C. Parker, *et al.* (2012) Csnk1e is a genetic regulator of sensitivity to psychostimulants and opioids. *Neuropsychopharmacology* **37**(4): 1026–35.

Cano-Cebrian, M.J., T. Zornoza-Sabina, *et al.* (2003) Acamprosate blocks the increase in dopamine extracellular levels in nucleus accumbens evoked by chemical stimulation of the ventral hippocampus. *Naunyn Schmiedebergs Arch Pharmacol* **368**(4): 324–7.

Chen, C.P., P. Kuhn, *et al.* (2004) Chronic ethanol consumption impairs the circadian rhythm of pro-opiomelanocortin and period genes mRNA expression in the hypothalamus of the male rat. *J Neurochem* **88**(6): 1547–54.

Dahchour, A. and P. De Witte (2000) Ethanol and amino acids in the central nervous system: assessment of the pharmacological actions of acamprosate. *Prog Neurobiol* **60**(4): 343–62.

Dallmann, R., A.U. Viola, *et al.* (2012) The human circadian metabolome. *Proc Natl Acad Sci USA* **109**(7): 2625–9.

Davidson, A.J., S.L. Cappendijk, *et al.* (2000) Feeding-entrained circadian rhythms are attenuated by lesions of the parabrachial region in rats. *Am J Physiol Regul Integr Comp Physiol* **278**(5): R1296–304.

Dibner, C., U. Schibler, *et al.* (2010) The mammalian circadian timing system: organization and coordination of central and peripheral clocks. *Annu Rev Physiol* **72**: 517–49.

Doi, M., I. Yujnovsky, *et al.* (2006) Impaired light masking in dopamine D2 receptor-null mice. *Nat Neurosci* **9**(6): 732–4.

Dong, L., A. Bilbao, *et al.* (2011) Effects of the circadian rhythm gene period 1 (per1) on psychosocial stress-induced alcohol drinking. *Am J Psychiatry* **168**(10): 1090–8.

Feillet, C.A., J.A. Ripperger, *et al.* (2006) Lack of food anticipation in Per2 mutant mice. *Curr Biol* **16**(20): 2016–22.

Fonzi, S., G.P. Solinas, *et al.* (1994) Melatonin and cortisol circadian secretion during ethanol withdrawal in chronic alcoholics. *Chronobiologia* **21**(1-2): 109–12.

Fulton, S., P. Pissios, *et al.* (2006) Leptin regulation of the mesoaccumbens dopamine pathway. *Neuron* **51**(6): 811–22.

Gillman, A.G., J.K. Leffel, 2nd, *et al.* (2009) Fentanyl, but not haloperidol, entrains persisting circadian activity episodes when administered at 24- and 31-h intervals. *Behav Brain Res* **205**(1): 102–14.

Glass, J.D., A.J. Brager, *et al.* (2012) Cocaine modulates pathways for photic and nonphotic entrainment of the mammalian SCN circadian clock. *Am J Physiol Regul Integr Comp Physiol* **302**(6): R740–50.

Grant, D., L. Yin, *et al.* (2010) GSK4112, a small molecule chemical probe for the cell biology of the nuclear heme receptor Rev-erbalpha. *ACS Chem Biol* **5**(10): 925–32.

Gravotta, L., A.M. Gavrila, *et al.* (2011) Global depletion of dopamine using intracerebroventricular 6-hydroxydopamine injection disrupts normal circadian wheel-running patterns and PERIOD2 expression in the rat forebrain. *J Mol Neurosci* **45**(2): 162–71.

Hampp, G., J. A. Ripperger, *et al.* (2008) Regulation of monoamine oxidase a by circadian-clock components implies clock influence on mood. *Curr Biol* **18**(9): 678–83.

Hirota, T., J.W. Lee, *et al.* (2012) Identification of small molecule activators of cryptochrome. *Science* **337**(6098): 1094–7.

Hommel, J.D., R. Trinko, *et al.* (2006) Leptin receptor signaling in midbrain dopamine neurons regulates feeding. *Neuron* **51**(6): 801–10.

Honma, K., S. Honma, *et al.* (1986) Disorganization of the rat activity rhythm by chronic treatment with methamphetamine. *Physiol Behav* **38**(5): 687–95.

Honma, K., S. Honma, *et al.* (1987) Activity rhythms in the circadian domain appear in suprachiasmatic nuclei lesioned rats given methamphetamine. *Physiol Behav* **40**(6): 767–74.

Honma, S., T. Yasuda, *et al.* (2008) Circadian behavioral rhythms in Cry1/Cry2 double-deficient mice induced by methamphetamine. *J Biol Rhythms* **23**(1): 91–4.

Hood, S., P. Cassidy, *et al.* (2010) Endogenous dopamine regulates the rhythm of expression of the clock protein PER2 in the rat dorsal striatum via daily activation of D2 dopamine receptors. *J Neurosci* **30**(42): 14046–58.

Hood, S., P. Cassidy, *et al.* (2011) Daily morphine injection and withdrawal disrupt 24-h wheel running and PERIOD2 expression patterns in the rat limbic forebrain. *Neuroscience* **186**: 65–75.

Howe, R.C., F.W. Hegge, *et al.* (1980) Acute heroin abstinence in man: I. Changes in behavior and sleep. *Drug Alcohol Depend* **5**(5): 341–56.

Huang, M.C., C.W. Ho, *et al.* (2010) Reduced expression of circadian clock genes in male alcoholic patients. *Alcohol Clin Exp Res* **34**(11): 1899–904.

Iijima, M., T. Nikaido, *et al.* (2002) Methamphetamine-induced, suprachiasmatic nucleus-independent circadian rhythms of activity and mPer gene expression in the striatum of the mouse. *Eur J Neurosci* **16**(5): 921–9.

Iitaka, C., K. Miyazaki, *et al.* (2005) A role for glycogen synthase kinase-3beta in the mammalian circadian clock. *J Biol Chem* **280**(33): 29397–402.

Imatoh, N., Y. Nakazawa, *et al.* (1986) Circadian rhythm of REM sleep of chronic alcoholics during alcohol withdrawal. *Drug Alcohol Depend* **18**(1): 77–85.

Jackson, C.R., G.X. Ruan, *et al.* (2012) Retinal dopamine mediates multiple dimensions of light-adapted vision. *J Neurosci* **32**(27): 9359–68.

Jeyaraj, D., F.A. Scheer, *et al.* (2012) Klf15 orchestrates circadian nitrogen homeostasis. *Cell Metab* **15**(3): 311–23.

Johnsson, A., W. Engelmann, *et al.* (1983) Period lengthening of human circadian rhythms by lithium carbonate, a prophylactic for depressive disorders. *Int J Chronobiol* **8**(3): 129–47.

Jones, E.M., D. Knutson, *et al.* (2003) Common problems in patients recovering from chemical dependency. *Am Fam Physician* **68**(10): 1971–8.

Junker, U. and S. Wirz (2010) Review article: chronobiology: influence of circadian rhythms on the therapy of severe pain. *J Oncol Pharm Pract* **16**(2): 81–7.

Klemfuss, H. (1992) Rhythms and the pharmacology of lithium. *Pharmacol Ther* **56**(1): 53–78.

Kumar, N., L.A. Solt, *et al.* (2010) Regulation of adipogenesis by natural and synthetic REV-ERB ligands. *Endocrinology* **151**(7): 3015–25.

Kumar, N., D.J. Kojetin, *et al.* (2011) Identification of SR3335 (ML-176): a synthetic RORalpha selective inverse agonist. *ACS Chem Biol* **6**(3): 218–22.

Kumar, S., D. Chen, *et al.* (2012) Dopamine acts through Cryptochrome to promote acute arousal in Drosophila. *Genes Dev* **26**(11): 1224–34.

Lamia, K.A., S.J. Papp, *et al.* (2011) Cryptochromes mediate rhythmic repression of the glucocorticoid receptor. *Nature* **480**(7378): 552–6.

LeSauter, J., N. Hoque, *et al.* (2009) Stomach ghrelin-secreting cells as food-entrainable circadian clocks. *Proc Natl Acad Sci USA* **106**(32): 13582–7.

Li, J., W.Q. Lu, *et al.* (2012) Lithium impacts on the amplitude and period of the molecular circadian clockwork. *PLoS One* **7**(3): e33292.

Li, S.X., L.J. Liu, *et al.* (2009) Morphine withdrawal produces circadian rhythm alterations of clock genes in mesolimbic brain areas and peripheral blood mononuclear cells in rats. *J Neurochem* **109**(6): 1668–79.

Li, S.X., L.J. Liu, *et al.* (2010) Circadian alteration in neurobiology during protracted opiate withdrawal in rats. *J Neurochem* **115**(2): 353–62.

Liu, Y., Y. Wang, *et al.* (2005) The role of mPer1 in morphine dependence in mice. *Neuroscience* **130**(2): 383–8.

Liu, Y., Y. Wang, *et al.* (2007) The extracellular signal-regulated kinase signaling pathway is involved in the modulation of morphine-induced reward by mPer1. *Neuroscience* **146**(1): 265–71.

Lüscher, C. (2007) Drugs of abuse. *Basic and clinical pharmacology*. In: Basic and Clinical Pharmacology (ed. B.G. Katzung). McGraw Hill, New York, pp. 511–25.

Masubuchi, S., S. Honma, *et al.* (2001) Circadian activity rhythm in methamphetamine-treated Clock mutant mice. *Eur J Neurosci* **14**(7): 1177–80.

McClung, C.A., K. Sidiropoulou, *et al.* (2005) Regulation of dopaminergic transmission and cocaine reward by the Clock gene. *Proc Natl Acad Sci USA* **102**(26): 9377–81.

Meck, W.H. (2007) Acute ethanol potentiates the clock-speed enhancing effects of nicotine on timing and temporal memory. *Alcohol Clin Exp Res* **31**(12): 2106–13.

Mendoza, J., U. Albrecht, *et al.* (2010) Behavioural food anticipation in clock genes deficient mice: confirming old phenotypes, describing new phenotypes. *Genes Brain Behav* **9**(5): 467–77.

Meng, Q.J., E.S. Maywood, *et al.* (2010) Entrainment of disrupted circadian behavior through inhibition of casein kinase 1 (CK1) enzymes. *Proc Natl Acad Sci USA* **107**(34): 15240–5.

Mistlberger, R.E. (1992) Anticipatory activity rhythms under daily schedules of water access in the rat. *J Biol Rhythms* **7**(2): 149–60.

Motzkus, D., E. Maronde, *et al.* (2000) The human PER1 gene is transcriptionally regulated by multiple signaling pathways. *FEBS Lett* **486**(3): 315–9.

Nestler, E.J. and W.A. Carlezon Jr., (2006) The mesolimbic dopamine reward circuit in depression. *Biol Psychiatry* **59**(12): 1151–9.

Nikaido, T., M. Akiyama, *et al.* (2001) Sensitized increase of period gene expression in the mouse caudate/putamen caused by repeated injection of methamphetamine. *Mol Pharmacol* **59**(4): 894–900.

Partonen, T., J. Treutlein, *et al.* (2007) Three circadian clock genes Per2, Arntl, and Npas2 contribute to winter depression. *Ann Med* **39**(3): 229–38.

Pelissier, A.L., M. Gantenbein, *et al.* (1998) Nicotine-induced perturbations on heart rate, body temperature and locomotor activity daily rhythms in rats. *J Pharm Pharmacol* **50**(8): 929–34.

Perreau-Lenz, S., C. Sanchis-Segura, *et al.* (2010) Development of morphine-induced tolerance and withdrawal: involvement of the clock gene mPer2. *Eur Neuropsychopharmacol* **20**(7): 509–17.

Perreau-Lenz, S., V. Vengeliene, *et al.* (2012) Inhibition of the casein-kinase-1-epsilon/delta prevents relapse-like alcohol drinking. *Neuropsychopharmacology* **37**(9): 2121–31.

Plante, G.E. and T.B. VanItallie (2010) Opioids for cancer pain: the challenge of optimizing treatment. *Metabolism* **59**(Suppl 1): S47–52.

Raymond, R.C., M. Warren, *et al.* (1992) Periodicity of presentations of drugs of abuse and overdose in an emergency department. *J Toxicol Clin Toxicol* **30**(3): 467–78.

Rosenwasser, A.M., M.E. Fecteau, *et al.* (2005a) Circadian activity rhythms in selectively bred ethanol-preferring and nonpreferring rats. *Alcohol* **36**(2): 69–81.

Rosenwasser, A.M., M.E. Fecteau, *et al.* (2005b) Effects of ethanol intake and ethanol withdrawal on free-running circadian activity rhythms in rats. *Physiol Behav* **84**(4): 537–42.

Roybal, K., D. Theobold, *et al.* (2007) Mania-like behavior induced by disruption of CLOCK. *Proc Natl Acad Sci USA* **104**(15):6406–11.

Sanford, A.E., E. Castillo, *et al.* (2008) Cannabinoids and hamster circadian activity rhythms. *Brain Res* **1222**: 141–8.

Schmutz, I., J.A. Ripperger, *et al.* (2010) The mammalian clock component PERIOD2 coordinates circadian output by interaction with nuclear receptors. *Genes Dev* **24**(4): 345–57.

Shang, Y., P. Haynes, *et al.* (2011) Imaging analysis of clock neurons reveals light buffers the wake-promoting effect of dopamine. *Nat Neurosci* **14**(7): 889–95.

Shi, J., L.Y. Zhao, *et al.* (2007) Long-term methadone maintenance reduces protracted symptoms of heroin abstinence and cue-induced craving in Chinese heroin abusers. *Pharmacol Biochem Behav* **87**(1): 141–5.

Shibley, H.L., R.J. Malcolm, *et al.* (2008) Adolescents with insomnia and substance abuse: consequences and comorbidities. *J Psychiatr Pract* **14**(3): 146–53.

Shumay, E., J.S. Fowler, *et al.* (2012) Repeat variation in the human PER2 gene as a new genetic marker associated with cocaine addiction and brain dopamine D2 receptor availability. *Transl Psychiatry* **2**: e86.

Simerly, R. (2006) Feeding signals and drugs meet in the midbrain. *Nat Med* **12**(11): 1244–6.

Solt, L.A., Y. Wang, *et al.* (2012) Regulation of circadian behaviour and metabolism by synthetic REV-ERB agonists. *Nature* **485**(7396): 62–8.

Spanagel, R., G. Pendyala, *et al.* (2005) The clock gene Per2 influences the glutamatergic system and modulates alcohol consumption. *Nat Med* **11**(1): 35–42.

Spencer, S., M.I. Torres-Altoro, *et al.* (2012) A mutation in CLOCK leads to altered dopamine receptor function. *J Neurochem* **123**(1): 124–34.

Stephan, F.K., J.M. Swann, *et al.* (1979) Entrainment of circadian rhythms by feeding schedules in rats with suprachiasmatic lesions. *Behav Neural Biol* **25**(4): 545–54.

Stinus, L., C. Robert, *et al.* (1998) Continuous quantitative monitoring of spontaneous opiate withdrawal: locomotor activity and sleep disorders. *Pharmacol Biochem Behav* **59**(1): 83–9.

Tataroglu, O., A.J. Davidson, *et al.* (2006) The methamphetamine-sensitive circadian oscillator (MASCO) in mice. *J Biol Rhythms* **21**(3): 185–94.

Tsai, G. and J.T. Coyle (1998) The role of glutamatergic neurotransmission in the pathophysiology of alcoholism. *Annu Rev Med* **49**: 173–84.

Turek, F.W., C. Joshu, *et al.* (2005) Obesity and metabolic syndrome in circadian Clock mutant mice. *Science* **308**(5724): 1043–5.

Uz, T., R. Ahmed, *et al.* (2005) Effect of fluoxetine and cocaine on the expression of clock genes in the mouse hippocampus and striatum. *Neuroscience* **134**(4): 1309–16.

Vansteensel, M.J., M.C. Magnone, *et al.* (2005) The opioid fentanyl affects light input, electrical activity and Per gene expression in the hamster suprachiasmatic nuclei. *Eur J Neurosci* **21**(11): 2958–66.

Walther, S., R. Mahlberg, *et al.* (2006) Delta-9-tetrahydrocannabinol for nighttime agitation in severe dementia. *Psychopharmacology (Berl)* **185**(4): 524–8.

Walton, K.M., K. Fisher, *et al.* (2009) Selective inhibition of casein kinase 1 epsilon minimally alters circadian clock period. *J Pharmacol Exp Ther* **330**(2): 430–9.

Wang, X., K. Mozhui, *et al.* (2012) A promoter polymorphism in the Per3 gene is associated with alcohol and stress response. *Transl Psychiatry* **2**: e73.

Wasielewski, J.A. and F.A. Holloway (2001) Alcohol's interactions with circadian rhythms. A focus on body temperature. *Alcohol Res Health* **25**(2): 94–100.

Willoughby, J.O. and A. Medvedev (1996) Opioid receptor activation resets the hypothalamic clock generating growth hormone secretory bursts in the rat. *J Endocrinol* **148**(1): 149–55.

Witkovsky, P. (2004) Dopamine and retinal function. *Doc Ophthalmol* **108**(1): 17–40.

Wittmann, M., J. Dinich, *et al.* (2006) Social jetlag: misalignment of biological and social time. *Chronobiol Int* **23**(1-2): 497–509.

Wittmann, M., M. Paulus, *et al.* (2010) Decreased psychological well-being in late 'chronotypes' is mediated by smoking and alcohol consumption. *Subst Use Misuse* **45**(1-2): 15–30.

Xu, C.M., J. Wang, *et al.* (2011) Glycogen synthase kinase 3beta in the nucleus accumbens core is critical for methamphetamine-induced behavioral sensitization. *J Neurochem* **118**(1): 126–39.

Yamamoto, H., K. Imai, *et al.* (2005) Methamphetamine modulation of gene expression in the brain: analysis using customized cDNA microarray system with the mouse homologues of KIAA genes. *Brain Res Mol Brain Res* **137**(1-2): 40–6.

Yin, L., J. Wang, *et al.* (2006) Nuclear receptor Rev-erbalpha is a critical lithium-sensitive component of the circadian clock. *Science* **311**(5763): 1002–5.

Yin, L., N. Wu, *et al.* (2007) Rev-erbalpha, a heme sensor that coordinates metabolic and circadian pathways. *Science* **318**(5857): 1786–9.

Yuferov, V., T. Kroslak, *et al.* (2003) Differential gene expression in the rat caudate putamen after binge cocaine administration: advantage of triplicate microarray analysis. *Synapse* **48**(4): 157–69.

Yugar-Toledo, J.C., S.E. Ferreira-Melo, *et al.* (2005) Blood pressure circadian rhythm and endothelial function in heavy smokers: acute effects of transdermal nicotine. *J Clin Hypertens (Greenwich)* **7**(12): 721–8.

Yujnovsky, I., J. Hirayama, *et al.* (2006) Signaling mediated by the dopamine D2 receptor potentiates circadian regulation by CLOCK:BMAL1. *Proc Natl Acad Sci USA* **103**(16): 6386–91.

How a Disrupted Clock may Cause a Decline in Learning and Memory

16

Christopher S. Colwell

Laboratory of Circadian and Sleep Medicine, Department of Psychiatry and Biobehavioral Sciences, University of California Los Angeles, Los Angeles, CA, USA

16.1 Introduction

The circadian timing system through its regulation of the temporal profile of sleep (Chapter 4) and arousal (Chapter 5) is intimately involved in cognitive processes, including learning and memory (Kyriacou and Hastings, 2010). Many studies have documented daily rhythms in human cognitive performance (Blatter and Cajochen, 2007; Waterhouse, 2010) with obvious consequences for workplace accidents and errors (OTA, 1991). Broadly speaking, you do not want to be performing a delicate surgery or studying for an exam between the hours of 2 and 4 a.m. In an attempt to tease apart the relative roles of sleep and circadian rhythms in cognitive performance, researchers have taken advantage of the fact that human sleep–wake cycle can synchronize to non-24-hour cycle lengths (e.g., 20 or 28 h) that are beyond the range of entrainment of the circadian system. With this type of "forced desynchrony" protocol, the circadian system free-runs (lengthening by 30 min or so per cycle) as the sleep–wake cycle remains fixed to the light–dark (LD) cycle. After two weeks, the circadian and sleep systems should have aligned with all phase relationships and the relative contribution of these two processes can be extracted. These types of studies provide evidence that the circadian system regulates cognitive processes independently of sleep and that sleeping at the "wrong phase" of the circadian cycle will disrupt performance (Dijk and Czeisler, 1995; Wright *et al.*, 2006; Zhou *et al.*, 2011). A discussion of the complicated intersection of circadian phase, sleep inertia, and homeostatic drive as well as the forced desynchrony protocols, can be found elsewhere (Wright *et al.*, 2012).

Since circadian control of sleep and arousal mechanisms have already been discussed, this chapter instead presents evidence that "extra-SCN" (suprachiasmatic nucleus) circadian oscillators are common. Further, it will be shown that these oscillatory processes regulate cellular and molecular components that are known to be important for learning and memory. Finally, it will be argued that disruption of the circadian system has negative consequences on learning and memory. Since additive behavior can also be considered a form of learning, the material presented in Chapter 15 is very relevant for this chapter.

16.2 Molecular clockwork expressed in brain regions central to learning and memory including the hippocampus, amygdala, and cortex

As described in earlier chapters, clock genes including *Per2* are widely expressed in peripheral organs as well as in the nervous system (Abe *et al.*, 2002; Yoo *et al.*, 2004). In mammals, these circadian-related genes are found in brain regions that are critical for learned behaviors, such as the hippocampus

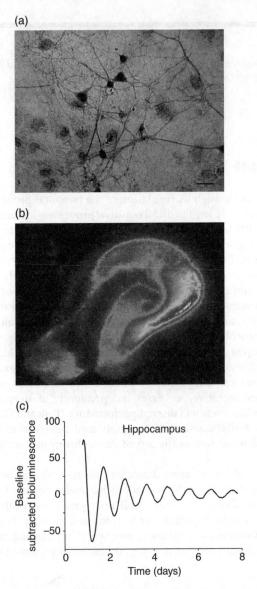

Fig. 16.1 The hippocampus is an "extra-SCN" circadian oscillator. (a) Expression of PER2 measured with immunohistochemical techniques in cultured hippocampal neurons. (b) Bioluminescence recorded from an organotypic hippocampal slice made from a PER2::LUC mouse. (c) The circadian rhythm in bioluminescence recorded from the hippocampal slice. Rhythmicity of bioluminescence damped over a period of several days (Modified from Wang *et al.*, 2009.) *(See insert for color representation of the figure.)*

(Wakamatsu et al., 2001; Lamont et al., 2005; Jilg et al., 2010; Wang et al., 2009; Duncan et al., 2013), the amygdala (Lamont et al., 2005), and the ventral tegmental area (McClung et al., 2005; Hampp et al., 2008) (Fig. 16.1). To provide one example, Amir's group used immunohistochemistry techniques to measure the expression of PER2 in the rat forebrain every 30 minutes throughout the 24-hour LD cycle. Over 18 distinct anatomical regions show significant expression of PER2 including parts of the amygdala, hippocampus, striatum, and cortex. These regions are known to be critical for learned behavior. Phase differences in these protein expression rhythms hint at an underlying temporal structure that can influence learning and memory (Harbour et al., 2013). In humans, it has been possible to document 24-hour diurnal rhythms in clock gene expression in cortical and limbic regions (Li et al., 2013).

This extra-SCN clock gene expression raises the possibility that a variety of brain regions may be able to generate circadian oscillations. It is also possible that "clock genes" like *Per2* may play functional roles as transcriptional regulators independent of circadian function. In this regard, the finding that PER2 expression is rhythmic when the hippocampus is isolated from the SCN in culture is an important observation (Wang et al., 2009; Fig. 16.1). This result demonstrates that the hippocampus is indeed capable of generating independent circadian oscillations. In mammals, neurons in the hippocampus (Wang et al., 2009), olfactory bulb (Abraham et al., 2005), and other brain regions (Abe et al., 2002) have been shown to generate independent oscillations in circadian gene expression. In many ways, the central nervous system is starting to look analogous to the state of affairs with peripheral oscillators as described earlier (Chapters 6–14), in which the central clock in the SCN has the function of synchronizing a network of oscillators found in all of the major organs. These local clocks would control the temporal patterning of biological processes important to the local environment. Thus, cell-autonomous circadian clocks are likely to operate in several regions within the nervous system but the neurons desynchronize in the absence of the SCN (Welsh et al., 2010).

Per2 mRNA and protein in the hippocampus appear to be in anti-phase with their expression in the SCN. Future studies will need to determine how these phase relationships are altered in response to environmental perturbations and disease (Duncan et al., 2013). The hippocampus is one of the brain regions strongly implicated in the pathophysiology of mood disorders (Drevets et al., 2008). The "social zeitgeber theory" of depression postulates that life stresses can produce a misalignment of the phase relationship between the central clock and the environment and that this misalignment could have a negative impact on nervous system function and health (McCarthy and Welsh, 2012; Chapter 17). Interestingly, these extra-SCN circadian rhythms highlight the importance of coupling between circadian oscillators within the nervous system. The fact that both the hippocampus and the SCN have distinct clockwork mechanisms raises the possibility that coupling between cell populations within the nervous system may impact cognitive function (i.e., properly synchronized clocks lead to improved cognitive performance while misaligned clocks result in decreased cognitive performance).

16.3 The circadian clockwork regulates intracellular signaling pathways known to be important to learning and memory

The molecular clockwork regulates the temporal pattern of gene expression and rhythmic changes can be expected in the transcriptome in the hippocampus, cortex, and amygdala. As described in Chapter 1, intracellular signaling pathways like those mediated by Ca^{2+} and cAMP are rhythmic in the SCN (Colwell, 2000; Fukuhara et al., 2004; O'Neill et al., 2008), the retina (McMahon et al., 2014), and pineal (Bustos et al., 2011). These pathways are likely to be rhythmic in other regions of the central nervous system (Table 16.1). In cultured cells, there is evidence that CRY1 can directly inhibit cAMP in response to G protein-coupled receptor activation through a G protein interaction (Zhang et al., 2010). In fact, there is a remarkable overlap in key elements of the signaling pathway thought to be involved with photic regulation of the SCN and those involved in synaptic plasticity, including key roles for NMDA receptor action, Ca^{2+} influx, and phosphorylation of CREB (cAMP response element-binding protein). Perhaps the nervous system only has a few mechanisms available to turn a brief environmental stimulus into

Table 16.1 Cellular/molecular processes involved in learning and memory rhythmically regulated in the hippocampus.

- Electrical activity
- BDNF
- cAMP
- MAPK
- CREB phosphorylation
- Histone modification

long-term changes. In the SCN, these elements are all rhythmically regulated and it is reasonable to hypothesize a similar regulation in other brain regions.

In terms of signaling pathways outside of the SCN, the MAPK (mitogen-activated protein kinase) pathway in the hippocampus provides perhaps the clearest example of a circadian regulated pathway. Previous work indicates that the levels of cAMP and MAPK activity in the hippocampus exhibit circadian oscillations (Eckel-Mahan *et al.*, 2008). The rhythms in the MAPK activation persist in the hippocampus when the mice are held in constant conditions and are lost upon ablation of the SCN (Phan *et al.*, 2011). A novel rhythmic protein (SCOP or suprachiasmatic nucleus circadian oscillatory protein) appears to be responsible for driving the rhythm in MAPK activation (Shimizu *et al.*, 2010). The inducible over-expression of SCOP in the mouse forebrain alters memory for novel objects (Shimizu *et al.*, 2007). These rhythms peak during the time that the nocturnal rodents would normally be sleeping and, thus, the data fit nicely with the suggestion that the consolidation of memory takes place during sleep. Previous work in *Aplysia* also implicates the circadian gating of the MAPK pathway as the mechanistic control point for circadian regulation of sensitization (Lyons, 2011; Michel *et al.*, 2013). Downstream from the MAPK pathway, circadian rhythms in CREB phosphorylation and histone modification have been described in the hippocampus (Rawashdeh *et al.*, 2014). A variety of evidence links the MAPK pathway and CREB and the consolidation of some forms of hippocampus-dependent memory (Kandel, 2012; Abel *et al.*, 2013).

16.4 The circadian system impacts electrical activity and synaptic plasticity

The electrical activity patterns in the brain change dramatically from day to night. Recorded extracellularly with electrodes on the surface of the skull, these changes in activity are picked up as rhythmic EEG patterns that are frequently used to define the sleep state in mammals (Chapter 4). Underlying these rhythmic electrical signals are changes in the temporal patterns of action potentials. In the SCN itself, the molecular clockwork drives rhythms in neural activity (Colwell, 2011). It is possible that clock genes play this type of role outside of the SCN. One of the leading theories on the function of sleep is the "synaptic homeostasis hypothesis", which proposes that sleep is a time in which synaptic strengths are homeostatically adjusted after leaning during the activity cycle (Tononi and Cirelli, 2014). Evidence for this hypothesis comes from sleep-associated changes in AMPA receptor trafficking, pre-synaptic release mechanisms, evoked responses and changes in dendritic spines. Broadly speaking, the contribution of the circadian system in these changes has not been carefully examined. In the hippocampus, *in vivo* electrophysiological studies describe a diurnal rhythm of synaptic excitability in the dentate gyrus of the rat (Barnes *et al.*, 1977; Winson and Abzug, 1978; West and Deadwyler, 1980; Cauller *et al.*, 1985). In addition, *in vivo* recordings from anesthetized rats have also reveal a diurnal rhythm in long-term potentiation (LTP) from hippocampal granule cells (Dana and Martinez, 1984). Finally, two studies report diurnal variations in the incidence and magnitude of LTP in the CA1 region of the rat hippocampus with the largest responses occurring in the day (Harris and Teyler, 1983; Raghavan *et al.*, 1999).

These latter two studies were done with brain slice preparations, demonstrating that the diurnal variation can be studied *in vitro*. In our own work (Chaudhury *et al.*, 2005), LTP was measured by stimulating

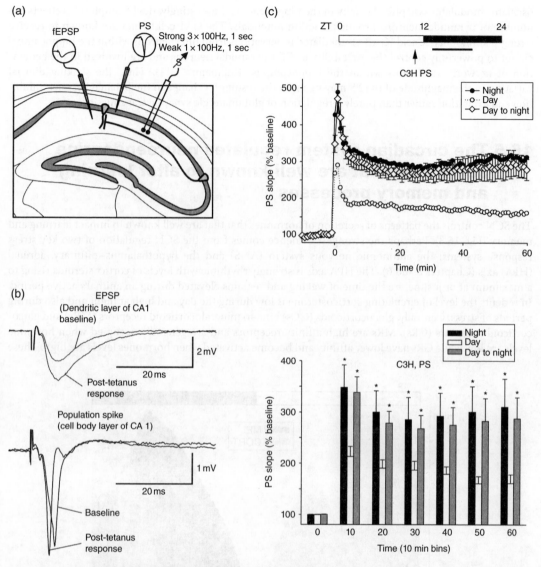

Fig. 16.2 (a) Schematic of the hippocampus illustrating electrode placement for stimulating as well as recording electrodes. (b) examples of fEPSP and fPS before and after tetanus. The increase in the magnitude of the evoked response illustrate what is known as long-term synaptic plasticity. (c) isolated hippocampal slices prepared in the day but recorded during the night exhibited a "night"-like profile. Typically in this study, the slices are prepared and measurements of LTP made in the day or in the night. For the experiments in this section, the tissue was prepared in the day but the recordings were made at night. C3H mice were kept in a LD cycle and killed in the day (1 h prior to lights off at ZT 11) and evoked responses were recorded at night (from ZT 13–18). The PS LTP of slices prepared during the day but recorded during the night had a profile remarkably similar to the night group. The magnitude of LTP was significantly larger in the transition group compared to the day group at all time points. (Modified from Chaudhury et al., 2005.)

the Schaffer collaterals (SC) and recording the field excitatory postsynaptic potential (fEPSP) from the CA1 dendritic layer or the population spike (PS) from the soma in brain slices (Fig. 16.2). The magnitude of the enhancement of the PS was significantly greater in LTP recorded from night slices compared to day slices of both C3H and C57 mice. These rhythms continued when mice were held in constant darkness prior to experimentation. These results provide the first evidence that an endogenous circadian oscillator modulates synaptic plasticity in the hippocampus. Interestingly, the PS amplitude reflects the number of pyramidal neurons producing action potentials. The CA1 cell bodies are known to receive strong γ-aminobutyric acid (GABA)–mediated innervations from interneurons within the hippocampal circuit to powerfully control the excitability of CA1 pyramidal neurons and are involved in the generation of network oscillations within the hippocampus (Kullmann, 2011). Thus, the striking diurnal variation in the magnitude of the PS may be more the result of a change in the balance between inhibition and excitation rather than purely a regulation of glutamatergic synaptic transmission.

16.5 The circadian system regulates neuroendocrine secretions that are well known to alter learning and memory processes

The SCN controls the patterns of secretion of hormones that that are well known to impact learning and memory (Fig. 16.3). Perhaps the strongest evidence comes from the SCN regulation of two key stress response systems: the autonomic nervous system (ANS) and the hypothalamus–pituitary–adrenal (HPA) axis (Chapters 3 and 6). The HPA axis is strongly rhythmic with levels of corticosteroids rising to a maximum at or just before the time of waking and remains elevated during an animal's active period. In rodents the level of circulating corticosterone is low during the day and high at night and also during periods of stress. Centrally, glucocorticoids (GCs) bind to mineralocorticoid receptors (MRs) and glucocorticoid receptors (GRs). MRs are high affinity receptors and are generally occupied when hormone levels are low while GRs have lower affinity and become activated when hormones levels are high. These

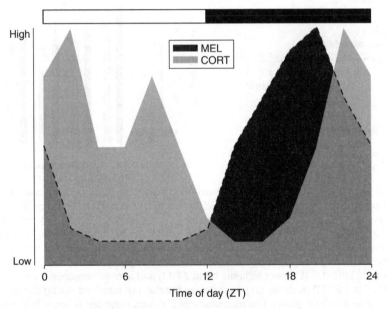

Fig. 16.3 The SCN controls the patterns of secretion of hormones that are well known to impact learning and memory. The HPA axis is strongly rhythmic with levels of corticosteroids (light green) rising to a maximum at or just before the time of waking and remains elevated during an animal's active period. Melatonin is another rhythmically secreted hormone that has been suggested to regulate learning functions. The SCN drives a daily rhythm in melatonin (dark green) secretion such that its levels are high during the night and low during the day. Both glucocorticoid and melatonin receptors are highly expressed in brain regions important for learned behavior and both hormones are known to impact learning and memory in a variety of species. For human data see Dijk *et al.*, 2012.

receptors are well known transcriptional regulators but also exert rapid membrane effects. Both receptors are localized in brain regions centrally involved in learning and memory, including the hippocampus, amygdala and prefrontal cortex. Many studies have documented the impact of GCs on learning and memory processes in both humans and animals (Luksys and Sandi, 2011; Roozendaal and McGaugh, 2011; McEwen and Morrison, 2013). In general, some levels of GC facilitate consolidation of memory while high levels interfere with the same processes. The mechanisms underlying these hormonally driven changes in learning and memory are not fully known but recent work stresses the impact of this hormone on pre-synaptic release of glutamate and AMPA receptor trafficking (Krugers *et al.*, 2010; Treccani *et al.*, 2014). GCs are a major regulator of the phase of the molecular clock in the liver (Chapter 6) and there is some evidence that GCs may play a similar role in the central nervous system (Segall and Amir, 2010). Thus, the possibility has to be considered that the rhythms in learning and memory that are so widely observed could be driven by rhythms in the levels of the adrenal stress hormones.

Melatonin is another rhythmically secreted hormone that has been suggested to regulate learning functions (Fig. 16.3). The circadian regulation of pineal gland secretion of melatonin is one of the best understood output pathways (Moore, 1996). In mammals, the pineal gland is not directly light sensitive but is photically regulated through a complicated neuronal pathway involving the SCN (Chapter 3). The SCN drives a daily rhythm in melatonin secretion such that its levels are high during the night and low during the day. Melatonin receptors are present in the hippocampus, subiculum and entorhinal cortex (Weaver *et al.*, 1989; Siuciak *et al.*, 1990; Adamah-Biassi *et al.*, 2014). Furthermore, several groups have found that melatonin can block the induction of LTP in the CA1 region of rat hippocampal slices (Collins and Davies, 1997; Wang *et al.*, 2005; Ozcan *et al.*, 2006; Takahashi and Okada, 2011). These observations suggest that the physiological rhythm of melatonin secretion may be responsible for daily rhythms in the induction of LTP and, consequently, learning. In one study, fear conditioning was compared between the C3H strain that secrete melatonin rhythmically and the C57 strain that does not (Chaudhury and Colwell, 2002). The strains performed very similarly on the measurements of recall and extinction. The only observable difference between the two strains of mice was found during acquisition (learning). Another study manipulated the duration of melatonin exposure by controlling the photoperiod or by melatonin implants and found that long duration melatonin signal impaired both Schaffer collateral LTP in the CA1 region of the hippocampus and spatial learning and memory (Walton *et al.*, 2013). To put it another way, high melatonin levels during the night could serve to regulate learning mechanisms and, thus, be partially responsible for rhythms in learned behavior. Evidence for this role of melatonin has also been found in Zebrafish (Rawashdeh *et al.*, 2007; Rawashdeh and Maronde, 2012). It is worth pointing out that melatonin, through activation of G(i)-coupled receptors, is a potent inhibitor of adenylyl cyclase. Maintenance of cAMP signals within an optimal range for memory (Pineda *et al.*, 2004) may well be part of the normal function of melatonin. While the pathways linking the SCN with neuroanatomical regions that underlie learning are not known, rhythmically driven hormones are likely candidates.

16.6 Disruptions of the circadian timing system alter learned behavior

Three lines of evidence link disruptions of circadian timing system with deficits in learning and memory. One obvious strategy to study the role of the circadian timing system is to lesion the master clock in the SCN. Early work established that without their SCN animals lose their rhythms in locomotor activity, body temperature, and secretion of corticosterone. The impact of SCN ablation on learning and memory has been inconsistent and perhaps varies with the particular learned task. Several studies have demonstrated that performance on learning tasks is optimal at 24-hour intervals from the time of training and is significantly worse at noncircadian intervals (Fig.16.4) (Holloway and Wansely, 1973; Chaudhury and Colwell, 2002; Cain *et al.*, 2004) and that SCN lesions interfere with the expression of this type of rhythm in recall (Stephan and Kovacevic, 1978). More recently, ablation of the SCN was shown to result in significant impairments in the acquisition of a sustained attention task in rats (Gritton *et al.*, 2013).

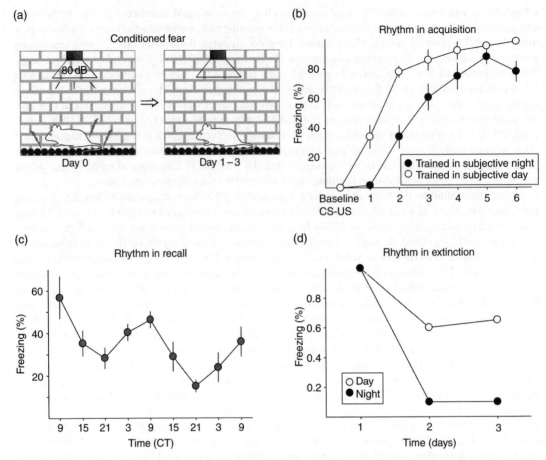

Fig. 16.4 Contextual or trace fear conditioning has been used to explore the circadian regulation of learning and memory. (a) Briefly, on the day of training (denoted as Day 0), mice were placed individually into cages and allowed to acclimatize to the new environment (conditioned stimulus; CS), after which time animals received a footshock (unconditioned stimulus; US). On the day of testing (Day 1 to 3), mice were placed individually into the same conditioning chamber. Experiments are carried out in normal light–dark cycle (LD), reverse light–dark cycle (DL) and constant darkness (DD). (b) Rhythms in acquisition in C-3H mice. Animals were trained either in the day (CT 3) or the night (CT 15). Percentage freezing following each tone-shock pairing in animals trained in the day was compared with percentage freezing following the equivalent tone-shock pairing in animals trained at night. Animals trained in the day acquired the conditioning better then mice trained at night. (c) Rhythms in recall in C-3H mice trained in the day (CT 3). In all experiments animals were first tested for context 24-hours post-training then repeatedly tested every 6 hours, for 3 days. Mice were maintained in DD. (d) Rhythms in long-term extinction for context. The degree of extinction in animals repeatedly tested at CT 3 or CT 15 was measured. (Modified from Chaudhury and Colwell, 2002.)

In contrast, the role of the SCN in time-place learning, in which the time of day is used as a discriminatory cue, is much less direct. Mammals can "time stamp" a memory without the SCN (Mistlberger *et al.*, 1996; Ko *et al.*, 2003).

Ralph and colleagues have come to the conclusion that neural representation of the time of day (time memory) in hamsters involves the setting of a 24-hour oscillator that is functionally and anatomically distinct from the SCN (Cain *et al.*, 2012; Ralph *et al.*, 2013). The SCN plays a role in synchronizing this undefined oscillator. Given the distributed nature of the circadian system as described throughout this book, the hypothesis that extra-SCN circadian oscillators may drive rhythms in learning and memory is appealing. In this regard, interpretation of the SCN lesion experiments has to consider evidence that

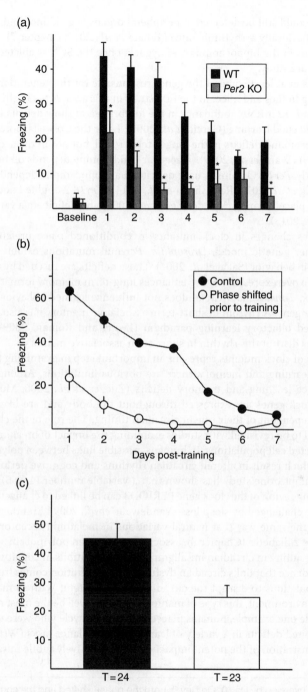

Fig. 16.5 Several types of evidence link circadian disruption with a decline in learning and memory. (a) Genetic mutations of circadian system can cause memory deficits. Levels of trace-fear conditioning recall in *Per2*-mutant mice tested at 24-h intervals post-training during the day (ZT 6) show severe deficits in their ability to recall learning. This same line of mice did not show deficits in conditioned fear when tone was used as the CS (data not shown) demonstrating that the deficits are selective to certain learned behaviors. (Modified from Wang *et al.*, 2009). (b) Environmental perturbation of the circadian system can cause memory deficits. In this experiment, adult male mice were entrained to a 12:12 LD cycle for at least 2 weeks. One group (open circles) was subjected to a 12-h extension of the dark phase on Day −1 to cause a phase

circadian oscillations could still be detected in peripheral organs (e.g., kidney and liver) in about half of the SCN-lesioned, behaviorally arrhythmic mice (Tahara *et al.*, 2012; Chapter 7). It is not known what happens to the rhythms in the hippocampus or amygdala once the SCN is ablated and this remains an important area for future study.

Secondly, mutations in at least some of the genes responsible for the generation of circadian oscillations can alter learning in flies and mice. In the first study in this area, *Npas2* deficient mice were found to lose their rhythm in *Per2* mRNA abundance in the forebrain and show deficits in long-term memory for both contextual and cued learning (Garcia *et al.*, 2000). Later the Colwell laboratory found that *Per2*-mutant mice exhibit profound deficits in the longer-term recall, but not in the acquisition, of trace fear conditioning (Fig. 16.5) (Wang *et al.*, 2009). Trace fear conditioning depends on both the hippocampus and amygdala. Similarly, *Per1* KO animals have deficits in a hippocampus-dependent long-term spatial learning paradigm (Jilg *et al.*, 2010; Rawashdeh *et al.*, 2014). *Cry1&2* double knock out mice show the loss of circadian time-place learning (Van der Zee *et al.*, 2008) and deficits in a variety of other learning tasks (De Bundel *et al.*, 2013).

Work that describes changes in clock mutants in conditioned place preference is described in Chapter 15. In another genetic model, *Drosophila*, *Per*-null mutations exhibit disrupted long-term memory for a courtship behavior (Sakai *et al.*, 2004). These deficits are rescued by the induction of a *Per* transgene, whereas the overexpression of *Per* enhances long-term memory formation. The loss of other circadian genes (*Clock*, *Timeless*, and *Cycle*) does not influence learned behavior in flies, suggesting a special role for the *Per* gene. A rhythm in short-term associative memory has also been described using a negatively reinforced olfactory learning paradigm (Lyons and Roman, 2009). Mutations in both *Timeless* and *Per* genes disrupt this rhythm in short-term associative memory.

While these studies of clock mutants represent an important step in examining the links between circadian rhythms and learning and memory, there are obvious limitations. Among other issues, not all clock mutants produce learning and memory deficits (Zueger *et al.*, 2006; Mulder *et al.*, 2013). In addition, circadian clock genes are expressed throughout the body and are likely to have regulatory functions that are independent of their role in circadian timing. The role of the clock genes in learning and memory will need to be revisited with studies examining the impact of breaking the molecular clock in anatomically restricted cell populations. In humans, possible links between polymorphisms in the circadian clock genes, which result in altered circadian rhythms and cognitive performance, appear to be understudied. For example, one study has shown that a variable number (4 or 5) tandem-repeat polymorphism in the coding region of the clock gene PERIOD3 can be linked to changes in executive function when the subjects are challenged by sleep loss (Vandewalle *et al.*, 2009). Still there has not been much work in this area. In the same way that natural variations in melatonin receptors are associated with increased risk for type 2 diabetes (Chapter 8), associations between polymorphisms might be expected in core clock genes, resulting in circadian misalignment and alterations in cognitive performance.

The third set of evidence that links circadian dysfunction to cognition comes from experiments using environmental manipulations to disrupt the circadian timing system. With so many people living in a temporally unstable environment, this type of manipulation may well be the most relevant to the general population. To provide one example, humans placed on a 24.6 T-cycle who were unable to synchronize to this LD cycle exhibited deficits in a variety of learning and vigilance tasks (Wright *et al.*, 2006). This provides a nice demonstration of the potent impact of even a relatively subtle misalignment in humans.

Fig. 16.5 (*continued*) inversion by Day 0. On Day 0, both the phase shifted and the control group (dark circles) were trained at ZT 3. 24 h after training, both groups of mice were returned to the same context for testing of the recall in once a day. Acquisition of the conditioned fear behavior was not altered by the phase shift. Freezing in response to CS-US 1 and CS-US 2 was not different between the control and phase shifted groups. Recall of the conditioned fear was dramatically reduced by the phase shift. (Data from Loh *et al.*, 2010.) (c) Placing organisms on different cycle lengths can also disturb learning and memory. In previous work, humans placed on a 24.6 T-cycle who were unable to synchronize to this LD cycle exhibited deficits in a variety of learning and vigilance tasks (Wright *et al.*, 2006). Mice held on T = 23 LD showed reduced acquisition of trace fear conditioning. (Data courtesy of Dr L. Wang.)

Similarly, fear conditioning after training for wild-type (WT) mice was notably lower when the mice were held on the T = 23 LD cycle (Wang *et al.*, 2009). In another example of this type of study (Karatsoreos *et al.*, 2011), housing mice in 20-hour LD cycles was used to chronically disrupt the circadian system. Just holding mice on this short T-cycle, caused a decrease in dendritic length and decreased complexity of neurons in the prefrontal cortex as well as caused performance decrease in cognitive tasks.

In addition to the chronic disruption caused by T-cycle experiments, several studies have demonstrated that desynchronizing the circadian system by phase shifting the LD cycle impairs retention of learned behaviors (Tapp and Holloway, 1981; Fekete *et al.*, 1985; Devan *et al.*, 2001; Loh *et al.*, 2010). Of course, most of us are familiar with the impact of these rapid changes in the LD cycle; it is called "jet lag." In the later study (Loh *et al.*, 2010), Loh and colleagues found that the jet lag did not alter baseline levels of corticosterone nor did it result in overall sleep deprivation. One piece of good news for those frequent travelers is that prior experience of jet lag helps to compensate for the reduced recall due to acute phase shifts. In addition, exposing a diurnal rodent (Nile grass rat) to light at night was sufficient to both reduce dendritic length in DG and basilar CA1 neurons but also to impaired learning and memory in the Barnes maze (Fonken *et al.*, 2012). Finally, there has been some really interesting work in Siberian hamsters by Rudy and Heller (Ruby *et al.*, 2008; 2013). This group has developed a single light treatment that disrupts circadian rhythms in behavior. This noninvasive treatment causes the loss of performance in a novel object recognition task. Sleep manipulations had no effect on the performance of this task; however, the GABA antagonist pentylenetetrazol restored learning without restoring circadian rhythms. SCN ablation also completely rescues memory deficits in this model (Fernandez *et al.*, 2014). The authors speculate that the circadian influence on learning may be exerted via cyclic GABA output from the SCN to target sites involved in learning. Overall, this data suggests that a synchronized circadian system may be broadly important for normal cognition and that the consolidation of memories may be particularly sensitive to disruptions of circadian timing.

16.7 Conclusions

The circadian timing system has intimate relationship with cognitive processes including learning and memory. Some of this regulation is the result of control over temporal processes of sleep and arousal as described in previous chapters. The circadian system also regulates cellular and molecular processes critical to the mechanisms underlying learned behavior. Certainly, disruptions of the circadian system produce decline in learning and memory functions. Therefore, in patient groups whose symptoms include cognitive decline, careful attention should be paid to environmental factors, such as light and scheduled sleep, activity, and meals, that can improve or cause deterioration of circadian timing.

References

Abe M, Herzog ED, Yamazaki S, *et al.* 2002. Circadian rhythms in isolated brain regions. *J Neurosci* **22**:350–356.

Abel T, Havekes R, Saletin JM, Walker MP. 2013. Sleep, plasticity and memory from molecules to whole-brain networks. *Curr Biol* **23**(17):R774–788.

Abraham U, Prior JL, Granados-Fuentes D, *et al.* 2005. Independent circadian oscillations of Period1 in specific brain areas in vivo and in vitro. *J Neurosci* **25**:8620–8626.

Adamah-Biassi EB, Zhang Y, Jung H, *et al.* 2014. Distribution of MT1 melatonin receptor promoter-driven RFP expression in the brains of BAC C3H/HeN transgenic mice. *J Histochem Cytochem* **62**(1):70–84.

Barnes CA, McNaughton, BL, Goddard GV, *et al.* 1977. Circadian rhythm of synaptic excitability in rat and monkeys CNS. *Science* **197**:91–92

Blatter K, Cajochen C. 2007. Circadian rhythms in cognitive performance: methodological constraints, protocols, theoretical underpinnings. *Physiol Behav* **90**(2–3):196–208.

Bustos DM, Bailey MJ, Sugden D, *et al.* 2011. Global daily dynamics of the pineal transcriptome. *Cell Tissue Res* **344**(1):1–11.

Cain SW, Chalmers JA, Ralph MR. 2012. Circadian modulation of passive avoidance is not eliminated in arrhythmic hamsters with suprachiasmatic nucleus lesions. *Behav Brain Res* **230**(1):288–290.

Cain SW, Chou T, Ralph MR. 2004. Circadian modulation of performance on an aversion-based place learning task in hamsters. *Behav Brain Res* **150**:201–205.

Cauller LJ, Boulos Z, Goddard GV. 1985. Circadian rhythms in hippocampal responsiveness to perforant path stimulation and their relation to behavioral state. *Brain Res* **329**(1–2):117–130.

Chaudhury D, Colwell CS. 2002. Circadian modulation of learning and memory in fear-conditioned mice. *Behavioral Brain Res* **133**:95–108.

Chaudhury D, Wang LM, Colwell CS. 2005. Circadian regulation of hippocampal long-term potentiation. *J Biol Rhythms* **20**(3):225–236.

Collins DR, Davies SN. 1997. Melatonin blocks the induction of long-term poteniation in an NMDA independent manner. *Brain Res* **767**:162–165.

Colwell CS. 2000. Circadian modulation of calcium levels in cells in the suprachiasmatic nucleus. *Eur J Neurosci* **12**(2):571–576.

Colwell CS. 2011. Linking neural activity and molecular oscillations in the SCN. *Nat Rev Neurosci* **12**(10):553–569.

Dana RC, Martinez JL. 1984. Effect of adrenalectomy on the circadian rhythm of LTP. *Brain Res* **308**(2):392–395.

De Bundel D, Gangarossa G, Biever A, *et al.* 2013. Cognitive dysfunction, elevated anxiety, and reduced cocaine response in circadian clock-deficient cryptochrome knockout mice. *Front Behav Neurosci* **7**:152.

Devan BD, Goad EH, Petri HL, *et al.* 2001. Circadian phase-shifted rats show normal acquisition but impaired long-term retention of place information in the water task. *Neurobiol Learn Mem* **75**:51–62.

Dijk DJ, Czeisler CA. 1995. Contribution of the circadian pace-maker and the sleep homeostat to sleep propensity, sleep structure, electroencephalographic slow waves, and sleep spindle activity in humans. *J Neurosci* **15**:3526–3538.

Dijk DJ, Duffy JF, Silva EJ, *et al.* 2012. Amplitude reduction and phase shifts of melatonin, cortisol and other circadian rhythms after a gradual advance of sleep and light exposure in humans. *PLoS One* **7**(2):e30037.

Drevets WC, Price JL, Furey ML. 2008. Brain structural and functional abnormalities in mood disorders: implications for neurocircuitry models of depression. *Brain Struct Funct* **213**:93–118.

Duncan MJ, Prochot JR, Cook DH, *et al.* 2013. Influence of aging on Bmal1 and Per2 expression in extra-SCN oscillators in hamster brain. *Brain Res* **1491**:44–53.

Eckel-Mahan KL, Phan T, Han S, *et al.* 2008. Circadian oscillation of hippocampal MAPK activity and cAMP: implications for memory persistence. *Nat Neurosci* **11**(9):1074–1082.

Fekete M, van Ree JM, Niesink RJ, de Wied D. 1985. Disrupting circadian rhythms in rats induces retrograde amnesia. *Physiol Behav* **34**:883–887.

Fernandez F, Lu D, Ha P, *et al.* 2014. Circadian rhythm. Dysrhythmia in the suprachiasmatic nucleus inhibits memory processing. *Science* **346**(6211):854–7.

Fonken LK, Kitsmiller E, Smale L, Nelson RJ. 2012. Dim nighttime light impairs cognition and provokes depressive-like responses in a diurnal rodent. *J Biol Rhythms* **27**(4):319–327.

Fukuhara C, Liu C, Ivanova TN, *et al.* 2004. Rhythmic expression of the gene encoding adenylyl cyclase 1 (Adcy1) in the SCN and retina. *J Neurosci* **24**:1803.

Garcia JA, Zhang D, Estill SJ, *et al.* 2000. Impaired cued and contextual memory in NPAS2-deficient mice. *Science* **88**:2226–2230.

Gritton HJ, Stasiak AM, Sarter M, Lee TM. 2013. Cognitive performance as a zeitgeber: cognitive oscillators and cholinergic modulation of the SCN entrain circadian rhythms. *PLoS One* **8**(2):e56206.

Hampp G, Ripperger JA, Houben T, *et al.* 2008. Regulation of monoamine oxidase A by circadian-clock components implies clock influence on mood. *Curr Biol* **18**:678–683.

Harbour VL, Weigl Y, Robinson B, Amir S. 2013. Comprehensive mapping of regional expression of the clock protein PERIOD2 in rat forebrain across the 24-h day. *PLoS One* **8**(10):e76391

Harris KM, Teyler TJ. 1983. Age differences in a circadian influence on hippocampal LTP. *Brain Res* **261**: 69–73.

Holloway FA, Wansley R. 1973. Multiphasic retention deficits at periodic intervals after passive-avoidance learning. *Science* **180**(4082):208–10.

Jilg A, Lesny S, Peruzki N, *et al.* 2010. Temporal dynamics of mouse hippocampal clock gene expression support memory processing. *Hippocampus* **20**(3):377–388.

Kandel ER. 2012. The molecular biology of memory: cAMP, PKA, CRE, CREB-1, CREB-2, and CPEB. *Mol Brain* **5**:14.

Karatsoreos IN, Bhagat S, Bloss EB, *et al.* 2011. Disruption of circadian clocks has ramifications for metabolism, brain, and behavior. *Proc Natl Acad Sci USA* **108**(4):1657–1662.

Ko CH, McDonald RJ, Ralph MR. 2003. The suprachiasmatic nucleus is not required for temporal gating of performance on reward-based learning and memory task. *Biol Rhythm Res* **34**:177–192.

Krugers HJ, Hoogenraad CC, Groc L. 2010. Stress hormones and AMPA receptor trafficking in synaptic plasticity and memory. *Nat Rev Neurosci* **11**(10):675–681.

Kullmann DM. 2011. Interneuron networks in the hippocampus. *Curr Opin Neurobiol* **21**(5):709–716.

Kyriacou CP, Hastings MH. 2010. Circadian clocks: genes, sleep, and cognition. *Trends Cogn Sci* **14**(6):259–267.

Lamont EW, Robinson B, Stewart J, Amir S. 2005. The central and basolateral nuclei of the amygdala exhibit opposite diurnal rhythms of expression of the clock protein Period2. *Proc Natl Acad Sci USA* **102**:4180–4184.

Li JZ, Bunney BG, Meng F, et al. 2013. Circadian patterns of gene expression in the human brain and disruption in major depressive disorder. *Proc Natl Acad Sci USA* **110**:9950–9955.

Loh DH, Navarro J, Hagopian A, et al. 2010. Rapid changes in the light/dark cycle disrupt memory of conditioned fear in mice. *PLoS One* **5**(9):e12546.

Luksys G, Sandi C. 2011. Neural mechanisms and computations underlying stress effects on learning and memory. *Curr Opin Neurobiol* **21**(3):502–508.

Lyons LC. 2011. Critical role of the circadian clock in memory formation: lessons from Aplysia. *Front Mol Neurosci* **4**:52.

Lyons LC, Roman G. 2009. Circadian modulation of short-term memory in Drosophila. *Learn Mem* **16**:19–27.

McCarthy MJ, Welsh DK. 2012. Cellular circadian clocks in mood disorders. *J Biol Rhythms* **27**(5):339–352.

McClung CA, Sidiropoulou K, Vitaterna M, et al. 2005. Regulation of dopaminergic transmission and cocaine reward by the Clock gene. *Proc Natl Acad Sci USA* **102**:9377–9381.

McEwen BS, Morrison JH. 2013. The brain on stress: vulnerability and plasticity of the prefrontal cortex over the life course. *Neuron* **79**(1):16–29.

McMahon DG, Iuvone PM, Tosini G. 2014. Circadian organization of the mammalian retina: from gene regulation to physiology and diseases. *Prog Retin Eye Res* **39**:58–76.

Michel M, Gardner JS, Green CL, et al. 2013. Protein phosphatase-dependent circadian regulation of intermediate-term associative memory. *J Neurosci* **33**(10):4605–4613.

Mistlberger RE, de Groot MHM, Bossert JM, Marchant EG. 1996. Discrimination of circadian phase in intact and suprachiasmatic nuclei-ablated rats. *Brain Res* **739**:12–18.

Moore RY. 1996. Neural control of the pineal gland. *Behav Brain Res* **73**(1–2):125–130.

Mulder C, Van Der Zee EA, Hut RA, Gerkema MP. 2013. Time-place learning and memory persist in mice lacking functional Per1 and Per2 clock genes. *J Biol Rhythms* **28**(6):367–379.

O'Neill JS, Maywood ES, Chesham JE, et al. 2008. cAMP-dependent signaling as a core component of the mammalian circadian pacemaker. *Science* **320**(5878):949–953.

Ozcan M, Yilmaz B, Carpenter DO. 2006. Effects of melatonin on synaptic transmission and long-term potentiation in two areas of mouse hippocampus. *Brain Res* **1111**(1):90–94.

Phan TX, Chan GC, Sindreu CB, et al. 2011. The diurnal oscillation of MAP (mitogen-activated protein) kinase and adenylyl cyclase activities in the hippocampus depends on the suprachiasmatic nucleus. *J Neurosci* **31**(29):10640–10647.

Pineda VV, Athos JI, Wang H, et al. 2004. Removal of G(ialpha1) constraints on adenylyl cyclase in the hippocampus enhances LTP and impairs memory formation. *Neuron* **41**(1):153–163.

Raghavan AV, Horowitz JM, Fuller CA. 1999. Diurnal modulation of long-term potentiation in the hamster hippocampal slice. *Brain Res* **833**:311–314.

Ralph MR, Sam K, Rawashdeh OA, et al. 2013. Memory for time of day (time memory) is encoded by a circadian oscillator and is distinct from other context memories. *Chronobiol Int* **30**(4):540–547.

Rawashdeh O, Maronde E. 2012. The hormonal Zeitgeber melatonin: role as a circadian modulator in memory processing. *Front Mol Neurosci* **5**:27.

Rawashdeh O, de Borsetti NH, Roman G, Cahill GM. 2007. Melatonin suppresses nighttime memory formation in zebrafish. *Science* **318**:1144–1146.

Rawashdeh O, Jilg A, Jedlicka P, et al. 2014. PERIOD1 coordinates hippocampal rhythms and memory processing with daytime. *Hippocampus* **24**(6):712–723.

Roozendaal B, McGaugh JL. 2011. Memory modulation. *Behav Neurosci* **125**(6):797–824.

Ruby NF, Hwang CE, Wessells C, et al. 2008. Hippocampal-dependent learning requires a functional circadian system. *Proc Natl Acad Sci USA* **105**(40):15593–15598.

Ruby NF, Fernandez F, Garrett A, et al. 2013. Spatial memory and long-term object recognition are impaired by circadian arrhythmia and restored by the GABA$_A$ antagonist pentylenetetrazole. *PLoS One* **8**(8):e72433.

Sakai T, Tamura T, Kitamoto T, Kidokoro Y. 2004. A clock gene, *period*, plays a key role in long-term memory formation in Drosophila. *Proc Natl Acad Sci USA* **101**:16058–16063.

Segall LA, Amir S. 2010. Glucocorticoid regulation of clock gene expression in the mammalian limbic forebrain. *J Mol Neurosci* **42**(2):168–175.

Shimizu K, Phan T, Mansuy IM, Storm DR. 2007. Proteolytic degradation of SCOP in the hippocampus contributes to activation of MAP kinase and memory. *Cell* **128**(6):1219–1229.

Shimizu K, Mackenzie SM, Storm DR. 2010. SCOP/PHLPP and its functional role in the brain. *Mol Biosyst* **6**(1):38–43.

Siuciak JA, Fang J-M, Dubocovich ML. 1990. Autoradiographic localization of 2-[125I]iodomelatonin binding sites in the brains of C3H/HeN and C57BL/6J strains of mice. *Eur J Pharmacol* **180**:387–390.

Stephan FK, Kovacevic NS. 1978. Multiple retention deficit in passive avoidance in rats is eliminated by suprachiasmatic lesions. *Behav Biol* **22**(4):456–462.

Tahara Y, Kuroda H, Saito K, *et al.* 2012. *In vivo* monitoring of peripheral circadian clocks in the mouse. *Curr Biol* **22**(11):1029–1034.

Takahashi Y, Okada T. 2011. Involvement of the nitric oxide cascade in melatonin-induced inhibition of long-term potentiation at hippocampal CA1 synapses. *Neurosci Res* **69**(1):1–7.

Tapp WN, Holloway FA. 1981. Phase shifting circadian rhythms produces retrograde amnesia. *Science* **211**:1056–1058.

Tononi G, Cirelli C. 2014. Sleep and the price of plasticity: from synaptic and cellular homeostasis to memory consolidation and integration. *Neuron* **81**(1):12–34.

Treccani G, Musazzi L, Perego C, *et al.* 2014. Stress and corticosterone increase the readily releasable pool of glutamate vesicles in synaptic terminals of prefrontal and frontal cortex. *Mol Psychiatry* **19**(4):433–443.

OTA (Office of Technology Assessment). 1991. *Biological Rhythms: Implications for the Worker.* OTA-BA-463, US Congress, Office of Technology Assessment (US Government Printing Office, Washington, DC).

Van der Zee EA, Havekes R, Barf RP, *et al.* 2008. Circadian time-place learning in mice depends on Cry genes. *Curr Biol* **18**(11):844–848.

Vandewalle G, Archer SN, Wuillaume C, *et al.* 2009. Functional magnetic resonance imaging-assessed brain responses during an executive task depend on interaction of sleep homeostasis, circadian phase, and PER3 genotype. *J Neurosci* **29**(25):7948–7956.

Wakamatsu H, Yoshinobu Y, Aida R, *et al.* 2001. Restricted-feeding-induced anticipatory activity rhythm is associated with a phase-shift of the expression of mPer1 and mPer2 mRNA in the cerebral cortex and hippocampus but not in the suprachiasmatic nucleus of mice. *Eur J Neurosci* **13**:1190–1196.

Walton JC, Chen Z, Travers JB, Nelson RJ. 2013. Exogenous melatonin reproduces the effects of short day lengths on hippocampal function in male white-footed mice, Peromyscus leucopus. *Neurosci* **248C**:403–413.

Wang LM, Suthana NA, Chaudhury D, *et al.* 2005. Melatonin inhibits hippocampal long-term potentiation. *Eur J Neurosci* **22**(9):2231–7.

Wang LM, Dragich JM, Kudo T, *et al.* 2009. Expression of the circadian clock gene Period2 in the hippocampus: possible implications for synaptic plasticity and learned behaviour. *ASN Neuro* **1**(3):e00012.

Waterhouse J. 2010. Circadian rhythms and cognition. *Prog Brain Res* **185**:131–153.

Weaver DR, Rivkees SA, Reppert SM. 1989. Localization and characterization of melatonin receptors in rodent brain by in vitro autoradiography. *J. Neurosci* **9**:2581–2590.

Wright KP Jr., Hull JT, Hughes RJ, *et al.* 2006. Sleep and wakefulness out of phase with internal biological time impairs learning in humans. *J Cogn Neurosci* **18**:508–521.

Wright KP, Lowry CA, Lebourgeois MK. 2012. Circadian and wakefulness-sleep modulation of cognition in humans. *Front Mol Neurosci* **5**:50.

Welsh DK, Takahashi JS, Kay SA. 2010. Suprachiasmatic nucleus: cell autonomy and network properties. *Annu Rev Physiol* **72**:551–77.

West MO, Deadwyler S. 1980. Circadian modulation of granule cell response to perforant path synaptic input in the rat. *Neurosci* **5**:1597–1602.

Winson J, Abzug C. 1978. Neural transmission through hippocampal pathway is dependent on behavior. *J Neurophysiol* **41**:716–732.

Yoo SH, Yamazaki S, Lowrey PL, *et al.* 2004. PERIOD2::LUCIFERASE real-time reporting of circadian dynamics reveals persistent circadian oscillations in mouse peripheral tissues. *Proc Natl Acad Sci USA* **101**:5339–5346.

Zhang EE, Liu Y, Dentin R, *et al.* 2010. Cryptochrome mediates circadian regulation of cAMP signaling and hepatic gluconeogenesis. *Nat Med* **16**(10):1152–1156.

Zhou X, Ferguson SA, Matthews RW, *et al.* 2011. Sleep, wake and phase dependent changes in neurobehavioral function under forced desynchrony. *Sleep* **34**:931–941.

Zueger M, Urani A, Chourbaji S, *et al.* 2006. mPer1 and mPer2 mutant mice show regular spatial and contextual learning in standardized tests for hippocampus dependent learning. *J Neural Transmission* **113**:1435–1463.

Circadian Rhythms in Mood Disorders

17

Colleen A. McClung

Department of Psychiatry, University of Pittsburgh School of Medicine, Pittsburgh, PA, USA

17.1 Introduction

There are few diseases that have a greater impact on health, families, and society as mood and affective disorders. According to the National Institute of Mental Health (NIMH) nearly 21% of the adults in the United States will be diagnosed with a mood disorder in their lifetime. These disorders often lead to loss of productivity or employment, loss of family and friends and can ultimately lead to additional health problems and suicide. The estimated cost of serious mental illness to the United States in 2002 was in excess of $300 billion per year. Moreover, the rate of antidepressant use has almost tripled in the last 15 years and only one-third of patients attain remission. Thus, it is important to understand how these disorders develop and to design better treatments for these illnesses.

The link between mood disorders (particularly the episodic nature of these disorders) and abnormal rhythmicity has been described for decades. In the 1950s, Curt Richter (the man who created the phrase "biological clock") described the fact that depressive episodes occurred with particular times of day, times of year, more frequently in areas of the world with little sunlight, and correlated with sleep disturbances. In fact, one of the major diagnostic criteria in the DSM-IV for any mood disorder involves changes in the sleep–wake cycle. Moreover, sleep disruptions increase the risk of relapse into a new depressive episode (Pigeon *et al.*, 2008). In addition, shortened latency to rapid eye movement (REM) sleep, increased REM density and increased REM sleep are predictive endophenotypes for depression (Wulff *et al.*, 2010). Individuals with major depressive disorder (MDD) often have insomnia with early morning wakening or other problems that prevent a full night of sleep. This is particularly characteristic of those with typical or "melancholic" depression, which usually also involves severe weight loss and overall anhedonia. However, people with either atypical depression or Seasonal Affective Disorder (SAD) often sleep too much, gain weight, and feel that they are chronically fatigued. Thus, both too little and too much sleep is associated with altered mood. Bipolar disorder (BD), a disease in which individuals cycle through periods of depression and mania, also involves dramatic and often cyclic changes in the sleep–wake cycle. Posttraumatic stress disorder (PTSD) is also characterized by difficulties in falling asleep and staying asleep. The DSM-IV criteria for a depressive or manic episode are outlined in Table 17.1. Features of SAD are given in Table 17.2.

In addition to sleep–wake abnormalities, depression symptoms seem to have a diurnal component with the worst symptoms typically occurring in the morning and then tapering off throughout the day. In 1968, Franz Halberg suggested that some of the internal circadian rhythms in bipolar patients were

Circadian Medicine, First Edition. Edited by Christopher S. Colwell.
© 2015 John Wiley & Sons, Inc. Published 2015 by John Wiley & Sons, Inc.

Table 17.1 DSM IV criteria for depression and mania.

Depression	Mania
Depressed mood	Persistently elevated or irritable mood for 1 week
Loss of interest or pleasure in nearly all activities	Excessive involvement in pleasurable activities with a high potential for painful consequences
Weight loss or gain	Racing thoughts
Insomnia or hypersomnia	Little need for sleep
Psychomotor agitation or retardation	Increased goal directed behavior or agitation
Fatigue or loos of energy	Racing thoughts
Feelings of worthlessness/guilt	Inflated self-esteem
Diminished ability to think or concentrate	Lack of attention/ distractibility
Suicidal thoughts	More talkative than usual or pressure to keep talking

Five or more symptoms should be present for at least two consecutive weeks (including either depressed mood or loss of interest in pleasurable activities) to constitute a major depressive episode. Three or more symptoms must be present for at least one week (including elevated mood to constitute a manic episode. Four additional symptoms must be present if the mood is only irritable. One or more episodes of mania is sufficient for a diagnosis of bipolar disorder.

Table 17.2 Features of seasonal affective disorder (SAD), a specifier for major depression.

Increased sleep
Increased appetite and carbohydrate cravings
Weight gain
Irritability
Interpersonal difficulties, rejection sensitivity, social withdrawal
Heavy, leaden feelings in the arms or legs

The criteria for the seasonal specifier focuses on the appearance of symptoms only in the fall and winter months. However, SAD is generally characterized by the symptoms often seen with atypical depression.

not synchronized with the 24-hour day/night cycle. Halberg's theory was that the interaction between the unsynchronized, "free-running" rhythms and the normally synchronized "entrained" rhythms causes switches back and forth between mania and depression (Halberg, 1968). Then, in 1975, Papousek postulated that the risk for a depressive episode could arise from a *tempora minoris resistentiae* or in other words, a temporal disturbance that disrupts the inner and/or outer synchronization in predisposed individuals (Papousek, 1975). Later Wehr, Goodwin, Wirz-Justice (1980) and then Kripke (1983) proposed a more refined theory that mood disorders may result from a phase advance of the circadian rhythm governing temperature, cortisol, and REM sleep relative to other circadian rhythms such as sleep–wakefulness (Wehr et al., 1979; Kripke, 1984). This theory was later labeled the "internal phase coincidence model," which suggests that when awakening occurs at an abnormally early or "sensitive" phase of circadian rhythms this leads to depressive symptoms. Then, in the late 1980s, Ehlers, Frank and Kupfer developed the "Social Zeitgeber Theory" of mood disorders, which postulates that in susceptible individuals (i.e., those with a genetically abnormal clock) stressful life events lead to disruptions to the sleep–wake cycle, which then lead to changes in biological rhythms and processes governed by these rhythms, culminating in a mood-related episode (Ehlers *et al.*, 1988).

Since the early 1970s, a multitude of animal and plant studies have identified the key components of the molecular clock and located the suprachiasmatic nucleus (SCN) as the central pacemaker in mammals (Chapter 3). These molecular components of the clock are reviewed in detail in other chapters (Chapters 1 and 2). Today psychiatric researchers are trying to identify the precise role of the molecular clock in mood regulation and learn how specific types of rhythm disruptions lead to and/or exacerbate mood-related phenotypes.

17.2 Categories of rhythm disruptions

There are four features of rhythms that may be disrupted in individuals with mood disorders. Studies have found evidence that all of these types of disruptions can influence mood.

17.2.1 Entrainment

Circadian rhythms can be entrained to light or other nonphotic stimuli. These other "Zeitgebers" or "time givers" include food, drugs of abuse and social interaction. The ability to entrain to a certain environmental cue (like food or light) is an evolutionary strength, since it allows an animal to take advantage of resources that are temporally restricted and avoid predators. Likewise, after a period of rhythm disruption, the ability to re-entrain to a light–dark cycle is important. This is very evident for anyone who has traveled overseas and experienced prolonged jet lag. One robust feature of bipolar disorder is that manic episodes are very often precipitated by a change to the normal sleep–wake cycle (Malkoff-Schwartz *et al.*, 1998). This suggests an inability to affectively adapt to a change in schedule. One interesting retrospective study of 186 patients admitted to a psychiatric hospital near London's Heathrow airport found a double dissociation between the direction of travel and the type of mood episode experienced. Depression was more common in patients after westward travel while hypomania was more common in those flying eastward (Jauhar and Weller, 1982). Interpersonal and Social Rhythm therapy (IPSRT) developed at the University of Pittsburgh is designed to help keep individuals with bipolar disorder entrain to a specific sleep–wake and social schedule (Frank *et al.*, 2000). This helps to prevent the precipitation of mood-related episodes due to a change in schedule.

In addition, shift workers, particularly those that work varied schedules, are more prone to a host of health problems, including cancer, diabetes, and depression. This is termed "shift workers syndrome" and it has become quite prevalent in our modern society. These chronic environmental alterations to the normal sleep–wake cycle do not allow proper entrainment and are deleterious in many ways to human health.

17.2.2 Amplitude

Blunted rhythms in activity and other physiological processes are very commonly seen in individuals with mood disorders. These include rhythms in body temperature, plasma cortisol, norepinephrine, thyroid stimulating hormone, melatonin, pulse and blood pressure (reviewed in Wirz-Justice, 2006). Moreover, when molecular rhythms are measured in fibroblast samples taken from bipolar subjects and controls, the magnitude of the rhythms are blunted in the tissue taken from bipolar subjects, suggesting an overall dampened or less robust rhythm. Interestingly, an increase in amplitude of several physiological rhythms often accompanies remission of depressive symptoms with treatment (Souetre *et al.*, 1988a, 1988b). Recent studies also suggest that the mood stabilizing drugs lithium and valproic acid both increase molecular rhythm amplitude (Johansson *et al.*, 2011; Li *et al.*, 2012).

17.2.3 Period

Most individuals have a rhythm that is slightly greater than 24 hours. Some people have rhythms which are too short (less than 24 hours) or too long (greater than 24 hours). Early studies of subjects with mood disorders suggested that their rhythms were running too fast. Indeed, studies of bipolar subjects put into temporal isolation in the late 1970s found that several of them had fast running body temperature rhythms. Interestingly, lithium has an extremely robust period lengthening effect, which occurs in a host of organisms from fruit flies on up to humans. In these early studies only the bipolar subjects with a fast running rhythm were responsive to lithium treatment while those with normal or long periods were not responsive (Kripke *et al.*, 1978). These studies have been difficult to reproduce given new human research regulations. Moreover, recent studies of fibroblast samples or dim light melatonin onset (DLMO) do not consistently find changes in period length in bipolar subjects or in subjects with MDD. Therefore, the role of period changes in mood disorders is still controversial.

17.2.4 Phase

Certain individuals have a chronotype indicative of a delayed phase (preference for evening) or an advanced phase (preference for early morning). In the extreme case, these phase differences become disorders themselves. Familial Advanced Sleep Phase Syndrome (FASPS) is characterized by an extremely early wake time and early bed time while Delayed Sleep Phase Syndrome (DSPS) is characterized by a late wake time and sleep time. Preference for the morning or evening is genetic and controlled by the central circadian genes, particularly *Clock* and *Per2*. Interestingly, early studies suggested that depression was often associated with a phase advance as indicated in the internal coincidence model put forth in the early 1980s. However, many of the early studies of phase were not well controlled.

The most important confound is the "masking effects" that could result from behavioral and environmental factors, such as sleep changes that are not due to circadian factors. Moreover, early morning awakening, which is often seen in depression, alters light exposure and can lead to clock shifting. However, in one study of depressed individuals under constant conditions (temporal isolation for a period of weeks), 80% of depressed patients were phase advanced compared to 25% of normal controls (Wehr *et al.*, 1979), so there may be some validity to the phase advance model. The vast majority of recent studies, however, have found that rhythms are more often phase delayed in individuals with MDD and the extent of the delay correlates with the severity of depressive symptoms (Emens *et al.*, 2009; Buckley and Schatzberg, 2010; Abe *et al.*, 2011). This is consistent with an evening preference that is strongly associated with depression. The phase of rhythms is also important in the concept of "social jet lag," which was recently described (Wittmann *et al.*, 2006). Essentially, individuals with an evening preference are forced during the week to wake up early due to school or work obligations. Then they sleep late on the weekends in accordance with their natural preference. Thus, their body is in a perpetual state of jet lag, as if they are traveling overseas and back every week. Higher rates of social jet lag are associated with a higher body mass index (BMI) and increased depression.

In seasonal depression, rhythms are generally phase delayed (in approximately 70% of patients) and bright light therapy in the morning is very effective in advancing rhythms to alleviate depressive symptoms (as is discussed in more detail later). Bipolar subjects are also overwhelmingly phase delayed and mania is more common in phase delayed subjects than controls. In a recent study of young people with bipolar disorder, 62% had delayed sleep phase compared to 10% of controls (Robillard *et al.*, 2012). Thus, mood dysregulation seems to be most commonly associated with a phase delay.

17.3 Seasonal affective disorder

SAD is perhaps the best characterized disorder that appears to arise from a desynchronization of the internal clock with the environment. In fact, the symptoms of SAD (Table 17.2) are often anecdotally compared to those of animal hibernation in the winter months. Several studies have suggested that the circadian hormone, melatonin, is centrally involved in the development of SAD (Lewy *et al.*, 2009). Melatonin is released primarily by the pineal gland in the evening and can bind to the G-protein coupled receptors, MT1 and MT2 (Pandi-Perumal *et al.*, 2006). These receptors are expressed at high levels in the SCN and upon stimulation they modulate SCN transmission and circadian rhythms. Melatonin is strongly suppressed by light and seasonal variations in melatonin are commonly seen in mammals.

The role of melatonin rhythms in SAD is controversial. In some studies, SAD is associated with a pronounced seasonal melatonin rhythm, or more daytime melatonin specifically in the winter, whereas healthy control subjects have little seasonal alterations in their melatonin rhythms (Danilenko *et al.*, 1994; Wehr *et al.*, 2001). However, other studies have found greater melatonin in the summer months in subjects with SAD, or they have seen significant seasonal changes in melatonin rhythms in healthy, unaffected individuals. Much of this variability in melatonin measurements likely comes from the variations in seasonal changes between different areas of the world in which these studies were conducted. For example, studies done in the arctic, which have extreme seasonal differences in day/night light intensity and duration, generally find stronger seasonal rhythms in melatonin. However, studies done in more temperate or tropical climates do not find pronounced seasonal rhythms, particularly in individuals who are exposed to artificial light in the evening.

Several studies have suggested that the later dawn in winter leads to a phase delay in circadian rhythms in sensitized individuals, causing a desynchronization of the molecular rhythms of the SCN and the sleep–wake cycle. This idea is the basis of the phase shift hypothesis of SAD. This theory is supported by research demonstrating that early morning bright light therapy (BLT) is the most effective in treating SAD, whereas evening light therapy is very often not effective (Wirz-Justice and Terman, 2012). Therefore, the early morning light leads to a phase advance in the circadian system putting it back on track with the sleep–wake cycle.

17.4 Treatments for mood disorders alter rhythms

Essentially all of the commonly used treatments for mood disorders have effects on the circadian clock. Some of these have already been mentioned but additional details are given below.

17.4.1 Bright light therapy (BLT)

Light therapy has been used for more than 30 years in the treatment of SAD but is now also being utilized for other mood disorders. The exposure to bright light early in the morning leads to a dramatic phase advance in rhythms. In 2005, the American Psychiatric Association recognized BLT as a first line treatment for both seasonal and nonseasonal depression. In particular, the use of light therapy over medications has grown in popularity for pregnant women, children and adolescents, elderly patients, and women with postpartum depression, since the potential side effects are very minor compared with most antidepressant medications. However, BLT is not ideal for bipolar patients, since it can shift them into a manic state.

Initially researchers thought that light therapy would be most effective if it mimicked the longer day length of the summer months, thus they gave light at the end of the day. However, this strategy was not as successful as those that gave light as a short pulse (about 30 minutes) only in the morning to mimic the earlier dawn of spring/summer. Normal room lighting falls in the range of 100–300 lx. In comparison, noontime sunlight can reach upwards of 100,000 lx. Usually, BLT is administered at 10,000 lx via a light box to mimic what is typical of natural sunlight without causing unnecessary stress to the eyes. While light therapy at the time of awakening is preferable for most people with SAD or other mood disorders, recent studies suggest an individual variability in the optimal timing of BLT based on dim light melatonin onset (DLMO) readings. By customizing the timing of BLT, remission rates can reach upwards of 80% for SAD. Generally the greater the phase advance of DLMO (up to 2.5 h) the better the therapeutic response.

17.4.2 Melatonin

Most studies find low levels of nocturnal melatonin secretion in individuals with MDD. Furthermore, several animal studies have shown that melatonin can have an antidepressant effect in behavioral models (Manda and Reiter, 2010; Ramirez-Rodriguez et al., 2009). However, while melatonin treatment in the evening seems to help promote better sleep in subjects with MDD, it does not significantly alter depressive symptoms on its own. Agomelatine, a melatonin receptor (MT1/MT2) agonist and weak 5-HT2c receptor antagonist, has been approved for the treatment of depression in most countries and has clear clinical efficacy when compared to placebo (De Berardis et al., 2011). Moreover, as compared with other antidepressant drugs, agomelatine promotes coalesced sleep leading to greater daytime alertness. Agomelatine treatment in the evening produces a significant entrainment and phase advance of rhythms. Several studies in animal models suggest that the synergistic interaction between the melatonin and serotonin signaling changes are required for the antidepressant effects of agomelatine. Agomelatine produces a distinctive EEG profile when compared to melatonin, a selective MT1/MT2 agonist (ramelteon) or a 5-HT2c antagonist (S32006). Moreover, increased *Brain Derived Neurotrophic factor* (BDNF) mRNA expression in the mPFC (an effect very often seen with antidepressant treatment) is produced with agomelatine treatment but not with melatonin or 5-HT2c antagonists, and this increase can be prevented with pretreatment of melatonergic antagonists (Molteni *et al.*, 2010). Thus, a combination of melatonin and serotonin signaling changes produce clear antidepressant effects which may (or may not) be a direct result of better entrained and phase shifted clock function. Interestingly, the 5-HT2c receptors are strongly expressed in the SCN where they have a circadian rhythm in expression. Along with melatonin, serotonin input to the SCN is keenly involved in SCN entrainment.

As mentioned previously, most studies find a delayed melatonin phase or exaggerated rhythm in melatonin in individuals with SAD. Studies from Lewy and colleagues suggest that melatonin administration in the evening can be beneficial for the treatment of SAD. In a 2006 study they identified an optimal phase angle difference (PAD) of six hours between the DLMO and the midpoint of sleep which correlated with normal mood (Lewy *et al.*, 2006). Melatonin was given to SAD patients at particular times of the evening to produce a six-hour PAD based on the individual's DLMO readings. The response to treatment correlated with a corrected circadian alignment and those that were given an incorrectly timed melatonin treatment did not have a significant therapeutic response. Thus, as opposed to MDD, melatonin treatments at times that produce an optimal PAD may be therapeutically beneficial for the treatment of SAD.

17.4.3 Sleep deprivation therapy (SDT)

Sleep deprivation therapy (SDT) was first proposed as a method to quickly reduce depressive symptoms in the late 1960s to early 1970s by Schulte, Pflug and Tolle (Schulte, 1966; Pflug and Tolle, 1971; Pflug, 1976). One whole night of total sleep deprivation (TSD – 36–40 continuous hours of wakefulness) improves depressive symptoms in 40–60% of patients (Giedke and Schwarzler, 2002). This effect can last for weeks, although 50–80% of patients suffer a complete or partial relapse after recovery sleep. The positive effects of SDT can be extended following a combined treatment with morning BLT, sleep phase advances (SPA), as well as pharmacological treatments. In particular, lithium appears to have a synergistic effect with SDT, leading to longer times before relapse. As with BLT, SDT must be used with caution in the case of bipolar patients, since it can switch them into a hypomanic or manic state. However, the rate of switches is relatively low (4–6%) and this can often be prevented with mood stabilizer treatment. Partial sleep deprivation (PSD) involves about 20 hours of wakefulness with sleep deprivation occurring in either the first (early) or second (late) half of the night. Studies are mixed as to whether PSD can be as effective as TSD. SDT may also be administered repeatedly as TSD over alternating nights for 3–7 days or PSD for 3–6 consecutive nights.

One study of bipolar subjects compared the effects of a "chronotherapy group," which is one that received sleep deprivation, light therapy, sleep phase advances, plus medications (antidepressants and lithium) to a traditional medication alone group. A significant decrease in depression ratings within 48 hours in the chronotherapy group over the medication alone group was found (Wu *et al.*, 2009). Moreover, after a seven week trial, 63% of the chronotherapy group had fulfilled criteria for remission.

It is unclear as to how SDT alters mood. One theory is that SDT may normalize the sensitivity to light stimuli and modulate light-induced phase-shifting responses. Evidence for this comes from data demonstrating that some depressed patients are supersensitive to light stimuli (Lewy *et al.*, 1981; Seggie *et al.*, 1989). Moreover, clinical improvement in SDT responders is correlated with changes in light–dark adaptation (i.e., the greater the response to TSD, the larger the changes in light sensitivity). This is an effect not seen in SDT nonresponders or in healthy controls who were also deprived of sleep (Sokolski *et al.*, 1995). SDT has also been viewed as a rhythm "reset button" and sleep deprivation without exercise in hamsters can bring on large phase advances and rapidly reset the molecular clock (Antle and Mistlberger, 2000).

A study by Benedetti and colleagues measured wrist actigraphy in bipolar subjects treated for one week with repeated SDT and morning BLT (Benedetti *et al.*, 2007). Two thirds of the patients responded to treatment (i.e., had a 50% or greater reduction in depression symptoms) and these subjects showed a phase advance in rhythms of 57 min compared to pretreatment baseline. Nonresponders did not show significant changes in their rhythms, suggesting that the phase advance in rhythms is crucial for therapeutic success (Benedetti *et al.*, 2007). SDT is also associated with enhanced dopaminergic transmission, however. The role of this enhanced dopamine in the therapeutic effects of SDT is controversial and genetic studies have failed to find an association between polymorphisms in dopamine receptor subtypes and SDT response.

17.4.4 Interpersonal and social rhythm therapy (IPSRT)

IPSRT is a psychotherapeutic intervention developed from the Social Zeitgeber Theory put forward by Ehlers and colleagues (Ehlers *et al.*, 1988). IPSRT specifically attempts to stabilize and entrain daily routines for individuals with bipolar disorder. Social contacts and regular sleep–wake routines can function as powerful Zeitgebers to entrain rhythms. A daily log or Social Rhythm Metric (SRM) is kept which measures five endpoints: (i) time out of bed, (ii) first contact with another person, (iii) start of work/school/volunteer/family care, (iv) dinner time, and (v) bed time. IPSRT also involves some aspects of traditional psychotherapy, such as helping the patient come to terms with the loss of their "healthy self" and creating support networks for patients. The more days an individual can stick to a constant routine, the better their chances of avoiding a manic or depressive episode. IPSRT is done in conjunction with pharmacological treatments such as lithium or antidepressants. Studies have found that IPSRT in combination with medication leads to a faster therapeutic response than medication alone or medication in combination with traditional psychotherapy (Frank *et al.*, 2005). The routine schedule of IPSRT also helps patients adhere to their medication schedules and reduce everyday life stressors that often come with a hectic schedule.

17.4.5 Antidepressant and mood stabilizing drugs

As mentioned previously, agomelatine is the first antidepressant drug that is specifically aimed at altering the circadian system for a therapeutic effect. However, essentially all known drugs currently used to treat mood disorders have some measurable effect on circadian rhythms. Besides agomelatine the most well studied medication in terms of its circadian effects is lithium. Lithium leads to a phase delay in rhythms and a lengthening of the circadian period. Recent studies find that lithium can also increase rhythm amplitude, an effect seen as well with the mood stabilizing drug, valproic acid (Li *et al.*, 2012). The exact mechanism by which lithium alters circadian rhythms is unclear. It had been suggested for several years that these effects were mediated through the direct inhibition of GSK3β by lithium. GSK3β phosphorylates several members of the core molecular clock, including BMAL1, CRY2, PER2 and REV-ERBα. However, several studies have now found that specific GSK3β inhibitors, or knock-down of GSK3β expression, leads to a shortened rather than a lengthened period in cell culture and tissue slices (Hirota *et al.*, 2008; Li *et al.*, 2012). So the rhythm lengthening effect is likely not due to the inhibition of GSK3β. The increased rhythm amplitude with lithium treatment, however, may be due to the inhibition of GSK3β since GSK3β specific inhibitors can also increase molecular rhythm amplitude in the SCN and peripheral tissues.

In contrast to lithium, which is primarily an antimanic drug, treatment with antidepressant, selective serotonin reuptake inhibitors (SSRIs) such as fluoxetine (Prozac) generally produce a phase advance in SCN neuronal firing rhythms and shorten the circadian period (Sprouse *et al.*, 2006). These effects are likely mediated by the 5-HT1A and 5-HT7 receptors, since treatment with agonists for these receptors in hamster SCN yield similar effects. Importantly, 5-HT stimulation via a 5-HT receptor agonist or SSRI treatment leads to behavioral phase advances in rhythms under constant conditions in both diurnal and nocturnal rodent species (Cuesta *et al.*, 2008). Interestingly, monoamine oxidase inhibitors (MAOIs) (another class of antidepressant drugs) also alter the magnitude of light-induced phase advances via increased 5-HT levels. Monoamine oxidase A itself is also a direct transcriptional target of the NPAS2 and BMAL1 genes (Hampp *et al.*, 2008) and, as discussed later, this association may be a mechanism by which mood is regulated by circadian genes.

Results with older, tricyclic antidepressants are mixed. The tricyclic antidepressant imipramine produces a desynchronization between activity rhythms and body temperature rhythms resulting in a phase advance of temperature rhythms compared to activity rhythms (Nagayama, 1996). There are also some indications that imipramine enhances rhythm amplitude. However, other studies find that it has minimal if any effect on rhythms. There are also studies that find that imipramine's rhythm altering effects are more pronounced in animals with a depressive-like phenotype compared to wild-type animals. Research on tricyclics in humans is lacking, since today these antidepressants are rarely used clinically due to their serious side effects.

There is strong evidence from multiple studies which suggest that antidepressant efficacy (regardless of the class of drug) is dependent upon levels of brain BDNF. BDNF and its receptor TrkB are both expressed in the SCN and levels of BDNF fluctuate rhythmically. Both BDNF and TrkB-deficient mice have a reduction in the phase shifting effects of light on circadian rhythms, thus BDNF secretion appears to be necessary for light-induced phase shifts. Interestingly, both amplitude and frequency of SCN spontaneous excitatory currents are increased with BDNF and decreased with the neurotrophin receptor inhibitor, K252a. The magnitude of currents evoked by application of N-methyl-d-aspartate (NMDA) and amino-methyl proprionic acid (AMPA) are also increased with BDNF application (Kim *et al.*, 2006; Michel *et al.*, 2006). Moreover, K252a reduces the magnitude of phase shifts of SCN activity rhythms generated by glutamate. BDNF on its own can also cause phase shifts in SCN activity, which can be blocked by K252a. Given the general phase advancing properties of most antidepressant medications, and the apparent role of BDNF in both antidepressant efficacy and phase shifts in SCN activity, it is tempting to speculate that the phase shifting of the SCN is important in antidepressant efficacy and that this might be mediated by both 5-HT and BDNF.

17.4.6 Future drugs

In recent years, several compounds have been identified through reporter screens that alter circadian rhythms in particular ways. A casein kinase $1\varepsilon/\delta$ inhibitor (PF-670462) was isolated in one such screen; it produces a dose-dependent phase delay in rhythms of both nocturnal rats and diurnal monkeys (Badura *et al.*, 2007; Sprouse *et al.*, 2009). Chronic treatment also produces cumulative and lasting phase delays in rhythms (Sprouse *et al.*, 2010). Interestingly, when this compound and others like it were given to mice with disrupted rhythms due to either a mutation in the *Vipr2* gene, or constant light, daily treatment with these compounds elicited robust 24-hour activity rhythms that persisted throughout the treatment (Meng *et al.*, 2010). In addition, a similar compound to PF-670462 was able to partially reverse the bipolar mania-like phenotype of mice with a mutation in the *Clock* gene (*Clock*Δ19) and prevent relapse-like alcohol drinking in mice with prior alcohol exposure (Arey and McClung, 2012; Perreau-Lenz *et al.*, 2012). These results are very exciting and suggest that CK1 inhibitors may be viable agents for the treatment of mood and addictive disorders.

Additional compounds that alter circadian rhythms are under investigation. Hirota and colleagues identified several small molecule activators of cryptochrome proteins that dose dependently lengthen the circadian period (Hirota *et al.*, 2012). Interestingly, one of these compounds, KL001, inhibits glucagon-induced gluconeogenesis in primary hepatocytes, suggesting it might be useful in the treatment of metabolic disorders. Even though this compound has reduced potency in the SCN and does not cross the blood–brain barrier (BBB), it's structure gives chemists a starting point for the development of other compounds that target the CRY proteins.

A large screen of 200,000 small molecules was undertaken by Chen and colleagues who used fibroblasts from *Per2::*luciferase mice to screen for compounds that alter molecular rhythms (Chen *et al.*, 2012). They identified several new molecules that alter rhythms in particular ways, creating a "tool box" for researchers to utilize for drug development studies. The most interesting of these might be the Clock Enhancing Molecules (CEMs), which increase rhythm amplitude even in a *Clock*Δ19 heterozygous background.

Recently, synthetic REV-ERB agonists that alter circadian rhythmicity were also described. Rev-erbα and β both are both involved in regulating circadian rhythms in a mostly redundant manner

(Liu *et al.*, 2008). These proteins are thought to mediate a direct link between the circadian and metabolic systems (Cho *et al.*, 2012). Interestingly, these drugs enhance the amplitude of *Per2* and *Clock* expression in the hypothalamus but suppress rhythms in *Cry2*. The phase of the molecular rhythms in certain clock genes is also altered by these compounds. Impressively, these compounds decrease fat mass and plasma lipids in mice fed a high fat diet, indicating that these drugs also may be efficacious in the treatment of metabolic diseases. Whether these drugs have any efficacy in mood disorder treatment has not been determined. Intriguingly, Rev-erbα is rapidly degraded in response to lithium treatment (Yin *et al.*, 2006). Thus, both Rev-erb agonists and antagonists should perhaps be considered as favorable targets for the development of novel antidepressant or mood stabilizing compounds.

17.5 Human genetic studies

At least 50 human genetic studies to date have identified single nucleotide polymorphisms (SNPs) or haplotypes in several of the circadian genes that associate with various psychiatric diseases using candidate gene approaches. These include polymorphisms in the core clock genes, clock gene modifiers (like the microRNA, miR-182) and genes involved in melatonin synthesis (reviewed in Etain *et al.*, 2011). However, to date very few genome-wide association studies (GWAS) have identified a circadian gene that significantly associates with any psychiatric disorders. Part of the discrepancy between the candidate gene studies and GWAS studies could come from the fact that these disorders most certainly arise from multiple gene mutations.

Furthermore, there are significant gene–environment interactions and the stringent tests for multiple comparisons used in GWAS studies remove most statistical hits when looking at more than a million SNPs. This is evident in a study from the Major Depressive Disorder Working Group of the Psychiatric GWAS Consortium (2013), which performed the largest GWAS study of MDD to date, examining more than 1.2 million SNPs in 18,759 subjects, followed by replication studies (57,478 subjects) and cross-disorder meta-analysis with the bipolar consortium data (32,050 subjects). No SNPs in any gene achieved genome-wide significance in any of their analyses. Thus, large GWAS approaches may not be particularly fruitful when it comes to psychiatric disorders, and more targeted and focused approaches may prove more insightful.

McCarthy and colleagues performed a survey of multiple GWAS studies to determine if there is a significant association between the circadian system as a whole and either bipolar disorder, lithium responsiveness, schizophrenia, depression, or ADHD (McCarthy *et al.*, 2012). Essential "core" clock genes, upstream circadian clock modulators, and downstream clock controlled genes were considered in their statistical analysis (McCarthy *et al.*, 2012). They determined that both bipolar disorder and lithium responsiveness were significantly associated with core clock genes and rhythmic clock-controlled genes (as a group) but not upstream clock modulators or nonrhythmic clock controlled genes. This suggests a fundamental association between the central clock and mood, rather than a shared upstream process that regulates both circadian rhythms and mood.

In addition, an epistasis network centrality analysis of two GWAS cohorts for bipolar disorder revealed an enrichment for genes in the circadian rhythm pathway (along with other pathways including Wnt signaling, axon guidance and cadherin signaling) (Pandey *et al.*, 2012). Thus, more detailed pathway and survey types of analyses of GWAS information do reveal significant associations between mood disorders and the circadian system as whole.

17.6 Animal studies

Animal models of depression, reward and anxiety-related phenotypes have given us great insight into the molecular mechanisms and neurobiology that underlies the development of mood disorders and the changes in the brain that occur to facilitate treatment.

17.6.1 Light–dark manipulations

In order to better understand the role of daily light–dark disruptions and seasonal changes on mood, many researchers have turned to the use of animal models (reviewed in McClung, 2007)). Since many of the effects of light are mediated by alterations in melatonin, it is important to have an intact melatonin system in the model organism for these types of studies. Unfortunately, most laboratory mouse strains lack a functional melatonin system, due to inbred mutations through domestication in genes involved in the melatonin synthesis pathway. Therefore, laboratories that are interested in seasonal mood changes, or effects of light on mood, have turned to other rodent models, such as rats and hamsters. It is also important to keep in mind that most laboratory mice and rats are nocturnal while humans are diurnal; this may be a confounding factor in studies involving changes in light. However, nocturnal rodents also show mood-related phenotypes when exposed to altered photoperiods. Einat and colleagues have argued that diurnal rodents like the fat sand rat (*Psammommys Obesus*) and the unstriped Nile grass rat (*Arvicanthis niloticus*) are compelling models for studies of seasonal depression (Kronfeld-Schor and Einat, 2012). In both species, six weeks in a very short photoperiod (5 h light/19 h dark) results in increased depression-like behavior in the forced swim test (FST) and saccharin preference test compared with animals kept on a traditional 12/12 light–dark cycle. Moreover, after three weeks in a short photo-period, when these rats are treated with one hour daily 3000 lx morning light therapy for three weeks, the rats experience reduced anxiety-related and depression related behavior in the elevated plus maze (EPM) and FST.

Nocturnal rats and Siberian hamsters kept in a short photoperiod also have altered behavior consistent with greater depression-related behavior. Even a brief exposure to constant darkness at an early developmental time period can have long-lasting effects on mood. Prolonged dark phase conditions (6 h light/18 h dark) administered from postnatal day 2 to day 14 in Sprague-Dawley rats results in increased anxiety, decreased social interaction, and decreased object recognition memory later in life.

How does prolonged darkness affect mood? Scientists do not know for sure, but constant darkness for six weeks or more in rats results in profound apoptosis in a number of brain regions and a decrease in the number of cortical nucleus accumbens boutons. Chronic treatment with the antidepressant desipramine can reverse the behavioral effects of light depravation and reverse the changes in apoptosis in noradrenergic neurons. Prolonged constant darkness also results in a decrease in the amplitude of SCN-dependent sleep-wake rhythms and loss of locus coeruleus (LC) terminals in the frontal cortex. Thus, a prolonged absence of light seems to modify the influence of the SCN over monaminergic structures and lead to a loss of noradrenergic signaling.

Other animal studies have found deleterious effects of constant light exposure on mood-related behaviors. These studies are particularly relevant now in the modern world, where artificial light exposure at night is prominent. Constant light has interesting effects on circadian rhythms in mice. Unlike constant darkness where mice maintain a robust circadian rhythm in activity with a period that is slightly shorter than 24 hours, in constant light they generally display an initial long period and then become arrhythmic with overall reduced locomotor activity. Three weeks of constant light exposure in Swiss Weber mice produces an increase in depression-like behavior in the FST and in sucrose preference; however, they also showed reduced anxiety in the open field (OF) and EPM. Interestingly, chronic constant light also impairs spatial memory in rats and affects long-term depression (LTD) in the hippocampus. Thus, altered mood-related behaviors are produced with prolonged darkness and prolonged light.

17.6.2 The SCN and mood

The few studies that have examined the impact of SCN lesions on mood-related behavior have provided mixed results. Somewhat surprisingly, bilateral SCN lesions in rats leads to a reduction in depression-related behavior in the FST (Tataroglu *et al.*, 2004). However, a study by Tuma and colleagues found that lesions of the SCN had no effect on depression and anxiety-related behavior following social defeat stress, but instead SCN integrity was necessary for the effective antidepressant actions of agomelatine

(Tuma *et al.*, 2005). Thus, in certain paradigms, destruction of the SCN leads to an antidepressant phenotype, and in others it is necessary for an antidepressant response. These results may not be completely at odds with each other, since agomelatine is known to inhibit SCN neuronal firing, so a reduction in SCN activity could prove to be antidepressant.

17.6.3 Circadian gene mutations

Interestingly, in general (with some exceptions), most of the mice that carry mutations in circadian genes that have been tested thus far have a decrease in depression or anxiety-related behavior rather than an increase in these responses. This is consistent with some of the SCN lesion studies, which found that this produces less behavioral despair in the FST. However, not all circadian gene mutations produce the same effect on behavior, which shows that there is some specificity to their actions, perhaps in brain regions outside of the SCN.

More recent studies have examined the influence of single circadian gene knockouts or mutations in the regulation of mood and anxiety-related behavior. The best characterized of these is the *Clock*Δ19 mouse. The *Clock*Δ19 mutant mice were created through ENU mutagenesis by Joe Takahashi and colleagues and contain a point mutation that results in the removal of exon 19 and a protein with a dominate-negative function (King *et al.*, 1997). In constant conditions, these mice have either an extremely long circadian period or are arrhythmic (Vitaterna *et al.*, 2006). When tested in a variety of behavioral measures, the *Clock*Δ19 homozygous mice are hyperactive in a novel environment, display lowered anxiety or greater "risk-taking" behavior on the EPM, OF and dark–light measures, display less depression-related behavior in both the FST and learned–helplessness measures, show an increase in sucrose preference, increased cocaine preference, and an increase in goal directed behavior measured by intracranial self-stimulation and cocaine self-administration (Easton *et al.*, 2003; McClung *et al.*, 2005; Roybal *et al.*, 2007; Ozburn *et al.*, 2012). In addition, these mice show a reduction in all phases of sleep (Naylor *et al.*, 2000). Taken together, the behavioral profile of these mice looks remarkably like that of bipolar patients specifically in the manic state. When these mice are given the mood stabilizing drug, lithium, the majority of their behavioral responses are normalized towards those of wild-type mice (Roybal *et al.*, 2007).

Similar to the *Clock*Δ19 mice, *Per2* knock-out mice (*Per2*[Brdm1]) also have reduced immobility in the FST and an increase in alcohol preference (Spanagel *et al.*, 2005; Hampp *et al.*, 2008). However, the *Per2*[Brdm1] mice are not hyperactive in response to novelty like the *Clock*Δ19 mice. Moreover, mice with mutations in both *Per1* and *Per2* (*Per1; Per2* double mutant) have increased anxiety-related behavior (Spencer *et al.*, 2013). Mice with single mutations in either *Per1* or *Per2* showed inconsistent results across anxiety measures suggesting that the two genes can compensate for one another to some extent. Interestingly, *Per1* knock-out mice (*Per1*[Brdm1]) display decreased conditioned cocaine preference and normal levels of alcohol intake unless chronically stressed, suggesting some specificity in function between the *Per1* and *Per2* genes (Abarca *et al.*, 2002; Dong *et al.*, 2011).

Investigators have started to examine other circadian gene mutants to determine if they have altered mood and anxiety-related behavior. Transgenic mice overexpressing GSK3β are hyperactive and have reduced immobility in the FST (Prickaerts *et al.*, 2006). This supports the idea that the therapeutic response to lithium may involve the inhibition of GSK3β. It has been reported that the circadian period mutant, *afterhours*, an ENU induced mutant in the gene *Fbxl3* with a long period of about 27 hours, has reduced anxiety and depression-related behavior similar to the *Clock*Δ19 mice (Keers *et al.*, 2012). Moreover, three separate human data sets revealed a genome-wide association between a polymorphism in FBXL3 and bipolar disorder.

SIRT1, is a histone deacetylase (HDAC) protein that interacts with CLOCK/BMAL1 to inhibit its transcriptional activity. SIRT1 knockout mice also have a decrease in anxiety-related behavior at baseline and lowered depression-related behavior following chronic social defeat (Libert *et al.*, 2011). Overexpression of SIRT1 leads to the opposite effect on behavior. Additional studies of other circadian gene mutants (including conditional and tissue-specific mutations) are just beginning and it will be interesting to determine the specific importance of each circadian gene in these responses.

17.7 SCN output-rhythmic hormones and peptides

The potential role of melatonin in mood regulation has already been discussed. However, melatonin is only one of several direct and indirect output signals thast are rhythmically regulated and involved in peripheral and central timing of biological processes. The identification of these various molecules is covered in other chapters and they include arginine vasopressin (AVP), vasoactive intestinal peptide (VIP), glucocorticoids, tumor necrosis factor-α (TNF-α), and prokinetican 2 (PK2) among others. Some of these other clock-controlled outputs may be prominently involved in mood regulation. For example, PK2, a molecule involved in transmitting signal from the SCN to other brain regions, appears to be involved in anxiety and depressive-behaviors. Brain-wide infusion of PK2 increases anxiety-like and depressive-like behavior in mice (Li *et al.*, 2009). Conversely, PK2 knockout mice have reduced anxiety and depression-like behaviors similar to the *Clock*Δ19 mice. However, unlike the *Clock*Δ19 mice, PK2 null mice are hypoactive and do not have an increase in reward-related behaviors.

Another class of circadian regulated hormones, glucocorticoids, are particularly important in the response to stress. Glucocorticoids are multifunctional adrenal steroid hormones that are associated with arousal. Glucocorticoids have a strong circadian rhythm in expression and peak in expression just prior to the onset of awakening to prepare the body for daily activity (Chapter 6). This is mediated through signaling of the SCN to the paraventricular nucleus (PVN) which then signals the pituitary to synthesize and release adrenocorticotropin (ACTH), signaling the adrenal gland to release glucocorticoid (GC) (Fig. 17.1). Moreover, GC can feed back and inhibit activity of the pituitary and PVN via the glucocorticoid receptor (GR). GR activity is also regulated by circadian proteins like CLOCK and CRY, leading to a complex feedback pathway. Acute stressful events lead to a sharp increase in glucocorticoids by activation of the hypothalamus–pituitary–adrenal (HPA) axis. Chronic stress can lead to long-term glucocorticoid dysregulation, which is very often seen in individuals with mood disorders. Interestingly, the type of dysregulation of this system can be quite different depending upon the type of mood disorder (i.e., MDD versus BPD versus PTSD) as well as the amount of early life trauma the individual has experienced (Frodl and O'Keane, 2012). The exact role of glucocorticoids in the development of mood disorders is uncertain but there is evidence to suggest that antidepressant treatment helps to stabilize HPA axis function via the serotonergic system. Thus, it seems that restoration of the circadian rhythm of HPA axis function in individuals with mood disorders should be beneficial to mood stabilization, although this has not been systematically tested.

Metabolic disorders are very highly comorbid with mood disorders (reviewed in Schellekens *et al.*, 2012). Moreover, mood disorders are often associated with changes in appetite. Peptides involved in metabolism, including ghrelin, orexin (also known as hypocretin), leptin, and cholecystokinin (CCK), all display a circadian rhythm in expression (Fig. 17.1). In human blood samples, leptin is increased during the night, orexin A levels are increased during the active phase, and ghrelin and CCK levels are increased prior to meals and during the night. Leptin and CCK are involved in the inhibition of appetite and feeding behavior while ghrelin stimulates appetite.

Leptin (which is produced in adipose tissue) and ghrelin (produced in the stomach) both signal through orexin neurons, which enhance wakefulness when stimulated by ghrelin and promote sleep when inhibited by leptin. In fact, narcolepsy, a condition where individuals experience sudden sleep bouts, is caused by a dysfunctional orexin system, linking regulation of feeding and sleep to this small population of hypothalamic neurons. CCK is more widely expressed throughout the brain and gut, including high levels of expression in GABAergic interneurons of the prefrontal cortex, dopaminergic neurons of the VTA, and the shell of the SCN. Interestingly, in the SCN, CCK neurons do not express vasopressin or VIP, they do not respond to light, and are not involved in photic shifting of the clock. However, the CCK-expressing neurons are innervated by VIPergic neurons in the SCN and they have synaptic connections via their process with both VIP and vasopressin neurons (Hannibal *et al.*, 2011). CCK increases activity in the PVN and acts on the vagal afferent neurons to inhibit food intake. These peptides and several others involved in feeding behaviors are arrhythmic in the *Clock*Δ19 mice, demonstrating that their expression is regulated by the core molecular clock (Turek *et al.*, 2005).

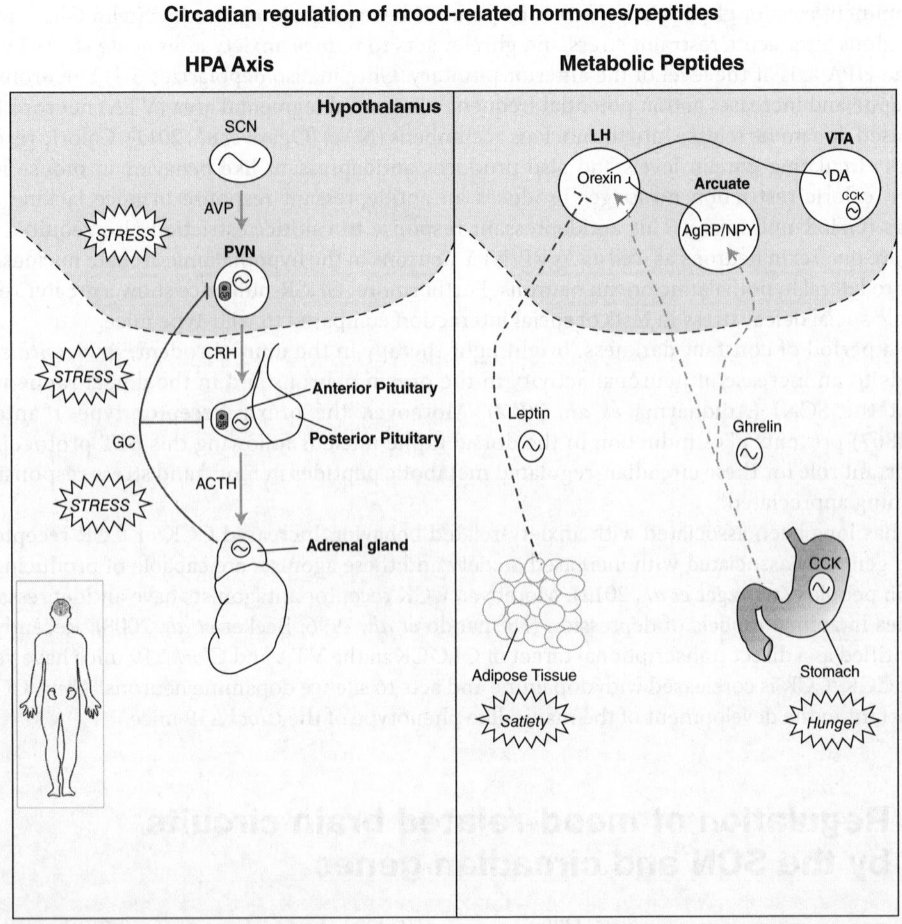

Fig. 17.1 The circadian system regulates many hormones and peptides in the brain and periphery that impact mood and reward. *(left panel)* The circadian control of the hypothamo–pituitary–adrenal (HPA) axis originates in the suprachiasmatic nucleus (SCN), which projects to the paraventricular nucleus (PVN) with arginine vaso-pressin (AVP) synthesizing neurons, causing the release of corticotropin-releasing hormone (CRH). Subsequently, CRH stimulates the synthesis and release of adrenocorticotropin hormone (ACTH) from the anterior pituitary, which travels through the blood stream and stimulates the release of glucocorticoids (GC) from the adrenal gland. Glucocorticoids negatively feedback to multiple sites via interaction with the intracellular glucocorticoid receptor (GR) in order to maintain basal stress hormone levels within a homeostatic range. Rhythmic clock gene expression coordinates incoming hormonal signals to rhythms in local receptor expression at the level of the PVN, pituitary and adrenal gland. *(right panel)* The circadian system regulates multiple peptides that detect, and respond to, changes in energy balance, which also impact mood and arousal. The hormone leptin is expressed in adipose tissue and is a satiety signal conveying a positive energy balance to the brain. Leptin levels also fluctuate on a daily basis, as clock genes are expressed in adipose tissue, and lead to circadian rhythms in hunger and satiety. Leptin is sleep-inducing and may alter mood by inhibiting orexin neurons in the lateral hypo-thalamus (LH). An opposing metabolic signal, ghrelin, is released by the stomach to convey a negative energy balance to the brain by stimulating orexigenic Agouti-Related peptide (AgRP)/ Neuropeptide Y (NPY)-secreting neurons in the arcuate nucleus of the hypothalamus. Additionally, ghrelin directly stimulates orexinergic neurons in the LH, which induces arousal and feeding behavior. The effects of ghrelin on orexin neurons in the LH may have an additional antidepressant-like effect and contribute to motivated behavior, as these orexigenic neurons project directly to dopaminergic neurons in the ventral tegmental area (VTA). Finally, cholecystokinin (CCK) is a ubiquitously expressed, circadian regulated peptide that is synthesized in the gut and contributes to feeding behavior, as well as the VTA, which contributes to motivated behavior and reward sensitivity.

A prominent role for ghrelin in the stress response is becoming appreciated. Ghrelin Ghr$^{-/-}$ mice are more anxious after acute restraint stress and ghrelin acts to reduce anxiety after acute stress by stimulating the HPA axis at the level of the anterior pituitary. Ghrelin also depolarizes 5-HT neurons in the dorsal raphe and increases action potential frequency in ventral tegmental area (VTA) neurons leading to increased dopamine release into the nucleus accumbens (NAc) (Ogaya *et al.*, 2011). Caloric restriction increases circulating ghrelin levels and also produces antidepressant-like behavior in mouse models. However, caloric restriction no longer produces an antidepressant response in mice lacking ghrelin receptors (GHSR-null mice). This antidepressant response to caloric restriction also requires orexin. GHSRs are on orexin neurons as well as AgRP/NPY neurons in the hypothalamic arcuate nucleus, which projects to lateral hypothalamic orexin neurons. Furthermore, GHSR-null mice show a greater response to chronic social defeat stress in tests of social interaction compared to wild-type mice.

After a period of constant darkness, bright light therapy in the diurnal rodent, *Arvicanthis niloticus,* leads to an increase in neuronal activity in the orexin neurons and in the dorsal raphe nucleus (but not the SCN) (Adidharma *et al.*, 2012). Moreover, the orexin receptor type 1 antagonist (SB-334867) prevents cFos induction in the dorsal raphe nucleus following this BLT protocol. Thus, an important role for these circadian-regulated metabolic peptides in mood and stress responsiveness is becoming appreciated.

CCK has long been associated with anxiety-related behavior. Increased CCK or CCK receptor agonists are generally associated with increased anxiety and these agonists are capable of producing panic attacks in people (Zwanzger *et al.*, 2012). Moreover, CCK receptor antagonists have antidepressant-like properties in animal models of depression (Hernando *et al.*, 1996; Becker *et al.*, 2008). Recently, CCK was identified as a direct transcriptional target of CLOCK in the VTA and *Clock*Δ19 mice have very low levels of CCK. CCK is coreleased with dopamine and acts to silence dopamine neurons. Thus, CCK may be important in the development of the manic-like phenotype of the *Clock*Δ19 mice.

17.8 Regulation of mood-related brain circuits by the SCN and circadian genes

The monoaminergic (i.e., serotonin (5-HT), dopamine (DA) and norephinephrine (NE)) hypothesis of mood regulation is largely based on the fact that antidepressant and mood stabilizing medications directly impact levels and release of these neuromodulators (reviewed in Delgado, 2004). For example, the major class of antidepressant drugs used today is selective serotonin reuptake inhibitors (SSRIs). Drugs of abuse like cocaine, morphine, alcohol and nicotine all lead to large increases in monoamine transmission, and dopamine and 5-HT are crucial for the rewarding or pleasurable properties of these drugs (Chapter 15). Moreover, subjects with mood disorders typically have altered neuronal circuitry involving these systems in brain imaging studies.

Numerous studies have found that 5HT, NE and DA all have a circadian rhythm in their levels, release, and synthesis related enzymes (reviewed in McClung, 2011). There are also circadian rhythms in the expression and activity of several of the receptors that bind these neurotransmitters, suggesting that these entire circuits are under circadian control. Since these systems are chiefly involved in arousal, motivation, and reward, it makes sense from an evolutionary prospective for these circuits to have a diurnal rhythm, so that the motivation to find a mate or look for food is not in temporal conflict with the drive for sleep. Some of the rhythms in these circuits arise from indirect connections with the SCN (Fig. 17.2). For example, an indirect projection from the SCN to the locus coeruleus appears to regulate the circadian rhythm in noradrenergic neuronal activity (Aston-Jones *et al.*, 2001). Moreover, the SCN indirectly projects to the VTA via the medial preoptic nucleus (MPON) (Luo and Aston-Jones, 2009).

All of these neuronal populations also express circadian genes, which may directly regulate expression of genes involved in monoamine synthesis and release. MAOA, a gene important in dopamine metabolism is a direct transcriptional target of NPAS2, BMAL1 and PER2 in the striatum (an area innervated by dopamine terminals from the VTA and substantia nigra) (Hampp *et al.*, 2008). Moreover,

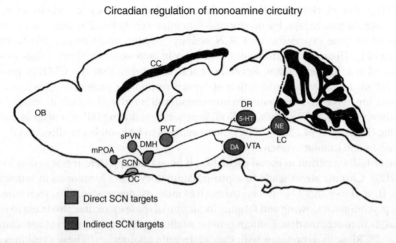

Circadian regulation of monoamine circuitry

Fig. 17.2 The circadian system regulates multiple monoaminergic brain regions that control mood, anxiety and motivated behaviors, through local expression of clock genes as well as indirect connections originating from the master pacemaker in the suprachiasmatic nucleus (SCN). The SCN projects monosynaptically to multiple hypothalamic nuclei (in blue), which subsequently communicate with regions (in red) that synthesize dopamine (DA), serotonin (5-HT) and norepinephrine (NE). As a result, serotonin, norepinephrine and dopamine all have a circadian rhythm in their levels, release, and synthesis-related enzymes. Abbreviations: medial preoptic area (mPOA), subparaventricular nucleus of the hypothalamus (sPVN), dorsomedial hypothalamus (DMH), paraventricular nucleus of the thalamus (PVT), dorsal raphe (DR), ventral tegmental area (VTA), locus coeruleus (LC), optic chiasm (OC), corpus callosum (CC), olfactory bulb (OB). (*See insert for color representation of the figure.*)

a mutation in *Per2* leads to increased dopamine levels and altered neuronal activity in the striatum, which may explain some of their abnormal behavioral phenotypes in measures of mood, reward and anxiety. In addition, *Per1* and *Per2* mRNA levels are altered in the ventral striatum (nucleus accumbens (NAc))in response to chronic stress and drugs of abuse. Selective knock-down of both *mPer1* and *mPer2* via RNA interference (RNAi) in the NAc is sufficient to produce an increase in anxiety, suggesting prominent roles for the *Per* genes outside of the SCN. *Clock*Δ19 mice have a profound increase in dopaminergic activity in the VTA. Further, many, but not all, of the manic-like phenotypes of the *Clock*Δ19 mice are rescued by expression of a functional CLOCK protein specifically in the VTA where dopamine neurons are prevalent (Roybal *et al.*, 2007). Interestingly, knock-down of Clock expression only in the VTA of otherwise wild-type mice leads to a "mixed state" where mice are less anxious and hyperactive but have greater levels of depression-related behavior (Mukherjee *et al.*, 2010). This is particularly interesting given the fact that bipolar subjects cycle through periods of depression and mania, but can also experience similar mixed states. The regulation of dopaminergic activity by CLOCK is so fundamental that even fruit flies with a mutation in the *Clock* gene (*Clk*[jrk]) have an increase in brain dopamine levels (Kumar *et al.*, 2012). Thus, circadian genes appear to have a prominent role in the VTA–NAc circuit as well as other monoaminergic regions in the regulation of anxiety and mood-related behavior.

17.9 Neuroinflammation

Alterations in the immune system are thought to underlie a number of health problems, including rheumatoid arthritis, autoimmune diseases, inflammatory bowel disease and asthma (Chapter 14). Circadian rhythm disruption leads to an increase in pro-inflammatory cytokines including TNF-α, macrophage inflammatory protein 2 (MIP-2) and leukemia inhibitory factor (LIF) in human and rodent studies (reviewed in Logan and Sarkar, 2012). In turn, pro-inflammatory cytokines, such as TNF-α, interferon (IFN)-γ, and interleukin 6 (IL-6), modulate the sleep–wake cycle and circadian gene expression via NF-κB signaling pathways. Furthermore, a lipopolysaccharide (LPS)-induced immune challenge modulates circadian gene expression and SCN activity (Beynon and Coogan, 2010). Interestingly, a central infusion of IL-1β causes a significant phase delay in locomotor rhythms, a state often associated with an increased risk for depression. Recently, it was discovered that the CLOCK protein interacts directly with NF-κB to activate transcription at NF-κB responsive promoters (Spengler *et al.*, 2012). Moreover, activation of NF-κB in response to immunostimuli is reduced in cells in which *Clock* has been knocked-out. Interestingly, RORα inhibits NF-κB function by inducing IκB-α, a protein that antagonizes NF-κB signaling (Delerive *et al.*, 2001). Thus, there appears to be complex bi-directional cross talk between the circadian and immune systems.

A role for neuroinflammation in mood regulation is becoming apparent (reviewed in Krishnadas and Cavanagh, 2012)). Chronic stress leads to a pro-inflammatory state. Moreover, in humans, cytokines, such as IL-1β, IL-6, IFN-γ and TNF-α, can themselves induce a depression-like syndrome with feelings of anhedonia, psychomotor slowing and fatigue. Induction of these cytokines also leads to robust depression-like behavior in rodent models. Human genetic studies have found significant associations between TNF-a, IL-6 and CRP with depression with candidate gene approaches. These cytokines are hypothesized to enter the brain through several different humoral, neural, and cellular pathways (reviewed in Eyre and Baune, 2012)). Pro-inflammatory cytokines in the brain lead to reduced neurogenesis, synaptic plasticity, andlong-term potentiation(LTP) in the hippocampus, which is similar to effects often seen with chronic stress. They can also impact monoamine signaling, leading to reductions in 5-HT and DA release, as well as altered HPA axis function. Thus, a scenario could be proposed where genetic or environmental disruptions of circadian rhythms lead to a pro-inflammatory response in the brain, which alters monoamine signaling, SCN function, and neuroplasticity, ultimately leading to a depression-like state.

Certain antidepressant medications do appear to reduce neuroinflammation. However, there is little clinical evidence to suggest that anti-inflammatory drugs themselves are efficacious in the treatment of depression. In fact, some studies find that drugs like ibuprofen can actually hinder the effects of antidepressants. Records from the STAR*D trial (a large multicenter study of antidepressant efficacy) found that the remission rate fell from 54% to 40% in patients taking SSRIs when they were also taking an anti-inflammatory drug (Warner-Schmidt *et al.*, 2011). Thus the role of a pro-inflammatory response in the development of depression is still far from clear.

17.10 Cell cycle regulation/neurogenesis

While most parts of the brain do not generate new neurons after development, the dentate gyrus of the hippocampus is consistently producing new cells throughout adulthood. The neurogenic hypothesis of depression stems from animal studies showing that chronic stress reduces hippocampal neurogenesis while antidepressants enhance neurogenesis (reviewed in Tang *et al.*, 2012). While studies have been mixed regarding the role of neurogenesis in the development of depression, most point towards a significant role for neurogenesis in the therapeutic effects of antidepressants. Hippocampal neurons have molecular rhythms in circadian gene expression and neurogenesis varies over the circadian cycle (Guzman-Marin *et al.*, 2007; Gilhooley *et al.*, 2011). The molecular clock directly regulates many genes involved in cell cycle regulation including c-Myc, P21, XPA, and Wee1 (Sancar *et al.*, 2010; Chapter 12). Moreover, chronic disruption in circadian rhythms via weekly phase shifts inhibits hippocampal neurogenesis; the degree of reduction in neurogenesis depends upon the direction and duration of the shifts (Kott *et al.*, 2012). Furthermore, circadian rhythms in cotricosterone are necessary for proper BDNF signaling and the proliferation of progenitor cells in the dentate gyrus in response to the antidepressant, fluoxetine (Huang and Herbert, 2006). These results suggest that the diurnal rhythm of corticosterone regulates the stimulating action of antidepressants on neurogenesis in the dentate gyrus. This might be mediated by circadian gene expression in the hippocampus, but more work needs to be done in this area.

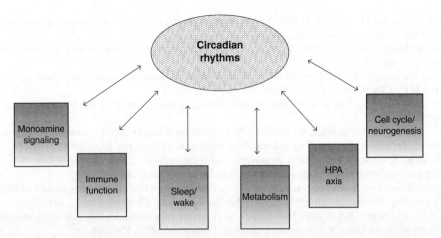

Fig. 17.3 Multiple hypotheses have been put forth in an attempt to understand the development of mood disorders. Circadian rhythm disruptions (both genetic and environmental) have an impact on virtually all of the systems that are thought to underlie mood regulation. In turn, the systems tend to influence the circadian clock leading to bidirectional regulation.

17.11 Conclusions

Though lots of work remains, our understanding of the circadian clock and how it is involved in the development of mood disorders has come a long way from the initial hypotheses put forth in the 1960s and 1970s. We know considerably more about molecular rhythms and how they are regulated. We also now know that circadian genes are not only found in the SCN, but rather they are expressed widely throughout the brain and body. They appear to have some independent functions outside of the central clock in various brain regions. Multiple pathways which are hypothesized to underlie the development of depression and other mood disorders are strongly influenced by the circadian system (Fig. 17.3). The SCN sends outputs to mood-related regions of the brain both through indirect neuronal projections and by circulating peptides and hormones. Ongoing clinical studies are beginning to determine the specific types of rhythm disruptions that occur in people with mood disorders on an individual basis and how these relate to the pathophysiology of their particular disease. This is part of a greater trend towards personalized medicine. Moreover, our understanding of how antidepressant and mood stabilizing drugs work is developing and should allow more targeted approaches to treatment in the future. The development of new compounds that alter rhythms in specific ways is very exciting and holds a lot of promise for the treatment of multiple diseases including mood disorders.

Acknowledgement

I would like to acknowledge Dr Trey Williams for assistance with the figures.

References

Major depressive disorder working group of the psychiatric GWAS consortium (2013). A mega-analysis of genome-wide association studies for major depressive disorder. *Mol Psychiatry* **18**(4):497–511.

Abarca, C., Albrecht, U., and Spanagel, R. (2002). Cocaine sensitization and reward are under the influence of circadian genes and rhythm. *Proc Natl Acad Sci USA* **99**, 9026–30.

Abe, T., Inoue, Y., Komada, Y., *et al.* (2011). Relation between morningness-eveningness score and depressive symptoms among patients with delayed sleep phase syndrome. *Sleep Med* **12**, 680–4.

Adidharma, W., Leach, G., and Yan, L. (2012). Orexinergic signaling mediates light-induced neuronal activation in the dorsal raphe nucleus. *Neuroscience* **220**, 201–7.

Antle, M.C. and Mistlberger, R.E. (2000). Circadian clock resetting by sleep deprivation without exercise in the Syrian hamster. *J Neurosci* **20**, 9326–32.

Arey, R. and McClung, C.A. (2012). An inhibitor of casein kinase 1 epsilon/delta partially normalizes the manic-like behaviors of the ClockDelta19 mouse. *Behav Pharmacol* **23**, 392–6.

Aston-Jones, G., Chen, S., Zhu, Y., and Oshinsky, M.L. (2001). A neural circuit for circadian regulation of arousal. *Nature Neurosci* **4**, 732–8.

Badura, L., Swanson, T., Adamowicz, W., *et al.* (2007). An inhibitor of casein kinase I epsilon induces phase delays in circadian rhythms under free-running and entrained conditions. *J Pharmacol Exp Ther* **322**, 730–8.

Becker, C., Zeau, B., Rivat, C., *et al.* (2008). Repeated social defeat-induced depression-like behavioral and biological alterations in rats: involvement of cholecystokinin. *Mol Psychiatry* **13**, 1079–92.

Benedetti, F., Dallaspezia, S., Fulgosi, M. C., *et al.* (2007). Phase advance is an actimetric correlate of antidepressant response to sleep deprivation and light therapy in bipolar depression. *Chronobiol Int* **24**, 921–37.

Beynon, A.L. and Coogan, A.N. (2010). Diurnal, age, and immune regulation of interleukin-1beta and interleukin-1 type 1 receptor in the mouse suprachiasmatic nucleus. *Chronobiol Int* **27**, 1546–63.

Buckley, T.M. and Schatzberg, A.F. (2010). A pilot study of the phase angle between cortisol and melatonin in major depression - a potential biomarker? *J Psychiatr Res* **44**, 69–74.

Chen, Z., Yoo, S.H., Park, Y.S., *et al.* (2012). Identification of diverse modulators of central and peripheral circadian clocks by high-throughput chemical screening. *Proc Natl Acad Sci USA* **109**, 101–6.

Cho, H., Zhao, X., Hatori, M., *et al.* (2012). Regulation of circadian behaviour and metabolism by REV-ERB-alpha and REV-ERB-beta. *Nature* **485**, 123–7.

Cuesta, M., Mendoza, J., Clesse, D., *et al.* (2008). Serotonergic activation potentiates light resetting of the main circadian clock and alters clock gene expression in a diurnal rodent. *Exp Neurol* **210**, 501–13.

Danilenko, K.V., Putilov, A. A., Russkikh, G. S., *et al.* (1994). Diurnal and seasonal variations of melatonin and serotonin in women with seasonal affective disorder. *Arctic Med Res* **53**, 137–45.

De Berardis, D., Di Iorio, G., Acciavatti, T., *et al.* (2011). The emerging role of melatonin agonists in the treatment of major depression: focus on agomelatine. *CNS Neurol Disord Drug Targets* **10**, 119–32.

Delerive, P., Monte, D., Dubois, G., *et al.* (2001). The orphan nuclear receptor ROR alpha is a negative regulator of the inflammatory response. *EMBO Rep* **2**, 42–8.

Delgado, P.L. (2004). How antidepressants help depression: mechanisms of action and clinical response. *J Clin Psychiatry* **65**(Suppl 4), 25–30.

Dong, L., Bilbao, A., Laucht, M., *et al.* (2011). Effects of the circadian rhythm gene period 1 (per1) on psychosocial stress-induced alcohol drinking. *Am J Psychiatry* **168**, 1090–8.

Easton, A., Arbuzova, J., and Turek, F.W. (2003). The circadian Clock mutation increases exploratory activity and escape-seeking behavior. *Genes Brain Behav* **2**, 11–9.

Ehlers, C.L., Frank, E., and Kupfer, D.J. (1988). Social zeitgebers and biological rhythms. A unified approach to understanding the etiology of depression. *Arch Gen Psychiatry* **45**, 948–52.

Emens, J., Lewy, A., Kinzie, J.M., *et al.* (2009). Circadian misalignment in major depressive disorder. *Psychiatry Res* **168**, 259–61.

Etain, B., Milhiet, V., Bellivier, F., and Leboyer, M. (2011). Genetics of circadian rhythms and mood spectrum disorders. *Eur Neuropsychopharmacol* **21**(Suppl 4), S676–82.

Eyre, H. and Baune, B.T. (2012). Neuroimmunomodulation in unipolar depression: a focus on chronobiology and chronotherapeutics. *J Neural Transm* **119**, 1147–66.

Frank, E., Swartz, H. A., and Kupfer, D.J. (2000). Interpersonal and social rhythm therapy: managing the chaos of bipolar disorder. *Biol Psychiatry* **48**, 593–604.

Frank, E., Kupfer, D.J., Thase, M.E., *et al.* (2005). Two-year outcomes for interpersonal and social rhythm therapy in individuals with bipolar I disorder. *Arch Gen Psychiatry* **62**, 996–1004.

Frodl, T. and O'Keane, V. (2012). How does the brain deal with cumulative stress? A review with focus on developmental stress, HPA axis function and hippocampal structure in humans. *Neurobiol Dis* **52**, 24–37.

Giedke, H. and Schwarzler, F. (2002). Therapeutic use of sleep deprivation in depression. *Sleep Med Rev* **6**, 361–77.

Gilhooley, M. J., Pinnock, S.B., and Herbert, J. (2011). Rhythmic expression of per1 in the dentate gyrus is suppressed by corticosterone: implications for neurogenesis. *Neurosci Lett* **489**, 177–81.

Guzman-Marin, R., Suntsova, N., Bashir, T., *et al.* (2007). Cell proliferation in the dentate gyrus of the adult rat fluctuates with the light-dark cycle. *Neurosci Lett* **422**, 198–201.

Halberg, F. (1968). Physiological considerations underlying rhythmometry with special reference to emotional illness. In: Cycles Biologiques et Psychiatrie (ed. J. de Ajuriaguerra). Masson et Cie, Paris.

Hampp, G., Ripperger, J.A., Houben, T., *et al.* (2008). Regulation of monoamine oxidase A by circadian-clock components implies clock influence on mood. *Curr Biol* **18**, 678–83.

Hannibal, J., Hsiung, H.M., and Fahrenkrug, J. (2011). Temporal phasing of locomotor activity, heart rate rhythmicity, and core body temperature is disrupted in VIP receptor 2-deficient mice. *Am J Physiol Regul Integr Comp Physiol* **300**, R519–30.

Hernando, F., Fuentes, J. A., Fournie-Zaluski, M.C., *et al.* (1996). Antidepressant-like effects of CCK(B) receptor antagonists: involvement of the opioid system. *Eur J Pharmacol* **318**, 221–9.

Hirota, T., Lewis, W.G., Liu, A.C., *et al.* (2008). A chemical biology approach reveals period shortening of the mammalian circadian clock by specific inhibition of GSK-3beta. *Proc Natl Acad Sci USA* **105**, 20746–51.

Hirota, T., Lee, J.W., St John, P., *et al.* (2012). Identification of small molecule activators of cryptochrome. *Science* **337**, 1094–7.

Huang, G.J. and Herbert, J. (2006). Stimulation of neurogenesis in the hippocampus of the adult rat by fluoxetine requires rhythmic change in corticosterone. *Biol Psychiatry* **59**, 619–24.

Jauhar, P. and Weller, M.P. (1982). Psychiatric morbidity and time zone changes: a study of patients from Heathrow airport. *Br J Psychiatry* **140**, 231–5.

Johansson, A.S., Brask, J., Owe-Larsson, B., *et al.* (2011). Valproic acid phase shifts the rhythmic expression of Period2::Luciferase. *J Biol Rhythms* **26**, 541–51.

Keers, R., Pedroso, I., Breen, G., *et al.* (2012). Reduced anxiety and depression-like behaviours in the circadian period mutant mouse afterhours. *PLoS One* **7**, e38263.

Kim, Y.I., Choi, H.J., and Colwell, C.S. (2006). Brain-derived neurotrophic factor regulation of N-methyl-D-aspartate receptor-mediated synaptic currents in suprachiasmatic nucleus neurons. *J Neurosci Res* **84**, 1512–20.

King, D.P., Zhao, Y., Sangoram, A.M., *et al.* (1997). Positional cloning of the mouse circadian clock gene. *Cell* **89**, 641–53.

Kott, J., Leach, G., and Yan, L. (2012). Direction-dependent effects of chronic "jet-lag" on hippocampal neurogenesis. *Neurosci Lett* **515**, 177–80.

Kripke, D.F. (1984) Critical interval hypothesis for depression. *Chronobiol Int* **1**, 73–80.

Kripke, D.F., Mullaney, D.J., Atkinson, M., and Wolf, S. (1978). Circadian rhythm disorders in manic-depressives. *Biol Psychiatry* **13**, 335–51.

Krishnadas, R. and Cavanagh, J. (2012). Depression: an inflammatory illness? *J Neurol Neurosurg Psychiatry* **83**, 495–502.

Kronfeld-Schor, N. and Einat, H. (2012). Circadian rhythms and depression: human psychopathology and animal models. *Neuropharmacology* **62**, 101–14.

Kumar, S., Chen, D., and Sehgal, A. (2012). Dopamine acts through Cryptochrome to promote acute arousal in Drosophila. *Genes Dev* **26**, 1224–34.

Lewy, A.J., Wehr, T.A., Goodwin, F.K., *et al.* (1981). Manic-depressive patients may be supersensitive to light. *Lancet* **1**, 383–4.

Lewy, A.J., Lefler, B.J., Emens, J.S., and Bauer, V.K. (2006). The circadian basis of winter depression. *Proc Natl Acad Sci USA* **103**, 7414–9.

Lewy, A.J., Emens, J.S., Songer, J.B., *et al.* (2009). Winter Depression: Integrating mood, circadian rhythms, and the sleep–wake and light/dark cycles into a bio-psycho-social-environmental model. *Sleep Med Clin* **4**, 285–99.

Li, J.D., Hu, W.P., and Zhou, Q.Y. (2009). Disruption of the circadian output molecule prokineticin 2 results in anxiolytic and antidepressant-like effects in mice. *Neuropsychopharmacology* **34**, 367–73.

Li, J., Lu, W.Q., Beesley, S., *et al.* (2012). Lithium impacts on the amplitude and period of the molecular circadian clockwork. *PLoS One* **7**, e33292.

Libert, S., Pointer, K., Bell, E.L., *et al.* (2011). SIRT1 activates MAO-A in the brain to mediate anxiety and exploratory drive. *Cell* **147**, 1459–72.

Liu, A.C., Tran, H.G., Zhang, E.E., *et al.* (2008). Redundant function of REV-ERBalpha and beta and non-essential role for Bmal1 cycling in transcriptional regulation of intracellular circadian rhythms. *PLoS Genet* **4**, e1000023.

Logan, R.W. and Sarkar, D.K. (2012). Circadian nature of immune function. *Mol Cell Endocrinol* **349**, 82–90.

Luo, A.H. and Aston-Jones, G. (2009). Circuit projection from suprachiasmatic nucleus to ventral tegmental area: a novel circadian output pathway. *Eur J Neurosci* **29**, 748–60.

Malkoff-Schwartz, S., Frank, E., Anderson, B., *et al.* (1998). Stressful life events and social rhythm disruption in the onset of manic and depressive bipolar episodes: a preliminary investigation. *Arch Gen Psychiatry* **55**, 702–7.

Manda, K. and Reiter, R.J. (2010). Melatonin maintains adult hippocampal neurogenesis and cognitive functions after irradiation. *Prog Neurobiol* **90**, 60–8.

McCarthy, M.J., Nievergelt, C.M., Kelsoe, J.R., and Welsh, D.K. (2012). A survey of genomic studies supports association of circadian clock genes with bipolar disorder spectrum illnesses and lithium response. *PLoS One* **7**, e32091.

McClung, C.A. (2007). Circadian genes, rhythms and the biology of mood disorders. *Pharmacol Ther* **114**, 222–32.

McClung, C.A. (2011). Circadian rhythms and mood regulation: insights from pre-clinical models. *Eur Neuropsychopharmacol* **21**(Suppl 4), S683–93.

McClung, C.A., Sidiropoulou, K., Vitaterna, M., *et al.* (2005). Regulation of dopaminergic transmission and cocaine reward by the Clock gene. *Proc Natl Acad Sci USA* **102**, 9377–81.

Meng, Q.J., Maywood, E.S., Bechtold, D.A., *et al.* (2010). Entrainment of disrupted circadian behavior through inhibition of casein kinase 1 (CK1) enzymes. *Proc Natl Acad Sci USA* **107**, 15240–5.

Michel, S., Clark, J.P., Ding, J.M., and Colwell, C.S. (2006). Brain-derived neurotrophic factor and neurotrophin receptors modulate glutamate-induced phase shifts of the suprachiasmatic nucleus. *Eur J Neurosci* **24**, 1109–16.

Molteni, R., Calabrese, F., Pisoni, S., *et al.* (2010). Synergistic mechanisms in the modulation of the neurotrophin BDNF in the rat prefrontal cortex following acute agomelatine administration. *World J Biol Psychiatry* **11**, 148–53.

Mukherjee, S., Coque, L., Cao, J.L., *et al.* (2010). Knockdown of Clock in the ventral tegmental area through RNA interference results in a mixed state of mania and depression-like behavior. *Biol Psychiatry* **68**, 503–11.

Nagayama, H. (1996). Chronic administration of imipramine and lithium changes the phase-angle relationship between the activity and core body temperature circadian rhythms in rats. *Chronobiol Int* **13**, 251–9.

Naylor, E., Bergmann, B.M., Krauski, K., *et al.* (2000). The circadian clock mutation alters sleep homeostasis in the mouse. *J Neurosci* **20**, 8138–43.

Ogaya, M., Kim, J., and Sasaki, K. (2011). Ghrelin postsynaptically depolarizes dorsal raphe neurons in rats in vitro. *Peptides* **32**, 1606–16.

Ozburn, A.R., Larson, E.B., Self, D.W., and McClung, C.A. (2012). Cocaine self-administration behaviors in ClockDelta19 mice. *Psychopharmacology (Berl)* **223**, 169–77.

Pandey, A., Davis, N.A., White, B.C., *et al.* (2012). Epistasis network centrality analysis yields pathway replication across two GWAS cohorts for bipolar disorder. *Transl Psychiatry* **2**, e154.

Pandi-Perumal, S.R., Srinivasan, V., Maestroni, G.J., *et al.* (2006). Melatonin: Nature's most versatile biological signal? *FEBS J* **273**, 2813–38.

Papousek, M. (1975). Chronobiologische Aspekte der Zyklothymie. *Fortschr Neurol Psychiatr* **43**, 381–440.

Perreau-Lenz, S., Vengeliene, V., Noori, H.R., *et al.* (2012). Inhibition of the casein-kinase-1-epsilon/delta prevents relapse-like alcohol drinking. *Neuropsychopharmacology* **37**, 2121–31.

Pigeon, W.R., Hegel, M., Unutzer, J., *et al.* (2008). Is insomnia a perpetuating factor for late-life depression in the IMPACT cohort? *Sleep* **31**, 481–8.

Pflug, B. (1976) The effect of sleep deprivation on depressed patients. *Acta Psychiat Scand* **53**, 148–58.

Pflug, B. and Tolle, R. (1971) Therapy of endogenous depression by sleep deprivation: practical and theoretical considerations. *Nervenarzt* **42**, 117–24.

Prickaerts, J., Moechars, D., Cryns, K., *et al.* (2006). Transgenic mice overexpressing glycogen synthase kinase 3beta: a putative model of hyperactivity and mania. *J Neurosci* **26**, 9022–9.

Ramirez-Rodriguez, G., Klempin, F., Babu, H., *et al.* (2009). Melatonin modulates cell survival of new neurons in the hippocampus of adult mice. *Neuropsychopharmacology* **34**, 2180–91.

Robillard, R., Naismith, S.L., Rogers, N.L., *et al.* (2012). Delayed sleep phase in young people with unipolar or bipolar affective disorders. *J Affect Disord* **145**(2):260–3.

Roybal, K., Theobold, D., Graham, A., *et al.* (2007). Mania-like behavior induced by disruption of CLOCK. *Proc Natl Acad Sci USA* **104**, 6406–11.

Sancar, A., Lindsey-Boltz, L.A., Kang, T.H., *et al.* (2010). Circadian clock control of the cellular response to DNA damage. *FEBS Lett* **584**, 2618–25.

Schellekens, H., Finger, B.C., Dinan, T.G., and Cryan, J.F. (2012). Ghrelin signalling and obesity: at the interface of stress, mood and food reward. *Pharmacol Ther* **135**, 316–26.

Schulte, W. (1966). Kombinierte Psycho und Pharmakotherapie bei melancholikern: In: Probleme der pharmakopsychiatrichen kombinations und langzeitbehandlung (eds H.H. Kranz and N. Petrilowitsch). Rothenburger Gesparach, Karger, pp. 150–69.

Seggie, J., Canny, C., Mai, F., *et al.* (1989). Antidepressant medication reverses increased sensitivity to light in depression: preliminary report. *Prog Neuropsychopharmacol Biol Psychiatry* **13**, 537–41.

Sokolski, K.N., Reist, C., Chen, C.C., and DeMet, E.M. (1995). Antidepressant responses and changes in visual adaptation after sleep deprivation. *Psychiatry Res* **57**, 197–207.

Son, G.H., Chung, S., and Kim, K. (2011). The adrenal peripheral clock: glucocorticoid and the circadian timing system. *Front Neuroendocrinol* **32**, 451–65.

Souetre, E., Salvati, E., Rix, H., *et al.* (1988a). Effect of recovery on the cortisol circadian rhythm of depressed patients. *Biol Psychiatry* **24**, 336–40.

Souetre, E., Salvati, E., Wehr, T.A., *et al.* (1988b). Twenty-four-hour profiles of body temperature and plasma TSH in bipolar patients during depression and during remission and in normal control subjects. *Am J Psychiatry* **145**, 1133–7.

Spanagel, R., Pendyala, G., Abarca, C., *et al.* (2005). The clock gene Per2 influences the glutamatergic system and modulates alcohol consumption. *Nat Med* **11**, 35–42.

Spencer, S., Falcon, E., Kumar, J., *et al.* (2013). Circadian genes Period 1 and Period 2 in the nucleus accumbens regulate anxiety-related behavior. *Eur J Neurosci* **37**(2):242–50.

Spengler, M L., Kuropatwinski, K.K., Comas, M., *et al.* (2012). Core circadian protein CLOCK is a positive regulator of NF-kappaB-mediated transcription. *Proc Natl Acad Sci USA* **109**, E2457–65.

Sprouse, J., Braselton, J., and Reynolds, L. (2006). Fluoxetine modulates the circadian biological clock via phase advances of suprachiasmatic nucleus neuronal firing. *Biol Psychiatry* **60**, 896–9.

Sprouse, J., Reynolds, L., Swanson, T.A., and Engwall, M. (2009). Inhibition of casein kinase I epsilon/delta produces phase shifts in the circadian rhythms of Cynomolgus monkeys. *Psychopharmacology (Berl)* **204**, 735–42.

Sprouse, J., Reynolds, L., Kleiman, R., *et al.* (2010). Chronic treatment with a selective inhibitor of casein kinase I delta/epsilon yields cumulative phase delays in circadian rhythms. *Psychopharmacology (Berl)* **210**, 569–76.

Tang, S.W., Helmeste, D., and Leonard, B. (2012). Is neurogenesis relevant in depression and in the mechanism of antidepressant drug action? A critical review. *World J Biol Psychiatry* **13**, 402–12.

Tataroglu, O., Aksoy, A., Yilmaz, A., and Canbeyli, R. (2004). Effect of lesioning the suprachiasmatic nuclei on behavioral despair in rats. *Brain Res* **1001**, 118–24.

Tuma, J., Strubbe, J.H., Mocaer, E., and Koolhaas, J.M. (2005). Anxiolytic-like action of the antidepressant agomelatine (S 20098) after a social defeat requires the integrity of the SCN. *Eur Neuropsychopharmacol* **15**, 545–55.

Turek, F.W., Joshu, C., Kohsaka, A., *et al.* (2005). Obesity and metabolic syndrome in circadian Clock mutant mice. *Science* **308**, 1043–5.

Vitaterna, M.H., Ko, C.H., Chang, A.M., *et al.* (2006). The mouse Clock mutation reduces circadian pacemaker amplitude and enhances efficacy of resetting stimuli and phase-response curve amplitude. *Proc Natl Acad Sci USA* **103**, 9327–32.

Warner-Schmidt, J.L., Vanover, K.E., Chen, E.Y., *et al.* (2011). Antidepressant effects of selective serotonin reuptake inhibitors (SSRIs) are attenuated by antiinflammatory drugs in mice and humans. *Proc Natl Acad Sci USA* **108**, 9262–7.

Wehr, T.A., Wirz-Justice, A., Goodwin, F.K., *et al.* (1979). Phase advance of the circadian sleep-wake cycle as an antidepressant. *Science* **206**, 710–3.

Wehr, T.A., Duncan, W.C. Jr., Sher, L., *et al.* (2001). A circadian signal of change of season in patients with seasonal affective disorder. *Arch Gen Psychiatry* **58**, 1108–14.

Wirz-Justice, A. (2006). Biological rhythm disturbances in mood disorders. *Int Clin Psychopharmacol* **21**(Suppl 1), S11–5.

Wirz-Justice, A. and Terman, M. (2012). Chronotherapeutics (light and wake therapy) as a class of interventions for affective disorders. *Handb Clin Neurol* **106**, 697–713.

Wittmann, M., Dinich, J., Merrow, M., and Roenneberg, T. (2006). Social jetlag: misalignment of biological and social time. *Chronobiol Int* **23**, 497–509.

Wu, J.C., Kelsoe, J.R., Schachat, C., *et al.* (2009). Rapid and sustained antidepressant response with sleep deprivation and chronotherapy in bipolar disorder. *Biol Psychiatry* **66**, 298–301.

Wulff, K., Gatti, S., Wettstein, J.G., and Foster, R.G. (2010). Sleep and circadian rhythm disruption in psychiatric and neurodegenerative disease. *Nat Rev Neurosci* **11**, 589–99.

Yin, L., Wang, J., Klein, P.S., and Lazar, M.A. (2006). Nuclear receptor Rev-erbalpha is a critical lithium-sensitive component of the circadian clock. *Science* **311**, 1002–5.

Zwanzger, P., Domschke, K., and Bradwejn, J. (2012). Neuronal network of panic disorder: the role of the neuropeptide cholecystokinin. *Depress Anxiety* **29**, 762–74.

Sleep and Circadian Rhythm Disruption in Psychosis

18

Stuart N. Peirson and Russell G. Foster

Nuffield Department of Clinical Neurosciences (Nuffield Laboratory of Ophthalmology), John Radcliffe Hospital, Oxford, UK

18.1 Introduction

Circadian rhythms are near-24-hour cycles in physiology and behavior that occur in nearly all life on Earth. These internally-generated rhythms persist in the absence of external time cues, enabling an organism to anticipate the predictably changing environment rather than passively responding to it. Here the basic mechanisms underlying mammalian circadian rhythms are considered, before considering perhaps the most familiar such rhythm – the sleep–wake cycle.

In mammals, the primary circadian pacemaker is located in the suprachiasmatic nuclei (SCN) of the anterior hypothalamus (Chapter 3). The SCN regulate circadian rhythms in locomotor activity and coordinate circadian rhythms throughout the body via neural, hormonal and behavioral signals (Albrecht, 2012). Rhythmic SCN neuronal activity is synchronized (*entrained*) to the external light–dark cycle as a result of light detected by retinal photoreceptors and conveyed to the SCN via the retinohypothalamic tract (RHT). These photoreceptors include the classical rods and cones, as well as the recently identified photosensitive retinal ganglion cells (pRGCs) expressing the photopigment melanopsin (Hughes *et al.*, 2012). In addition to neuronal rhythms within the SCN, circadian oscillators occur in other regions of the brain (Guilding and Piggins, 2007) as well as other organs and tissues throughout the body (Fig. 18.1a). However, communication between these independent cellular networks is necessary to ensure that they are aligned to an appropriate circadian phase. Rhythms in many peripheral tissues dampen rapidly when isolated, as their constituent individual cellular oscillators become desynchronized (Albrecht, 2012).

Intracellular rhythms are the product of a transcriptional-translational feedback loop (TTFL), involving a number of core clock genes (Chapters 2 and 3). This mechanism is depicted in Fig. 18.1b, and briefly summarized below. Whilst space precludes a detailed overview of this molecular mechanism, this involves a core loop comprised of CLOCK:BMAL1 dimers which bind to E-box elements to drive the expression of *Period* (*Per*) and *Cryptochrome* (*Cry*) transcription. PER and CRY proteins form homo- and hetero-dimers which undergo various posttranslational modifications before re-entering the nucleus and inhibiting the CLOCK:BMAL1 transcriptional drive. In addition, an auxiliary loop involving RORα and REV-ERBα regulate the expression of *Bmal1* via retinoic acid receptor-related orphan receptor-binding elements (RRE), stabilizing the core oscillator loop. This core clock mechanism is linked into other cellular processes via the regulation of clock-controlled genes (CCGs). These do not form part of

Circadian Medicine, First Edition. Edited by Christopher S. Colwell.
© 2015 John Wiley & Sons, Inc. Published 2015 by John Wiley & Sons, Inc.

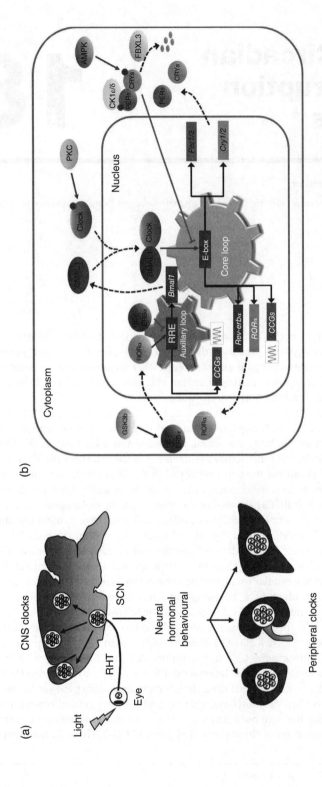

Fig. 18.1 The mammalian circadian system and the molecular clock. (a) The mammalian circadian system consists of intracellular oscillators found in both central nervous system and peripheral tissues throughout the body. These clocks are synchronized via neural, hormonal and behavioral time cues. The central circadian pacemaker is located in the suprachiasmatic nuclei (SCN) in the hypothalamus, which is entrained to the external light–dark cycle via light detected by retinal photoreceptors and conveyed via the retinohypothalamic tract (RHT). These peripheral clocks provide temporal regulation of local physiology. (b) Intracellular circadian oscillations are the product of a transcriptional-translational feedback loop (TTFL) comprised of core clock genes. This involves two interloping feedback loops – a core loop consisting of *Clock*, *Bmal1*, *Per1-2* and *Cry1-2* and auxiliary loop consisting of *Rev-erbα* and *Rorα* driving *Bmal1* expression. Various posttranslational modifications regulate the rate of the TTFL. Disruption of the components making up the TTFL may result in a change in circadian period (*tau*) or even complete arrhythmia. (TTFL figure based on that of Son et al., 2011). (*See insert for color representation of the figure.*)

the core oscillator mechanism, but provide outputs by which tissue-specific cellular processes can be temporally regulated.

The regular cycle of sleep and wakefulness is perhaps the most obvious 24-hour rhythm. Sleep is regulated by a range of internal and external drivers, most notably homeostatic and circadian processes (Chapter 4). The homeostatic process describes the increase in the requirement for sleep as a function of the duration of wakefulness. As a result, prolonged wakefulness gives rise to an increasing drive for sleep. By contrast, the circadian process provides a rhythmic drive for wakefulness and the active maintenance of sleep. The correct phasing of these two processes is therefore necessary for normal sleep (Fig. 18.2). Whilst there has been considerable progress in our understanding of the circadian system, far less is known regarding the molecular and cellular processes underlying sleep homeostasis and its interaction with the circadian timing system. Sleep is a complex physiological process involving the interaction of multiple neurotransmitter systems and a diverse network of both arousal and sleep-promoting brain nuclei (Fig. 18.2). This coordinated neural activity drives alternating patterns of behavior characterized by changes in rest/activity, body posture and responsiveness to stimuli (Tobler, 1995).

18.2 Psychosis

Psychosis is a term applied to a range of conditions characterized by a loss of contact with reality, typically presenting with delusions and/or hallucinations. Diagnosis of psychosis is based upon a range of criteria set out in the Diagnostic and Statistical Manual of Mental Disorders IV (DSM-IV) and the 10th International Classification of Diseases (ICD-10). These criteria include duration; dysfunction; associated substance abuse; the nature of the delusions; presence of depression or mania; and the presence of other somatic disorders. In the DSM-IV, for example, this gives rise to four broad categories: (i) nonaffective psychotic disorders, including schizophrenia and schizoaffective disorder; (ii) affective psychosis, including bipolar disorder with psychotic features and major depressive disorders with psychotic features; (iii) substance induced psychotic disorders, including alcohol- or drug-induced psychosis; and (iv) psychotic disorder due to a general medical condition (van Os and Kapur, 2009).

It has been suggested that the fundamental defect underlying psychosis may be an abnormality of attention and sensorimotor gating. This stimulus salience model emphasizes the role of attention in determining the importance of internally- and externally-generated stimuli. When this process is affected, inappropriate relevance is attached to such stimuli, resulting in delusions due to abnormal interpretation of thought processes, or paranoia due to abnormal interpretation of the external environment or misattribution of internal thoughts to an external source (Kapur, 2003; Kapur *et al.*, 2005). This model provides an important framework for the study of psychosis, especially in rodent models. Whilst it is not possible to study hallucinations and delusions in animal models, attention and sensorimotor gating can be readily measured using a range of behavioral assays.

18.2.1 The psychosis spectrum

This chapter focuses primarily on schizophrenia and bipolar disorder. However, as described above these disorders form part of a broader psychosis spectrum. This may be depicted as a group of personality traits including mood elevation/instability, anxiety/neuroticism and paranoia/abnormal salience, which occur as a continuum within the general population (Fig. 18.3). The presence of these traits places an individual at risk of developing illness. Such a model may account for the range of subtypes of psychotic disorder, as well as the complex genetic and environmental contributions to these disorders, which may account for why individuals who may be at risk of illness never go on to develop psychosis. The extent of the different traits will determine whether an individual is diagnosed as having bipolar disorder – characterized by mood elevation and instability (affective psychosis) – or schizophrenia – characterized by paranoia and abnormal salience (nonaffective psychosis). Whilst it is difficult to review the existing literature without resorting to the division of psychoses into conditions such as schizophrenia and bipolar disorder, consideration of psychosis as a spectrum of severity and type may provide a greater understanding of the traits which are associated with features such as sleep and circadian rhythm disruption (SCRD).

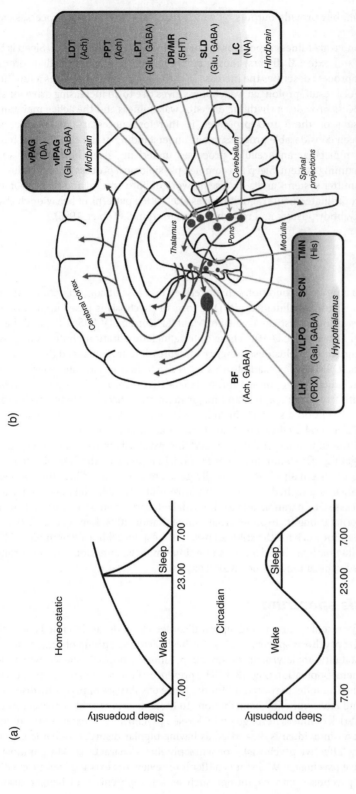

Fig. 18.2 Mechanisms involved in the regulation of sleep. (a) The homeostatic drive for sleep increases sleep propensity with prolonged wakefulness. Sleep pressure declines following sleep but increases again at waking. The circadian regulation of sleep creates a drive for wakefulness during the day, which declines at night. As such, sleep propensity is low during the day, but increases at night. (Figure based on that of Borbely, 1982.) (b) Sleep is the product of multiple brain regions and neurotransmitters. Abbreviations for brain regions: BF = Basal forebrain; DR/MR = Dorsal/medial raphe nucleus; LC = Locus coeruleus; LDT = Laterodorsal tegmental nuclei; LH = Lateral hypothalamus; LPT = Lateral pontine tegmentum; PPT = Pedunculopontine tegmental nuclei; SCN = Suprachiasmatic nuclei; SLD = Sublaterodorsal nucleus; TMN = Tuberomammillary nucleus; VLPO = Ventrolateral preoptic nuclei; vPAG = Ventral periaqueductal grey; vlPAG = Ventrolateral periaqueductal grey. Abbreviations for neurotransmitters: 5HT = Serotonin; Ach = Acetylcholine; DA = Dopamine; GABA = γ-Aminobutyric acid; Gal = Galanin; Glu = Glutamate; His = Histamine; NA = Noradrenaline; ORX = Orexin. (Figure based on that of Lockley and Foster, 2012.) (See insert for color representation of the figure.)

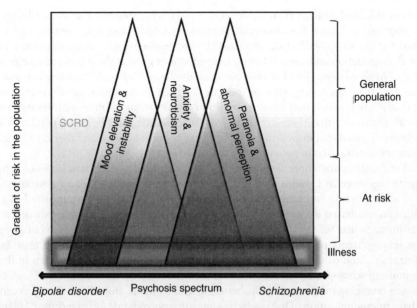

Fig. 18.3 The psychosis spectrum within the general population. Psychosis can be considered as a product of three personality traits, mood elevation/instability, anxiety/neuroticism and paranoia/abnormal salience which occur as a continuum in the general population (y axis). The presence of a high level of these traits places an individual at risk, though only a subset of those at risk go on to develop illness. The level of the individual personality traits will determine where an individual lies on the psychosis spectrum, ranging from those with predominant mood elevation/instability (Bipolar disorder) to those with predominant paranoia/abnormal salience (Schizophrenia).

18.2.2 The social and economic impact of psychosis

Psychosis is a major disease burden in both the developed and developing world. In Europe alone, it is estimated that psychosis affects around six million people at any one time, with an estimated annual cost of around €30billion. In addition to the financial, personal and social costs, these illnesses are associated with a major reduction in life expectancy, estimated at 12–15 years on average (Saha *et al.*, 2007). As prevention is currently not possible, patients typically face prolonged treatment with powerful antipsychotic drugs (Gustavsson *et al.*, 2011). These striking figures have driven research into alternative approaches to alleviating this disease burden.

18.3 Sleep and circadian rhythm disruption in psychosis

The relationship between SCRD and mental health has been the subject of recent attention (Lamont *et al.*, 2007, 2010; Wulff *et al.*, 2010; Menet and Rosbash, 2011; Pritchett *et al.*, 2012). Here the key evidence for the links between these seemingly disparate disorders is summarized.

18.3.1 Schizophrenia

The relationship between schizophrenia and abnormal sleep was first considered in detail in 1883 by one of the founding fathers of psychiatry, Emil Kraepelin (Manoach and Stickgold, 2009). In recent studies, SCRD has been reported in 30–80% of patients with schizophrenia. As a result, SCRD can be considered one of the most common and consistent features of the disorder (Cohrs, 2008). Whilst such links have been attributed to the use of antipsychotics, such disturbances have been shown to be a common feature in previously unmedicated patients (Van Cauter *et al.*, 1991). Schizophrenia is associated with significant circadian disruption, including the abnormal phasing, instability and fragmentation of rest-activity rhythms (Martin *et al.*, 2001; Wulff *et al.*, 2006, 2012). Specific sleep disturbances found in schizophrenia include poor sleep initiation and consolidation, and reductions in total sleep time, sleep efficiency, REM sleep latency, REM sleep density and slow-wave sleep duration (Cohrs, 2008; Manoach and Stickgold, 2009). These data have been suggested to indicate a deficit in the homeostatic regulation of sleep (Chouinard *et al.*, 2004), which may occur in addition to the circadian abnormalities described above. Consistent with the theory that there are underlying mechanistic links between psychosis and SCRD, recent data have suggested that improving sleep by use of cognitive behavioral therapy may improve the psychotic symptoms (paranoia) in patients with schizophrenia (Myers *et al.*, 2011).

At the level of genetic association, several studies have identified associations between schizophrenia and clock genes (reviewed in Lamont *et al.*, 2010). There is some evidence of an association with *Per3* and *Tim* with schizophrenia and schizoaffective disorder, and *Cry1* has been suggested as a candidate gene for schizophrenia based on its location near a linkage hotspot for schizophrenia on chromosome 12q24. A transmission bias for the *Clock* 3111C/T polymorphism has been suggested in a population of 145 Japanese schizophrenia patients. This polymorphism has been associated with aberrant dopaminergic neurotransmission to the SCN. Elevated *Per1* expression has also been shown in the temporal lobe of post-mortem schizophrenic brains (Lamont *et al.*, 2010).

There are also emerging mechanistic links between schizophrenia and SCRD. Firstly, recent evidence has shown that a microduplication of the vasoactive intestinal polypeptide (VIP) receptor 2 (*Vipr2*) confers a significant risk for schizophrenia (Vacic *et al.*, 2011). VIPR2 is known to play a critical role in the SCN in synchronizing neuronal oscillations (Maywood *et al.*, 2006) and *Vipr2* knockout mice have reduced clock gene expression, blunted SCN electrical activity and show a range of circadian phenotypes, from relatively normal to arrhythmic (Hughes and Piggins, 2008). Further evidence comes from work on the *Blind-drunk* mutant mouse, which carries a mutation in *Snap25*, a gene encoding an exocytotic synaptic protein. This mouse model of schizophrenia displays behavioral phenotypes that are modulated by environmental stress and corrected by antipsychotics (Jeans *et al.*, 2007; Oliver and Davies, 2009). Furthermore, these mice display phase advanced and fragmented circadian rhythms in locomotor activity (Oliver *et al.*, 2012). Further, there is plausible mechanistic evidence to suggest that many more genes associated with schizophrenia may be linked to SCRD, including *Nrg1*, *Tcf4*, *Pde4d* and *Cckar* (Pritchett *et al.*, 2012).

18.3.2 Bipolar disorder

In bipolar disorder, sleep disturbances have been shown to be triggers for manic episodes, including irregular sleep timing and reduced total sleep time (Lamont *et al.*, 2007; McClung, 2007). Disruption of the sleep–wake cycle, for example, as caused by travel across multiple time zones, can cause relapses into mania (Plante and Winkelman, 2008). Circadian disturbances include phase-advanced melatonin and cortisol rhythms, whereas sleep disturbances include insomnia or hypersomnia, early morning waking, reduced sleep efficiency and altered REM latency (Lamont *et al.*, 2010; Murray and Harvey, 2010).

There is now quite compelling genetic evidence for links between bipolar disorder and SCRD. Based on analysis of 46 SNPs of eight clock genes (*Bmal1*, *Clock*, *Per1-3*, *Cry1-2*, *Tim*), *Bmal1* and *Tim* were found to be associated with bipolar disorder or schizophrenia (Mansour *et al.*, 2006). The association of *Bmal1* has been confirmed in separate study (Nievergelt *et al.*, 2006). Further evidence comes from patients carrying the long allele variant of the clock gene *Per3* (*PER3⁵/⁵*), which has been linked to early onset of bipolar disorder (Benedetti *et al.*, 2008).

Further mechanistic evidence for a link between the circadian system and bipolar disorder comes from work on animal models. Firstly, the serine/threonine protein kinase GSK3B is known to phosphorylate elements of the TTFL (Fig. 18.1b), and is a target of the mood stabilizer lithium (Yin *et al.*, 2006). Additional evidence has come from behavioral phenotyping of clock mutant mice. Mice carrying a mutation of the TTFL component *Clock* show hyperactivity, reduced sleep, lower anxiety and increased risk-taking behavior and increased reward value for cocaine, sucrose or medial forebrain stimulation. Chronic administration of lithium returned these responses to wild-type levels. These behaviors are analogous to those seen in patients with mania. The *Clock* mutant animals also showed elevated dopamine function in the ventral tegmental area (VTA), and the behavioral phenotype could be rescued by expressing functional CLOCK protein in this region alone (Roybal *et al.*, 2007). Moreover, *in vivo* gene silencing in the VTA alone has been shown to produce such mania-related behaviors (Mukherjee *et al.*, 2010). It is possible that role of CLOCK in the VTA that gives rise to the mania phenotype described in these studies may occur as a result of a deficit in circadian function, but it could also occur via an unrelated role of this protein in the VTA. Certainly, silencing this gene in the VTA results in changes in the expression of other genes, including ion channels and genes involved in dopamine synthesis (Mukherjee *et al.*, 2010). Further evidence comes from the *Myshkin* mouse mutant, which is caused by a mutation in the neuron-specific sodium, potassium ATPase α3 (*Atp1a3*). Similar to Clock mutant mice, these animals are both a mania and SCRD phenotype, with a reduction in REM and NREM sleep, reduced sleep bouts and increased waking (Kirshenbaum *et al.*, 2011). Work on the *Afterhours* (*Afh*) mutant again shows a phenotype consistent with mania, with reduced anxiety and depression. Moreover, this study also showed an association between variation in *Fbxl3* and bipolar disorder in three separate human data sets (Keers *et al.*, 2012). Remarkably, *Clock*, *Myshkin* and *Afterhours* mutants all show a long circadian period (27 h, 25 h and 27 h, respectively), suggesting that a long circadian period may be associated with the mania-related behavior observed in these animal models.

18.3.3 Relationship between psychosis and SCRD

As the above evidence shows, there are clearly links between psychosis and SCRD. However, the exact nature of these links is currently unclear. Whilst some genetic association studies have addressed the role of clock genes, such SNPs reflect only around 5–10% of all SNPs linked to neuropsychiatric disease and these associations often require further validation (Menet and Rosbash, 2011). However, it is evident that the sleep–wake cycle plays a vital role in regulating mood and cognition, which, in turn, impact upon mental health. Defects in any of the mechanisms regulating the sleep–wake cycle may give rise to impaired emotional, cognitive or somatic consequences (Wulff *et al.*, 2010). As a result, abnormalities in circadian clock function (including both central and peripheral clocks), HPA axis or pineal melatonin production, defects in homeostatic sleep regulation, changes in social behavior or abnormal light exposure could all act to destabilize the sleep–wake cycle with resulting effects on mood and cognition. This provides a simplistic model to account for the broad relationship between psychosis and SCRD (Fig. 18.4).

18.4 Possible mechanisms underlying SCRD in psychosis

Because the molecular and anatomical basis of psychosis is not clearly understood, and little is known about how genes and environment interact to give rise to these illnesses, mechanistic associations between SCRD and psychosis are problematic. However, a number of potential mechanisms that are associated with psychosis may enable the mechanistic basis to be further understood. It seems unlikely that SCRD itself is directly causative. Instead, it could reflect a distinct comorbidity that may be viewed as a hallmark symptom of psychotic disorders. By contrast, given that environmental factors clearly contribute to the onset of psychosis, SCRD may provide an additional environmental stressor that contributes to disease onset and may lead to further cognitive impairments in this susceptible group. It should not be overlooked that given the psychosis spectrum, different mechanisms may give rise to SCRD in different cases. Another factor that should be considered in this context is that circadian rhythms and sleep are mechanistically different, albeit interacting, processes. Circadian rhythms are the product of an intracellular transcriptional-translational feedback loop resulting in a network of oscillators that must correctly aligned to prevent internal desynchrony. Moreover, internal time must be correctly entrained to the external environment. By contrast, sleep is the product of a network of brain nuclei using a wide range of neurotransmitters, which the circadian system modulates. As such, any hypothesis as to specific mechanisms should account for both circadian and sleep phenotypes. A number of potential mechanisms that may account for SCRD in psychosis are summarized in Fig. 18.5 and discussed in more detail in the following sections.

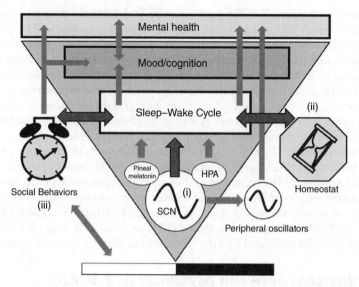

Fig. 18.4 Links between SCRD and mental health. The circadian clock in the SCN (i) is entrained to the light–dark cycle and directly regulates the sleep–wake cycle. Sleep is also regulated by a homeostatic process (ii) and social behavior (iii). The SCN also regulates the hypothalamic-pituitary adrenal (HPA) axis and pineal melatonin synthesis, which also influence sleep. The sleep–wake cycle in turn modulates mood and cognition, which are important for mental health. In turn, peripheral oscillators, particularly clocks in other regions of the CNS (extra-SCN oscillators) are thought to be important for mood/cognition and mental health.

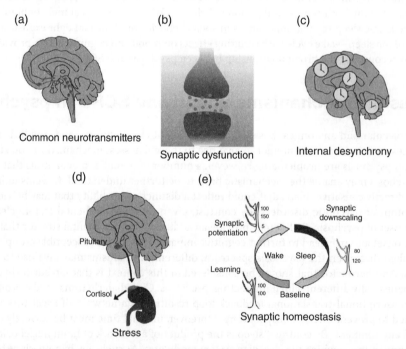

Fig. 18.5 Possible mechanisms underlying SCRD in psychosis may include defects in common neurotransmitter systems (A), dysfunction of specific synaptic processes (B), internal desynchrony between oscillators found throughout the brain (C), stress responses mediated via the hypothalamic–pituitary–adrenal axis (D), or abnormalities in synaptic homeostasis (E). (See text for further details.)

18.4.1 Common neurotransmitters

Sleep is the product of a complex interaction between numerous brain regions, neurotransmitter systems and regulatory hormones (Section 18.3). As such, abnormalities in any of these neurotransmitter systems in disease may give rise to sleep disturbances (Wulff *et al.*, 2010). The positive symptoms of schizophrenia have been attributed to dopaminergic hyperfunction, although given that atypical antipsychotics act upon serotonin and acetylcholine, this may be an oversimplification. Whilst these neurotransmitter systems are also involved in the regulation of sleep–wake timing, evidence for a mechanistic overlap is limited. However, transgenic mice with hyperdopaminergic function do show REM-like intrusions during wakefulness, which can be blocked by haloperidol (Dzirasa *et al.*, 2006). A common neurotransmitter mechanism would predict that pharmacological manipulation of these neurotransmitter systems would similarly result in SCRD. In support of this hypothesis, many drugs affecting neurotransmitters, such as dopamine, histamine, serotonin, GABA, glutamate, or acetylcholine, do indeed affect sleep and arousal (Szabadi, 2006). However, such effects are critically associated with actions on specific neurotransmitter receptors in defined neuroanatomical targets (Fig. 18.2b). As such, a future challenge for this model would be to provide evidence for defects in specific receptor systems and brain regions that are affected in both psychosis and SCRD. Clearly, this may be very challenging in human subjects and is likely to depend upon the use of animal models.

18.4.2 Synaptic dysfunction

Schizophrenia has been considered a disease of the synapse, or synaptopathy (Grant, 2012). Certainly, many of the genes associated with psychosis appear to be involved in synaptic function. As a result, defects in the function of specific synapses may underlie SCRD. Given the interaction of different brain regions in the production and maintenance of sleep, abnormal synaptic function in these pathways would be expected to result in sleep disturbances. Moreover, as neuronal communication within the SCN is also critical for coordinated pacemaker output, synaptic defects at this level could account for circadian abnormalities. At first appearance, such a model may provide a rather broad, nonspecific mechanism, which would suggest that virtually all aspects of central nervous system function should be impaired in psychosis. However, synapses are not homogeneous and the genetic and proteomic complexity of synapses may account for deficits in specific pathways. Evidence from *Bdr* mice, which carry a mutation in *Snap25*, a protein involved in synaptic exocytosis, provides support for such a model (Oliver *et al.*, 2012). Future work on animal models of the synaptic processes associated with psychosis is clearly required.

18.4.3 Internal desynchrony

The uncoupling of central and peripheral oscillator networks has been implicated in neuropsychiatric disease (Barnard and Nolan, 2008; Menet & Rosbash 2011). The SCN controls both endocrine and behavioral output rhythms via both neuronal connections and paracrine signals, which may in turn provide synchronizing feedback. Loss of the SCN results in arrhythmic behavior and loss of such circadian outputs. However, such rhythms are not abolished but instead simply become desynchronized, resulting in different tissues exhibiting different circadian phases. This phenomenon is termed internal desynchrony. As described above (Section 18.1), clock genes are expressed in other areas of the CNS as well as the SCN (Guilding and Piggins, 2007), including brain regions associated with neuropsychiatric disease, such as the prefrontal cortex (PFC), ventral tegmental area (VTA), hippocampus and amygdala (Menet and Rosbash, 2011). Data from *Clock* mutant mice support a role of internal desynchrony in mania, and more specifically a role of a circadian oscillator in the dopaminergic VTA (see Section 18.3.2 for details). However, studies on the *Bdr* mouse model of schizophrenia provided no evidence of internal desynchrony (Oliver *et al.*, 2012). This may provide an example of the range of conditions in the psychotic spectrum. If internal desynchrony is indeed involved, it would suggest that environmental, lesion and genetic models of circadian disruption that result in internal desynchrony should give rise to psychosis-relevant behaviors in animal models. Recent work on the *Fbxl3 Afterhours* mutant appears to support this (Keers *et al.*, 2012). However, further work is clearly required in this area to separate clock and non-clock functions of such genes.

18.4.4 Stress

Elevated cortisol levels have been reported in patients with schizophrenia (Corcoran *et al.*, 2003). However, it is unclear if elevated cortisol levels reflect a disruption of the hypothalamic–pituitary–adrenal (HPA) axis caused by circadian dysfunction. It appears likely that the symptoms of psychosis, such as delusions and hallucinations, produce a primary source of stress that results in elevated cortisol or abnormal cortisol profiles, which may, in turn, give rise to SCRD. Elevated cortisol may also be associated with anxiety and neuroticism, considered as one of the personality traits associated with the psychotic spectrum (Fig. 18.3). In support of a role for stress, sleep disturbances have been shown to be associated with elevated HPA axis hormones (Steiger, 2002) and abnormal cortisol rhythms have been linked to sleep abnormalities, with low morning cortisol being associated with anxiety and exhaustion and elevated evening cortisol associated with stress (Steiger, 2002). Furthermore, data from mouse models of high trait anxiety and stress reactivity demonstrate sleep abnormalities (Touma *et al.*, 2009; Jakubcakova *et al.*, 2012). Whilst such data suggest that stress may result in SCRD, as yet it is unclear as to whether this is the primary mechanism underlying SCRD in psychosis. If this were the case, treatment of psychotic symptoms may be expected to simultaneously reduce stress and result in improvements in SCRD. Clearly, understanding the impact of SCRD and psychosis on the HPA axis is critical in understanding how these disorders are mechanistically linked.

18.4.5 Synaptic homeostasis

There is considerable support for a role of sleep in the process of synaptic homeostasis (Tononi and Cirelli, 2006). This model proposes that as synaptic weightings increase during wakefulness due to synaptic potentiation, this process is downregulated during sleep. Otherwise, with prolonged wakefulness this process would become inefficient due to increasing energy and space costs and would eventually saturate. As a result, during slow wave sleep a process of synaptic downscaling occurs, reducing the synaptic weightings to save energy and space and to improve signal–noise. Due to the synaptic abnormalities that occur in psychosis, this process may be impaired. If this process is affected by disease, possibly arising through abnormal neurotransmission or synaptic dysfunction, it would lead to impaired synaptic homeostasis, evident as sleep deficits. The deficits in homeostatic sleep described in schizophrenia may relate to an impairment of this process. A prediction of this model is that a deficit in synaptic downscaling would lead to inefficient increases in synaptic weighting to the point of saturation, which may relate to the abnormal salience seen in psychosis, as well as the disorganized thought processes and cognitive symptoms which often occur in such illnesses (Section 18.2). This model would predict that psychosis may be the result of a failure of synaptic homeostasis, and that improved sleep should affect psychotic symptoms. Data from CBT to improve sleep in schizophrenia would support this model (Myers *et al.*, 2011). The sleep homeostasis model may also account for the cognitive deficits observed following sleep deprivation in healthy subjects. Another prediction of this hypothesis would be that animal models of psychosis should show specific deficits in homeostatic sleep. Further studies are clearly needed to evaluate the role of sleep homeostasis in psychosis, though it may help to mechanistically link some of the seemingly unrelated data in this field.

18.5 Conclusions

There is an emerging consensus that SCRD and psychosis are linked, arising from a broad literature based upon extended characterization of specific patient groups. However, understanding the specific mechanistic basis of such a link remains a considerable challenge. Work in animal models is essential to this endeavor, as it enables molecular, cellular and anatomical pathways to be evaluated in a manner that is either not possible or unethical in human patients. This work cannot be carried out in isolation and parallel research in animal models and human patients will be critical to ensure progress in this field. Moreover, having specific theories as to the specific mechanisms underlying these links is essential to advance this field, as this enables hypotheses to be rigorously tested. Several potential mechanisms are described here, which are by no means exhaustive. Moreover, these are not mutually exclusive, and the complex etiology and progression of psychosis may result in SCRD via a range of mechanisms. Addressing the underlying SCRD in these conditions provides an alternative approach to intervention in these disorders, and may even provide future targets for treatment.

Acknowledgements

This work was funded by a Wellcome Trust Strategic Award to Russell G. Foster and Stuart N. Peirson. The authors would also like to thank David Pritchett and Carina Pothecary for commenting on the manuscript and figures, and our colleagues in the SCNi for many stimulating discussions which have greatly contributed to the content of this chapter.

References

Albrecht U. 2012. Timing to perfection: the biology of central and peripheral circadian clocks. *Neuron* 74:246–60.

Barnard AR, Nolan PM. 2008. When clocks go bad: neurobehavioural consequences of disrupted circadian timing. *PLoS Genet* 4:e1000040.

Benedetti F, Dallaspezia S, Colombo C, *et al*. 2008. A length polymorphism in the circadian clock gene Per3 influences age at onset of bipolar disorder. *Neurosci Lett* 445:184–7.

Borbely AA. 1982. A two process model of sleep regulation. *Hum Neurobiol* 1:195–204.

Chouinard S, Poulin J, Stip E, Godbout R. 2004. Sleep in untreated patients with schizophrenia: a meta-analysis. *Schizophr Bull* 30:957–67.

Cohrs S. 2008. Sleep disturbances in patients with schizophrenia: impact and effect of antipsychotics. *CNS Drugs* 22:939–62.

Corcoran C, Walker E, Huot R, *et al*. 2003. The stress cascade and schizophrenia: etiology and onset. *Schizophr Bull* 29:671–92.

Dzirasa K, Ribeiro S, Costa R, *et al*. 2006. Dopaminergic control of sleep-wake states. *J Neurosci* 26:10577–89.

Grant SG. 2012. Synaptopathies: diseases of the synaptome. *Curr Opin Neurobiol* 22:522–9.

Guilding C, Piggins HD. 2007. Challenging the omnipotence of the suprachiasmatic timekeeper: are circadian oscillators present throughout the mammalian brain? *Eur J Neurosci* 25:3195–216.

Gustavsson A, Svensson M, Jacobi F, *et al*. 2011. Cost of disorders of the brain in Europe 2010. *Eur Neuropsychopharmacol* 21:718–79.

Hughes AT, Piggins HD. 2008. Behavioral responses of Vipr2−/− mice to light. *J Biol Rhythms* 23:211–9.

Hughes S, Hankins MW, Foster RG, Peirson SN. 2012. Melanopsin phototransduction: slowly emerging from the dark. *Prog Brain Res* 199:19–40.

Jakubcakova V, Flachskamm C, Landgraf R, Kimura M. 2012. Sleep phenotyping in a mouse model of extreme trait anxiety. *PLoS One* 7:e40625.

Jeans AF, Oliver PL, Johnson R, *et al*. 2007. A dominant mutation in Snap25 causes impaired vesicle trafficking, sensorimotor gating, and ataxia in the blind-drunk mouse. *Proc Natl Acad Sci USA* 104:2431–6.

Kapur S. 2003. Psychosis as a state of aberrant salience: a framework linking biology, phenomenology, and pharmacology in schizophrenia. *Am J Psychiatry* 160:13–23.

Kapur S, Mizrahi R, Li M. 2005. From dopamine to salience to psychosis-linking biology, pharmacology and phenomenology of psychosis. *Schizophr Res* 79:59–68.

Keers R, Pedroso I, Breen G, *et al*. 2012. Reduced anxiety and depression-like behaviours in the circadian period mutant mouse afterhours. *PLoS One* 7:e38263.

Kirshenbaum GS, Clapcote SJ, Duffy S, *et al*. 2011. Mania-like behavior induced by genetic dysfunction of the neuron-specific Na+,K+-ATPase alpha3 sodium pump. *Proc Natl Acad Sci USA* 108:18144–9.

Klein DC, Moore RY, Reppert SM. 1991. *Suprachiasmatic Nucleus: The Mind's Clock*. Oxford University Press.

Lamont EW, Legault-Coutu D, Cermakian N, Boivin DB. 2007. The role of circadian clock genes in mental disorders. *Dialogues Clin Neurosci* **9**:333–42.

Lamont EW, Coutu DL, Cermakian N, Boivin DB. 2010. Circadian rhythms and clock genes in psychotic disorders. *Isr J Psychiatry Relat Sci* **47**:27–35.

Lockley SW, Foster RG. 2012. *Sleep: A Very Short Introduction*. Oxford University Press.

Manoach DS, Stickgold R. 2009. Does abnormal sleep impair memory consolidation in schizophrenia? *Front Hum Neurosci* **3**:21.

Mansour HA, Wood J, Logue T, *et al.* 2006. Association study of eight circadian genes with bipolar I disorder, schizoaffective disorder and schizophrenia. *Genes Brain Behav* **5**:150–7.

Martin J, Jeste DV, Caliguiri MP, *et al.* 2001. Actigraphic estimates of circadian rhythms and sleep–wake in older schizophrenia patients. *Schizophr Res* **47**:77–86.

Maywood ES, Reddy AB, Wong GK, *et al.* 2006. Synchronization and maintenance of timekeeping in suprachiasmatic circadian clock cells by neuropeptidergic signaling. *Curr Biol* **16**:599–605.

McClung CA. 2007. Circadian genes, rhythms and the biology of mood disorders. *Pharmacol Ther* **114**:222–32.

Menet JS, Rosbash M. 2011. When brain clocks lose track of time: cause or consequence of neuropsychiatric disorders. *Curr Opin Neurobiol* **21**:849–57.

Mukherjee S, Coque L, Cao JL, *et al.* 2010. Knockdown of Clock in the ventral tegmental area through RNA interference results in a mixed state of mania and depression-like behavior. *Biol Psychiatry* **68**:503–11.

Murray G, Harvey A. 2010. Circadian rhythms and sleep in bipolar disorder. *Bipolar Disord* **12**:459–72.

Myers E, Startup H, Freeman D. 2011. Cognitive behavioural treatment of insomnia in individuals with persistent persecutory delusions: a pilot trial. *J Behav Ther Exp Psychiatry* **42**:330–6.

Nievergelt CM, Kripke DF, Barrett TB, *et al.* 2006. Suggestive evidence for association of the circadian genes PERIOD3 and ARNTL with bipolar disorder. *Am J Med Genet B Neuropsychiatr Genet* **141B**:234–41.

Oliver PL, Davies KE. 2009. Interaction between environmental and genetic factors modulates schizophrenic endophenotypes in the Snap-25 mouse mutant blind-drunk. *Hum Mol Genet* **18**:4576–89.

Oliver PL, Sobczyk MV, Maywood ES, *et al.* 2012. Disrupted circadian rhythms in a mouse model of schizophrenia. *Curr Biol* **22**:314–9.

Plante DT, Winkelman JW. 2008. Sleep disturbance in bipolar disorder: therapeutic implications. *Am J Psychiatry* **165**:830–43.

Pritchett D, Wulff K, Oliver PL, *et al.* 2012. Evaluating the links between schizophrenia and sleep and circadian rhythm disruption. *J Neural Transm* **119**:1061–75.

Reppert SM, Weaver DR. 2002. Coordination of circadian timing in mammals. *Nature* **418**:935–41.

Roybal K, Theobold D, Graham A, *et al.* 2007. Mania-like behavior induced by disruption of CLOCK. *Proc Natl Acad Sci USA* **104**:6406–11.

Saha S, Chant D, McGrath J. 2007. A systematic review of mortality in schizophrenia: is the differential mortality gap worsening over time? *Arch Gen Psychiatry* **64**:1123–31.

Son GH, Chung S, Kim K. 2011. The adrenal peripheral clock: glucocorticoid and the circadian timing system. *Front Neuroendocrinol* **32**:451–65.

Steiger A. 2002. Sleep and the hypothalamo-pituitary-adrenocortical system. *Sleep Med Rev* **6**:125–38.

Szabadi E. 2006. Drugs for sleep disorders: mechanisms and therapeutic prospects. *Br J Clin Pharmacol* **61**:761–6.

Tobler I. 1995. Is sleep fundamentally different between mammalian species? *Behav Brain Res* **69**:35–41.

Tononi G, Cirelli C. 2006. Sleep function and synaptic homeostasis. *Sleep Med Rev* **10**:49–62.

Touma C, Fenzl T, Ruschel J, *et al.* 2009. Rhythmicity in mice selected for extremes in stress reactivity: behavioural, endocrine and sleep changes resembling endophenotypes of major depression. *PLoS One* **4**:e4325.

Vacic V, McCarthy S, Malhotra D, *et al.* 2011. Duplications of the neuropeptide receptor gene VIPR2 confer significant risk for schizophrenia. *Nature* **471**:499–503.

Van Cauter E, Linkowski P, Kerkhofs M, *et al.* 1991. Circadian and sleep-related endocrine rhythms in schizophrenia. *Arch Gen Psychiatry* **48**:348–56.

van Os J, Kapur S. 2009. Schizophrenia. *Lancet* **374**:635–45.

Wulff K, Joyce E, Middleton B, *et al.* 2006. The suitability of actigraphy, diary data, and urinary melatonin profiles for quantitative assessment of sleep disturbances in schizophrenia: a case report. *Chronobiol Int* **23**:485–95.

Wulff K, Gatti S, Wettstein JG, Foster RG. 2010. Sleep and circadian rhythm disruption in psychiatric and neurodegenerative disease. *Nat Rev Neurosci* **11**:589–99.

Wulff K, Dijk DJ, Middleton B, *et al.* 2012. Sleep and circadian rhythm disruption in schizophrenia. *Br J Psychiatry* **200**:308–16.

Yin L, Wang J, Klein PS, Lazar MA. 2006. Nuclear receptor Rev-erbalpha is a critical lithium-sensitive component of the circadian clock. *Science* **311**:1002–5.

Alzheimer's Disease and the Mistiming of Behavior

19

Roxanne Sterniczuk[1] and Michael Antle[2]

[1] Department of Psychology and Neuroscience, Dalhousie University, Halifax, NS, Canada

[2] Departments of Psychology, Physiology & Pharmacology, Hotchkiss Brain Institute, University of Calgary, Calgary, AB, Canada

19.1 Introduction

Changes to circadian rhythms in individuals with Alzheimer's disease (AD) are more pronounced than those observed in normal aging (Chapter 22). The attenuation of these rhythms may be due to a reduction in environmental zeitgebers, loss of functionality within the circadian clock, or disrupted output from the pacemaker. Alterations to any of these components at the neurological level may result in the behavioral and physiological disturbances that AD patient's exhibit.

19.2 Behavioral changes

Individuals with AD exhibit prominent behavioral changes in both their sleep–wake and rest–activity patterns (Weldemichael and Grossberg, 2010). AD patients can exhibit bouts of both insomnia and hypersomnia throughout the 24-hour day, which are an exaggeration of changes seen in normal healthy aging. These changes occur more frequently, and with greater severity, particularly in those with moderate to severe AD. In fact, the level of sleep disruption is strongly correlated with dementia severity (Bonanni et al., 2005; Ju et al., 2013; Lim et al., 2013). Daytime activity levels are lower in AD patients and activity tends to be more fragmented. Up to 50% of AD patients report fragmentation of their sleep–wake cycle, with daytime napping, increased total sleep time, and early awakenings, being the most common alterations. However, the severity of fragmentation can vary greatly, ranging from a complete loss of rest–activity rhythms, to no disruption at all (Fig. 19.1; Paavilainen et al., 2005). Sleep problems are frequently observed in people exhibiting mild cognitive impairment (the prodromal stage of AD). Although not fully understood, the declines in sleep indices observed in the preclinical stages of AD may contribute to inadequate memory consolidation and an increased risk of dementia (Tranah et al., 2011).

Environmental conditions appear to play an important role in the severity of altered daytime and nighttime activity levels. Daytime activity levels are higher for AD patients housed at home rather than in an institution, providing evidence for an increase in circadian disruptions due to institutionalization. Particularly true of institutionalized patients, there is a rapid cycling between sleep and wakefulness, since most of the 24-hour day is spent in bed. Sleep disruption may be so pronounced and fragmented that an individual may not even experience more than one full hour in a sleep state. Increased time spent in bed also contributes to a general decline in health status and has been shown to increase the rate of

Circadian Medicine, First Edition. Edited by Christopher S. Colwell.

© 2015 John Wiley & Sons, Inc. Published 2015 by John Wiley & Sons, Inc.

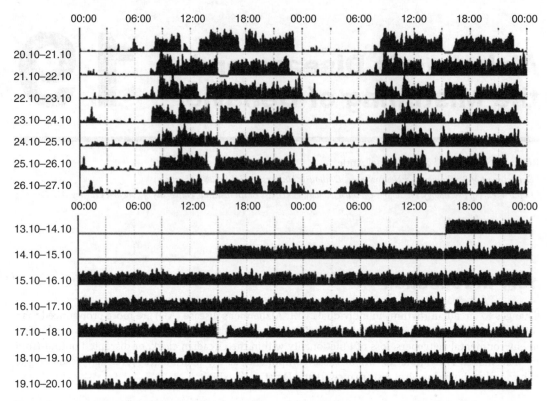

Fig. 19.1 Data from actigraphy watches. Top panel: Example of a normal sleep–wake cycle in a nonde-mented subject with a clear circadian rhythm. Botton panel: Example of a disrupted sleep–wake pattern in a demented subject, which displays a decreased amplitude, higher frequency of overall activity, and no clear circadian pattern (Paavilainen *et al.*, 2005).

cognitive deterioration in AD. In addition, an increase in pacing behavior is also observed in institution-alized AD patients, which may contribute to circadian disruptions. However, an increase in activity levels through pacing may act as a mechanism to preserve circadian organization, as it keeps an individual active and can promote better health.

Various underlying conditions in AD patients may contribute to the severity of the changes in sleep parameters. Psychiatric comorbidities, such as depression, anxiety and delirium, are common in AD, and are important factors contributing to insomnia. In addition, the presence of restless leg syndrome may directly interfere with sleep onset and increase activity in the evening hours. During the daytime, other neurological conditions, such as narcolepsy, Parkinson's disease or dementia, and Lewy body dementia, contribute to hypersomnia in the elderly and may add to excessive daytime sleepiness.

Medication use can also interfere with the maintenance of a stable sleep–wake cycle. Medications pre-scribed for treating AD itself, specifically acetylcholinesterase inhibitors (ChEIs), have different effects depending on the timing of administration. Cholingeric stimulation typically causes awakenings and decreases sleep time and efficiency; however, this primarily affects non-REM sleep. During REM sleep, the cholinergic system can be enhanced due its increased activity at this time. These effects are visible at doses considerably lower than those needed to treat AD. Because the cholingeric system is responsible for inhibiting sleep-inducing regions during the daytime (i.e., ventrolateral preoptic area), restoring cho-linergic functioning via ChEIs during the daytime has the greatest beneficial effect on AD patients. Cholinesterase inhibition before bed tends to interfere with sleep, as well as verbal and spatial memory consolidation (Davis and Sadik, 2006).

19.2.1 Sundowning behavior

Although not recognized as a formal psychiatric condition, one frequently reported behavioral disturbance in those with AD is a phenomenon described as "sundowning" (Khachiyants *et al.*, 2011). The term comes from the observation of increased neuropsychiatric symptoms in the late afternoon and/or evening hours. These behaviors can include agitation, confusion, pacing, yelling, suspiciousness, mood swings, aggression and both visual and auditory hallucinations. Anywhere between 2 and 66% of AD patients can experience this phenomenon, with environmental conditions and cognitive status being important predisposing factors. Symptoms also tend to worsen during the fall and winter months, and have been linked to a decrease in the duration and amount of sunlight. "Sundowners" typically exhibit decreased diurnal activity, a higher percentage of nocturnal activity, a higher mesor and amplitude of core body temperature (CBT), as well as a delayed acrophase of both activity and CBT; these alterations are associated with the severity of sundowning (Volicer *et al.*, 2001). These behaviors and shifts in circadian rhythms typically peak in the moderate stage of AD and diminish as the disease progresses. Despite its name, individuals with AD can exhibit sundowning symptoms at any time of the day. Finally, certain people tend to be sundowners more than others; this has been related to the number of sedatives that a patient administers daily, as well as the duration of institutionalized.

Often these behaviors are a common cause of institutionalization due to increased caregiver stress at home. "Sundowners" are more likely to be individuals with dementia who have been recently institutionalized and are experiencing a great deal of confusion, especially during the evening hours. The appearance of sundowning may be due to maladaptive responses to various environmental factors, such as nurse shift changes, which cause noise and overstimulation, or the decrease in staff-to-patient ratio, which may lead to boredom, decreased environmental structure, and distress from diminishing independence. As well, afternoon fatigue from higher activity levels in the morning and disturbed nighttime sleep may all contribute to the severity of sundowning symptoms. Next to wandering, sundowning is the second most common behavioral disturbance in institutionalized dementia patients. Many doubt the existence of this phenomenon, however, stating that symptoms such as irritation and confusion may occur at any point in the day/night, and that some individuals show these symptoms throughout the whole day with no discernible pattern. Future research is required in order to understand the role of the circadian pacemaker in the occurrence of sundowning.

19.3 Physiological changes

In addition to altered behavioral patterns, AD patients exhibit changes to various aspects of physiology that are under circadian control. Physiological fluctuations may underlie, or contribute to, the disruptions observed with regards to sleep and wakefulness. The most prominent changes include altered sleep architecture, shifted core body temperature (CBT), and diminished melatonin secretion.

19.3.1 Sleep architecture

Not only does AD create disruptions in one's sleep–wake cycle, but it also significantly alters sleep architecture (Chapter 4). Changes to sleep architecture appear to contribute to an overall decrease in sleep maintenance and efficiency, determined by the ratio of total sleep time to total time in bed. As well, a greater arousal index is also observed in AD patients, characterized by multiplying the number of spontaneous arousals from sleep by the number of hours slept.

Due to an increase in awakenings, both in frequency and duration, there is also an increase in the amount of time spent in stage 1 sleep. It becomes more difficult to differentiate between stages 1 and 2, since sleep spindles and K complexes are much lower in amplitude, shorter in duration, and less numerous. These EEG characteristics diminish as the severity of AD increases. The most consistently reported change in mild-to-moderate AD is a greater decrease in slow wave sleep (SWS). Not only do sleep spindles and K complexes diminish but the delta waves characteristic of slow wave sleep (SWS) become virtually eliminated (Petit *et al.*, 2004).

Typically stable in normal aging, the percentage of time spent in REM sleep also significantly decreases in AD. As well, a decrease in the mean REM sleep episode duration is observed. EEG measures show marked slowing of REM rhythms, when compared to wakefulness, as well as to control patients, which may make REM sleep a better diagnostic measurement of AD development and severity. REM sleep is dependent upon the nucleus basalis of Meynert, which suppresses non-REM sleep generation from the nucleus reticularis of the thalamus. It also depends on the integrity of the cholinergic system, which, as previously mentioned, is related to disrupted REM sleep in AD. The deterioration of these systems, the basal forebrain, raphe nucleus, or reticular formation, may all contribute to altered sleep architecture and abnormal circadian rhythms in AD patients.

19.3.2 Core body temperature

Numerous studies have examined the effects of AD on CBT because it is a readily obtained endogenous measure of the circadian cycle and one of the best estimates of human circadian phase. However, a reliable characterization of CBT can be cofounded by various external factors, such as light, body posture and movement, and even social interaction. Both the temperature amplitude and mesor of CBT appear to be significantly higher in AD patients, when compared to controls. However, CBT amplitude rhythms are reduced and phase delayed in probable AD patients when compared to younger controls (age 18–32). Interestingly, there tends to be an advance in body temperature seen in normal aging, whereas the opposite is observed in AD with delayed CBT rhythms. Low body temperature may hit its nadir later in the morning (e.g., 6 a.m.), or in extreme cases closer to the afternoon. Reduced CBT amplitude may also simply be an artifact of abnormal aging, since normal aging is characterized by a 40% reduction in amplitude, whereas AD patients typically demonstrate a 50% reduction. However, daytime sleepiness is related to increased skin temperature in AD patients and is suggestive of impaired thermoregulation (Most *et al.*, 2012).

19.3.3 Melatonin secretion

Another measurable marker of circadian rhythms is melatonin secretion. Melatonin is produced by the pineal gland under circadian regulation. Just as in normal aging, melatonin levels rise during the night and are suppressed at the onset of daylight. The SCN exhibits a reduction in melatonin receptors and an altered rhythmicity in their production. Profound reductions in secretion are observed in AD and are dependent on the severity of neuronal degeneration. As AD neuropathology progresses, cerebrospinal fluid melatonin levels decrease, such that as little as one-fifth of normal melatonin levels may be present in AD patients. Declines in secretion are present at the very earliest stages of neuropathological development and the disappearance of daily melatonin rhythms and decreased cerebrospinal fluid can serve as an early marker for the first stages of AD (Wang and Wang, 2006).

19.4 Neurological changes

Distinct neurological changes accompany AD, which are different from those observed in normal aging. The most salient physical change to the brain is progressive cortical atrophy, which is characterized by a narrowing of the gyri and widening of the sulci, as well as atrophy of the hippocampus and dilation of the lateral ventricle. The entorhinal cortex is the first to show a change in volume, and declines of equal magnitude are observed in the hippocampus. The basal forebrain is most severely affected, as it is the primary site of cholinergic innervation. In addition, accelerated temporal lobe volume reduction has been shown to be a better predictor of early AD, which corresponds to long-term memory impairment. Neuronal loss is not characteristic of normal aging, suggesting that alterations to these AD afflicted regions, visible via neuroimaging or biomarkers, may provide early cues to the onset of the disease.

In addition to cortical atrophy, there are two distinctive neuropathological hallmarks associated with AD: the accumulation of amyloid-β plaques (Aβ) and hyperphosphorylated microtubule-associated tau protein causing neurofibrillary tangles (NFTs). Plaques first appear in low densities within the basal portions of the frontal, temporal and occipital lobes. Moderate densities appear in the neocortical regions, sparing the sensory and motor areas, which are eventually affected in later stages of AD. Within the hypothalamus, the nucleus basalis of Meynert contains a greater amount of pretangles in women and is highly affected by AD. The opposite is seen in the infundibular nucleus of the mediobasal hypothalamus, where neurofibrillary tangles are identified in up to 90% of males with AD versus 8–10% of females. The progression of NFTs occurs in a similar manner, spreading from the entorhinal region to hippocampal formation to the temporal, frontal and parietal cortices, and finally to the primary sensory and motor areas.

Altered sleep–wake patterns may influence the expression of AD neuropathology. For example, chronic sleep deprivation has been shown to significantly increase the level of hippocampal Aβ plaque formation, whereas time spent asleep negatively correlates with the amount of Aβ (Kang *et al.*, 2009). Conversely, increased Aβ neuropathology has been shown to contribute to disrupted sleep–wake cycles (Roh *et al.*, 2012). Importantly, the elimination of Aβ deposits in the mouse brain by immunization with Aβ(42) normalized the sleep–wake cycle in the mouse model. Thus, sleep and AD may influence each other (Ju *et al.*, 2014) raising the possibility of treatments for AD that focus on stabilizing the circadian system (also see Chapter 23).

19.4.1 The circadian pacemaker

Alterations to the SCN (Chapter 3) have been speculated to be the primary cause for circadian rhythm disruption in AD patients. The SCN exhibits both NFT formation and rare diffuse plaques, although to a lesser extent than surrounding hypothalamic regions; neuritic plaques do not appear to form within the SCN (Stopa *et al.*, 1999). In addition to AD neuropathology, there is marked neuronal degeneration within the SCN, including a decrease in the volume and total cell count of SCN neurons, suggesting organic deterioration of the circadian oscillator. Levels of vasopressin (VP)-expressing neurons are significantly reduced within the SCN, when compared to those lost in normal aging, which may be due to degeneration of the visual system. The decrease in VP-expressing neurons is three times lower in AD patients than age and time-of-death matched controls (Liu *et al.*, 2000). However, there does not appear to be significant VP cell loss within surrounding regions, such as the paraventricular nucleus or the supraoptic nucleus. The number of vasoactive intestinal polypeptide (VIP)-expressing neurons also decreases dramatically in presenile AD patients, particularly in females, by about 52% when compared to controls. Both the number and volume of VIP-expressing neurons decline in the SCN in AD patients (Zhou *et al.*, 1995).

Little is known regarding changes to the molecular clockwork of the circadian pacemaker (Chapters 1 and 2). It is presumed that altered clock gene and protein expression underlie abnormal circadian oscillations and, in turn, may cause the behavioral disruptions observed in AD patients. Variations in the expression of clock genes have been noted between AD patients and controls. Postmortem studies have demonstrated that AD patients that exhibit an altered monoamine oxidase A promoter polymorphism, which plays a role in sleep regulation, appear to be at a greater predisposition to sleep disturbances (Craig *et al.*, 2006). Circadian fluctuations of gene expression in the SCN may make the controlled examination of these clock components quite challenging.

Altered input to, and output from, the circadian pacemaker may also contribute to disturbed rhythms in behavior and physiology. Individuals with AD have been shown to exhibit degenerated optic nerves and retinal ganglion cells, making it difficult to transmit photic information to the SCN. Extra-SCN regions (i.e., pineal gland, bed nucleus of the stria terminalis and cingulate cortex) exhibit rhythmic 24-hour expression in *Clock, Per1, Per2* and *Bmal1* gene expression in AD patients. However, the temporal synchrony is lost between the individual oscillating cells, suggesting that output signals from the SCN are impaired in the disease (Thome *et al.*, 2011).

19.4.2 Sleep regulatory regions

Brain regions that are involved in regulating sleep (Chapter 4) are susceptible to AD pathology, especially those that encompass the hypocretin, cholinergic, or serotonergic and noradrenergic signaling systems. Disruption to any of these regions may impair the normal expression and 24-hour fluctuation of sleep and wakefulness (Rothman and Mattson, 2012). The accumulation of Aβ, specifically, has been linked to the dysfunction of these various neurotransmitter systems (Fig. 19.2).

Hypocretins (a.k.a. orexins), are excitatory neurotransmitters secreted from the hypothalamus that promote wakefulness. Individuals that suffer from narcolepsy, or a difficulty in maintaining wakefulness, exhibit decreased levels of hypocretin signaling. Patients with AD exhibit a 40% reduction in the number of hypothalamic hypocretin-1 neurons, as well as a 14% reduction in hypocretin-1 levels in their cerebrospinal fluid (CSF). Patients with increased levels of daytime sleepiness appear to have the lowest concentrations of CSF hypocretin-1. In addition, sleep–wake fragmentation exhibits an inverse relationship with CSF hypocretin levels. As with chronic sleep deprivation, increased hypocretin signaling has also been linked to elevated Aβ plaque formation, suggesting that alterations to this system may be directly involved in AD pathogenesis.

The cholinergic system experiences possibly the greatest deficits in AD. As mentioned, cholinergic signaling plays an important role in the regulation of sleep. There is a plethora of research demonstrating a loss of cholinergic neurons and decreased choline acetyltransferase activity in AD, particularly in the basal forebrain. Because the initiation and maintenance of REM sleep is dependent upon the cholinergic system, loss of cholinergic neurons is speculated to be one of the main culprits for causing sleep disturbances in AD patients.

There are also marked decreases to the noradrenergic and serotonergic systems in AD, which are primarily secreted from the locus coeruleus and raphe nucleus, respectively. Both regions exhibit marked neuronal loss; as well, there is a reduction in circulating cortical levels of each neurotransmitter. Increasing serotonin levels via the prescription of selective serotonin reuptake inhibitors has been shown to improve cognitive function in AD patients and decrease levels of Aβ plaques. Because of the behavioral

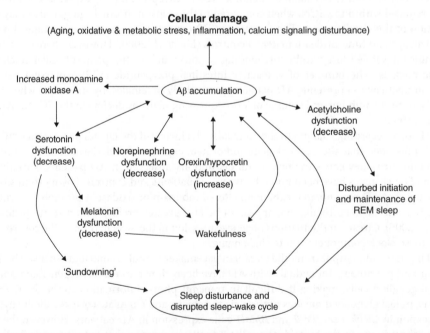

Fig. 19.2 Potential pathways of dysfunction that may lead to the development of sleep disturbances in AD patients. Arrow indicates established directionality of the relationship between the accumulation of Aβ plaques and various neurotransmitter systems (adapted from Rothman and Mattson, 2012).

(e.g., emotion, mood, sleep) and psychological (e.g., agitation, confusion, depression) symptoms observed in early AD, and the presence of AD neuropathology in the raphe nucleus at this time, it has been speculated that the brainstem is one of the first regions afflicted by the disease (Simic *et al.*, 2009).

Less understood is the role of the noradrenergic system in AD, although profound loss is visible in the hippocampus and may be related to impaired learning and memory. In addition, depletion of norepinephrine causes an increase in Aβ deposition. It is still unclear, however, whether altered norepinephrine levels are directly involved in sleep disruption and cognitive deterioration in AD.

19.5 Modeling AD

The identification of several genes that are directly linked to AD has allowed for the generation of various animal models that mimic the pathology of human AD, the most commonly used being mouse models. Transgenic animal models permit both a time and cost effective way of characterizing the cellular and biochemical origins leading to the observed abnormalities in AD brains. There are over a dozen AD mouse models, which exhibit amyloid pathology from the overexpression of amyloid precursor protein (APP), but less than half of these express familial AD-associated presenilin mutations and/or tauopathies (Elder *et al.*, 2010). Delineating the mechanisms that underlie AD through these models will aid in the identification of therapeutic targets and the formulation of novel treatments.

Transgenic mouse models of AD are most often chosen for understanding the effects of the disease on circadian rhythms. Currently, two models are available that express both the aggregation of Aβ and formation of NFTs, namely the triple transgenic mouse model of AD (3xTg-AD) and PLB1 mice. Since review of all the mouse models is beyond the scope of this chapter, only alterations to circadian rhythms in these two models are summarized here.

Developed in 2003, the 3xTg-AD model was generated by crossing APP_{swe} and human tau_{P301L}, controlled by the murine Thy1 promoter, into a single-cell embryo harvested from mutant $PS1_{M146V}$ knockin mice (Oddo *et al.*, 2003). Intraneuronal Aβ immunoreactivity is visible in the neocortex at three months and in the CA1 region at six months. Extracellular Aβ deposits are first apparent at six months, predominantly in layers 4 and 5 of the frontal cortex, and by 12 months in the hippocampus and other cortical regions. In contrast, tau immunoreactivity is first apparent at about 12 months in pyramidal neurons in the CA1 region. Tau-reactive neurons are also found in the amygdala and hippocampus, and an age-related progression towards higher cortical structures is observed. Both Aβ and tau show age- and regional-dependent formation, with Aβ manifesting prior to tangles, pathology which is very similar to that seen in human AD patients. By six months, synaptic dysfunction and impairment in long-term potentiation are apparent and correlate heavily with memory and cognitive deficits.

Initial findings regarding circadian rhythmicity demonstrated similar total daily activity in these mice at two and six months. However, more recently it was shown that by four months of age male 3xTg-AD mice have significantly altered activity patterns. The transgenics exhibit elevated levels of activity during their subjective day, as well as shorter free-running periods. Diminished percentage of nighttime activity is also visible in the males, although the amplitude of early night activity is increased. Older female mice, however, spend less time in an active state during the subjective night (Fig. 19.3; Sterniczuk *et al.*, 2010). However, at four months these mice exhibit phase advanced core body temperature rhythms, which by six months increase in amplitude (Knight *et al.*, 2013). Thus, there are noncognitive changes that occur prior to the development AD pathology, specifically extracellular Aβ, with an exacerbation of disruptions in rhythmicity once extracellular Aβ depositions are formed. As is observed postmortem in human patients, these mice exhibit diminished VP- and VIP-expression within the SCN prior to the development of NFTs (Fig. 19.4; Sterniczuk *et al.*, 2010) but no difference in the number of retinorecipient gastrin-releasing neuropeptide-expressing cells. No AD neuropathology has been noted in the hypothalamus of these mice. Also, the photic pathway to the SCN does not appear to be affected in these mice, since there are no alterations to photic phase shifting ability. These findings suggest that deterioration to the circadian clock may be an early indicator of AD progression. Understanding these changes may provide useful cues to aid in the early diagnosis of the future AD development.

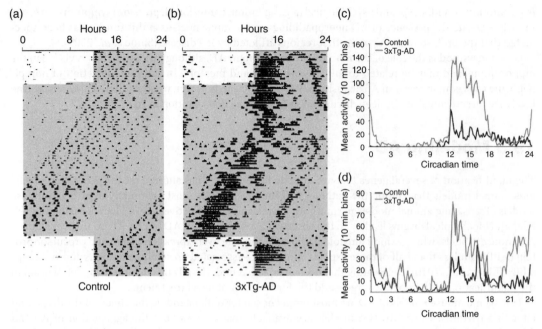

Fig. 19.3 Activity patterns of a representative (a) control and (b) 3xTg-AD male mouse over the course of three months. (c) Mean activity waveform for all male mice prior to Aβ patholoy (<6 months of age) for 10 days in a 12:12 LD cycle indicated by the top vertical bar. (d) Mean activity waveform for all male mice post-Aβ pathology (>6 months of age) for 10 days in a 12:12 LD cycle indicated by the lower vertical bar (Sterniczuk *et al.*, 2010).

In 2011, the PLB1 model was generated using a single-copy knock-in of mutated APP and Tau (Platt *et al.*, 2011). Both proteins are preferentially visible within the hippocampus and cortex, around 5–6 months of age. Much less is known regarding the expression of circadian rhythms in this model. These mice appear to have a normal pattern of circadian activity over the 24-hour day. However, they experience lower levels of activity at five months and higher activity at 12 months, which does not reflect the normal decrease in activity due to aging that is observed in wild types. In addition, these mice exhibit altered sleep–wake EEG architecture, characterized by increased delta power during wakefulness and REM sleep. A delay in sleep onset and NREM fragmentation is visible at 12 months.

19.6 Chronobiological treatment of AD symptomology

Depending on the severity of the disease, either an acetylcholinesterase inhibitor or NMDA receptor antagonist is prescribed to alleviate AD symptoms. Hypnotics are typically prescribed for insomnia and circadian rhythm disorders. However, they quickly lose their effectiveness over time and provide little help for chronic sleeping problems in AD patients. In addition, none of these drugs is capable of regulating the circadian clock and resynchronizing disrupted rhythms. That said, both pharmacological and nonpharmacological approaches have been considered as modulators of the circadian timing system and potential treatments for circadian disruptions in AD (Wu and Swaab, 2007; Deschenes and McCurry, 2009; Weldemichael and Grossberg, 2010).

19.6.1 Melatonin

Due to the observed decrease and dysregulation of melatonin in AD, the most popular pharmacological treatment for circadian disruption is to use melatonin as a chronobiotic. Melatonin has been suggested to be a powerful anti-aging and anti-oxidant agent by preventing the formation of free

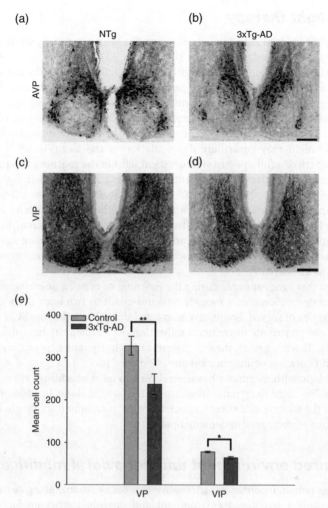

Fig. 19.4 Representative SCN tissue slices of (a, b) VP and and (c, d) VIP fluorescent immunocytochemistry staining. Male controls (a, c) exhibited significantly more VP- and VIP-containing cells than 3xTg-AD mice (b, d). (E) Scale bar = 100 μm; * Significant at $p < 0.05$ and ** at $p < 0.01$ (Sterniczuk et al., 2010).

radicals. Decreased levels of melatonin have been found to lead to excessive oxidation and neurotoxicity, resulting in neuronal death. Transgenic mice engineered to exhibit AD pathology demonstrate a reduction in Aβ generation and tau hyperphosphorylation following melatonin treatment. It can be hypothesized that by supplementing lost melatonin levels, normal sleep–wake rhythms can be restored. There are conflicting results, however, as to the efficacy of melatonin replacement. Several recent studies have demonstrated improved sleep quality, and reduced sundowning behavior, nighttime activity, and sleep latency, as well as slower progression of cognitive impairments in AD patients. However, other well-controlled, randomized studies of AD patients did not find an improvement in sleep–wake rhythms. The administration of melatonin seems most effective when administered either: before naps during the wakeful period when melatonin levels are low or before melatonin levels begin to rise several hours before the regular bedtime. Overall, the effectiveness of melatonin in alleviating sleep disturbances and circadian dysfunction in AD is still debatable. However, the ability for melatonin to prevent or ameliorate Aβ and tau pathology suggests that melatonin may serve as a potential treatment for AD, and consequently the symptoms that accompany the disease.

19.6.2 Bright light therapy

Light, being the most prominent mammalian zeitgeber, has been extensively studied as a nonpharmacological treatment for disrupted sleep–wake rhythms in AD. In theory, presenting a bright light pulse (e.g., 2000–10,000 lux) to an individual with AD at specific times of the day should result in an advance or delay in activity, and possibly realign the sleep–wake cycle. Old rats that are exposed to bright light appear to reverse age-related alterations in sleep–wake disturbances, as well as prevent a decrease in the number of VP-expressing neurons in the SCN. Although more common in institutionalized residents, AD patients typically receive very little bright light exposure during the day, and light throughout the night may contribute dysregulation of the sleep–wake cycle. Administering roughly two hours' worth of a full-spectrum fluorescent light in the morning to a patient can alleviate sundowning symptoms and improve sleep quality. This effect is visible when light is approximately one meter away, and it does not have to be direct (i.e., it is effective when administered while the person is engaging in other activities). Improvements in daytime sleepiness have also been observed following a bright light pulse in the morning, whereby daytime wakefulness may increase by about 30 minutes in those with dementia. However, vision deteriorates with increasing age and the light presented may not be as effective as it could be upon healthy eyes. As with melatonin, the effectiveness of light therapy is also inconclusive.

Others have shown that light exposure during the morning or evening does not improve measures of nighttime or daytime sleep. However, a roughly one-and-a-half to two hour delay in the acrophase of circadian rhythms may be observed. Some have suggested that stimulating the SCN as early as possible in the course of AD may contribute to greater stabilization of circadian rhythms, due to some preservation of SCN plasticity. Taken together, the effectiveness of light therapy depends on the severity of AD, as well as the level and duration of illumination one is exposed to.

Combining bright light with melatonin has been shown to have an additive effect by increasing daytime activity and the day–night sleep ratio, when compared to light alone. In addition, this combination can alleviate some of the adverse side effects associated with melatonin (e.g., dysphoric mood) and may even improve cognitive performance in dementia patients.

19.6.3 Structured environment and behavioral modification

Although the findings remain inconsistent, alternative approaches to realigning circadian rhythms have been examined. Creating a structured environment and providing strict guidance to patients with regards to daily behavior may aid in diminishing the impact that disrupted circadian rhythms have on AD patients. A consistent sleep–wake schedule helps to reinforce time cues and promotes rhythmicity by preventing sleep disturbances at night. This may be done by limiting daytime napping (to a shorter period) and increasing daytime physical activity, as well as creating a relaxing, "sleep friendly" environment by minimizing noise, light, and the distraction of others (e.g., hospital staff, family members). During the evening hours, it is also important for caregivers to limit patient exposure to activities and events that might disrupt sleep, such as television viewing (i.e., violent events may be particularly distressing to cognitively impaired individuals). A combination of social activity and low intensity physical exercise during the morning and afternoon can even increase SWS in older adults. Consistency is key to effective treatment; maintaining regular daytime light exposure, meal times, and daily routines (e.g., avoiding or planning ahead for novelties like family get-togethers) can all help to ease or slow the progression of disruptions in circadian rhythms as well as decrease symptoms of sundowning.

19.7 Conclusion

Recognizing the subtle behavioral, neurological and physiological variations in the developing stages of AD may aid in earlier and more accurate diagnosis. This, in turn, would guide treatment that is appropriate for restabilizing disturbed circadian rhythms and prevent, or delay, early institutionalization and exacerbation of symptoms. There is no "right" form of treatment for AD. Alleviating symptoms and slowing progression of this disease is based on many factors, such as the type and severity of dementia, as well as visual deterioration and the surrounding environment. In most cases, a combination of pharmacological and nonpharmacological treatments is necessary to restore normal functioning (as much as it is possible).

References

Bonanni, E. *et al.* 2005. Daytime sleepiness in mild and moderate Alzheimer's disease and its relationship with cognitive impairment. *J Sleep Res* **14**(3):311–7.

Craig D. *et al.* 2006. Genetically increased risk of sleep disruption in Alzheimer's disease. *Sleep* **29**(8):1003–7.

Davis, B. and Sadik, K. 2006. Circadian cholingergic rhythms: Implications for cholinesterase inhibitor therapy. *Dement Geriatr Cogn Disord* **21**(2):120–9.

Deschenes, C.L. and McCurry, S.M. 2009. Current treatments for sleep disturbances in individuals with dementia. *Curr Psychiatry Rep* **11**(1):20–6.

Elder, G.A. *et al.* 2010. Transgenic mouse models of Alzheimer's disease. *Mt Sinai J Med* **77**(1):69–81.

Ju, Y.E. *et al.* 2013. Sleep quality and preclinical Alzheimer disease. *JAMA Neurol.* **70**(5):587–93.

Ju, Y.E. *et al.* 2014. Sleep and Alzheimer disease pathology--a bidirectional relationship. *Nat Rev Neurol.* **10**(2):115–9.

Kang, J-E. *et al.* 2009. Amyloid-β dynamics are regulated by orexin and the sleep–wake cycle. *Science* **326**(5955): 1005–7.

Khachiyants, N. *et al.* 2011. Sundown syndrome in person with dementia: An update. *Psychiatry Investig* **8**(4):275–87.

Knight, E.M. *et al.* 2013. Age-related changes in core body temperature and activity in triple-transgenic Alzheimer's disease (3xTgAD) mice. *Dis Model Mech* **6**(1):160–70.

Lim, A.S. *et al.* 2013. Sleep fragmentation and the risk of incident Alzheimer's disease and cognitive decline in older persons. *Sleep* **36**(7):1027–32.

Liu, R-Y. *et al.* 2000. Decreased vasopressin gene expression in the biological clock in Alzheimer disease patients with and without depression. *J Neuropathol Exp Neurol* **59**(4):314–22.

Most, E.I. *et al.* 2012. Increased skin temperature in Alzheimer's disease is associated with sleepiness. *J Neural Transm* **119**(10):1185–94.

Oddo, S. *et al.* 2003. Triple-transgenic model of Alzheimer's disease with plaques and tangles: intracellular Abeta and synaptic dysfunction. *Neuron* **39**(3):409–21.

Paavilainen, P. *et al.* 2005. Circadian activity rhythm in demented and non-demented nursing-home residents measured by telemetric actigraphy. *J Sleep Res* **14**(1):61–8.

Petit, D. *et al.* 2004. Sleep and quantitative EEG in neurodegenerative disorders. *J Psychosom Res* **56**(5):487–96.

Platt, B. *et al.* 2011. Abnormal cognition, sleep, EEG and brain metabolism in a novel knock-in Alzheimer mouse, PLB1. *PLoS One* **6**(11):e27068.

Roh, J.H. *et al.* 2012. Disruption of the sleep–wake cycle and diurnal fluctuation of β-amyloid in mice with Alzheimer's disease pathology. *Sci Transl Med* **5**;4(150):150ra122.

Rothman, S.M. and Mattson, M.P. 2012. Sleep disturbances in Alzheimer's and Parkinson's disease. *Neuromolecular Med* **14**(3):194–204.

Simic, G. *et al.* 2009. Does AD begin in brainstem? *Neuropathol Appl Neurobiol* **35**(6):532–54.

Sterniczuk, R. *et al.* 2010. Characterization of the 3xTg-AD mouse model of Alzheimer's disease: part 1. Circadian changes. *Brain Res* **1348**:149–55.

Stopa, E. *et al.* 1999. Pathologic evaluation of the human suprachiasmatic nucleus in severe dementia. *J Neuropathol Exp Neurol* **58**(1):29–39.

Thome, J. *et al.* 2011. CLOCK genes and circadian rhythmicity in Alzheimer disease. *J Aging Res* **2011**:383091.

Tranah, G.J. *et al.* 2011. Circadian activity rhythms and risk of incident dementia and mild cognitive impairment in older women. *Ann Neurol* **70**(5):722–32.

Volicer, L. *et al.* 2001. Sundowning and circadian rhythms in Alzheimer's disease. *Am J Psychiatry* **158**(5):704–11.

Wang, J. and Wang, Z. 2006. Role of melatonin in Alzheimer-like neurodegeneration. *Acta Pharmacol Sin* **27**(1)41–9.

Weldemichael, D.A. and Grossberg, G.T. 2010. Circadian rhythm disturbances in patients with Alzheimer's disease: a review. *Int J Alzheimers Dis* **pii**:716453.

Wu, Y-H. and Swaab, D. 2007. Disturbance and strategies for reactivation of the circadian system in aging and Alzheimer's disease. *Sleep Med* **8**(6):623–36.

Zhou, J-N. *et al.* 1995. VIP neurons in the human SCN in relation to sex, age, and Alzheimer' disease. *Neurobiol Aging* **16**(4):571–6.

Circadian Dysfunction in Parkinson's Disease

20

Christopher S. Colwell

Laboratory of Circadian and Sleep Medicine, Department of Psychiatry and Biobehavioral Sciences, University of California Los Angeles, Los Angeles, CA, USA

20.1 Introduction

Parkinson's disease (PD) is one of the most common neurodegenerative disorders and is a leading cause of cognitive decline and dementia (Pontone *et al.*, 2012). The classical triad of clinical features in PD consists of worsening resting tremor, rigidity, and bradykinesia. Pathologically, PD patients exhibit a progressive loss of dopaminergic neurons and the formation of Lewy bodies in the substantia nigra pars compacta (SNpc). Until relatively recently, it had been thought that it was this loss of dopaminergic neurons in the SNpc that accounted for the symptoms of the disease. However, it is increasingly clear that PD is a multisystem disorder in which numerous brain structures are affected during the course of the illness (Braak *et al.*, 2006; Jain, 2011). The neuropsychiatric aspects of PD are particularly prominent, including cognitive impairment that progresses to dementia and depression in up to 40% of patients. Anxiety, personality changes, and sleep disorders are also common (Blonder and Slevin, 2011). Other well established nonmotor symptoms of PD include metabolic abnormalities, altered olfaction, cardiovascular dysfunction, gastrointestinal problems and sleep disturbances (Chaudhuri and Odin, 2010). One of the most interesting aspects of these nonmotor symptoms of PD is that they develop many years prior to the onset of motor symptoms.

Sleep disorders are extremely common in PD, with most patients reporting primary insomnia, restless legs syndrome, hypersomnia, or rapid eye movement (REM) sleep disorder. These sleep disturbances occur well in advance of the motor symptoms of PD (Schenck *et al.*, 1996; Boeve *et al.*, 2007, 2010; Claassen *et al.*, 2010). The sleep disorders in PD patients are due to multiple causes, including motor disability, loss of function in the sleep control centers located in the brain stem, off-target effects of the drugs used to treat the motor symptoms, and possibly circadian dysfunction (Diederich and McIntyre, 2012; Videnovic and Golombek, 2012). Sleep is generally viewed as being regulated by the combination of two predominant, sometimes competing processes (Chapter 4): (i) the homeostatic sleep drive, representing the accumulated sleep need based on the time elapsed since the last sleep episode, termed "Process S"; and (ii) the circadian-controlled rhythm in wakefulness and sleep, termed "Process C". The potential impact of a disrupted circadian system in PD, has received relatively little attention in the literature. In this chapter, the focus is on the potential role of disrupted circadian rhythms in the pathogenesis of the nonmotor symptoms in PD. Circadian disruption is likely to contribute to the severity of the symptoms. Since circadian disruptions are likely early in the disease progression, improved understanding of this aspect of PD could have important implications for improving early diagnosis and treatment.

Circadian Medicine, First Edition. Edited by Christopher S. Colwell.

20.2 Dysfunction in the circadian system may contribute to the nonmotor symptoms of PD

As described in previous chapters, the circadian system is made up of a network of oscillators. This network controls the temporal patterning of molecular, cellular, and physiological processes throughout the body and the potential disruption of this timing system in PD would be expected to produce widespread symptoms (Table 20.1). Several of the prominent nonmotor symptoms of PD have a diurnal, temporal component that suggests an underlying circadian dysfunction. Most striking are the various types of sleep disruptions reported by PD patients: increased sleep latency, decreased sleep maintenance, fragmented sleep, and excessive daytime sleepiness. All of these symptoms may reflect alterations in the temporal patterning of sleep(Chapters 4 and 5). Therefore, circadian disruption should be considered one of the factors that contributes to the insomnia and hypersomnia experienced by PD patients. Other sleep disorders seen so commonly in PD are less likely to involve the circadian system. In patients with REM sleep disorder, there is a loss of somatic muscle atonia during the REM phase of sleep which is thought to be due to damage to the medullar and pontine structures. Without this inhibition of muscular tone, patients with REM sleep disorder exhibit abnormal motor behavior during REM, usually resulting in minor repetitive limb movements that can be ameliorated to some degree with melatonin or clonazepam (Kunz and Mahlberg, 2010; Arnulf *et al.*, 2012). While the circadian system controls the timing of REM sleep, we do not believe that there is any direct evidence that the SCN is directly involved in inhibiting motor tone during REM sleep. As far as we know, the possibility of this link has not been explored experimentally.

PD patients commonly exhibit disruption in other physiologic processes like the cardiovascular system (Chapters 8 and 9) that are known to be influenced by the circadian system. For example, the autonomic nervous system is subject to circadian regulation; the balance between sympathetic and parasympathetic tone varies in synchrony with the daily circadian cycle (Jain and Goldstein, 2012). In healthy individuals, parasympathetic tone predominates during nighttime/sleep and acts to reduce heart rate and blood pressure. Mechanistically, the central circadian clock in the SCN projects to the pre-autonomic neurons in the paraventricular nucleus (PVN) to effect these changes in autonomic tone (Buijs *et al.*, 2003). Numerous studies have found that the autonomic nervous system is disrupted in PD patients and this disruption drives changes in blood pressure and heart rate. Approximately 30–40% of PD patients have orthostatic hypotension, which has been linked with cardiac sympathetic denervation as well as combined sympathetic/parasympathetic dysfunction of the arterial baroreflex (Jain, 2011). These cardiac symptoms are independent of the motor problems associated with SNpc deterioration, are associated with Lewy body deposition in catecholaminergic neurons. Disruptions in the circadian system (Scheer *et al.*, 2009) may well act in concert with the loss of the catecholaminergic neurons to cause the autonomic symptoms seen in PD.

To provide another example, urinary tract symptoms, such as nocturia, increased urgency and frequency of urination, and incontinence are nearly as common in PD patients as are sleep disturbances (Yeo *et al.*, 2012; Chapter 10). Circadian disruption of sleep architecture contributes to more frequent nighttime waking, which alone might increase the likelihood that a patient will decide to urinate. The

Table 20.1 Overlap of symptoms seen in PD and as a result of circadian disruption.

Some of the shared symptoms include:
- Difficult with sleep onset and maintenance
- Fragmented sleep
- Fatigue
- Cognitive dysfunction including memory problems
- Affective disorders
- Cardiovascular dysfunction
- Urinary tract problems.

See Chapters 4, 5, 8, 9, 16, 17 for references and more discussion.

SCN is also known to regulate the osmotic pressure sensing cells that are responsible for the nocturnal increase in arginine vasopression (also known as anti-diuretic hormone) secretion, which, in turn, reduces the volume of nighttime urine production (Trudel and Bourque, 2010). In addition, disruption of the circadian control of the autonomic nervous system, which normally promotes nocturnal relaxation of the bladder wall and increased urethral sphincter tone, might lead to abnormal bladder contraction and relaxation of the urethral sphincter, resulting in an increased risk of nocturia and urinary incontinence.

While it is often challenging to parse the relative contributions of insomnia, circadian dysfunction, and motor disturbances to a particular PD-associated symptom, little clinical attention has been directed toward normalizing circadian-controlled physiologic functions. A better appreciation of the broad effects that result from circadian rhythm dysregulation in PD patients might offer new insights into the etiology of nonmotor symptoms and suggest novel therapeutic interventions. The circadian system represents a compelling target as a powerful potential modulator of disease progression and patient quality of life.

20.3 Dopaminergic treatments for the motor symptoms of PD may contribute to circadian disruption

Central dopamine (DA) is generally associated with arousal (Chapters 5 and 15) and a variety of evidence suggests that this transmitter is involved in the regulation of the sleep–wake cycle at multiple circuits. Overall, levels of DA appear to exhibit a low amplitude, daily rhythm in humans (Poceta *et al.*, 2009) and in mice (Hampp *et al.*, 2008). Centrally, DA levels are modulated by monoamine oxidase A (MAO-A) and monoamine oxidase B (MAO-B), which are key enzymes that regulate the breakdown of several different monoamine neurotransmitters. Importantly, MAO-A appears to be a clock-controlled gene. A mutation in the circadian clock gene *Period2* (*Per2*) in mice leads to reduced expression and activity of MAO-A in the mesolimbic dopaminergic system, which results in increased DA levels and changes in electrical activity in the striatum (Hampp *et al.*, 2008). So any disruption of the circadian clockwork could be expected to alter levels of DA via MAO-A activity.

Since the motor symptoms are driven by the loss of dopaminergic neurons in the SNpc, the general treatment strategy has been to provide a blood–brain barrier-permeable metabolic precursor in the dopamine biosynthetic pathway with the goal of increasing synaptic concentrations of DA in the SNpc and striatum. DA and dopaminergic drugs, including L-DOPA, are well known to modulate clock gene expression (Imbesi *et al.*, 2009; Hood *et al.*, 2010). Furthermore, there is an extensive literature of rodent studies documenting the powerful circadian effects of dopaminergic drugs such as cocaine and methamphetamine, including profound disruption of sleep (Honma and Honma 2009; Ironside *et al.*, 2010; Glass *et al.*, 2012). For example, continuous administration of methamphetamine in drinking water alters the rhythm of circadian activity in rats and mice (Honma *et al.*, 1986; Tataroglu *et al.*, 2006). Interestingly, methamphetamine treatment can even restore robust circadian activity in mice whose SCN had been ablated (Honma *et al.*, 1987), demonstrating that dopaminergic drugs can modulate the circadian system even without a functional central circadian clock in the SCN.

Taken together, it seems likely that the very drugs that are prescribed to alleviate the motor symptoms of PD (or related disorders like restless leg syndrome, which is similarly treated with dopamine agonists) are themselves contributing to the sleep disturbances in these patients (Santiago *et al.*, 2010). Specifically, the data suggests that low doses of pharmacological agents that increase DA can improve sleep while higher doses delay the onset of sleep and decrease total sleep time (Schafer and Greulich, 2000; Diederich and McIntyre 2012). Further work will be required to see if controlling the timing of the dosing of the L-DOPA and related compounds can minimize the undesirable sleep disruptions caused by dopaminergic medications (Wailke *et al.*, 2011). For example, one simple prediction is that using pharmacological tools to reinforce the normal daily rhythm of DA with higher levels of DA activity during the day and lower levels at night may improve motor function without disrupting sleep or circadian function.

20.4 PD models show sleep and possible circadian disruption

The loss of DA neurons may play a role in the circadian disruption observed in nonhuman primates. One of the most developed models of PD involves treating primates with the toxin MPTP (1-methyl-4-phenyl-1,2,3,6-tetrahydropyridine), which produces a set of symptoms that resemble PD (Fox and Brotchie, 2010) and can be treated with dopaminergic drugs. The MPTP-treated primates exhibit an immediate disruption of the sleep–wake cycle as well as alteration in REM sleep and increased daytime sleepiness (Barraud et al., 2009; Verhave et al., 2011; Vezoli et al., 2011; Fifel et al., 2014). Interestingly, mice treated with MPTP exhibit a significant loss of dopaminergic neurons (approximately 50%) without disruption of the circadian rhythms (Laloux et al., 2008; Tanaka et al., 2012). The injection with the toxin 6-hydroxydopamine produces a larger loss of neurons that does disrupt behavioral and clock gene expression rhythms in the rat (Gravotta et al., 2011).

Loss of function in dopaminergic cells has also been linked to nonmotor symptoms, including sleep and circadian disruptions. For example, mice deficient in vesicular monoamine transporter expression (VMAT2) exhibit severely diminished levels of the major monoamines, including DA, 5-HT and NE (Taylor et al., 2009, 2011). These mice exhibit many of the nonmotor symptoms associated with PD, including altered latency to sleep and reduced amplitude of their diurnal rhythm. It would be interesting to examine the circadian behavior of these mice. In *Drosophila*, the targeted expression of mutant α-synuclein to monoamine (5HT, DA) expressing neurons resulted in altered sleep and circadian activity (Gajula Balija et al., 2011). It is worth noting that sleep disturbances have been reported in patients with mutations in the *Parkin* and *DJ-1* genes (Kumru et al., 2004; Limousin et al., 2009; Lo Coco et al., 2009; Nishioka et al., 2009), which again highlight the importance of rigorously examining a range of PD models for possible circadian dysfunction.

One of the best studied models of PD and other synucleinopathies is a line of transgenic mice expressing human α-synuclein (aSyn) under the Thy-1 promoter: the α-synuclein overexpressing (Thy1-aSyn) mice (Rockenstein et al., 2002). Genetic mutations in, and duplication of, α-synuclein are strongly associated with familial forms of PD; and polymorphisms in this gene are associated with increased PD risk. Prior work has shown that at 2–3 months of age, Thy1-aSyn mice begin to exhibit progressive impairments in motor and nonmotor symptoms that are analogous to those experienced by human PD patients; these include deficits in olfaction, cognition, and control of the autonomic nervous system (Fleming and Chesselet, 2009). Thus, the Thy1-aSyn transgenic mouse provides an excellent model system to improve our understanding of the basic pathophysiologic mechanisms that cause PD, possibly including the early nonmotor symptoms and circadian-related symptoms.

As measured by wheel running activity under either a standard 12 hour light and 12 hour dark cycle (LD), or under a continuous dark cycle (DD), the observed circadian cycle of all Thy1-αSyn mice initially appeared to be grossly rhythmic (Kudo et al., 2011). However, the Thy1-αSyn mice exhibited fragmented, weak (low power) rhythms under both LD and DD conditions (Fig. 20.1). These deficits are clearly illustrated when the mice are placed in a skeleton photoperiod consisting of two 1-hour light exposures every 24 hours. The mice synchronize nicely and these lighting conditions allow us to see the clock driven locomotor output without the direct activity-suppressing influence of light. The peak amplitude of the behavioral rhythms and coherence (measured by fragmentation) under both LD and DD conditions progressively declined over the lifespan of both Thy1-αSyn and control wild-type (WT) mice. The core of the oscillatory clock that generates circadian rhythms has been previously described (Chapters 1 and 2). Surprisingly, the Thy1-αSyn mice show a normal pattern of oscillating PER2 expression. Elimination of dopaminergic neurons by administration of the neurotoxin 6-hydroxydopamine has been shown to alter clock gene expression in the forebrain (Gravotta et al., 2011). Thus, possible alterations in clock gene expression later in disease progression or in brain areas outside the SCN should be evaluated in the Thy1-αSyn line at a time when changes in DA are observed. Still, our characterization of the Thy1-αSyn mice suggests that, at least during the early

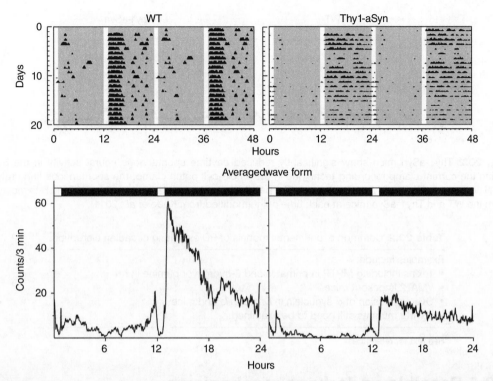

Fig. 20.1 Thy1-aSyn mice show an age-related decline in daily and circadian rhythms. Top panels show representative examples of wheel-running activity records from WT (left) and Thy1-aSyn (right) mice. Animals were initially entrained to 12:12 LD, then placed into a skeleton photoperiod (1:11:1:11 LD). Each horizontal row represents the activity record for a 24-hour day that is then double plotted. Successive days are plotted from top to bottom. Gray shaded area represents darkness. Bottom panels show examples of average wave-forms that illustrate the distribution of activity for WT (left) and Thy1-aSyn (right) mice. Besides the striking reduction in the amplitude of activity, the Thy1-aSyn mice exhibited a decrease in precision of the beginning of the nightly activity cycle and an increase in fragmentation of their activity (modified from Kudo *et al.*, 2011).

stages of disease, disruptions in periodicity are not the result of deficits in the molecular oscillations in the circadian system or its inputs, but in the downstream outputs of this system.

SCN neurons are spontaneously active and generate action potentials with peak activity during the day (Colwell, 2011). In the daytime, we found that the excitability of SCN neurons was significantly reduced in the Thy1-αSyn mice (Fig. 20.2) (Kudo *et al.*, 2011). At this age (3 months) we did not see evidence of cell loss within the SCN; however, we have not yet looked at older mice. In the Thy1-αSyn model, firing rate is also dramatically reduced in the striatal medium spiny neurons (Wu *et al.*, 2010), so decreased electrical activity may be a common feature of this model. Neurons in the SCN drive the rhythmic output of the circadian system via regulation of the autonomic nervous system and other neural and hormonal pathways (Chapter 3). The decrease in the daytime electrical activity that we observe in the SCN of Thy1-αSyn mice would be expected to weaken the temporal patterning of both the neural and hormonal outputs. Our observations are consistent with the hypothesis that decreased amplitude of efferent signals from the SCN could contribute to the nonmotor symptoms in PD. It will be important to extend this work on Thy1-αSyn mice to other models. Mutations in the human leucine-rich repeat kinase 2 (LRRK2) are the most common genetic cause of PD and new mouse models of LRRK2 mutations are starting to become available. Thus, many of the experimental models of PD exhibit circadian disruption (Table 20.2).

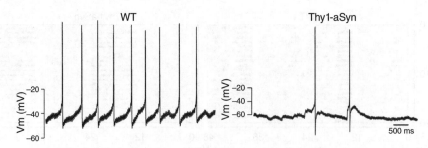

Fig. 20.2 Thy1-aSyn mice show significantly reduced daytime spontaneous neural activity in the SCN. Using the current-clamp recording technique in the whole-cell patch clamp, the spontaneous firing rate in SCN neurons during the day was measured. The panels show representative examples of firing rate recorded from the WT and Thy1-aSyn mice at each time point (modified from Kudo *et al.*, 2011).

Table 20.2 Common experimental models of PD exhibiting circadian disruption.

Examples include:
- Toxins including MPTP in primates and 6-hydroxydopamine in rat
- VMAT2 knockout mice
- Overexpression of α-synuclein in *Drosophila* and mice
- LRRK2 mutants still need to be examined.

See text for references

20.5 Possible underlying mechanisms

One mechanism by which aSyn overexpression could reduce SCN neural output is through changes in synaptic transmission. αSyn is a presynaptic protein that regulates synaptic vesicle release, and its misexpression alters synaptic transmission (Burré *et al.*, 2010). Recent work in a variety of mouse models of other neurodevelopmental and psychiatric disorders suggests that alterations in the balance between synaptic excitation and inhibition are a core pathophysiologic feature of these conditions (Shepherd and Katz, 2011). Within the SCN circuit, the neurotransmitter used is gamma-aminobutyric acid (GABA); most SCN neurons receive a constant flux of GABA signaling. The circadian symptoms of the Thy1-aSyn mice could be explained if aSyn overexpression tilted the balance toward increased inhibition within the SCN circuit.

An alternate explanation lies with the currents that underlie daily rhythms of spontaneous electrical activity in the SCN (Colwell, 2011). During the day, SCN neurons are relatively depolarized to keep them near the threshold for generating an action potential (−45 mV). This relatively depolarized resting potential is the result of excitatory drive provided by multiple cation currents. Changes in these currents could underlie the decreased daytime firing observed in the Thy1-aSyn mice. In response to this depolarized membrane potential, SCN neurons exhibit sustained discharge for 4–6 hours in the subjective day without spike adaptation. Prior work suggests that three potassium (K⁺) currents, including fast delayed rectifier (FDR), subthreshold-operating A-type (I_A) and large-conductance Ca^{2+} activated (BK), all play a critical role in the regulation of spontaneous action potential firing in SCN neurons during the day. Reduction in magnitude of the FDR and the BK currents would have the consequence of decreasing the daytime firing rate in the SCN. Interestingly, aging selectively impacts K⁺ (I_A and FDR) currents in the SCN, which reduces the synchrony of the SCN cell population (Chapter 22).

Although αSyn is primarily thought to be important for synaptic vesicle release and recycling, there is increasing evidence of its colocalization with the mitochondrial membrane (Li *et al.*, 2007, Nakamura *et al.*, 2008). Furthermore, mitochondrial function can be impaired upon misexpression of aSyn (Xie and Chung, 2012) and, conversely, the mitochondrial toxin MPTP leads to aSyn accumulation (Purisai *et al.*, 2005). Other mouse genetic models of PD also show altered mitochondrial function and increased oxidative stress (Trancikova *et al.*, 2012). SCN neurons require an energy-demanding sodium–potassium pump (Na$^+$/K$^+$-ATPase) to maintain the resting membrane potential during daytime peak firing (Wang and Huang, 2006). Without sufficient ATP, the neural membrane would depolarize, be unable to generate action potentials, thus dampening the output signals from the SCN. These data support the hypothesis that one cause of decreased electrical activity in the SCN is a decrease in mitochondrial function (Martin *et al.*, 2006; Schapira 2012).

One likely consequence of the circadian disruption seen in the Thy1-αSyn mice is an increase in oxidative stress and inflammation. Cellular metabolism results in the generation of byproducts of oxygen (O$_2$) known as reactive oxygen species (ROS). The reduction of O$_2$ to H$_2$O gives rise to a superoxide anion, hydrogen peroxide, and an hydroxyl radical, which can all be damaging to the cell. Therefore, cells control the production of ROS and manage the negative consequences by the production of anti-oxidants. A long body of work from both plants and animals indicates that both the production of ROS as well as cellular anti-oxidants is temporally controlled by the circadian system (Chapter 1). Deletion of the critical clock gene BMAL1 leads to mitochondrial dysfunction, including increases in ROS in peripheral organs (Kondratova and Kondratov, 2012). Mitochondrial ROS and oxidative stress have been consistently implicated in disease and age-related decline in tissues throughout the body. Although the molecular oscillator does not appear to be disrupted in the SCN of Thy1-aSyn mice, the effects of the overexpression of aSyn may disrupt ROS levels to affect neuronal firing. While oxidative stress damages a range of cellular processes, it is worth noting that K$^+$ channels can be quite sensitive to oxidative damage (Sesti *et al.*, 2010; Cotella *et al.*, 2012). Therefore, in the SCN, an increase in oxidative damage to K$^+$ channels may underlie the decrease in daytime firing observed in Thy1-αSyn mice.

Likewise, many immune parameters show daily and circadian variation, including levels of cytokines (Chapter 14). The molecular clock is found in many of the key cells involved in the immune response and disruption of the circadian system alters the immune response. Clock proteins can directly regulate the expression of proinflammatory cytokines through the NF-κB signaling pathway (Narasimamurthy *et al.*, 2012; Spengler *et al.*, 2012). Therefore, we speculate that a second consequence of circadian disruption in the Thy1-aSyn mice is changes in the NF-κB pathway, which will result in pathological inflammation throughout the body. Within the SCN, increases in cytokines are known to disrupt rhythms in firing rate (Lundkvist *et al.*, 2010).

Increases in oxidative stress and inflammation due to circadian dysfunction in combination with αSyn aggregation could accelerate the pathology of PD. If this hypothesis is correct, circadian disruption may be a risk factor for PD. Many PD models consider a two-hit model in which genetic risk factors coincide with environmental perturbations to lead to the disease (Hawkes *et al.*, 2007; Boger *et al.*, 2010). We propose that circadian disruption and the resulting increase in chronic inflammation, mitochondrial dysfunction, oxidative stress, and DNA damage may be an environmental risk factor for developing PD, and may also serve to accelerate the pathology of the disease.

20.6 Conclusion

Disruptions of the circadian system as seen in PD are likely to have profound consequences on patient health. There is mounting evidence that robust circadian rhythms are a necessary component to optimum health. In recent years, a wide range of studies have demonstrated that disruption of the circadian system leads to a cluster of symptoms, including cognitive deficits and psychiatric symptoms (Chapters 16 and 17), metabolic deficits (Chapter 11), cardiovascular problems (Chapters 8 and 9), gastrointestinal problems (Chapters 6 and 7), and increased risk for certain cancers (Chapters 12 and 13). Many of these same symptoms are described in patients with PD (Table 20.1). Our results from the analysis of Thy1-αSyn mice support these observations. This, combined with the observation that many of the symptoms predate the appearance of PD-related motor symptoms by years, raises the possibility that circadian dysfunction is not merely a symptom of PD but rather is a core component of the disease. (Fig. 20.3)

Our hypothesis suggests that placing a greater emphasis on the development of pharmacological tools and behavioral interventions that can boost circadian output and synchrony of the SCN may be

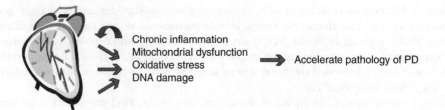

Fig. 20.3 Potential mechanisms by which circadian dysfunction could accelerate the pathology of PD. The molecular clockwork regulates mitochondrial function, reactive oxygen species homeostasis, DNA repair and immune response. Dysfunction of this timing system is likely to contribute to chronic inflammation, mitochondrial dysfunction, and DNA damage. These processes are all thought to contribute to the pathology of PD and contribute to age-related changes in the brain. Therefore, we suggest the possibility that circadian dysfunction due to genetic or environmental perturbations can accelerate the pathology of PD.

therapeutic in PD patients, perhaps especially in PD patients in early stages of the disease. Interventions should be designed to strengthen output and resynchronize the central and peripheral circadian clocks, that is, focus on the amplitude of the circadian output. New work suggests that the circadian system may be targeted with pharmacologic therapies and that high-throughput chemical screens can be applied to develop these potential treatments (Chapter 23). We would suggest that candidate molecules that boost amplitude may be particularly useful to counter the circadian dysfunction associated with PD. Together, the optimization of these strategies already in use and the development of new, targeted interventions aimed at restoring circadian functioning will provide promising avenues toward improving the prognosis of patients with PD. These same interventions are under discussion for AD (Chapter 19), HD (Chapter 21), and aging (Chapter 22).

References

Arnulf I. 2012. REM sleep behavior disorder: Motor manifestations and pathophysiology. *Mov Disord* **27**: 677–89.

Barraud Q, Lambrecq V, Forni C, *et al.* 2009. Sleep disorders in Parkinson's disease: the contribution of the MPTP non-human primate model. *Exp Neurol* **219**(2): 574–82.

Blonder LX, Slevin JT. 2011. Emotional dysfunction in Parkinson's disease. *Behav Neurol* **24**: 201–17.

Boeve BF. 2010. Predicting the future in idiopathic rapid-eye movement sleep behaviour disorder. *Lancet Neurol* **9**: 1040–2.

Boeve BF, Silber MH, Saper CB, *et al.* 2007. Pathophysiology of REM sleep behaviour disorder and relevance to neurodegenerative disease. *Brain* **130**: 2770–88.

Boger HA, Granholm AC, McGinty JF, Middaugh LD. 2010. A dual-hit animal model for age-related parkinsonism. *Prog Neurobiol* **90**: 217–29.

Braak H, Bohl JR, Müller CM, *et al.* 2006. The staging procedure for the inclusion body pathology associated with sporadic Parkinson's disease reconsidered. *Mov Disord* **21**: 2042–51.

Buijs RM, La Fleur SE, Wortel J, *et al.* 2003. The suprachiasmatic nucleus balances sympathetic and parasympathetic output to peripheral organs through separate preautonomic neurons. *J Comp Neurol* **464**: 36–48.

Burré J, Sharma M, Tsetsenis T, *et al.* 2010. Alpha-synuclein promotes SNARE-complex assembly *in vivo* and *in vitro*. *Science* **329**: 1663–7.

Chaudhuri KR, Odin P. 2010. The challenge of nonmotor symptoms in Parkinson's disease. *ProgBrain Res* **184**: 325–41.

Claassen DO, Josephs KA, Ahlskog JE, *et al.* 2010. REM sleep behavior disorder preceding other aspects of synucleinopathies by up to half a century. *Neurology* **75**: 494–9.

Colwell CS. 2011. Linking neural activity and molecular oscillations in the SCN. *Nat Rev Neurosci* **12**: 553–69.

Cotella D, Hernandez-Enriquez B, Wu X, *et al.* 2012. Toxic role of K+ channel oxidation in mammalian brain. *J Neurosci* **32**: 4133–44.

Diederich NJ, McIntyre DJ. 2012. Sleep disorders in Parkinson's disease: many causes, few therapeutic options. *J Neurol Sci* **314**: 12–9.

Fifel K, Vezoli J, Dzahini K, *et al.* 2014. Alteration of daily and circadian rhythms following dopamine depletion in MPTP treated non-human primates. *PLoS One* **9**(1): e86240

Fleming SM, Chesselet MF. 2009. Modeling nonmotor symptoms of Parkinson's disease in genetic mouse models. In: *Basal Ganglia IX* (eds Groenewegen HJ, Voorn P, Berendse HW, *et al.*), Springer, New York, pp. 483–92.

Fox SH, Brotchie JM. 2010. The MPTP-lesioned non-human primate models of Parkinson's disease. Past, present, and future. *Prog Brain Res* **184**: 133–57

Gajula Balija MB, Griesinger C, Herzig A, *et al.* 2011. Pre-fibrillar alpha-synuclein mutants cause Parkinson's disease-like nonmotor symptoms in Drosophila. *PLoS One* **6**(9): e24701.

Glass JD, Brager AJ, Stowie AC, Prosser RA. 2012. Cocaine modulates pathways for photic and nonphotic entrainment of the mammalian SCN circadian clock. *Am J Physiol Regul Integr Comp Physiol* **302**: 740–50.

Gravotta L, Gavrila AM, Hood S, Amir S. 2011. Global depletion of dopamine using intracerebroventricular 6-hydroxydopamine injection disrupts normal circadian wheel-running patterns and PERIOD2 expression in the rat forebrain. *J Mol Neurosci* **45**: 162–71.

Hampp G, Ripperger JA, Houben T, *et al.* 2008. Regulation of monoamine oxidase A by circadian-clock components implies clock influence on mood. *Curr Biol* **18**: 678–83.

Hawkes CH, Del Tredici K, Braak H. 2007. Parkinson's disease: a dual-hit hypothesis. *Neuropathol Appl Neurobiol* **33**: 599–614.

Honma K, Honma S. 2009. The SCN-independent clocks, methamphetamine and food restriction. *Eur J Neurosci* **30**: 1707–17.

Honma K, Honma S, Hiroshige T. 1986. Disorganization of the rat activity rhythm by chronic treatment with methamphetamine. *Physiol Behav* **38**: 687–695.

Honma K, Honma S, Hiroshige T. 1987. Activity rhythms in the circadian domain appear in suprachiasmatic nuclei lesioned rats given methamphetamine. *Physiol Behav* **40**: 767–774.

Hood S, Cassidy P, Cossette MP, *et al.* 2010. Endogenous dopamine regulates the rhythm of expression of the clock protein PER2 in the rat dorsal striatum via daily activation of D2 dopamine receptors. *J. Neurosci* **30**: 14046–58.

Imbesi M, Yildiz S, Dirim Arslan A, *et al.* 2009. Dopamine receptor-mediated regulation of neuronal "clock" gene expression. *Neurosci* **158**: 537–44.

Ironside S, Davidson F, Corkum P. 2010. Circadian motor activity affected by stimulant medication in children with attention-deficit/hyperactivity disorder. *J Sleep Res* **19**: 546–51.

Jain S. 2011. Multi-organ autonomic dysfunction in Parkinson disease. *Parkinsonism Relat Disord* **17**: 77–83.

Jain S, Goldstein DS. 2012. Cardiovascular dysautonomia in Parkinson disease: From pathophysiology to pathogenesis. *Neurobiol Dis* **46**: 572–80.

Kondratova AA, Kondratov RV. 2012. The circadian clock and pathology of the ageing brain. *Nat Rev Neurosci* **13**(5): 325–35.

Kudo T, Loh DH, Truong D, *et al.* 2011. Circadian dysfunction in a mouse model of Parkinson's disease. *Exp Neurol* **232**: 66–75.

Kumru H, Santamaria J, Tolosa E, *et al.* 2004. Rapid eye movement sleep behavior disorder in parkinsonism with parkin mutations. *Ann Neurol* **56**(4): 599–603.

Kunz D, Mahlberg R. 2010. A two-part, double-blind, placebo-controlled trial of exogenous melatonin in REM sleep behaviour disorder. *J Sleep Res* **19**: 591–6.

Laloux C, Derambure P, Kreisler A, *et al.* 2008. MPTP-treated mice: long-lasting loss of nigral TH-ir neurons but not paradoxical sleep alterations. *Exp Brain Res* **186**(4): 635–42.

Li WW, Yang R, Guo JC, *et al.* 2007. Localization of alpha-synuclein to mitochondria within midbrain of mice. *Neuroreport* **18**: 1543–6.

Limousin N., Konofal E, Karroum E, *et al.* 2009. Restless legs syndrome, rapid eye movement sleep behavior disorder, and hypersomnia in patients with two parkin mutations. *Mov Disord* **24**(13): 1970–6.

Lo Coco D, Caruso G, Mattaliano A. 2009. REM sleep behavior disorder in patients with DJ-1 mutations and parkinsonism-dementia-ALS complex. *Mov Disord* **24**(10): 1555–6.

Lundkvist GB, Sellix MT, Nygård M, *et al.* 2010. Clock gene expression during chronic inflammation induced by infection with Trypanosoma brucei brucei in rats. *J Biol Rhythms* **25**(2): 92–102.

Martin LJ, Pan Y, Price AC, *et al.* 2006. Parkinson's disease alpha-synuclein transgenic mice develop neuronal mitochondrial degeneration and cell death. *J Neurosci* **26**: 41–50.

Nakamura K, Nemani VM, Wallender EK, *et al.* 2008. Optical reporters for the conformation of alpha-synuclein reveal a specific interaction with mitochondria. *J Neurosci* **28**: 12305–17.

Narasimamurthy R, Hatori M, Nayak SK, *et al.* 2012. Circadian clock protein cryptochrome regulates the expression of proinflammatory cytokines. *Proc Natl Acad Sci USA* **109**(31): 12662–7.

Nishioka K, Ross OA, Ishii K, *et al.* 2009. Expanding the clinical phenotype of SNCA duplication carriers. *Mov Disord* **24**(12): 1811–9.

Poceta JS, Parsons L, Engelland S, Kripke DF. 2009. Circadian rhythm of CSF monoamines and hypocretin-1 in restless legs syndrome and Parkinson's disease. *Sleep Med* **10**(1): 129–33.

Pontone GM, Palanci J, Williams JR, Bassett SS. 2012. Screening for DSM-IV-TR cognitive disorder NOS in Parkinson's disease using the Mattis Dementia Rating Scale. *Int J Geriatr Psychiatry* **28**(4): 364–71.

Purisai MG, McCormack AL, Langston WJ, *et al.* 2005. Alpha-synuclein expression in the substantia nigra of MPTP-lesioned non-human primates. *Neurobiol Dis* **20**(3):898–906.

Rockenstein E, Mallory M, Hashimoto M, *et al.* 2002. Differential neuropathological alterations in transgenic mice expressing alpha-synuclein from the platelet-derived growth factor and Thy-1 promoters. *J Neurosci Res* **68**: 568–78.

Santiago PL, Rossi M, Cardinali DP, Merello M. 2010. Activity-rest rhythm abnormalities in Parkinson's disease patients are related to dopaminergic therapy. *Int J Neurosci* **120**: 11–6.

Schafer D, Greulich W. 2000. Effects of Parkinsonian medication on sleep. *J Neurol* **247**(Suppl 4): 24–7.

Schapira AH. 2012. Mitochondrial diseases. *Lancet* **379**: 1825–34.

Scheer FA, Hilton MF, Mantzoros CS, Shea SA. 2009. Adverse metabolic and cardiovascular consequences of circadian misalignment. *Proc Natl Acad Sci USA* **106**: 4453–8.

Schenck CH, Bundlie SR, Mahowald MW. 1996. Delayed emergence of a parkinsonian disorder in 38% of 29 older men initially diagnosed with idiopathic rapid eye movement sleep behaviour disorder. *Neuroloy* **46**: 388–93.

Sesti F, Liu S, Cai SQ. 2010. Oxidation of potassium channels by ROS: a general mechanism of aging and neurodegeneration? *Trends Cell Biol* **20**: 45–51.

Shepherd, G.M., Katz, D.M. 2011. Synaptic microcircuit dysfunction in genetic models of neurodevelopmental disorders: focus on Mecp2 and Met. *Curr Opin Neurobiol* **21**: 827–33.

Spengler ML, Kuropatwinski KK, Comas M, *et al.* 2012. Core circadian protein CLOCK is a positive regulator of NF-κB-mediated transcription. *Proc Natl Acad Sci USA* **109**(37): E2457–65.

Tanaka M, Yamaguchi E, Takahashi M, *et al.* 2012. Effects of age-related dopaminergic neuron loss in the substantia nigra on the circadian rhythms of locomotor activity in mice. *Neurosci Res* **74**(3–4): 210–5.

Tataroglu O, Davidson AJ, Benvenuto LJ, Menaker M. 2006. The methamphetamine-sensitive circadian oscillator (MASCO) in mice. *J Biol Rhythms* **21**: 185–94.

Taylor TN, Caudle WM, Shepherd KR, *et al.* 2009. Nonmotor symptoms of Parkinson's disease revealed in an animal model with reduced monoamine storage capacity. *J Neurosci* **29**(25): 8103–13.

Taylor TN, Caudle WM, Miller GW. 2011. VMAT2-deficient mice display nigral and extranigral pathology and motor and nonmotor symptoms of Parkinson's disease. *Parkinsons Dis* **2011**: 124165.

Trudel E, Bourque CW. 2010. Central clock excites vasopressin neurons by waking osmosensory afferents during late sleep. *Nat Neurosci* **13**: 467–74.

Trancikova A, Tsika E, Moore DJ. 2012. Mitochondrial dysfunction in genetic animal models of Parkinson's disease. *Antioxid Redox Signal* **16**: 896–919.

Verhave PS, Jongsma MJ, Van den Berg RM, *et al.* 2011. REM sleep behavior disorder in the marmoset MPTP model of early Parkinson disease. *Sleep* **34**(8): 1119–25.

Vezoli J, Fifel K, Leviel V, *et al.* 2011. Early presymptomatic and long-term changes of rest activity cycles and cognitive behavior in a MPTP-monkey model of Parkinson's disease. *PLoS One* **6**(8): e23952.

Videnovic A, Golombek D. 2012. Circadian and sleep disorders in Parkinson's disease. *Exp Neurol* **243**: 45–56.

Wailke S, Herzog J, Witt K, *et al.* 2011. Effect of controlled-release levodopa on the microstructure of sleep in Parkinson's disease. *Eur J Neurol* **18**(4): 590–6.

Wang YC, Huang RC. 2006. Effects of sodium pump activity on spontaneous firing in neurons of the rat suprachiasmatic nucleus. *J Neurophysiol* **96**: 109–18.

Wu N, Joshi PR, Cepeda C, *et al.* 2010. Alpha-synuclein overexpression in mice alters synaptic communication in the corticostriatal pathway. *J Neurosci Res* **88**: 1764–76.

Xie W, Chung KK. 2012. Alpha-synuclein impairs normal dynamics of mitochondria in cell and animal models of Parkinson's disease. *J Neurochem* **122**(2): 404–14.

Yeo L, Singh R, Gundeti M, *et al.* 2012. Urinary tract dysfunction in Parkinson's disease: a review. *Int Urol Nephrol* **44**: 415–24.

Zarranz JJ, Fernández-Bedoya A, Lambarri I, *et al.* 2005. Abnormal sleep architecture is an early feature in the E46K familial synucleinopathy. *Mov Disord* **20**(10): 1310–5.

Circadian Dysfunction in Huntington's Disease

21

A. Jennifer Morton

Department of Physiology, Development and Neuroscience, University of Cambridge, Cambridge, UK

21.1 Introduction

Huntington's disease (HD) is a complex neurological disorder that starts insidiously with motor, cognitive or psychiatric disturbances and progresses through a distressing range of symptoms to end with a devastating loss of function, both motor and cognitive (Bates *et al.*, 2002). HD is a dominant genetic disease. It is caused by an abnormal expansion of the CAG repeat in *HTT*, the gene that codes for huntingtin. It typically starts in the 4th decade of life, although there is a juvenile variant. HD is a rare disorder, affecting 1 in 8000–12,000 people. However, the time from diagnosis to the inevitable death of the patient can be 20–25 years, and for many of those years the patient is highly dependent on other people for their daily care. Thus, is it is a costly illness, with a large burden on both healthcare systems and families.

The classical description of HD is that it is a motor disorder characterized by involuntary choreiform movements, with an increasing occurrence of bradykinesia, rigidity, postural instability, and dystonia as the disease progresses. However, nonmotor symptoms, such as cognitive impairment, depression, irritability and other psychiatric symptoms, are prominent causes of disability in HD patients. In addition to the neurological symptoms, HD patients have a number of other symptoms, including circadian and sleep disturbances. There is a growing awareness of the possibility that, given what we know about the deleterious effects of sleep and circadian disruption in normal subjects, even mild sleep abnormalities might exacerbate neurological deficits in HD patients. Many of these nonmotor symptoms are similar to those that are present in neurologically normal individuals who are chronically sleep deprived and/or have severe circadian disruption.

21.2 Mechanisms underlying sleep and circadian rhythm generation

Circadian rhythms are orchestrated by an endogenous "master" oscillator/pacemaker located in the SCN of the hypothalamus (Reppert and Weaver, 2002; Chapter 3). A sophisticated molecular machinery drives the neuronal pacemaker (Chapter 1 and 2). Interestingly, the molecular machinery is not confined to the suprachiasmatic nucleus (SCN) but is also present in other brain regions, as well as peripheral tissues including liver, kidney, pancreas, spleen, thymus and skin (Chapters 6–13). The SCN is driven by entrainment agents (Zeitgebers) such as light and locomotor activity, and the role of the SCN is to keep the local clocks synchronized both with each other, and with the solar cycle. The SCN plays an important

Circadian Medicine, First Edition. Edited by Christopher S. Colwell.
© 2015 John Wiley & Sons, Inc. Published 2015 by John Wiley & Sons, Inc.

role in coordinating the physiological and behavioral output pathways (Dibner *et al.*, 2010). Although the sleep–wake cycle is the most obvious circadian-regulated behavior, the SCN plays a critical role in many different physiological processes. Circadian-regulated mechanisms include hormonal release, cardiovascular function, body temperature, feeding behavior, electrolyte balance and metabolism; for reviews see (Reddy *et al.*, 2006; Albrecht, 2012). It is particularly notable that abnormalities in nearly all of these domains are presented as symptoms in HD at one stage or another (Bates *et al.*, 2002).

21.3 Circadian disruption in HD

Breakdown of circadian rhythms caused by lifestyle changes (e.g., jet lag or shift work) are commonplace in the normal population. Daily clinical fluctuations of symptoms and signs associated with neurodegenerative diseases such as Alzheimer's disease (AD) and Parkinson's disease (PD) are now well recognized (Chapter 15). However, despite the frequent occurrence of disrupted sleep and alertness in the HD population, circadian rhythms have not been reported in HD until recently.

The first description of circadian behavioral abnormalities in HD came from an Actiwatch study that showed that there was an overall loss of form and definition in the rest–activity profiles in patients (Morton *et al.*, 2005)(Fig. 21.1). HD patients exhibited abnormal night/day ratios, although interestingly they did not report any major sleep difficulties. Nevertheless, when asked specifically about sleep disruption via the means of HD-specific questionnaires, sleep–wake disturbance was found to be commonplace (Goodman and Barker, 2010; Goodman *et al.*, 2010). Up to 90% of patients acknowledge having sleep problems, including daytime fatigue (Chapter 5), that were rated by about 60% of patients as either very important or moderately important contributors to their overall health problems = Identifying sleep or circadian disturbances through self-reporting of sleep problems in HD might be problematic because HD patients can lack insight. It is interesting that 10 years ago a similar underreporting of sleep problems was seen in PD (Askenasy, 2001; Shulman *et al.*, 2002), whereas now sleep disruption in PD is a well-recognized symptom.

While direct evidence for circadian dysfunction in HD patients is scant, indirect evidence is mounting. There is a delayed sleep phase, and increased rapid eye movement (REM) latency in HD (Aziz *et al.*, 2010) that is consistent with a phase-delayed circadian rhythm. Postmortem pathological changes have been reported in the SCN (van Wamelen *et al.*, 2013) and circadian changes in melatonin have been reported in HD (Aziz *et al.*, 2009b). Melatonin synthesis is directly regulated by the SCN and plays a major role in the regulation of sleep and other circadian rhythms. Dysregulation of melatonin is thought to be important in other neurodegenerative diseases as well as aging (Wu and Swaab, 2005, 2007; Cardinali *et al.*, 2013). It is possible that a delayed sleep phase syndrome-like circadian rhythm disorder is present in HD patients at an early stage.

21.4 Circadian disruption in animal models of HD

The first direct evidence of circadian rhythm disruption came from studies using a line of transgenic mice carrying the HD mutation in a fragment of the gene (R6/2 line; Morton *et al.*, 2005; Kudo *et al.*, 2011). These mice showed disturbed night–day activity that worsened with disease progression (Fig. 21.2). The sleep–wake activity disturbance was accompanied by a marked disruption of expression of the circadian clock genes in the SCN and other parts of the brain (e.g., motor cortex and striatum; Morton *et al.*, 2005). These changes correlated with decline in cognitive function. Surprisingly, given the profound breakdown in behavior, when the SCN was removed from the animal and studied *in vitro,* the molecular machinery driving circadian rhythms in the SCN was found to be intact (Pallier *et al.*, 2007). So on the molecular level, the circadian clockwork appears normal (Fig. 21.3) although physiologically SCN neurons in some HD lines show decreased neural activity rhythms (Kudo *et al.*, 2011). It is not known whether this type of pathophysiology is seen in the R6/2 line.

Circadian abnormalities in mouse models of HD have now been confirmed by a number of different laboratories (Morton, 2013). Additionally, there is growing evidence for changes in circadian measures

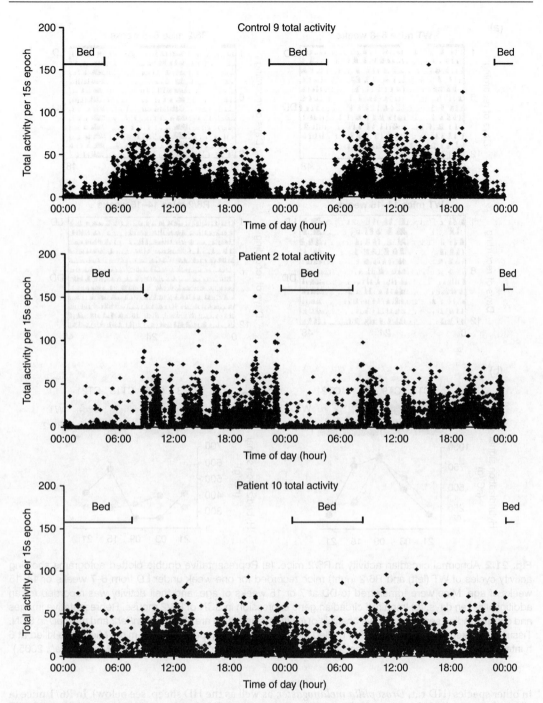

Fig. 21.1 Abnormal circadian activity in HD patients. Actimetry was monitored over 48 h in a neurologically normal control subject (top), an HD patient with an independence score of 90% (patient 2, middle), and an HD patient with an independence score of 60% (patient 10, bottom). The circadian rhythm is disrupted in the more severely affected patient. [Note that choreic movement is not included in these activity profiles.] (Taken from Morton *et al.*, 2005.)

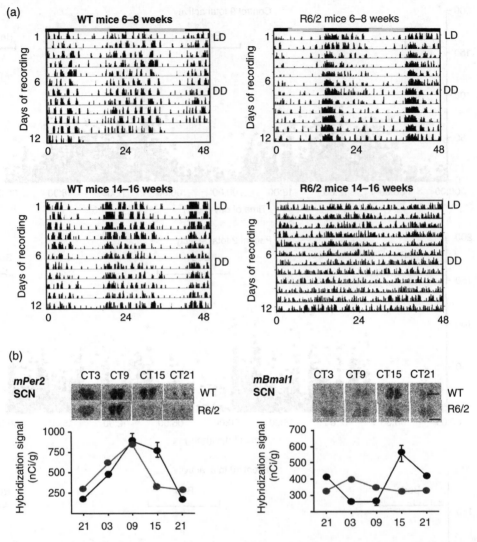

Fig. 21.2 Abnormal circadian activity in R6/2 mice. (a) Representative double-plotted actograms showing activity cycles of WT (left) and R6/2 (right) mice recorded for one week under LD from 6–7 weeks or 14–15 weeks of age. Mice were transferred to DD at 7 or 15 weeks of age, and their activity was recorded for an additional seven days. (b) Impaired circadian gene expression in SCN of R6/2 mouse. Representative images and corresponding semiquantitative analysis of *in situ* hybridization are shown for *mPer2* and *mBmal1* in SCN. Tissue was taken from 16-week-old WT (filled symbols) and R6/2 (open symbols) mice. Mice were killed at 6 h intervals over one 24-h period in the second cycle after release to DD. (Adapted from Morton *et al.*, 2005.)

in other species (HD rat, *Drosophila melanogaster*, as well as the HD sheep, see below). In R6/1 mice (a line similar to, but more slowly progressing, than R6/2), mild abnormalities have been seen in circadian behavior. Several studies have found evidence of circadian abnormalities in a bacterial artificial chromosome (BAC) mouse model of HD, including changes in daytime blood pressure, loss of circadian control of heart rate and motor activity (Kudo *et al.*, 2011; Schroeder *et al.*, 2011). The loss of circadian control of cardiac function in BACHD mice is particularly interesting, given the desynchronization in peripheral clocks reported in R6/2 mice (Maywood *et al.*, 2010) and the fact that R6/2 mice have progressive abnormalities in cardiac function (Wood *et al.*, 2012). This raises the possibility that

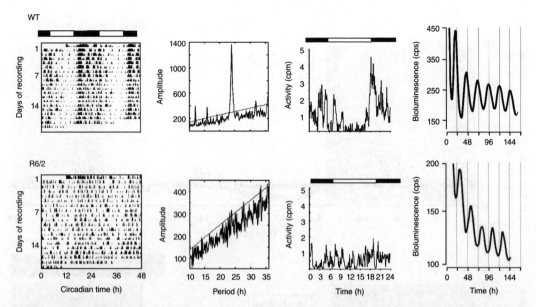

Fig. 21.3 R6/2 mutation disrupts activity–rest cycles in mPer1::Luciferase reporter mice used to analyze molecular time keeping in SCN *in vitro*. Representative actograms of WT (top) and R6/2 (bottom) mice held under 12 h light/dark cycle from 12 weeks of age onwards show a progressive deterioration of activity profile in R6/2 mice. Periodogram analyses of mice with circadian behavior show a highly significant peak in the WT but not in R6/2 mice. Mean daily activity profile of mice indicates more daytime and less nocturnal activity. Circadian bioluminescence recordings from SCN explants were obtained from two mice (one R6/2, one WT), whose activity is depicted in the actograms. The SCN from both R6/2 and WT mice showed functional molecular time keeping, as revealed by *in vitro* by bioluminescence gene expression. (Adapted from Pallier *et al.*, 2007.) *(See insert for color representation of the figure.)*

autonomic dysfunction seen in HD patients, particularly abnormalities of autonomic control of the cardiovascular system (Andrich *et al.*, 2002; Aziz *et al.*, 2010; Kobal *et al.*, 2010), may be due, at least in part, to circadian dysfunction. It would be interesting to see if there were changes in circadian rhythm of blood pressure, body temperature or changes in circadian control of heart rate variability in HD patients, since these are easily measured output of physiological function that are under circadian control.

Behavioral disruption that manifests as circadian abnormality has been shown in a transgenic HD sheep that carries a full length transgene with a CAG repeat in the juvenile range for HD (Fig. 21.4). These sheep (OVT73) express the full-length human huntingtin protein but show no overt symptoms and have very limited brain pathology up to five years of age (Jacobsen *et al.*, 2010; Reid *et al.*, 2013). Behavioral field testing using actigraphy showed that at the earliest time of testing (18 months of age), HD sheep display an increased period of restlessness after sunset compared to normal sheep. Interestingly, this behavior is reminiscent of the "sundowning" behavior that is seen in AD patients. The behavioral abnormalities worsened with age. By five years of age, there was a clear difference in nocturnal behavior of normal and HD sheep groups, with increased evening restlessness, significant nighttime disturbance and a phase advance in nocturnal activity pattern. It is particularly notable that the behavioral abnormalities were only detected in sheep kept in an "HD-only" flock. This suggests that HD sheep are capable of responding correctly to flock cues about nighttime behavior but that in the HD-only flock such cues are either not generated, or are generated incorrectly. Behavior of HD sheep kept mixed with normal sheep was relatively normal, with only a small disturbance at sunset. It is interesting that this small abnormal behavior was reflected throughout the flock, with both normal and HD animals showing the disturbance compared to sheep kept in a normal-only flock; this is reminiscent of the knock-on effects of disturbed HD patient behavior on carers (Morton *et al.*, 2005). The phase advance in the older sheep may signal the

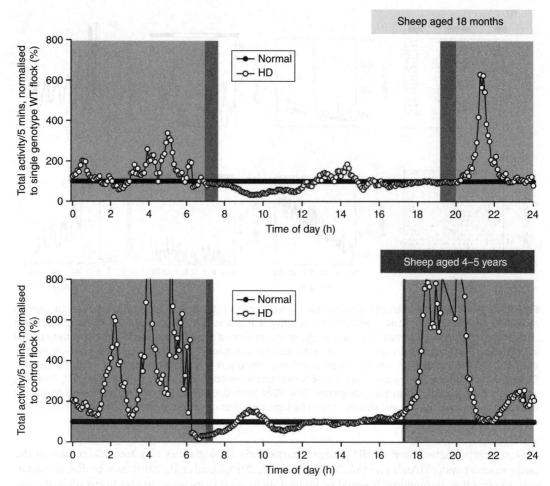

Fig. 21.4 Daily activity patterns differ in HD and normal sheep and worsen progressively with age. Total activity was collected from 20 normal (closed symbols) and 20 HD (open symbols) sheep from separate flocks, at two different ages (18 months (upper panel) and 4–5 years (lower panel)) using Actiwatches. Data were collected over several weeks at the end of summer. Mean daily activity of the HD sheep (kept in an HD-only flock) was normalized to data from normal sheep (kept in a normal-only flock). The differences in activity patterns can be seen clearly in both groups, with the 5-year-old sheep showing a more exaggerated change. Nighttime is shown as light grey, and the period including the range of sunrise/sunset times over the data collection period is shown in dark grey. Note that activity between 11 a.m. and 3 p.m. is contaminated by artefacts related to farm activity (feeding supplementary feed). (The figure has been modified from Morton et al., 2014.)

onset of explicit circadian behavioral symptoms and is consistent with the phase advance reported in melatonin secretion in HD patients (Aziz et al., 2009a).

The finding of behavioral disturbances in sleep–wake activity in sheep is particularly interesting for a number of reasons. Firstly, finding circadian behavioral abnormalities in another species, particularly one that is diurnal, suggests that the abnormalities seen in the HD mice are not mouse-specific. Secondly, the fact that the behavioral abnormalities are hidden when the HD animals are living in mixed genotype groups suggests that sleep–wake abnormalities in HD patients are also likely to be hidden, and may precede overt symptoms by many years. Thirdly, the abnormalities were progressive, which is consistent with them being part of the spectrum of HD symptoms. Fourthly, the abnormalities appeared very early. In 5-year-old sheep there is aggregate pathology, but it is very sparse, and there is no frank neurodegeneration. Yet, by

18 months, a significant behavioral disorder was present in the HD sheep. This supports the idea that the HD mutation causes circuitry changes many years before neurodegeneration is seen. Thus, circadian disorder may serve as a very useful readout for determining the onset of subtle behavioral disorder in HD.

21.5 Circadian disruption of peripheral clocks and metabolism in HD

Peripheral clocks exist in most tissues (Chapters 6–9). Although their function is not known, they are likely to be important parts of an information system that allows metabolism to be adjusted according to environmental conditions (Green *et al.*, 2008; Asher and Schibler, 2011), such as the availability of food, and temperature (Chapters 6 and 7). Studies using the R6/2 mouse model of HD showed that the peripheral clock(s) are uncoupled from the control of the SCN, and that this results in desynchronization of metabolism as shown by loss of circadian control of clock-controlled liver output (Maywood *et al.*, 2010). The consequences of such uncoupling are unknown, since the mechanisms controlling coordination of brain and peripheral rhythms are not fully understood (Albrecht, 2012). But if the timing of different physiological rhythms is altered so that there are changes in the phase relationship of rhythms to each other, then internal desynchronization would occur, as is seen in the R6/2 mouse brain and peripheral organs (Maywood *et al.*, 2010; Fig. 21.3). It is likely that the consequences of such disruption will be deleterious (Kyriacou and Hastings, 2010). For example, uncoupling liver metabolism from circadian drives would reduce metabolic efficiency (Chapters 6 and 7). This might be particularly important in HD where metabolic dysregulation has long been thought to be part of the disease process (Bates *et al.*, 2002). Given that some liver abnormalities are clearly associated with sleep disturbance (De Cruz *et al.*, 2012) and neurological dysfunction (Maywood *et al.*, 2010), it is possible that even subtle inefficiencies of liver metabolism may exacerbate neurological symptoms of HD.

21.6 Pharmacological manipulation of circadian disruption in HD mice

The fact that in a mouse with severely disrupted circadian rhythms, the cells in the SCN are capable of normal function is particularly interesting. If the machinery is not broken, then, in theory, malfunctions in behavioral output mediated via dysfunctional circuitry might be preventable, if the pathways can be reactivated/re-entrained correctly. This possibility was confirmed by a study showing that both cognitive decline and molecular dysregulation could be prevented with pharmacological treatments that manipulated the sleep–wake cycle (Pallier and Morton, 2009). This was a critically important study for the HD field, because cognitive symptoms are extremely disruptive and frequently coincide with the "beginning-of-the-end" of a fully functional life in HD patients. The possibility that cognitive decline can be improved by manipulation of the sleep–wake cycle makes circadian rhythms a compelling target for both drug and behavioral therapy. It is particularly relevant that improvements in cognitive function were seen in the R6/2 mouse, because disease onset and decline is very rapid in this line. If cognitive output could be modulated beneficially in R6/2 mice, then it is possible that this strategy might also be successful in HD patients.

21.7 Environmental modulation of circadian disruption in HD mice

Circadian rhythms of R6/2 mice can be modulated through nonpharmacological means as well as with drug treatments. The disruption to the circadian system that is a consequence of jet lag or shift work in humans can have significant impact on cognitive performance and health as a result of desynchronization between Zeitgebers and the endogenous clockwork. It has also been shown in mice that inducing experimental jet lag has deleterious effects on age at death, and that phase advances have a more profound effect on the mice than phase delays (Davidson *et al.*, 2006). Interestingly, R6/2 mice subjected to a jet-lag paradigm (six-hour delay or advance in light onset, then reversal after two weeks) could adapt well to the original shift but they could not adjust accurately to the reversal (Wood *et al.*, 2013). If similar abnormalities are present in HD patients, they may suffer exaggerated jet lag. Since the underlying molecular clock mechanism remains intact, light therapy may be a useful treatment for circadian dysfunction in HD.

21.8 Clinical changes in sleep in HD

Sleep is one of the most important circadian-controlled behaviors, and probably the most obvious one (Chapter 4). Sleep is generated and regulated by molecular mechanisms that are independent of those generating circadian rhythms. Different aspects of what we think of as "sleep" (sleep onset, staging, maintenance, and wakefulness) are themselves generated independently, via different (albeit interacting) brain systems (Cirelli, 2009; Saper *et al.*, 2010; España and Scammell, 2011). Disorders of nocturnal sleep are common in the general population and are one of the most common reasons for medication in the normal population. However, sleep dysfunction in HD is likely to be underdiagnosed by clinicians and underreported by patients because it seems that HD patients rarely complain to their doctors about sleep disturbance (Goodman *et al.*, 2011).

21.9 Disturbance in sleep architecture in HD

The only way of determining definitively whether or not sleep disorder is present is by using electroencephalography (EEG). Sleep is defined electrophysiologically by specific patterns of brain activity that can be measured by electroencephalography. EEG measurements carried out at the same time as electrooculography and electromyography are collectively known as polysomnography, and are typically used to define sleep stages. There are five stages of sleep that can be distinguished clearly: historically, these were four phases of nonrapid eye movement (NREM) sleep that progress from Stage 1 (light sleep) to Stage 4 (deep sleep) and one phase of REM sleep. (Note that the 4 NREM stages have been reclassified as N1–N3 by the American Academy of Sleep Medicine). After a bout of REM sleep, the brain cycles back through the NREM sleep stages. It takes 60–90 minutes to cycle through all stages of NREM sleep. In normal subjects, this sleep cycle is repeated 4–5 times a night. Early in the night, NREM sleep is usually deeper and longer, later in the night, a higher proportion of each cycle is made up of REM sleep. REM and NREM sleep are controlled separately (Morris *et al.*, 2012; Chapter 4). Recent work has raised the exciting possibility that there may be an EEG signature for HD. Pilot data in the three premanifest HD subjects reported that EEG abnormalities may be detectable even in premanifest gene carriers (Hunter *et al.*, 2010). In an important set of studies, abnormal EEG gamma activity (30–40 Hz) has been reported in R6/2 mice irrespective of sleep states (Kantor *et al.*, 2013; Fisher *et al.*, 2013).

Sleep disturbance is often reflected as disorders of daytime alertness (Chapter 5). HD patients report insomnia and have a tendency towards increased daytime somnolence (Videnovic *et al.*, 2009; Goodman *et al.*, 2010). Over the past 25 years or so, there have been a number of polysomnography studies looking at sleep and sleep-related disorder in HD (Morton, 2013). They showed that patients with HD had impairments in multiple aspects of sleep, although there was no "characteristic" sleep deficit signature for HD, and none of the studies reported all of the changes seen. Patients in moderate stages of disease spend more time in NREM sleep stages and less time in REM sleep or slow wave sleep (SWS). HD patients showed impaired initiation and maintenance of sleep, reduced sleep efficiency and reduced total sleep time compared to normal subjects. HD patients also showed a high percentage of wakefulness after sleep onset. Given the findings of abnormal EEG in HD patients, changes in sleep–wake activity patterns should be considered to be a part of the repertoire of HD symptoms (Morton, 2013).

One of the difficulties of conducting clinical studies before the cloning of the gene in 2003 made gene testing possible was that the definitive diagnostic criterion for HD was the presence of chorea. Thus, patients without chorea were never studied and, in fact, early-stage HD patients were thought to have no clinical sleep disturbance. However, since the cloning of the HD gene, investigators have had the advantage of being able to study early-stage HD patients as well as later-stage patients. Recent studies show that early in their disease, HD patients have mild polysomnography abnormalities, with increased interspersed wakefulness and a longer time to first REM episode (Arnulf *et al.*, 2008). The progressively worsening sleep disorder appeared to be independent of CAG repeat length.

Many of the changes seen in HD patients resemble changes in sleep that take place as part of the normal aging process in humans, including a decreased amount of total sleep time, sleep efficiency changes in percentages of SWS and REM sleep, with increases in sleep latency and Stages 1 and 2, and sleep fragmentation (Ohayon *et al.*, 2004). Although the average age of HD patients at onset of disease is considerably younger than that at which age-related changes in sleep typically present, it is an interesting possibility to consider that some of the changes seen in HD patients resemble accelerated aging.

21.10 Pathology underlying changes in sleep and circadian activity in HD

The characteristic pathology in HD is atrophy and degeneration of neostriatum (caudate nucleus, putamen, and globus pallidus) and cortex that eventually involves the whole brain, including subcortical structures (Bates *et al.*, 2002). Sleep disturbances in HD were originally reported to be correlated with the degree of atrophy of the caudate nucleus and the severity of clinical symptoms, although more recent finding showed that this correlation is weak (Arnulf *et al.*, 2008). A correlation of frontal lobe dysfunction and changes in sleep latency was also described (Cuturic *et al.*, 2009), but again the significance of this correlations is not clear, since few early stage and no presymptomatic patients were included in this study. The striatum is an important area for the control of locomotion and voluntary activity but it is not thought to be involved directly in the generation of sleep, although some striatal lesion studies suggested a possible involvement of the striatum in modulating wakefulness (Mena-Segovia *et al.*, 2002).

The hypothalamus is crucial for the regulation of circadian rhythms, sleep and metabolism, as well as for the regulation of automatic functions such as breathing and heartbeat. The anterior, ventral region of the hypothalamus contains the SCN. There is evidence of neurodegeneration in these areas (Petersén and Björkqvist, 2006) and it is thought that these changes may occur as much as a decade before clinical diagnosis of HD. Hypothalamic dysfunction in HD patients would not only have an impact on circadian rhythm and daytime sleepiness but would affect other relevant functions that have an impact on sleep. Although evidence from MRI studies suggests that neurodegeneration in the hypothalamus occurs very early in HD, it is only recently that the structure and function of the SCN have been examined to date in postmortem brains. A recent postmortem study showed that compared with control subjects, the SCN in patients with HD contained 85% fewer neurons immunoreactive for vasoactive intestinal polypeptide and 33% fewer neurons for arginine vasopressin, although the total amount of vasoactive intestinal polypeptide and arginine vasopressin messenger RNA was unchanged and there was no change in the number of melatonin 1 or 2 receptor immunoreactive neurons (van Wamelen *et al.*, 2013). These findings suggest that sleep and circadian rhythm disorders in these patients may at least partly arise from SCN dysfunction. Other parts of the hypothalamus have been given more attention. For example, significant atrophy and loss of orexin/hypocretin neurons has been identified in HD (Roos and Aziz, 2007; Aziz *et al.*, 2007, 2009b; Hult *et al.*, 2010). The thalamus is also crucially important for generation of sleep and wakefulness. It degenerates in HD but it is not how thalamic pathology impacts on sleep in HD.

21.11 The orexin system in HD

Orexins have been heavily implicated in sleep and circadian changes in HD, although cerebrospinal fluid levels of this peptide appear to be normal in HD patients (Gaus *et al.*, 2005; Meier *et al.*, 2005). In R6/2 mice, the size of an electrically distinct subpopulation of orexin neurons is reduced, as is the number of orexin-immunopositive cells in some hypothalamic regions (Williams *et al.*, 2011). R6/2 orexin cells display altered glutamatergic inputs and have an abnormal circadian profile of activity, despite normal circadian rhythmicity of the SCN. Nevertheless, even at advanced stages of HD, intrinsic firing properties of orexin cells remain normal and suppressible by serotonin, noradrenaline, and glucose. Furthermore, histaminergic neurons (key cells required for the propagation of orexin-induced arousal) also display normal responses to orexin. Together, these data suggest that the orexin system remains functional and modifiable in HD mice, although its circadian activity profile is disrupted and no longer follows that of the SCN.

There are a number of other neuropetides for which there is evidence implicating them in loss of control of sleep or circadian function. For example, melatonin is very important in sleep, and there is evidence of phase advance of melatonin cycles in HD (Aziz *et al.*, 2009a), although it has not been studied in detail in HD. There is also evidence for changes in the expression of two major regulatory neuropeptides, vasoactive intestinal polypeptide and arginine vasopressin (van Wamalen *et al.*, 2013). Finally, Shan and colleagues showed that there is clear evidence of diurnal fluctuation in histidine decarboxylase expression (the rate limiting enzyme for histamine production) as well as for disturbed diurnal fluctuation of neural histamine production in neurodegenerative diseases including HD (Shan *et al.*, 2012).

21.12 The role of non-SCN oscillators in HD

In addition to the SCN, there are at least two other independent circadian oscillators in the brain. These are the food-entrainable oscillator (FEO; Challet *et al.*, 2009; Verwey and Amir 2009; Mistlberger, 2011) and the methamphetamine-sensitive circadian oscillator (MASCO; Honma *et al.*, 1986, 1987; Tataroğlu *et al.*, 2006; Honma and Honma, 2009). The activity of the FEO persists even in the absence of the SCN and is thought to be located in the hypothalamus, but outside the SCN. However, it has not been well studied in humans. The activity of the MASCO is also independent of the SCN, since it is inducible in SCN-lesioned animals. Neither the site nor the functional role of the MASCO is known in rodents, and the relevance of the MASCO to circadian behavior in humans is completely unknown. In fact, the MASCO cannot be studied directly in humans (since the means of inducing it in mice is by keeping the mice in isolation in the dark and giving them low chronic dose of methamphetamine). Studies conducted using the R6/2 mouse model show that although the FEO remains intact (Maywood *et al.*, 2010) the MASCO is already dysfunctional at presymptomatic ages (Cuesta *et al.*, 2012). This oscillator, and its possible dysfunction, may, therefore, be important in HD. Why it becomes dysfunctional so early in R6/2 mice remains to be determined.

21.13 Consequences of sleep–wake disturbance in HD

The function of sleep remains unknown, but the consequences of sleep deprivation are well recognized in the neurologically normal population. Sleep is essential for optimal physical and mental performance. It is also important for the maintenance of general health and well-being. Even mild sleep deprivation for a few days causes a deterioration of performance. Sleep deprivation is common in modern society, with lifestyle choices, shift work and jet lag being the most common causes. Sleep deprivation is disruptive in the short term, and likely to be harmful in the long term. Experimental total sleep deprivation produces a syndrome in rats that includes metabolic dysregulation (including increased food intake, weight loss, increased energy expenditure and decreased body temperature; Rechtschaffen and Bergmann, 2002). Selective sleep stage deprivation (REM or SWS) resulted in similar findings (Kushida *et al.*, 1989). The effect of sleep deprivation on humans is not as dramatic as it is in rodents, perhaps because total sleep deprivation of humans in controlled conditions for long periods is extremely difficult to achieve. Nevertheless, sleep deprivation studies have revealed a broad range of impairments, including impaired memory and learning, reduced reaction times, irritability, depression, stress, increased susceptibility to illness, and metabolic abnormalities, and hormonal imbalances. Sleep deprivation can have a substantial impact on the health and quality of life of a normal individual – this may be even more significant in disease states such as HD. There is no study yet done, in either HD mouse models or in patients showing that sleep deprivation exacerbates cognitive dysfunction. Interestingly, the regions of the frontal cortex that degenerate in HD and are so critical for cognitive function are also key targets for neurochemical pathways regulating sleep. So, it is possible that degeneration in target regions causes not only the cognitive decline, but also a concomitant sleep disorder.

21.14 Cognitive dysfunction and mood disturbance in HD

Abnormalities in sleep and circadian rhythms have negative impacts upon cognitive, emotional and psychiatric function (Chapters 16–18). For example, sleep is thought to be important for memory consolidation, thus, the disruption of normal sleep patterns as a result of circadian clock ageing can be one of the contributors to memory impairment (Kyriacou and Hastings, 2010; Pace-Schott and Spencer, 2011; Pace-Schott *et al.*, 2012). Only circumstantial evidence exists to suggest a link between the HD-related symptoms and sleep deprivation. Nevertheless, this evidence is compelling. HD has a characteristic cluster of symptoms that may include a loss of motor control, changes in mood, and cognitive impairment. Sleep deprivation cause many of the same symptoms (Chapter 4). For example, hippocampus-dependent declarative memory consolidation is thought to occur during SWS. This may be relevant in HD, since impaired declarative memory has been found early in HD patients (Ghilardi *et al.*, 2008). It is possible, therefore, that the memory deficits found in HD are related, at least in part, to a reduction in SWS and/or circadian disturbances. Depression and anxiety are common in HD patients, even before disease onset. Given that depression in the neurologically normal population is associated with sleep problems, such as difficulty falling asleep, frequent nocturnal awakenings, early morning awakening, decreased total sleep and nonrestorative sleep, it is possible that many of the sleep abnormalities seen in the HD patients are due to depression. However, it is not clear if HD patients experience a "pure" sleep disorder or have sleep disruption that is a consequence of circadian disturbance. This is an important question to address, since many aspects of sleep disorder can be treated.

21.15 Management of circadian disturbance in HD

Pharmacological management of HD is poor (Bonelli and Wenning, 2006; Pidgeon and Rickards, 2012). Circadian dysfunction is only now emerging as part of the spectrum of symptoms in HD, and treatment strategies for sleep and/or circadian disorder in HD are poorly developed. Furthermore, it is not known how effective drugs that are typically used to treat sleep disorder are in HD patients. It is possible that drugs that are effective in normal people are either not effective or have different (and not necessarily beneficial) effects in patients with neurodegenerative disorder (Ellenbogen and Pace-Schott, 2012). Given the deleterious cognitive and psychiatric effects that arise with chronic sleep deprivation, all HD patients, whether or not they have a sleep problem severe enough to need medication, should be encouraged to establish good sleep hygiene (Morton, 2013). In particular, they should minimize their intake of caffeine, nicotine and alcohol, avoid napping during the daytime, and adopt a regular schedule that includes regular exercise. If it is suspected that they have a sleep disorder, patients should be referred to a sleep specialist. Detailed review of their medication should be carried out regularly, and timing of medications that impact sleep–wake cycles should be considered independently. Medications that disrupt sleep architecture should be prescribed with care. Drugs that might be prescribed for relief of symptoms in HD that may also cause sedation or drowsiness include tetrabenazine, clonazepam, riluzole, olanzapine, quetiapine, diazepam, dosulepin, venlafaxine. Those that may cause an increase in activation include sodium valproate, amantidine, and L-DOPA/carbidopa. If the patient has daytime sleepiness, the use of stimulants or wake-promoting agents, such as Modafinil, could be considered. Modafinil is a novel wake-promoting agent that has been promoted widely as a cognitive enhancer and is thought to have its effect through its action on sleep–wake activity. The effect of Modafinil has only been studied once in

HD patients, at a single dose given once. It did not improve either mood or cognition. However, it has been evaluated in open-label and controlled trials for the treatment somnolence in PD (Videnovic and Golembek, 2013). Modafinil was well tolerated, and did not affect the motor function of PD patients - this would be an important consideration of modafinil was to be used in HD patients- although its effects on sleep disorder in PD were mixed. Melatonin might also be useful. Melatonin is a neurohormone that

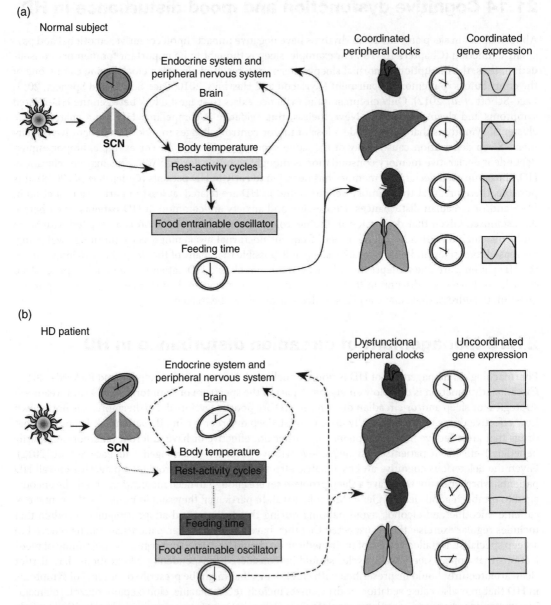

Fig. 21.5 Circadian control in HD subjects may be disturbed at multiple levels. In normal subjects, there is a sophisticated balance of feedback loops that regulates daily physiological function. Multiple aspects of this control system may be disturbed in HD patients, with the overall effect being either symptoms (such as abnormal daily activity) or hidden deficits (such as poorly coordinated metabolism). *(See insert for color representation of the figure.)*

has been shown to improve sleep disturbances in the elderly as well as in PD, and, again, although its efficacy is not well established, it is unlikely to have deleterious side-effects in HD patients.

Environmental enrichment has been shown to improve a number of aspects of disease progression including cognitive function in HD mice. It is possible that lifestyle modifications may be a useful therapy (Fig. 21.5; Chapter 23). This might include a regime of light therapy, or of regular exercise, since there is an association of regular exercise or physical activity with a lower prevalence of symptoms of disturbed sleep (Sherrill *et al.*, 1998).

One study using HD mice showed that pharmacological treatment aimed at improving circadian and sleep patterns, using alprazolam (at sedative doses to induce sleep) and Modafinil (to induce wakefulness) improved cognitive function and survival in the mice (Pallier and Morton, 2009). This is an approach that could be taken in HD patients, although it should be noted that while Alprazolam was used at a hypnotic dose to impose sleep on mice, it was chosen only because it had a short half-life and was, therefore, suitable for the experimental regime in the mice. It is a tantalizing possibility that, by treating sleep disturbance (with hynotics suitable for patients with neurodegenerative diseases) and/or circadian disorder (with, for example, melatonin, chronotherapy or light therapy) it might be possible to have beneficial knock-on effects on other aspects of HD. Using the R6/2 model, combinations of bright light therapy and voluntary exercise were used to delay disintegration of the rest–activity rhythm and improve behavioral synchronization to the light-dark cycle (Cuesta *et al.*, 2014). The best effects were observed in mice treated with a combination of bright light therapy and restricted periods of voluntary exercise. Neither the cause nor the consequence of deteriorating sleep–wake activity in HD patients is known. Nevertheless, these findings can be translated immediately to human patients with little cost or risk, since both light therapy and restricted exercise regimes are nonpharmacological interventions that are relatively easy to schedule. These approaches could be particularly important if they improve the cognitive deficits that are a core element of HD. These are a major problem for many patients and their families. There are currently no drug therapies that improve cognitive dysfunction caused by HD.

21.16 Conclusions

Sleep–wake disturbance in HD is likely to have an impact on patient well-being, and may play an important role in the disease process. There is a subset of symptoms seen in HD patients that in neurologically normal sleep-deprived subjects would be regarded as the predictable sequelae of chronic sleep deprivation or internal dysregulation relating to circadian dysfunction (Fig. 21.5). Some or all of these may arise in HD patients as a consequence of sleep deprivation. If this is the case, then sleep disturbance may exacerbate HD symptoms, particularly those in the cognitive and emotional domains. There is growing recognition that sleep and circadian disorders exist in the HD population and, correspondingly, increasing numbers of patients are seeking help for their problems, rather than accepting them as an inevitable part of the disease. However, the impact of sleep–wake disturbance in HD will not be known until systematic studies have been conducted. It remains to be determined whether or not symptoms that are part of the HD repertoire are secondary to sleep deprivation. If the latter is the case, then they may be treatable with conventional therapies. There are currently no specific therapeutic recommendations for the treatment of sleep disorder in HD. Furthermore, no study has been done to show that drugs used conventionally to treat sleep disorder are effective in HD patients. Ideally, controlled clinical trials of HD patients should be undertaken to determine both the efficacy and safety of therapies used for the treatment of sleep dysfunction in HD. The relationship between disruptions of the circadian system, sleep disturbance and other symptoms in HD should also be determined. Until this is done, we will not be in a position to know whether symptoms are a natural consequence of direct dysfunction caused by the HD gene, or if they are indirect consequences of HD-induced sleep deprivation. In the meantime, targeting the circadian clock as a means to strengthen homeostatic mechanisms that might reduce HD symptoms is a promising therapeutic approach. Knock-on effects of sleep abnormalities in HD may not only be critical for determining the care-plan of patients but may also may a have greater impact on quality of life than motor symptoms, as has been shown in other diseases.

References

Albrecht, U. 2012. Timing to perfection: The biology of central and peripheral circadian clocks. *Neuron* **74**, 246–60.

Andrich J., Schmitz T., Saft C., *et al.* 2002. Autonomic nervous system function in Huntington's disease. *J Neurol Neurosurg Psychiatry* **72**, 726–31.

Arnulf, I., Nielsen, J., Lohmann, E., *et al.* 2008. Rapid eye movement sleep disturbances in Huntington disease. *Arch Neurol* **65**, 482–8.

Asher, G., Schibler, U. 2011. Crosstalk between components of circadian and metabolic cycles in mammals. *Cell Metab* **2**, 125–37.

Askenasy, J.J. 2001. Approaching disturbed sleep in late Parkinson's disease: first step toward a proposal for a revised UPDRS. *Parkinsonism Relat Disord* **8**, 123–31.

Aziz, N.A., Swaab, D.F., Pijl, H., Roos, R.A. 2007. Hypothalamic dysfunction and neuroendocrine and metabolic alterations in Huntington's disease: clinical consequences and therapeutic implications. *Rev Neurosci* **18**, 223–51.

Aziz, N.A., Pijl, H., Frölich, M., *et al.* 2009a. Delayed onset of the diurnal melatonin rise in patients with Huntington's disease. *J Neurol* **256**, 1961–5.

Aziz, N.A., Pijl, H., Frölich, M., *et al.* 2009b. Increased hypothalamic-pituitary-adrenal axis activity in Huntington's disease. *J Clin Endocrinol Metab* **94**, 1223–8.

Aziz, N.A., Anguelova, G.V., Marinus, J., *et al.* 2010. Sleep and circadian rhythm alterations correlate with depression and cognitive impairment in Huntington's disease. *Parkinsonism Relat Disord* **16**, 345–50.

Bates, G.P., Harper, P.S., Jones, L. (eds) 2002. *Huntington's Disease*, 3rd edn. Oxford University Press, Oxford.

Bonelli, R.M., Wenning, G. K. 2006. Pharmacological Management of Huntington's Disease: An Evidence- Based Review. *Curr Pharm Design* **12**, 2701–20.

Cardinali, D.P., Pagano, E.S., Scacchi Bernasconi, P.A., *et al.* 2013. Melatonin and mitochondrial dysfunction in the central nervous system. *Horm Behav* **63**(2), 322–30.

Challet, E., Mendoza, J., Dardente, H., Pévet, P. 2009. Neurogenetics of food anticipation. *Eur J Neurosci* **30**, 1676–87.

Cirelli, C. 2009. The genetic and molecular regulation of sleep: from fruit flies to humans. *Nat Rev Neurosci* **10**, 549–60.

Cuesta, M., Aungier, J., Morton, A.J. 2012. The methamphetamine-sensitive circadian oscillator is dysfunctional in a transgenic mouse model of Huntington's disease. *Neurobiol Dis* **45**, 145–55.

Cuesta, M., Aungier, J., Morton, A.J. 2014. Behavioral therapy reverses circadian deficits in a transgenic mouse model of Huntington's disease. *Neurobiol Dis* **63**:85–91.

Cuturic, M., Abramson, R.K., Vallini, D., *et al.* 2009. Sleep patterns in patients with Huntington's disease and their unaffected first-degree relatives: a brief report. *Behav Sleep Med* **7**, 245–54.

Davidson, A.J., Sellix, M.T., Daniel, J., *et al.* 2006. Chronic jet-lag increases mortality in aged mice. *Curr Biol* **16**, R914–16.

De Cruz, S., Espiritu, J.R., Zeidler, M., Wang, T.S. 2012. Sleep disorders in chronic liver disease. *Semin Respir Crit Care Med* **33**, 26–35.

Dibner, C., Schibler, U., Albrecht, U. 2010. The mammalian circadian timing system:organization and coordination of central and peripheral clocks. *Annu Rev Physiol* **72**, 517–49.

Ellenbogen, J.M., Pace-Schott, E.F. 2012. Drug-induced sleep: theoretical and practical considerations. *Pflugers Arch* **463**, 177–86.

España, R.A., Scammell, T.E. 2011. Sleep neurobiology from a clinical perspective. *Sleep* **1**, 845–58.

Fisher, S.P., Black, S.W., Schwartz, M.D., *et al.* 2013. Longitudinal analysis of the electroencephalogram and sleep phenotype in the R6/2 mouse model of Huntington's disease. *Brain* **136**(Pt 7), 2159–72.

Gaus, S.E., Lin, L., Mignot, E. 2005. CSF hypocretin levels are normal in Huntington's disease patients. *Sleep* **28**, 1607–8.

Ghilardi, M.F., Silvestri, G., Feigin, A., *et al.* 2008. Implicit and explicit aspects of sequence learning in pre-symptomatic Huntington's disease. *Parkinsonism Relat Disord* **14**, 457–64.

Goodman, A.O., Barker, R.A. 2010. How vital is sleep in Huntington's disease? *J Neurol* **257**, 882–97.

Goodman, A.O., Morton, A.J., Barker, R.A. 2010. Identifying sleep disturbances in Huntington's disease using a simple disease-focused questionnaire. *PLoS Curr* **15**, 2.

Goodman, A.O., Rogers, L., Pilsworth, S., *et al.* 2011. Asymptomatic sleep abnormalities are a common early feature in patients with Huntington's disease. *Curr Neurol Neurosci Rep* **11**, 211–7.

Green, C.B., Takahashi, J.S., Bass, J. 2008. The meter of metabolism. *Cell* **134**, 728–42.

Honma, K., Honma, S. 2009. The SCN-independent clocks, methamphetamine and food restriction. *Eur J Neurosci* **30**, 1707–17.

Honma, K., Honma, S., Hiroshige, T. 1986. Disorganization of the rat activity rhythm bychronic treatment with methamphetamine. *Physiol Behav* **38**, 687–95.

Honma, K., Honma, S., Hiroshige, T. 1987. Activity rhythms in the circadian domain appear in suprachiasmatic nuclei lesioned rats given methamphetamine. *Physiol Behav* **40**, 767–74.

Hult, S., Schultz, K., Soylu, R., Petersén, A. 2010. Hypothalamic and neuroendocrine changes in Huntington's disease. *Curr Drug Targets* **11**, 1237–49.

Hunter, A., Bordelon, Y., Cook, I., Leuchter, A. 2010. QEEG Measures in Huntington's Disease: A Pilot Study. *PLoS Curr* **2**, RRN1192

Jacobsen, J.C, Bawden, C.S., Rudiger, S.R., *et al.* 2010. An ovine transgenic Huntington's disease model. *Hum Mol Gen* **19**, 1873–82.

Kantor, S., Szabo, L., Varga, J., *et al.* 2013. Progressive sleep and electroencephalogram changes in mice carrying the Huntington's disease mutation. *Brain* **136**(Pt 7), 2147–58.

Kobal, J., Melik, Z., Cankar, K., *et al.* 2010. Autonomic dysfunction in presymptomatic and early symptomatic Huntington's disease. *Acta Neurol Scand* **12**, 392–9.

Kudo, T., Schroeder, A., Loh, D.H., *et al.* 2011. Dysfunctions in circadian behavior and physiology in mouse models of Huntington's disease. *Exp Neurol* **228**, 80–90.

Kushida, C.A., Bergmann, B.M., Rechtschaffen, A. 1989. Sleep deprivation in the rat: IV. Paradoxical sleep deprivation. *Sleep* **12**, 22–30.

Kyriacou, C.P., Hastings, M.H. 2010. Circadian clocks: genes, sleep, and cognition. *Trends Cogn Sci* **14**, 259–67.

Maywood, E.S., Fraenkel, E., McAllister, C.J., *et al.* 2010. Disruption of peripheral circadian timekeeping in a mouse model of Huntington's disease and its restoration by temporally scheduled feeding. *J Neurosci* **28**, 10199–204.

Meier, A., Mollenhauer, B., Cohrs, S., *et al.* 2005. Normal hypocretin-1 (orexin-A) levels in the cerebrospinal fluid of patients with Huntington's disease. *Brain Res* **30**, 201–3.

Mena-Segovia, J., Cintra, L., Prospero-Garca, O., Giordano, M. 2002. Changes in sleep-waking cycle after striatal excitotoxic lesions. *Behav Brain Res* **15**, 475–81.

Mistlberger, R.E. 2011. Neurobiology of food anticipatory circadian rhythms. *Physiol Behav* **104**, 535–45.

Morris, C.J., Aeschbach, D., Scheer, F.A. 2012. Circadian system, sleep and endocrinology. *Mol Cell Endocrinol* **5**, 91–104.

Morton, A.J. 2013. Circadian and sleep disorder in Huntington's disease. *Exp Neurol* **243**, 34–44.

Morton, A.J., Wood, N.I., Hastings, M.H., *et al.* 2005. Disintegration of the sleep–wake cycle and circadian timing in Huntington's disease. *J Neurosci* **5**, 157–63.

Morton, A.J., Rudiger, S.R., Wood, N.I., *et al.* 2014. Early and progressive circadian abnormalities in Huntington's disease sheep are unmasked by social environment. *Hum Mol Gen* **23**(13), 3375–83.

Ohayon, M.M., Carskadon, M.A., Guilleminault, C., Vitiello, M.V. 2004. Meta-analysis of quantitative sleep parameters from childhood to old age in healthy individuals: developing normative sleep values across the human lifespan. *Sleep* **1**, 1255–73.

Pace-Schott, E.F., Spencer, R.M. 2011. Age-related changes in the cognitive function of sleep. *Prog Brain Res* **191**, 75–89.

Pace-Schott, E.F., Navem, G., Morgan, A., Spencer, R.M. 2012. Sleep-dependent modulation of affectively guided decision-making. *J Sleep Res* **21**, 30–9.

Pallier, P.N., Morton, A.J. 2009. Management of sleep/wake cycles improves cognitive function in a transgenic mouse model of Huntington's disease. *Brain Res* **7**, 90–8.

Pallier, P.N., Maywood, E.S., Zheng, Z., *et al.* 2007. Pharmacological imposition of sleep slows cognitive decline and reverses dysregulation of circadian gene expression in a transgenic mouse model of Huntington's disease. *J Neurosci* **18**, 7869–78.

Petersén, A., Björkqvist, M. 2006. Hypothalamic-endocrine aspects in Huntington's disease. *Eur J Neurosci* **24**, 961–7.

Pidgeon, C., Rickards, H. 2012. The pathophysiology and pharmacological treatment of Huntington disease. *Behav Neurol* **26**(4), 245–53.

Rechtschaffen, A., Bergmann, B.M. 2002. Sleep deprivation in the rat: an update of the 1989 paper. *Sleep* **1**, 18–24.

Reddy, A.B., Karp, N.A., Maywood, E.S., *et al.* 2006. Circadian orchestration of the hepatic proteome. *Curr Biol* **6**, 1107–15.

Reid, S. J., Patassini, S., Handley, R., *et al.* 2013. Further molecular characterisation of the OVT73 transgenic sheep model of Huntington's disease identifies cortical aggregates. *J Huntingtons Dis* **2**, 279–95.

Reppert, S.M., Weaver, D.R. 2002. Coordination of circadian timing in mammals. *Nature* **418**, 935–41.

Roos, R.A., Aziz, N.A. 2007. Hypocretin-1 and secondary signs in Huntington's disease. *Parkinsonism Relat Disord* **13**, S387–90.

Saper, C.B., Fuller, P.M., Pedersen, N.P., *et al.* 2010. Sleep state switching. *Neuron* **22**, 1023–42.

Schroeder, A.M., Loh, D.H., Jordan, M.C., *et al.* 2011. Baroreceptor reflex dysfunction in the BACHD mouse model of Huntington's disease. *PLoS Curr* **3**, RRN1266.

Shan, L., Hofman, M.A., van Wamelen, D.J., *et al.* 2012. Diurnal fluctuation in histidine decarboxylase expression, the rate limiting enzyme for histamine production, and its disorder in neurodegenerative diseases. *Sleep* **1**, 713–5.

Sherrill, D.L., Kotchou, K., Quan, S.F. 1998. Association of physical activity and human sleep disorders. *Arch Intern Med* **158**, 1894–8.

Shulman, L.M., Taback, R.L., Rabinstein, A.A., Weiner, W.J. 2002. Non-recognition of depression and other non-motor symptoms in Parkinson's disease. *Parkinsonism Relat Disord* **8**, 193–7.

Tataroğlu, O., Davidson, A.J., Benvenuto, L.J., Menaker, M. 2006. The methamphetamine-sensitive circadian oscillator (MASCO) in mice. *J Biol Rhythms* **21**, 185–94.

van Wamelen, D.J., Aziz, N.A., Anink, J.J., *et al.* 2013. Suprachiasmatic Nucleus Neuropeptide Expression in Patients with Huntington's Disease. *Sleep* **36**, 117–25.

Verwey, M., Amir, S. 2009. Food-entrainable circadian oscillators in the brain. *Eur J Neurosci* **30**, 1650–7.

Videnovic, A., Golembok, D. 2013. Circadian and sleep disorders in Parkinson's disease. *Exp Neurol* **243**, 45–56.

Videnovic, A., Leurgans, S., Fan, W., *et al.* 2009. Daytime somnolence and nocturnal sleep disturbances in Huntington disease. *Parkinsonism Relat Disord* **15**, 471–4.

Williams, R.H., Morton, A.J., Burdakov, D. 2011. Paradoxical function of orexin/hypocretin circuits in a mouse model of Huntington's disease. *Neurobiol Dis* **42**, 438–45.

Wood, N.I., Sawiak, S.J., Buonincontri, G., *et al.* 2012. Direct evidence of progressive cardiac dysfunction in a transgenic mouse model of Huntington's disease. *J Huntington's Dis* **1**, 65–72.

Wood, N.I., McAllister, C.J., Cuesta, M., *et al.* 2013. Adaptation to experimental jet-lag in R6/2 Mice despite circadian dysrhythmia. *PLoS One* **8**, e55036.

Wu, Y.H., Swaab, D.F. 2005. The human pineal gland and melatonin in aging and Alzheimer's disease. *J Pineal Res* **38**, 145–52.

Wu, Y.H., Swaab, D.F. 2007. Disturbance and strategies for reactivation of the circadian rhythm system in aging and Alzheimer's disease. *Sleep Med* **8**, 623–36.

The Aging Clock

22

Stephan Michel[1], Gene D. Block[2], and Johanna H. Meijer[1]

[1] Department of Molecular Cell Biology, Leiden University Medical Center, Leiden, The Netherlands
[2] Laboratory of Circadian and Sleep Medicine, Department of Psychiatry and Biobehavioral Sciences, University of California Los Angeles, Los Angeles, CA, USA

22.1 Introduction

There are many changes in physiology and behavior as humans and other mammals undergo healthy aging. Along with notable physical changes there are marked alterations in the sleep–wake cycle. One general observation about the effects of aging on circadian behaviors in both humans and higher animals is a significant amount of interindividual variability. On reflection, this should seem obvious. Humans appear to age at vastly different rates and degrees. Although the analysis of the effects of aging on the circadian system can be challenging due to interindividual variability, many empirical generalities have emerged. Nonetheless, changes associated with aging are common to humans and other species. Because of these common features, this review is focused on a range of organisms, taking a comparative approach that appears well justified. In addition, much that we know about the physiological and molecular changes associated with the aging process comes from the study of nonhuman models. Perhaps the most general mechanistic feature that emerges from this comparative approach is the observation that physiological changes in the expression of circadian rhythms begin prior to measurable changes in the underlying molecular clockwork. This important observation will help researchers focus on where to first look for age-related changes in the circadian timing system and also help inform strategies for treatment of age-related sleep disorders.

22.2 The effects of aging on rhythmic behaviors

22.2.1 Humans

There is a substantial literature documenting age-related alterations in the human circadian system. Reported changes include reduction in the quality and regularity of the sleep–wake cycle, changes in the phase of sleep with respect to the day–night cycle, increased difficulties with phase adjustments to changing light schedules or shift work, and changes in the free-running period of the sleep cycle. As pointed out by Monk (Monk, 2005), experimental support for these changes is far from consistent, often complicated by sample size, lack of appropriate gender balance and different experimental protocols. Perhaps the most commonly reported impact of aging on human circadian timing is on the quality and timing of sleep. Indeed, on surveys, more than half of older adults reported issues with sleep (Foley et al., 1995). For many older adults there is a reduction in the depth and quality of sleep, with decreased sleep duration and increased nocturnal awakenings (Dijk and Duffy, 1999). In addition, aged humans are more

Circadian Medicine, First Edition. Edited by Christopher S. Colwell.
© 2015 John Wiley & Sons, Inc. Published 2015 by John Wiley & Sons, Inc.

likely to be woken up by auditory stimuli, likewise suggesting that the depth of sleep is altered (Zepelin *et al.*, 1984). It is still uncertain, however, when, during aging, the changes in the sleep–wake cycle actually occur. A meta-analysis conducted by Ohayon and colleagues (Ohayon *et al.*, 2004) suggest that when comorbidities are controlled for, most of the alterations in sleep patterns occur from age 19 until 60, with more gradual changes thereafter. There may also be significant gender differences in age-related changes in sleep, with women being less affected (Redline *et al.*, 2004). Interestingly, many age-related changes in other organisms also appear to occur by middle age.

Aging also affects the phase of human circadian rhythms. There is a phase advance in the sleep–wake cycle. Between the ages of 20 and 80 the timing of sleep shifts by approximately two hours (Roenneberg *et al.*, 2007). In addition, there are phase advances in the rhythm of melatonin secretion (Duffy *et al.*, 2002), and the temperature rhythm (Duffy *et al.*, 1998). The relationship between the age-related changes in the phase of the central clock and the phase of the sleep cycle is complicated. The sleep–wake cycle appears to advance more than the melatonin rhythm, suggesting the possibility that other noncircadian factors may contribute to the onset of an early sleep time in addition to changes in the phase of the endogenous clock (Duffy *et al.*, 2002).

There is also evidence that phase shifting is impaired as humans age. The aged human circadian system is less sensitive to light (Duffy *et al.*, 2007; Sletten *et al.*, 2009), at least light at moderate intensities. In addition, aged humans seem less tolerant to phase shifts, such as those produced by jet lag or shift schedules. There is some evidence that older shift workers may be at additional risk of accidents in the workplace (Folkard, 2008).

Unlike what has been observed in several animal models and may be expected in humans, it appears that the circadian period length of the sleep–activity cycle does not alter appreciably as human's age (Czeisler *et al.*, 1999).

22.2.2 Rodents

Rodents exhibit a number of changes in circadian behaviors as they age. There are reductions in the amplitude of the circadian rhythm of locomotor activity in rats, hamsters and mice, although with considerable interindividual differences. This is also true for body temperature, although somewhat less consistent than activity (Weinert and Waterhouse, 2007). There is a tendency, too, for sleep–activity rhythms to become phase advanced with age, although at least one study failed to detect such changes in mice (Valentinuzzi *et al.*, 1997). Along with changes in rhythm amplitude, the range of entrainment becomes smaller – old hamsters lose entrainment to long T cycles more frequently than young animals (Morin, 1988). This is also true for mice but not monkeys (Weinert, 2000). In rodents there is a clear effect of aging on the speed of entrainment, although there is a good deal of variability among different studies as to whether advances and delays are affected similarly or differentially (Weinert, 2000).

22.2.3 Drosophila

As with humans and rodents, in *Drosophila*, circadian rhythms of sleep and activity are affected by aging and, similar to humans, there appear to be gender differences in the effects of aging. Young female flies sleep mostly at night and, as they age, nighttime sleep decreases and there is an increase in daytime sleep (Luo *et al.*, 2012). Males, which when young have peaks of activity at dawn and dusk and sleep in the middle of the day and night, as they age sleep more at dawn and dusk and less at mid-day and night. As with other species, the relative strength of the rhythm decreases with age. Sleep becomes fragmented but the amount of sleep does not decrease with age in *Drosophila* (Koh *et al.*, 2006). Surprisingly, a more recent study (Luo *et al.*, 2012) reveals that aged locomotor rhythms are weaker on LD (light–dark) cycles compared to constant darkness.

Interestingly, the rate at which sleep fragmentation occurs is dependent on ambient temperature and lifespan, suggesting it is part of the physiological aging process. Because an increase in oxidative stress disrupts sleep–wake cycles in a manner similar to that of aging, it has been proposed that the accumulation of oxidative damage with age accounts, in part, for the deterioration of sleep–wake cycles (Koh *et al.*, 2006).

22.3 The effects of aging on components of the circadian system

22.3.1 Ocular pacemaker of Aplysia

The eyes of *Aplysia* contain a circadian clock that modulates a rhythm in spontaneous optic nerve activity (Jacklet, 1969). The eye, when isolated and maintained in darkness, expresses a robust circadian rhythm in the production of compound action potentials, with most activity occurring during the time corresponding to daytime. The most prominent effect of aging is a marked reduction in the amplitude of the circadian rhythm. There are also age-related changes in the period and phase of entrainment of the eye, suggesting that the effects of aging are impacting the clock mechanism as well as the expression of the rhythm. Importantly, the reduction in amplitude of the ocular rhythm can be observed *in vivo*, demonstrating that the reduction in amplitude is not due to problems associated with *in vitro* viability of older tissues (Sloan *et al.*, 1999).

Some direct evidence for changes in the molecular components of the clock system comes from the work of Hattar and colleagues (Hattar *et al.*, 2002). The transcription factor, ApC/EBP (*Aplysia* CCAAT enhancer binding protein) is an immediate early gene that in the eye is under circadian control as well as modulated by serotonin and light. The authors point out that ApC/EBP is a candidate gene for a circadian transcription factor to mediate circadian responses activated by the cAMP and cGMP second messenger signaling pathways. The amplitude of the free-running rhythm in ApC/EBP decreases with age. Such changes could underlay alterations in the phase angle for entrainment.

22.3.2 In vivo *studies in rodents*

The deterioration of circadian rhythms observed with advancing age may arise from a decline in rhythmicity at the level of the suprachiasmatic nucleus (SCN), from attenuation of the output signal of the SCN, such as a decrease in neurotransmitter release at the synaptic terminals, or from a reduction in responsiveness of recipient areas. An age-related decrease in function at each of these levels can result in deterioration of rhythmicity, as observed in overt behavior and physiology. There is accumulating evidence that an age-related decline in the integrity of the SCN itself contributes strongly to the aging phenotype. The most convincing evidence comes from transplantation studies (Hurd and Ralph, 1998). Such studies allow determination of how effective young donor tissue can be in restoring a deteriorated behavioral activity pattern. Importantly, such experiments have revealed that young SCN grafts lead to improvement of the activity rhythm amplitude of aged mice. These results strongly support the view that the age-related phenotype is caused primarily by deterioration in the function of the SCN.

Several studies have shown cellular changes within the human, primate and rodent SCN that occur during aging. The SCN is a heterogeneous structure, and contains a large number of neurotransmitters, that are expressed in different parts of the nucleus (Morin, 2007; Chapter 3). The ventrolateral (or core) part of the SCN is light recipient and expresses mainly vasoactive intestinal polypeptide (VIP). The dorsomedial (or shell) part of the SCN expresses predominantly vasopressin. A significant reduction in several neurotransmitters, including VIP, vasopressin, gastrin releasing peptide, neurotensin, and GABA is observed with aging (Zhou *et al.*, 1995; Harper *et al.*, 2008; Palomba *et al.*, 2008; Duncan *et al.*, 2010). One of the prominent neurotransmitters in the SCN is GABA and aging has a profound effect on GABAergic connections. GABA is expressed throughout the SCN, and is also co-expressed with VIP. The number of GABAergic synapses and surface area are reduced in old rat SCN (Palomba *et al.*, 2008) and the amplitude of GABA mediated synaptic current is reduced in aged mice (Farajnia *et al.*, 2012). The changes in VIP and GABA are of particular importance, as these transmitters have been associated with neuronal communication and coupling within the SCN.

With advancing age, melatonin production decreases. Melatonin is produced by the pineal gland and is thought to promote coherence of SCN circadian rhythmicity (Wu *et al.*, 2007). It acts on G-protein coupled melatonin receptors MT1 and MT2, which are present in the SCN (Dubocovich, 2007). The decline in melatonin production with age may contribute to the decrement in rhythmicity of the central pacemaker.

Postmortem investigations in human SCN have documented the change in the number of VIP expressing neurons in senescence. In males, VIP cell count decreases in middle aged subjects, and remains low thereafter. In females, VIP containing cells show an increase with age. In Alzheimer patients the same tendencies were observed, but the changes in VIP cell number are larger than in normal aging (Zhou et al., 1995). In contrast, the number of vasopressin expressing neurons decrease only after the age of 80 (Swaab et al., 1985).

An important question is whether the decrease in neurotransmitter content is causal to the age-related changes in circadian timing. Alternatively, it could merely reflect a general decline in function within the central nervous system. This chicken and egg question is often raised in aging studies; it is difficult to answer, unless directed manipulations are carried out, which are possible in animal experiments only. In human studies a possible strategy is to perform longitudinal studies and compare the age-related changes in circadian parameters over time with the state of neurotransmitter systems postmortem. In an extensive study by Harper and colleagues (Harper et al., 2008), elderly end-stage dementia patients and normal elderly controls were followed longitudinally and recordings of core body temperature and locomotor activity were performed. Postmortem studies in the dementia patients were conducted to correlate the degree of degeneration in the SCN with patterns of core body temperature and behavioral activity rhythms. The data indicate that the functional consequence of the loss of neurons depends on the cell type. Reduction in the number of vasopressin expressing neurons in dementia patients is related to increased fragmentation of the activity rhythm, reflected in a decrease of consolidated sleep and in an increase in diurnal somnolescence. In contrast, a decrease in neurotensin is associated with a decline in the amplitude of rest–activity rhythm. The data indicate that specific loss of neurotransmitter systems contribute in different ways to the aging phenotype. Furthermore, the data suggest that the SCN clock in Alzheimer patients is compromised but still functional, providing a basis and entry point for potential chronotherapy.

The circadian rhythm of the SCN can be measured by recordings of spontaneous electrical activity in populations of neurons. Such multiunit recordings do not allow differentiation between cellular subtypes (i.e., vasopressin or VIP-containing cells), but are functionally interesting as they reflect the overall electrical rhythm that is generated in the SCN. In vivo multiunit activity recordings from the SCN of freely moving mice, versus middle aged mice (13–18 months), have revealed a strong reduction in the amplitude of the SCN rhythm (Nakamura et al., 2011; Fig. 22.1). The data confirm that the decline in neuronal activity rhythms, as observed in vitro (see below), occurs in the SCN of an intact animal. This is far from trivial, as it ensures that the recorded decline in rhythmicity with age is not the consequence of the aged tissue being less viable in a slice preparation, but is truly representative of the physiology of the aged SCN. Importantly, the in vivo data validate and justify the further use of slice preparations, which allow the advance to the single cell level.

The decrease in the amplitude of the electrical activity rhythm observed in middle-aged mice is about 50%. The decline in rhythm amplitude seems to stem mainly from a rise of neuronal activity during the nightly trough (Fig. 22.1). For nocturnal animals, increased SCN activity during the night is associated with decreased levels of behavioral activity and, thus, the SCN electrical activity is inversely related to behavioral activity. While recordings in aged diurnal animals remain to be performed, a similar age-related rise in SCN activity during the night of diurnal animals would translate into a decrease in sleep pressure and may explain defragmented sleep patterns in the elderly.

In addition to a reduction in rhythm amplitude, a significant increase in the variability of the multiunit activity was observed in middle-aged mice. The variability is not present in the SCN in vitro when it is isolated from the brain, neither in young nor old mice. The variability in the SCN electrical rhythm in vivo is thought to reflect input from other brain areas that mediate activity and sleep (Yamazaki et al., 1998; Deboer et al., 2003; Hughes and Piggins, 2012; van Oosterhout et al., 2012). The enhanced variability may reflect, therefore, an age-related change in the feedback of the central nervous system on the SCN clock (Nakamura et al., 2011).

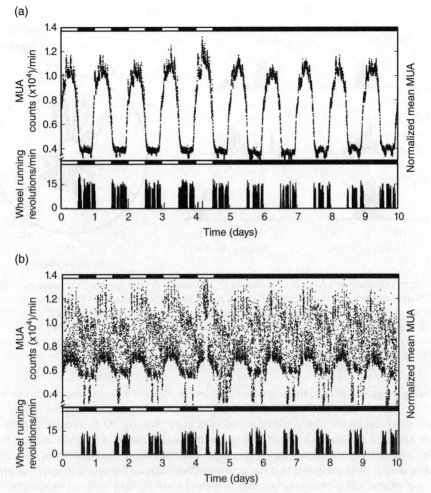

Fig. 22.1 Age affects the amplitude of the circadian timing signal generated in the mammalian central clock. Locomotor activity (bottom panels) and multiunit electrical activity (MUA) of the SCN measured *in vivo* (upper panels) in young (a; 4 month) and middle-aged mice (b; 15 month). Middle-aged mice have a more erratic MUA pattern with on average about 50% lower amplitude of the circadian rhythm as compared to young mice. Light conditions are indicated at the top of the figure (white/black bars = 12 h light/ 12 h dark; grey/ black bars: constant darkness) (modified from Nakamura *et al.*, 2011).

22.3.3 Rodent *in vitro work*

Studies in brain slices and cultured cells have shown that the circadian rhythm in spontaneous electrical activity persists in the isolated SCN. The viability of the circadian rhythm, *in vitro*, in slice preparation, provides a powerful tool to investigate the cellular changes that underlie the alterations in circadian timing during aging. Pioneering electrophysiological recordings from aged SCN tissue and dispersed SCN neurons demonstrated a decrease in the amplitude of the aged SCN (Satinoff *et al.*, 1993; Watanabe *et al.*, 1995; Aujard *et al.*, 2001; Biello, 2009; however, see Herzog *et al.*, 2004). In so far as electrical activity is a major output signal of the clock, and triggers the release of neurotransmitters and humoral factors, the decrease in electrical rhythm amplitude has potential functional relevance. The decrease in rhythm amplitude can result from deterioration at the single cell level, as well as from alterations in neuronal synchrony. There is evidence that both the cellular and network properties of the SCN are affected by age. In young mice, SCN neuronal activity is synchronized and most SCN neurons exhibit their

(a)   (b)

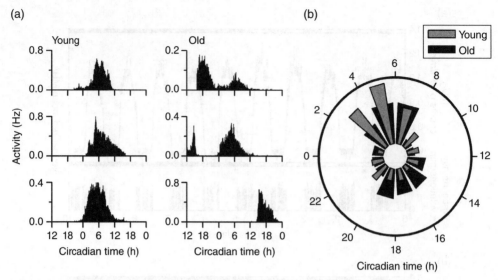

Fig. 22.2 Impact of aging on phase distribution of SCN neurons *in vitro*. (a) Temporal pattern of subpopulations of SCN neurons in hypothalamic brain slices is more dispersed in phase in old animals when compared to young animals. Electrical activity (in Hz) is plotted as a function of circadian time (CT with CT = 6 corresponds with the middle of the subjective day). (b) Radial plot of phase distribution of maximal activity shows that the majority of neurons in young mice are active during the day. In old mice, neuronal activity peaks either in the middle of the day or in antiphase in the middle of the night (modified from Farajnia *et al.*, 2012).

maximal firing frequency around the mid of the day. In old mice (24 months), the synchrony among the neurons is significantly affected (Farajnia *et al.*, 2012); while in young mice 71% of the neuronal subpopulations are active during the day, in old mice only 52% are active (Fig. 22.2). Remarkably, unlike young SCN where neuronal activity is clustered during the daytime, in old SCN a significant number of neurons exhibit peak activity clustering during the night, in antiphase to the majority of neurons that are active during the day. It is intriguing that the activity of the secondary group is in opposite phase, since antiphase is a second stable phase relationship that can be assumed by coupled oscillators. Antiphase oscillations of locomotor activity can be observed, for example, when hamsters are held in continuous light conditions which, similar to aging, acts as a desynchronizing factor. These results indicate that the neuronal network of the SCN, under certain conditions of decreased synchronization, shows a transition of a subpopulation of neurons to an antiphase relationship to the primary cluster of neurons. This observation may be important for the development of therapeutic interventions, aimed at restoring SCN rhythm amplitude.

The decrease in synchronization that was found in the aged SCN is consistent with the decrease in GABAergic and VIP activity, as these transmitters are integrally involved in communication and synchronization within the SCN. The antiphase populations can account for the increase in neuronal activity at night in the SCN. While these decrements in cellular communication are clearly age-related, functional cellular communication persists, as animals older than two years (up to 900 days) continue to express rhythmic behaviors and rhythmic electrical activity within the SCN network (Fig. 22.3).

22.3.4 Clock neuron physiology

The circadian rhythm in electrical activity observed in single pacemaker neurons is based on clock controlled modulations in ion channel activity (Brown and Piggins, 2007; Colwell, 2011). The ionic mechanism of circadian control of membrane potential seems to involve a K[+] conductance in SCN neurons, but further studies are required to identify the specific ion channels involved in producing a circadian rhythm in membrane potential. More is known about the voltage-dependent ion channels

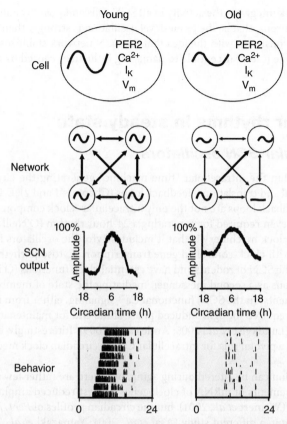

Fig. 22.3 Hierarchical levels of organization are differentially affected by aging. At the cellular level age can affect molecular and other intracellular rhythms as well as the proper circadian regulation of membrane properties. The neuronal network of the SCN seems to be more resilient to age and can partially compensate for the losses in cellular functions. The ensemble output from the SCN *in vitro* is still clearly rhythmic but shows a significant reduction in amplitude as a consequence of the weakening of coupling and the occurrence of antiphase oscillators. These results are comparable to observations *in vivo* (c.f. Fig. 23.1). On the behavioral level, aging results in changes of free-running period, decrease in activity, and increase in fragmentation.

controlling the circadian modulation of action potential frequency. Among them are the fast-delayed rectifier K^+ current (Itri *et al.*, 2005), the transient K^+ current (Itri *et al.*, 2010) and the large conductance calcium-activated K^+ current (Pitts *et al.*, 2006; Kent and Meredith, 2008). The activity of these currents is modulated by the circadian clock and blockage or removal of these conductances diminishes the rhythm in spike frequency leading to severe changes in circadian behavior (Meredith *et al.*, 2006; Kudo *et al.*, 2011).

Aging has differential effects on ion channel activity and expression in neurons of the CNS, which may depend on species, brain region, and cell type. Old SCN neurons in hypothalamic brain slices exhibited a more depolarized resting membrane potential at night and an increase in membrane leak conductance compared to young controls (Farajnia *et al.*, 2012). These data suggest that the circadian control of membrane potential and the underlying conductance is compromised by aging. In SCN neurons of old mice (>24 months of age) circadian control of voltage-dependent K^+ channels diminishes (Farajnia *et al.*, 2012). The decrease of activity in the transient K^+ current during the day may contribute to the dampening of the rhythm in electrical activity observed in old SCN neurons (Nygard *et al.*, 2005).

It is remarkable that circadian rhythm in individual cells (Aujard *et al.*, 2001) and membrane properties in the majority of SCN neurons (Farajnia *et al.*, 2012) are significantly affected by age, while the ensemble output of the clock is still functional and less affected by aging (Fig. 22.3). These data suggest that the neuronal network integrates the activity of all SCN cells and possibly enhances the contribution of still rhythmic SCN neurons, that is, the tissue-level oscillation is stronger than many of the individual aged oscillators. This is consistent with the idea that the SCN network stabilizes circadian functions of the central clock and make it less susceptible to damaging influences caused by different processes like aging (Welsh *et al.*, 2010).

22.4 Molecular rhythms in steady state

22.4.1 Intracellular SCN oscillators

Important elements within the intracellular "time machine" generating the circadian rhythm are the molecular transcriptional and translational feedback loops (Chapters 1 and 2). Evidence, however, shows that these molecular feedback loops are not the only intracellular "clock components" and, more importantly, in some cells not even required for generating a 24-hour rhythm (O'Neill and Reddy, 2011). The current view of cellular clock machinery is that it includes cytosolic oscillators for calcium and cAMP, which work in concert with clock-controlled gene transcription. Cytosolic rhythms in cAMP and Ca^{2+} have been described in the SCN of rodents and have essential clock functions (O'Neill and Reddy, 2012). Intracellular Ca^{2+} functions as a second messenger, mediating the state of membrane excitability to the molecular clock components. In the SCN, functional Ca^{2+} signaling, either from intracellular stores or a transmembrane flux, is required for light-induced phase shifts and for maintenance of a high amplitude molecular clock output (Lundkvist *et al.*, 2005; Antle *et al.*, 2009). Interestingly, early studies on marine snails already postulated a pivotal role for intracellular Ca^{2+} in circadian clock mechanisms (Khalsa *et al.*, 1993).

Clock gene transcription can be altered during aging, but there are rather few studies with somewhat conflicting data. Measurements of mRNA of clock genes suggest reduced amplitude rhythm of *Per2* in SCN neurons of old rats (Weinert *et al.*, 2001), but the circadian profiles of *Per1*, *Per2*, *Cyr1* mRNA were found unaltered by aging in a different study (Asai *et al.*, 2001; Yamazaki *et al.*, 2002). SCN neurons of old hamsters showed altered clock and *Bmal1* expression but no differences in *Per1* and *Per2* profiles (Kolker *et al.*, 2003). In mice, aging dampened the amplitude of expression of clock proteins CLOCK and BMAL1 in hippocampus, amygdala and the hypothalamus (Wyse and Coogan, 2010), the CLOCK expression in SCN, however, was only rhythmic in old mice.

Aging effects Ca^{2+} homeostasis (Foster, 2007) as well as cAMP mediated neuronal network interactions (Arnsten *et al.*, 2012) in neurons, leading to decline in cellular functions (e.g., working memory). Aging-associated dampening of cAMP rhythms have been found in the SCN (Gerhold *et al.*, 2005), which seems to be a consequence of the decline in VIP peptide in old SCN. The impact of age on Ca^{2+} signaling in the SCN neurons have not been studied to date, although many Ca^{2+}-dependent clock processes are altered in old SCN neurons (e.g., phase shift, molecular rhythms) and Ca^{2+} homeostasis is known to be altered in diseases with disturbed circadian rhythms (e.g., bipolar depression, Alzheimer's disease).

22.4.2 Peripheral oscillators

The primary function of the circadian clock is to regulate the timing of behavior and physiological processes within the organism (Chapters 6–14). This is achieved, in many instances, by control of the phase of the so-called peripheral oscillators (clocks in organs and tissues) by the central clock in the SCN (Mohawk *et al.*, 2012). It is assumed that if we stay in synchrony with the environmental cycles and eat and sleep at the biologically right time, our physiology and cognitive functions will perform best. Disruptions of this synchrony, for instance by shift work or jet lag, can lead to malfunctions and even development of serious diseases such as mood disorders or metabolic syndrome. Aging also affects the phase of peripheral oscillators in a number of tissues in rat, including kidney, the paraventricular nucleus, and pineal, as measured in rhythms of *Per1* gene expression (Yamazaki *et al.*, 2002).

In the case of lung and the arcuate nucleus, rhythmicity present in young tissue was absent in approximately half the samples of older tissue. Since the rhythm could be induced *in vitro* with a forskolin stimulus, it can be speculated that a decreased driving signal from the aged SCN permitted these tissues to damp *in vivo*.

Similar molecular rhythm studies in mouse, except using a PER2 as opposed to *Per1* reporter, revealed consistent phase advances between young and old peripheral oscillators in the lung, spleen, thymus, and esophageal tissue (Sellix *et al.*, 2012). The change in phase of the peripheral oscillators in rat and mouse may reflect a number of age-associated alterations occurring in both the peripheral tissues and other regulatory systems. However, an attractive hypothesis is that a reduction in coupling strength of the weakened aged SCN leads to a different, but stable, phase relationship between the driver (SCN) and driven (peripheral) oscillators. One approach to understanding the differential impact of impaired peripheral versus central clock function (e.g., associated with aging) is through the use of genetically modified mice with clock deficits affecting only the peripheral oscillators (Kennaway *et al.*, 2007). The loss of the circadian rhythm in a peripheral tissue such as the liver leads to disturbed metabolic homeostasis even with intact SCN signaling. Given the few studies looking at gender differences, it is noteworthy that male mice exhibited compromised insulin tolerance already at young age, while in females the impact of the peripheral clock disruption was only visible at greater age (24 month). While more research is needed to understand the temporal control of physiological functions, it is tempting to hypothesize that a strengthening of the SCN amplitude would rectify some of these dysfunctions caused by the aged clock.

22.5 The effects of aging on the resetting behavior of central and peripheral oscillators

Anticipation of dusk, dawn, food availability or other periodically occurring events is only possible if the endogenous clock, running at its own natural period, is properly synchronized to environmental cycles. The circadian clock receives information about the external time and these time cues are called zeitgebers. Among the cyclic parameters in the environment, light is the strongest zeitgeber. Light is received by the retina and transmitted to the SCN via specialized retinal ganglion cells. The information travels via glutamatergic nerve fibers of the retinohypothalamic tract to the SCN. Light stimulation leading to excitation of the SCN neurons will trigger a cascade of intracellular pathways that can eventually lead to phase adjustments of the clock (Antle *et al.*, 2009).

The aged circadian system is less sensitive to light and it is, for example, more difficult to reset the phase of the clock after a sudden shift in the light–dark cycle (e.g., during transmeridian flight). This deficit could be attributed to deficits at different levels of the light transduction pathway starting with the retina, glutamatergic transmission, the SCN intracellular signaling cascade, molecular components and also changed SCN network properties. Age-related changes in light transmission through the pupil and lens can alone reduce circadian photoreception by up to 90% in the elderly (Turner and Mainster, 2008). Behavioral experiments in rodents demonstrate the loss of sensitivity to light of the circadian system. *In vitro* experiments in rodents showed an age-related decrease in sensitivity of the SCN to neurotransmitters affecting the phase similar to light (e.g., glutamate, NMDA) (Biello, 2009). Light-induced induction of *Per1* and *Per2* in SCN neurons was reduced in old rats (Asai *et al.*, 2001) but only *Per1* induction was affected in old hamsters (Kolker *et al.*, 2003). Interestingly, the molecular machinery in the central clock within SCN neurons seems to be more robust in old age than the peripheral oscillators. After exposing old rats to sudden shifts in the light–dark cycle, the phase resetting of *Per1* rhythm in the SCN was not different compared to young controls, but resynchronization of the liver clock was strongly compromised by age (Davidson *et al.*, 2008). Supportive of this result, a recent study by Sellix and colleagues studying mouse reveal that a number of peripheral oscillators of aged animals are slowed in their resynchronization following a light schedule shift (Sellix *et al.*, 2012).

22.6 The effects of the circadian system on aging and age-related disease: Circadian misalignment and longevity

22.6.1 Drosophila

There is accumulating evidence that light schedules leading to disrupted synchronization or abnormal synchronization can have an adverse effect on lifespan. Pittendrigh and Minnis reared *Drosophila melanogaster*, under one of four conditions, normal 24-hour light cycles, 21 hour, 27 hour or constant light (Pittendrigh and Minis, 1972). They found that the flies on a 24-hour day lived significantly longer than the flies in the other environments. More recent research with *Drosophila* suggests that genetic disruption of circadian rhythms can adversely affect the aging process. It is now clear that a null mutation in the clock gene period (per^{01}) is associated with an increased susceptibility to oxidative challenge (Krishnan *et al.*, 2008) and increases their mortality risk (Krishnan *et al.*, 2009). In flies susceptible to neurodegenerative diseases, loss of the clock gene period accelerates the aging process (Krishnan *et al.*, 2012).

22.6.2 Circadian misalignment and longevity in rodents

Longevity in hamsters is increased by the implantation of fetal SCN tissue to aged adult hosts (Hurd and Ralph, 1998). The SCN graft recipients showed an increase in longevity of four months, which means that they lived more than twice as long as predicted from their age at the time of the transplantation (Hurd and Ralph, 1998). The authors suggest that manipulations that promote circadian temporal organization promote longevity and health, and predict that disruptions are potentially deleterious (Hurd and Ralph, 1998). Indeed, it has been shown that repetitive disturbance of the circadian system, by repeated advances or delays of the light–dark cycle, increases mortality in aged mice (Davidson *et al.*, 2006). The same is true for the effects of altered light schedules on the lifespan of cardiomyopathic hamsters (Penev *et al.*, 1998). An increasing number of studies now indicate that disturbed rhythms contribute to a variety of diseases. Rhythm disturbances can be introduced by specific clock gene mutations, repeated shifts of the light–dark cycle, or by exposure to continuous light (Fonken *et al.*, 2010; Coomans *et al.*, 2013).

What exactly is the relationship between robust SCN rhythmicity and longevity and health? One interpretation is that coherence between the SCN and peripheral oscillators, or even among peripheral oscillators, is crucial to health (Reddy and O'Neill, 2010). Peripheral oscillators are weak and require input from the SCN to stay synchronized in phase. Thus, while the SCN is considered a master clock, orchestrating other central and peripheral clocks, the other oscillatory structures are coordinated in time by the SCN and require mutual adjustment.

Loss of phase coherence among peripheral oscillators is thought to result in a variety of disorders, such as the metabolic syndrome, immune deficiencies, neurodegenerative disorders, bone and muscle weakness, and cardiovascular problems (Kondratova and Kondratov, 2012). The most prevalent neurodegenerative disorder in the elderly is Alzheimer's disease (AD), which accounts for 60–80% of dementia cases (Chapter 17). Circadian sleep disturbances such as "Sundowners Syndrome", which develop in many AD patients, present perhaps the greatest challenge to families attempting to avoid institutionalization of their loved ones (Pollak and Perlick, 1991). One benefit of chronotherapy for treatment of AD is a restoration of the disturbed sleep–wake pattern, which will enable the AD patient to stay longer in the care of the family. But there is also a potential effect on the progression of AD. The circadian clock is thought to be linked to neurodegeneration through multiple pathways and a dysfunctional clock may result in accelerated cell death and increased accumulation of aggregates in AD. The clock controls a number of defense mechanisms against oxidative stress, is involved in DNA repair, and may influence autophagy of extracellular aggregates (Kondratova and Kondratov, 2012).

Importantly, aging introduces a new challenge – a decrease in the rhythmic output of the SCN and, thus, enhances the probability for the development of many diseases, already by the age-associated decline in SCN rhythmicity. A decrease in the amplitude of the central pacemaker by 50% of the amplitude can be generated experimentally by exposure of animals to constant light. Constant light desynchronizes the neuronal activity patterns within the SCN, which leads at the population level to a decrease in rhythm amplitude with an increase in trough and decrease in peak value (Coomans *et al.*, 2013), corresponding closely to the SCN changes observed with aging (Nakamura *et al.*, 2011).

It has been shown that exposure to constant light leads to a loss of circadian rhythms in metabolic parameters and insulin sensitivity and also results in immediate gain of body weight (Coomans *et al.*, 2013; Chapter 11). In diabetes-prone HIP rats, the compromised circadian clock in constant light leads to earlier onset of diabetes (Gale *et al.*, 2011). Thus, the reduction in SCN rhythm amplitude *per se*, observed in normal aging in middle-aged mice, is a concern for health and may lead to secondary metabolic pathophysiology (Coomans *et al.*, 2013). This underscores the importance of treating age-related rhythm disturbances, as these treatments may also be effective in reducing the incidence of other diseases.

22.7 Therapeutic possibilities for age-related circadian disorders

While aging reduces the light sensitivity of the clock at many levels, light is still the first choice for chronotherapy in the elderly. Increasing light intensity and optimizing the wavelength of light can compensate for some of the shortcomings related to aging (Riemersma-van der Lek *et al.*, 2008). Bright light can promote synchrony between our endogenous clock with the environment. Additionally, the acute excitatory effect on SCN neurons during the day (Meijer *et al.*, 1998) will enhance the amplitude of the output of the central clock. Bright light may be required, especially since in the elderly a reduction in light sensitivity has been observed, as a consequence of yellowing of the lens and pupillary miosis (Monk, 2005; Turner and Mainster, 2008). The combination of light exposure during the day, with melatonin application in the evening, further improves the quality of sleep in the elderly (Riemersma-van der Lek *et al.*, 2008). The improvement observed was comparable with the improvement obtained with classical sleep medication but lacks the undesirable side effects, such as drowsiness and sleepiness in the daytime. The combination of light and melatonin treatment is also effective in the treatment of mild cognitive impairment (Cardinali *et al.*, 2010). Additionally, there is evidence that light treatment improves mood (Most *et al.*, 2010). Mood disturbances and depressive symptoms occur in about one-third of the elderly population, further supporting the relevance of sufficiently high light levels for the elderly (Alexopoulos, 2005).

There are several indications that behavioral activity and exercise lead to improvement of circadian rhythms at the behavioral level. For example, VIP-deficient mice show low amplitude rhythms due to a lack of synchronized activity among SCN neurons. However, when running wheels are introduced to the cages, the enhanced levels of activity lead to considerable improvement of the animals' circadian rhythms (Hughes and Piggins, 2012; Schroeder *et al.*, 2012). The influence of exercise on circadian rhythms is dependent on the timing of activity, suggesting that scheduled exercise may be one possibility for the treatment of rhythm disorders (Schroeder *et al.*, 2012).

In rodents, simultaneous recordings of SCN electrical activity and behavioral activity have revealed the direct influence of activity on the SCN. The effect of behavioral activity on the SCN is inhibitory (Yamazaki *et al.*, 1998; Schaap and Meijer, 2001). Video recordings of the animal's behavior indicated that different types of behavior lead to suppressions of the SCN, but that more intense behavior such as walking or running wheel activity has a stronger effect than milder forms of behavior such as eating (van Oosterhout *et al.*, 2012). It is notable, however, that mild forms of activity also appear to feed back on the SCN. Normally, behavioral activity of nocturnal rodents occurs during the trough of the SCN electrical activity profile. The suppressive influence of activity on the SCN thus leads to a further reduction in SCN electrical activity level, causing a positive feedback loop. Hence, behavioral activity during the animal's active phase generates an increase in the amplitude of the SCN, while activity during the resting phase results in a dampening of the SCN rhythm (van Oosterhout *et al.*, 2012).

For humans, too, it has been shown that behavioral activity or exercise influences the circadian system. Humans readjust more rapidly to an eight-hour phase advance of the light–dark cycle (as in eastward flights) when they are asked to take part in a two-hour interval training (Yamanaka *et al.*, 2010). Exercise by itself induces phase advances of the system, when scheduled in the afternoon or early night (Miyazaki *et al.*, 2001; Buxton *et al.*, 2003). In elderly patients with primary insomnia, structured physical activity during the day was part of a successful program to restore performance in insomniacs (Altena *et al.*, 2008). Moderate exercise training in patients with primary insomnia results in significant improvement of sleep and mood (Passos *et al.*, 2011). It is expected that the influence of exercise is acute (measurable on the same day) but not prolonged. Thus, daily activity would be required to keep the rhythm amplitude enhanced. Together, the results point to lifestyle recommendations that are structural but mild and involve a combination of sufficient levels of daily activity together with exposure to high levels of light during the day.

22.8 Conclusions

As discussed, in a wide range of organisms the aging process leads to reductions in the amplitude of circadian signals in behavior and physiology but less dramatic alterations in the core oscillator mechanism. There are also notable changes in the "temporal map", where various endogenous clocks assume new phase relationships with respect to one another. Future research will need to focus on which, if any, of these age-related changes are adaptive, making older organisms more able to cope with environmental challenges and which of these changes are pathological, making the older body and mind less fit. In those cases, interventions that restore the temporal profile of the younger organism may be advantageous. Whatever the outcome of these explorations, aging provides a dynamic and fascinating context in which to study biological timing.

References

Alexopoulos, G.S. 2005. Depression in the elderly. *Lancet* **365**(9475):1961–1970.

Altena, E., Y.D. Van Der Werf, R.L. Strijers, and E.J. Van Someren. 2008. Sleep loss affects vigilance: effects of chronic insomnia and sleep therapy. *Journal of Sleep Research* **17**(3):335–343.

Antle, M.C., V.M. Smith, R. Sterniczuk, *et al.* 2009. Physiological responses of the circadian clock to acute light exposure at night. *Reviews in Endocrine & Metabolic Disorders* **10**(4):279–291.

Arnsten, A.F., M.J. Wang and C.D. Paspalas. 2012. Neuromodulation of thought: flexibilities and vulnerabilities in prefrontal cortical network synapses. *Neuron* **76**(1):223–239.

Asai, M., Y. Yoshinobu, S. Kaneko, *et al.* 2001. Circadian profile of Per gene mRNA expression in the suprachiasmatic nucleus, paraventricular nucleus, and pineal body of aged rats. *Journal of Neuroscience Research* **66**(6):1133–1139.

Aujard, F., E.D. Herzog, and G.D. Block. 2001. Circadian rhythms in firing rate of individual suprachiasmatic nucleus neurons from adult and middle-aged mice. *Neuroscience* **106**(2):255–261.

Biello, S.M. 2009. Circadian clock resetting in the mouse changes with age. *Age* **31**(4):293–303.

Brown, T.M. and H.D. Piggins. 2007. Electrophysiology of the suprachiasmatic circadian clock. *Progress in Neurobiology* **82**(5):229–255.

Buxton, O.M., C.W. Lee, M. L'Hermite-Baleriaux, *et al.* 2003. Exercise elicits phase shifts and acute alterations of melatonin that vary with circadian phase. *American Journal of Physiology. Regulatory, Integrative and Comparative Physiology* **284**(3):R714–724.

Cardinali, D.P., A.M. Furio, and L.I. Brusco. 2010. Clinical aspects of melatonin intervention in Alzheimer's disease progression. *Current Neuropharmacology* **8**(3):218–227.

Colwell, C.S. 2011. Linking neural activity and molecular oscillations in the SCN. Nature reviews. *Neuroscience* **12**(10): 553–569.

Coomans, C.P., S.A.A. van den Berg, T. Houben, *et al.* 2013. Detrimental additive effects of nighttime light exposure and high-fat diet on circadian rhythms of energy metabolism and insulin sensitivity. *FASEB Journal* **27**(4):1721–1732.

Czeisler, C.A., J.F. Duffy, T.L. Shanahan, *et al.* 1999. Stability, precision, and near-24-hour period of the human circadian pacemaker. *Science* **284**(5423):2177–2181.

Davidson, A.J., M.T. Sellix, J. Daniel, *et al.* 2006. Chronic jet-lag increases mortality in aged mice. *Current Biology* **16**(21):R914–916.

Davidson, A.J., S. Yamazaki, D.M. Arble, *et al.* 2008. Resetting of central and peripheral circadian oscillators in aged rats. *Neurobiology of Aging* **29**(3):471–477.

Deboer, T., M.J. Vansteensel, L. Detari, and J.H. Meijer. 2003. Sleep states alter activity of suprachiasmatic nucleus neurons. *Nature Neuroscience* **6**(10):1086–1090.

Dijk, D.J. and J.F. Duffy. 1999. Circadian regulation of human sleep and age-related changes in its timing, consolidation and EEG characteristics. *Annals of Medicine* **31**(2):130–140.

Dubocovich, M.L. 2007. Melatonin receptors: role on sleep and circadian rhythm regulation. *Sleep Medicine* **8**(Suppl 3): 34–42.

Duffy, J.F., J.M. Zeitzer, D.W. Rimmer, *et al.* 2002. Peak of circadian melatonin rhythm occurs later within the sleep of older subjects. *American Journal of Physiology: Endocrinolology and Metabolism* **282**(2):E297–303.

Duffy, J.F., D.J. Dijk, E.B. Klerman, and C.A. Czeisler. 1998. Later endogenous circadian temperature nadir relative to an earlier wake time in older people. *American Journal of Physiology: Regulatory, Integrative and Comparative Physiology* **275**(5 Pt 2):R1478–1487.

Duffy, J.F., J.M. Zeitzer, and C.A. Czeisler. 2007. Decreased sensitivity to phase-delaying effects of moderate intensity light in older subjects. *Neurobiology of Aging* **28**(5):799–807.

Duncan, M.J., J.M. Hester, J.A. Hopper, and K.M. Franklin. 2010. The effects of aging and chronic fluoxetine treatment on circadian rhythms and suprachiasmatic nucleus expression of neuropeptide genes and 5-HT1B receptors. *European Journal of Neuroscience* **31**(9):1646–1654.

Farajnia, S., S. Michel, T. Deboer, *et al.* 2012. Evidence for neuronal desynchrony in the aged suprachiasmatic nucleus clock. *The Journal of Neuroscience* **32**(17):5891–5899.

Foley, D.J., A.A. Monjan, S.L. Brown, *et al.* 1995. Sleep complaints among elderly persons: an epidemiologic study of three communities. *Sleep* **18**(6):425–432.

Folkard, S. 2008. Shift work, safety, and aging. *Chronobiology International* **25**(2):183–198.

Fonken, L.K., J.L. Workman, J.C. Walton, *et al.* 2010. Light at night increases body mass by shifting the time of food intake. *Proceedings of the National Academy of Sciences of the United States of America* **107**(43):18664–18669.

Foster, T.C. 2007. Calcium homeostasis and modulation of synaptic plasticity in the aged brain. *Aging Cell* **6**(3): 319–325.

Gale, J.E., H.I. Cox, J. Qian, *et al.* 2011. Disruption of circadian rhythms accelerates development of diabetes through pancreatic beta-cell loss and dysfunction. *Journal of Biological Rhythms* **26**(5):423–433.

Gerhold, L.M., K.L. Rosewell, and P.M. Wise. 2005. Suppression of vasoactive intestinal polypeptide in the suprachiasmatic nucleus leads to aging-like alterations in cAMP rhythms and activation of gonadotropin-releasing hormone neurons. *The Journal of Neuroscience* **25**(1):62–67.

Harper, D.G., E.G. Stopa, V. Kuo-Leblanc, *et al.* 2008. Dorsomedial SCN neuronal subpopulations subserve different functions in human dementia. *Brain* **131**(Pt 6):1609–1617.

Hattar, S., L.C. Lyons, and A. Eskin. 2002. Circadian regulation of a transcription factor, ApC/EBP, in the eye of *Aplysia californica*. *Journal of Neurochemistry* **83**(6):1401–1411.

Herzog, E.D., S.J. Aton, R. Numano, *et al.* 2004. Temporal precision in the mammalian circadian system: a reliable clock from less reliable neurons. *Journal of Biological Rhythms* **19**(1):35–46.

Hughes, A.T. and H.D. Piggins. 2012. Feedback actions of locomotor activity to the circadian clock. *Progress in Brain Research* **199**:305–336.

Hurd, M.W. and M.R. Ralph. 1998. The significance of circadian organization for longevity in the golden hamster. *Journal of Biological Rhythms* **13**(5):430–436.

Itri, J.N., S. Michel, M.J. Vansteensel, *et al.* 2005. Fast delayed rectifier potassium current is required for circadian neural activity. *Nature Neuroscience* **8**(5):650–656.

Itri, J.N., A.M. Vosko, A. Schroeder, *et al.* 2010. Circadian regulation of A-type potassium currents in the suprachiasmatic nucleus. *Journal of Neurophysiology* **103**(2):632–640.

Jacklet, J.W. 1969. Circadian rhythm of optic nerve impulses recorded in darkness from isolated eye of *Aplysia*. *Science* **164**(3879):562–563.

Kennaway, D.J., J.A. Owens, A. Voultsios, *et al.* 2007. Metabolic homeostasis in mice with disrupted Clock gene expression in peripheral tissues. *American Journal of Physiology: Regulatory, Integrative and Comparative Physiology* **293**(4):R1528–1537.

Kent, J. and A.L. Meredith. 2008. BK channels regulate spontaneous action potential rhythmicity in the suprachiasmatic nucleus. *PloS One* **3**(12):e3884.

Khalsa, S.B., M.R. Ralph, and G.D. Block. 1993. The role of extracellular calcium in generating and in phase-shifting the *Bulla* ocular circadian rhythm. *Journal of Biological Rhythms* **8**(2):125–139.

Koh, K., J.M. Evans, J.C. Hendricks, and A. Sehgal. 2006. A *Drosophila* model for age-associated changes in sleep:wake cycles. *Proceedings of the National Academy of Sciences of the United States of America* **103**(37):13843–13847.

Kolker, D.E., H. Fukuyama, D.S. Huang, *et al.* 2003. Aging alters circadian and light-induced expression of clock genes in golden hamsters. *Journal of Biological Rhythms* **18**(2):159–169.

Kondratova, A.A. and R.V. Kondratov. 2012. The circadian clock and pathology of the ageing brain. *Nature Review Neuroscience* **13**(5):325–335.

Krishnan, N., A.J. Davis, and J.M. Giebultowicz. 2008. Circadian regulation of response to oxidative stress in *Drosophila* melanogaster. *Biochemical and Biophysical Research Communications* **374**(2):299–303.

Krishnan, N., D. Kretzschmar, K. Rakshit, *et al.* 2009. The circadian clock gene period extends healthspan in aging *Drosophila melanogaster. Aging* **1**(11):937–948.

Krishnan, N., K. Rakshit, E.S. Chow, *et al.* 2012. Loss of circadian clock accelerates aging in neurodegeneration-prone mutants. *Neurobiology of Disease* **45**(3):1129–1135.

Kudo, T., D.H. Loh, D. Kuljis, *et al.* 2011. Fast delayed rectifier potassium current: critical for input and output of the circadian system. *The Journal of Neuroscience* **31**(8):2746–2755.

Lundkvist, G.B., Y. Kwak, E.K. Davis, *et al.* 2005. A calcium flux is required for circadian rhythm generation in mammalian pacemaker neurons. *The Journal of Neuroscience* **25**(33):7682–7686.

Luo, W., W.F. Chen, Z. Yue, *et al.* 2012. Old flies have a robust central oscillator but weaker behavioral rhythms that can be improved by genetic and environmental manipulations. *Aging Cell* **11**(3):428–438.

Meijer, J.H., K. Watanabe, J. Schaap, *et al.* 1998. Light responsiveness of the suprachiasmatic nucleus: long-term multiunit and single-unit recordings in freely moving rats. *The Journal of Neuroscience* **18**(21):9078–9087.

Meredith, A.L., S.W. Wiler, B.H. Miller, *et al.* 2006. BK calcium-activated potassium channels regulate circadian behavioral rhythms and pacemaker output. *Nature Neuroscience* **9**(8):1041–1049.

Miyazaki, T., S. Hashimoto, S. Masubuchi, *et al.* 2001. Phase-advance shifts of human circadian pacemaker are accelerated by daytime physical exercise. *American Journal of Physiology. Regulatory, Integrative and Comparative Physiology* **281**(1):R197–205.

Mohawk, J.A., C.B. Green, and J.S. Takahashi. 2012. Central and peripheral circadian clocks in mammals. *Annual Review of Neuroscience* **35**:445–462.

Monk, T.H. 2005. Aging human circadian rhythms: conventional wisdom may not always be right. *Journal of Biological Rhythms* **20**(4):366–374.

Morin, L.P. 1988. Age-related changes in hamster circadian period, entrainment, and rhythm splitting. *Journal of Biological Rhythms* **3**(3):237–248.

Morin, L.P. 2007. SCN organization reconsidered. *Journal of Biological Rhythms* **22**(1):3–13.

Most, E.I., P. Scheltens, and E.J. Van Someren. 2010. Prevention of depression and sleep disturbances in elderly with memory-problems by activation of the biological clock with light--a randomized clinical trial. *Trials* **11**:19.

Nakamura, T.J., W. Nakamura, S. Yamazaki, *et al.* 2011. Age-related decline in circadian output. *The Journal of Neuroscience* **31**(28):10201–10205.

Nygard, M., R.H. Hill, M.A. Wikstrom, and K. Kristensson. 2005. Age-related changes in electrophysiological properties of the mouse suprachiasmatic nucleus in vitro. *Brain Research Bulletin* **65**(2):149–154.

O'Neill, J.S. and A.B. Reddy. 2011. Circadian clocks in human red blood cells. *Nature* **469**(7331):498–503.

O'Neill, J.S. and A.B. Reddy. 2012. The essential role of cAMP/Ca2+ signalling in mammalian circadian timekeeping. *Biochemical Society Transactions* **40**(1):44–50.

Ohayon, M.M., M.A. Carskadon, C. Guilleminault, and M.V. Vitiello. 2004. Meta-analysis of quantitative sleep parameters from childhood to old age in healthy individuals: developing normative sleep values across the human lifespan. *Sleep* **27**(7):1255–1273.

Palomba, M., M. Nygard, F. Florenzano, *et al.* 2008. Decline of the presynaptic network, including GABAergic terminals, in the aging suprachiasmatic nucleus of the mouse. *Journal of Biological Rhythms* **23**(3):220–231.

Passos, G.S., D. Poyares, M.G. Santana, *et al.* 2011. Effects of moderate aerobic exercise training on chronic primary insomnia. *Sleep Medicine* **12**(10):1018–1027.

Penev, P.D., D.E. Kolker, P.C. Zee, and F.W. Turek. 1998. Chronic circadian desynchronization decreases the survival of animals with cardiomyopathic heart disease. *American Journal of Physiology: Heart and Circulatory Physiology* **275**(6 Pt 2):H2334–2337.

Pittendrigh, C.S. and D.H. Minis. 1972. Circadian systems: longevity as a function of circadian resonance in *Drosophila melanogaster. Proceedings of the National Academy of Sciences of the United States of America* **69**(6):1537–1539.

Pitts, G.R., H. Ohta, and D.G. McMahon. 2006. Daily rhythmicity of large-conductance Ca^{2+}-activated K^+ currents in suprachiasmatic nucleus neurons. *Brain Research* **1071**(1):54–62.

Pollak, C.P. and D. Perlick. 1991. Sleep problems and institutionalization of the elderly. *Journal of Geriatric Psychiatry and Neurology* **4**(4):204–210.

Reddy, A.B. and J.S. O'Neill. 2010. Healthy clocks, healthy body, healthy mind. *Trends in Cell Biology* **20**(1):36–44.

Redline, S., H.L. Kirchner, S.F. Quan, *et al.* 2004. The effects of age, sex, ethnicity, and sleep-disordered breathing on sleep architecture. *Archives of Internal Medicine* **164**(4):406–418.

Riemersma-van der Lek, R.F., D.F. Swaab, J. Twisk, *et al.* 2008. Effect of bright light and melatonin on cognitive and noncognitive function in elderly residents of group care facilities: a randomized controlled trial. *JAMA* **299**(22):2642–2655.

Roenneberg, T., T. Kuehnle, M. Juda, *et al.* 2007. Epidemiology of the human circadian clock. *Sleep Medicine Reviews* **11**(6):429–438.

Satinoff, E., H. Li, T.K. Tcheng, *et al.* 1993. Do the suprachiasmatic nuclei oscillate in old rats as they do in young ones? *The American Journal of Physiology* **265**(5 Pt 2):R1216–1222.

Schaap, J. and J.H. Meijer. 2001. Opposing effects of behavioural activity and light on neurons of the suprachiasmatic nucleus. *European Journal of Neuroscience* **13**(10):1955–1962.

Schroeder, A.M., D. Truong, D.H. Loh, *et al.* 2012. Voluntary scheduled exercise alters diurnal rhythms of behavior, physiology and gene expression in wild-type and vasoactive intestinal peptide-deficient mice. *The Journal of Physiology* **590**(Pt 23):6213–6226.

Sellix, M.T., J.A. Evans, T.L. Leise, *et al.* 2012. Aging differentially affects the re-entrainment response of central and peripheral circadian oscillators. *The Journal of Neuroscience* **32**(46):16193–16202.

Sletten, T.L., V.L. Revell, B. Middleton, *et al.* 2009. Age-related changes in acute and phase-advancing responses to monochromatic light. *Journal of Biological Rhythms* **24**(1):73–84.

Sloan, M.A., J. Levenson, Q. Tran, *et al.* 1999. Aging affects the ocular circadian pacemaker of *Aplysia californica*. *Journal of Biological Rhythms* **14**(2):151–159.

Swaab, D.F., E. Fliers, and T.S. Partiman. 1985. The suprachiasmatic nucleus of the human brain in relation to sex, age and senile dementia. *Brain Research* **342**(1):37–44.

Turner, P.L. and M.A. Mainster. 2008. Circadian photoreception: ageing and the eye's important role in systemic health. *British Journal of Ophthalmology* **92**(11):1439–1444.

Valentinuzzi, V.S., K. Scarbrough, J.S. Takahashi, and F.W. Turek. 1997. Effects of aging on the circadian rhythm of wheel-running activity in C57BL/6 mice. *American Journal of Physiology: Regulatory, Integrative and Comparative Physiology* **273**(6 Pt 2):R1957–1964.

van Oosterhout, F., E.A. Lucassen, T. Houben, *et al.* 2012. Amplitude of the SCN clock enhanced by the behavioral activity rhythm. *PLoS One* **7**(6):e39693.

Watanabe, A., S. Shibata, and S. Watanabe. 1995. Circadian rhythm of spontaneous neuronal activity in the suprachiasmatic nucleus of old hamster in vitro. *Brain Research* **695**(2): 237–239.

Weinert, D. 2000. Age-dependent changes of the circadian system. *Chronobiology International* **17**(3):261–283.

Weinert, D. and J. Waterhouse. 2007. The circadian rhythm of core temperature: effects of physical activity and aging. *Physiology & Behavior* **90**(2–3):246–256.

Weinert, H., D. Weinert, I. Schurov, *et al.* 2001. Impaired expression of the mPer2 circadian clock gene in the suprachiasmatic nuclei of aging mice. *Chronobiology International* **18**(3):559–565.

Welsh, D.K., J.S. Takahashi, and S.A. Kay. 2010. Suprachiasmatic nucleus: cell autonomy and network properties. *Annual Review of Physiology* **72**:551–577.

Wu, Y.H., J.N. Zhou, J. Van Heerikhuize, *et al.* 2007. Decreased MT1 melatonin receptor expression in the suprachiasmatic nucleus in aging and Alzheimer's disease. *Neurobiology of Aging* **28**(8):1239–1247.

Wyse, C.A. and A.N. Coogan. 2010. Impact of aging on diurnal expression patterns of CLOCK and BMAL1 in the mouse brain. *Brain Research* **1337**:21–31.

Yamanaka, Y., S. Hashimoto, Y. Tanahashi, *et al.* 2010. Physical exercise accelerates reentrainment of human sleep-wake cycle but not of plasma melatonin rhythm to 8-h phase-advanced sleep schedule. *American Journal of Physiology. Regulatory, Integrative and Comparative Physiology* **298**(3):R681–691.

Yamazaki, S., M.C. Kerbeshian, C.G. Hocker, *et al.* 1998. Rhythmic properties of the hamster suprachiasmatic nucleus in vivo. *The Journal of Neuroscience* **18**(24):10709–10723.

Yamazaki, S., M. Straume, H. Tei, *et al.* 2002. Effects of aging on central and peripheral mammalian clocks. *Proceedings of the National Academy of Sciences of the United States of America* **99**(16):10801–10806.

Zepelin, H., C.S. McDonald, and G.K. Zammit. 1984. Effects of age on auditory awakening thresholds. *Journal of Gerontology* **39**(3):294–300.

Zhou, J.N., M.A. Hofman, and D.F. Swaab. 1995. VIP neurons in the human SCN in relation to sex, age, and Alzheimer's disease. *Neurobiology of Aging* **16**(4):571–576.

Can we Fix a Broken Clock?

23

Analyne M. Schroeder and Christopher S. Colwell

Laboratory of Circadian and Sleep Medicine, Department of Psychiatry and Biobehavioral Sciences, University of California Los Angeles, Los Angeles, CA, USA

23.1 Introduction

Because the circadian system interacts with so many aspects of our biology, it is not surprising that sleep and circadian disruptions develop as comorbid symptoms to many diseases and are a sensitive indicator of poor health. The presence of sleep and circadian disruptions may themselves contribute to disease pathology. Other times, the sleep problems are a direct result of poor "circadian hygiene" and are the cause for disease. By understanding the mechanisms of circadian regulation and identifying factors that lead to dysfunction, we can begin to develop effective therapies that predictably manipulate the circadian system to address the growing problems with sleep disturbances and disease (Fig. 23.1).

Circadian dysfunction can be triggered by inappropriately timed environmental and behavioral input. As previous chapters have elaborated, the circadian system is very sensitive to blue-light exposure and is one of the most potent external cues able to induce temporal changes in behavior, physiology, cell biology and gene expression. In this modern age, many people are exposed to this type of light during the night and are unknowingly disrupting their own clock. There is an inverse correlation between the cost of artificial lighting and the prevalence of sleep and circadian problems (Czeisler, 2013). Light at night alters the rhythms of circulating factors such as melatonin and cortisol that are responsible for mediating circadian information to various tissues (Lewy *et al.*, 1980; Jung *et al.*, 2010). Sleep architecture is also disrupted following light exposure at night and can lead to sleepiness the following day (Chang *et al.*, 2012; Chellappa *et al.*, 2013).

Behavioral factors such as the timing of feeding and activity modulate the circadian system and, when performed at the wrong time of day, can have detrimental effects on the body. For example, individuals who regularly consume calories late at night are at an increased risk of developing type 2 diabetes and obesity (Chapters 7, 11, and 13). Shift work is a prime example of circadian disruption, altering the timing of light exposure, meals and activity, which epidemiological studies have determined can significantly increase the risk of disease (Chapter 13). In some ways, the shift workers serve as early indicators or "canaries in the coal mine" of the long-term consequences of the circadian disruption experienced by a much broader segment of the population.

The effects of improper scheduled light and behaviors observed in humans have also been described and further explored in rodents. Following light exposure at night, the rhythms of melatonin and cortisol are dampened (Benshoff *et al.*, 1987; Kalsbeek *et al.*, 1999; Bedrosian *et al.*, 2013) and the oscillations of clock and clock-controlled genes are altered throughout the body, including the suprachiasmatic nucleus (SCN)

Circadian Medicine, First Edition. Edited by Christopher S. Colwell.
© 2015 John Wiley & Sons, Inc. Published 2015 by John Wiley & Sons, Inc.

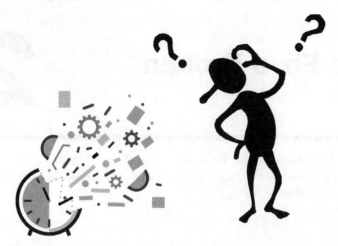

Fig. 23.1 Since the circadian system interacts with so many aspects of our biology, it is perhaps not surprising that circadian and sleep disorders can be caused by a number of factors. Many of the circadian problems experienced by people are the direct result of poor "circadian hygiene." This raises important questions about whether we can impose treatments to fix a broken clock.

(Sakamoto and Ishida, 2000; Szántóová *et al.*, 2011; Fonken *et al.*, 2013). Long-term exposures to irregular light–dark (LD) cycles or shift work paradigms cause imbalanced immune function, disrupt reproduction, induce depression and increase the incidence of obesity, cardiovascular disease and cancer (Chapters 6–13). Feeding at the wrong time of day triggers metabolic changes and disease in part by decoupling and mis-aligning the timing of gene expression rhythms of the liver and SCN (Chapters 6 and 7).

Depending on the survey, sleep disruptions are experienced by about 40–70% of aged individuals (Van Someren, 2000). As the population ages, we can expect to see more problems with sleep and the circadian system. As described in Chapter 22, fragmentation of sleep in older individuals is in part due to a weakening circadian system. Consistent with an earlier wake-up time in older individuals, rhythms in behavior and physiological processes, including the onset of activity, peak melatonin production, peak circulating cortisol levels and the acrophase of body temperature, are often advanced in phase. Disruptions in the timing and quality of sleep are also associated with neurodegenerative disorders such as Alzheimer's disease (AD) (Chapter 19), Parkinson's disease (PD) (Chapter 20), and Huntington's disease (HD) (Chapter 21). These disruptions could serve as early biomarkers because the onset of the sleep disruption occurs years before disease diagnosis.

The various mouse models of neurodegenerative diseases are helping to uncover mechanisms of pathology and the mounting evidence suggests that the circadian system is impacted. The timing of gene expression (including clock genes) is altered, suggesting a loss of circadian coordination and possible misalignment that may be an underlying factor leading to deficits in sleep. Finally, because circadian and sleep disruptions alone can increase oxidative stress and inflammation, the presence of these symptoms could initiate and/or accelerate pathology throughout the nervous system and peripheral tissues in aging and disease (Hardeland *et al.*, 2003; Antoch and Kondratov, 2010; Spengler *et al.*, 2012; Yu *et al.*, 2013). Targeting and strengthening circadian function may prove beneficial for aging and neurodegenerative diseases by delaying the course and ameliorating symptoms of disease.

A recurring theme throughout this book is that circadian disruption has detrimental health effects. This is very evident with patients and the caregivers who must adhere to their patient's fragmented internal schedule. This predicament demands effective interventions to boost circadian function in order to impose a temporally structured daily rhythm. Common strategies to alleviate circadian symptoms include the consumption of stimulants during the day to combat sleepiness and the treatment of insomnia and sleeplessness with sleep aids. These treatments, however, are acute in that they are taken to alleviate immediate symptoms but may have no or minimal benefits for the underlying circadian dysfunction. Furthermore, they may contribute to the problem. For example, stimulants (modafinil, amphetamines, nicotine and caffeine) can disrupt sleep (Boutrel and Koob, 2004) while prescription sleep aids (barbiturates, benzodiazepines and zolpidem), though able to induce sedation by enhancing GABA signaling and activating sleep centers, may not reinstate the normal restorative stages of sleep (Liu *et al.*, 2007). Another issue is that the principal neurotransmitter of the SCN is GABA and these drugs may have disruptive effects on neuronal signaling (Freeman *et al.*, 2013).

Melatonin may be the best-studied and most promising drug for circadian modulation. Recently, tasimelteon, a melatonin receptor 1 and 2 agonist, was approved by the FDA for the treatment of non-24 hour sleep–wake disorder and demonstrated to entrain the circadian system (Dhillon and Clarke, 2014). Still, melatonin and all other current treatment options require more work to determine their precise effects on circadian processes and health outcomes.

The current options for pharmacological treatments are limited but academic and industrial research are actively engaged in developing novel drugs with circadian efficacy that can be prescribed for the diverse group of diseases that present with circadian complications. In the remainder of this chapter, circadian targeted interventions with potential for realigning and reinstating circadian rhythms are discussed. These interventions include environmental and behavioral modifications as well as novel chemical targets of the circadian system. There is a growing demand for interventions that strengthen the circadian system and effective remedies would not only help improve the daily struggles of individuals experiencing circadian symptoms but may also have beneficial impact on disease.

23.2 Light therapy

Our modern inventions have granted us control over our lighting environment (Fig. 23.2). We can choose to stay awake and surf the Internet by peering into our blue backlit screens all night if we want, or to retreat into dark, cool shelters of Abercrombie shops or watch the game at a local bar during the day. The temporal restructuring of light can lead to a state of circadian disruption, exposing us to new health risks and disease. Light is the most potent environmental cue able to predictably phase shift the timing of behavior (Khalsa *et al.*, 2003). It is detected by the photopigment melanopsin localized in intrinsically

Fig. 23.2 Light is the most potent environmental cue for the circadian system and can predictably phase shift the timing of behavior. Light input at improper times can lead to circadian disruptions and disease. Knowing this, exposure to robust light–dark cycles is crucial for good health and may be particularly important in vulnerable populations.

photosensitive retinal ganglion cells (ipRGCs). Melanopsin is most sensitive to blue wavelengths of light and its activation leads to the release of glutamate onto the SCN via the retinohypothalamic tract (Schmidt *et al.*, 2011; Lucas *et al.*, 2012). The glutamate signaling causes immediate molecular and cellular changes in the SCN, including increases in firing rate and the induction of *c-fos* and *Per1* transcription that eventually lead to a shift in the timing of the molecular clock within the SCN and throughout the body (Chapters 1 and 2).

In diurnal animals, exposure to even low intensities of blue light during the night can interfere with sleep by inhibiting sleep-promoting neurons, acutely reducing melatonin levels, activating arousal-promoting orexin neurons and stimulating the sympathetic axis (Duffy and Czeisler, 2009; Ruger and Scheer, 2009; Adidharma *et al.*, 2012). In addition to poor sleep quality, light at night reduces daytime alertness the following day. Over a long period of time, these aberrant light cycles can increase the risk for serious diseases. Therefore, methods or behaviors that help reinforce the timing of natural, environmental light and maintain the normal variance of light intensities between night and day would reinstate a more robust and stable circadian system. Strengthening of the circadian network and enhancing circadian control of tissue function and physiology, will likely restore restorative sleep as well as daytime alertness helping to improve daily life and reducing the risk for disease.

In practice, light therapy has been demonstrated to ameliorate circadian symptoms in some conditions, including advanced/delayed sleep phase syndrome, jet lag, shift work, seasonal affective disorder and depression (Burgess *et al.*, 2002; Barion and Zee, 2007). The scheduled light exposure helped re-establish the daily sleep–wake cycle and improve mood (Magnusson and Boivin, 2003; Wirz-Justice *et al.*, 2004). The positive outcome is encouraging the use of light therapy for other conditions that present with circadian symptoms, including aging and neurodegenerative diseases. In these groups, light therapy improved daytime alertness and sleep (Lieverse *et al.*, 2011; Friedman *et al.*, 2012; Royer *et al.*, 2012; Rutten *et al.*, 2012) and enhanced motor and cognitive abilities (Yamadera *et al.*, 2000; Ancoli-Israel *et al.*, 2003; Riemersma-van der Lek *et al.*, 2008; Willis *et al.*, 2012). Individuals suffering from major depression show improvements in mood when light therapy is included in the treatment regimen (Benedetti, 2012; Chapter 17).

However, other studies show no or small changes in objective and subjective measures of sleep (Ancoli-Israel *et al.*, 2002; Friedman *et al.*, 2009). These discrepancies point out that a better understanding is needed of critical parameters such as light wavelength, intensity, and duration, as well as the timing of treatment, relative to the endogenous circadian rhythm. But it is worth re-emphasizing that even young, healthy individuals can be influenced by improved light exposure (Viola *et al.*, 2008). A study found that camping in the beautiful mountains of Colorado and exposure to natural lighting for several days was effective in advancing the phase of melatonin rhythms in young adults by two hours (Wright *et al.*, 2013). Thus lighting conditions provide one of our most powerful tools to influence the circadian system.

23.3 Scheduled meals

Obesity is a growing epidemic that requires attention and greater understanding (Chapters 11 and 13). One factor contributing to this health concern may be the constant availability of food and its consumption throughout the 24-hour day. In the previous chapters, the reciprocal interactions between the circadian system and metabolism enabling the timing and quality of food to modulate rhythms have been elaborated. It is, therefore, easy to imagine that an imbalance, such as mistimed or constant food consumption, can result in circadian and metabolic dysfunction that lead to diseases such as type 2 diabetes (Chapters 6 and 7).

Good health may, therefore, need to include a feeding schedule that preserves and reinforces the phase relationships of clock gene expression between the SCN and peripheral tissues (Fig. 23.3). In aging (Chapter 22) and neurodegenerative diseases (Chapters 19–21), where the communication between the SCN and peripheral tissues is deficient, scheduled feeding may provide the cues needed to reinforce and

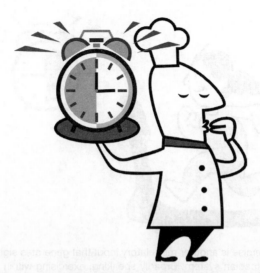

Fig. 23.3 The timing of meals is a critical signal for the peripheral circadian system and may even impact circadian clocks in the central nervous system. A variety of evidence suggests that eating at inappropriate times leads to weight gain and may contribute to metabolic syndrome. In contrast, restricting food consumption within the first 8–10 hours of being awake helps maintain a lean body mass and produce a more robust circadian cycle.

properly realign molecular rhythms of tissues with the LD cycle. In mouse models of circadian disruption (*Vipr2*–/–) and HD, scheduled feeding entrained the molecular rhythms of peripheral tissues (Sheward *et al.*, 2007; Maywood *et al.*, 2010). In humans, higher measures of daily routine, including mealtimes, is correlated with higher self-reported sleep quality in a variety of subjects (Monk *et al.*, 1994; Frank *et al.*, 1997; Câmara Magalhães *et al.*, 2005; Zisberg *et al.*, 2010).

Further testing and refinement in the scheduling of food consumption can determine whether there is an optimal time that leads to measureable improvements in circadian function, which may differ depending on the underlying condition or disease. In AD, for example, peak calorie intake in the early part of the active phase (morning) is correlated with lower body weights and worse cognitive and behavioral symptoms compared to food consumption later in the day (Young and Greenwood, 2001). Much more work will need to be done to clarify the benefits of scheduled feeding, but adjustments in mealtime seem to be a promising and relatively easy lifestyle choice to realign and improve circadian function.

23.4 Scheduled exercise

Exercise has a wealth of benefits, including promoting neurogenesis, enhancing immune function and improving mood. In addition, exercise may also be a tool to improve the function of the circadian system and strengthen its regulation of peripheral outputs when scheduled appropriately (Fig. 23.4). The daily patterning of activity is an output regulated by the circadian system. Studies have also demonstrated that stimulated activity or exercise feeds back and shifts the timing of the circadian system. For example, under constant dark conditions, a single, short bout of stimulated activity in the middle of the subjective day (the time when the animal perceives it is day despite the absence of light cues), causes the circadian system of rodents to shift, resulting in an earlier onset of wheel-running activity the following day, while stimulated activity during the end of the subjective night results in phase delays (Reebs and Mrosovsky, 1989).

Even under the strong entrainment effects of an LD cycle, daily scheduling of exercise during either the first or second half of the active period differentially alters properties of the molecular clock throughout the body, including the SCN, and reshapes the daily rhythms of behavior and physiological

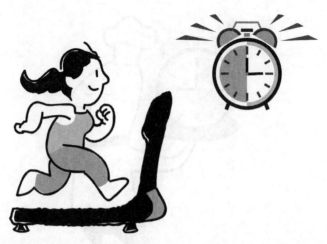

Fig. 23.4 The timing of exercise is another modulatory input that generates signaling cues altering the timing and amplitude of the circadian system. Broadly speaking, exercising within the active phase enhances the circadian output while exercising out of phase contributes to low amplitude rhythms.

processes (Schroeder *et al.*, 2012). Exercise or wheel availability aids in realignment of the circadian system following a 12-hour shift in the LD cycle only when it is scheduled in phase to the new lighting schedule (Dallmann and Mrosovsky, 2006; Castillo *et al.*, 2011). When access to exercise is maintained on the original schedule, the rate of re-entrainment is significantly slowed. These effects are likely mediated by the SCN because stimulated activity can induce direct and immediate changes in clock gene expression and neuronal firing activity in SCN neurons (Maywood *et al.*, 1999; Houben *et al.*, 2009).

The human circadian system is responsive to exercise as well. Although the effect of exercise is less robust in humans, evidence suggests that exercise is able to delay circadian timing as measured by shifts in the onset or peak time of melatonin rhythms (Buxton *et al.*, 2003; Yamanaka *et al.*, 2006; Atkinson *et al.*, 2007). The magnitude of this effect is dependent on the duration and intensity of exercise (Buxton *et al.*, 1997). Re-entrainment of the circadian system can also be hastened by exercise (Miyazaki *et al.*, 2001) and has been shown to aid in readjustments of schedule during shift work (Schmidt *et al.*, 1990; Eastman *et al.*, 1995). These studies demonstrate effective modulation of the circadian system brought about by exercise in rodents and humans.

Mounting evidence suggests that scheduled exercise can also be utilized to improve circadian function in aged and circadian compromised animals. In both the R6/2 mouse model of HD and in aged mice, scheduled wheel access boosted the amplitude and improved the temporal patterning of activity and rest when compared to animals without wheel access (Welsh *et al.*, 1988; Leise *et al.*, 2013; Cuesta *et al.*, 2014). Furthermore, the rate of re-entrainment of activity and clock gene expression rhythms following an 8-hour shift in the LD cycle was accelerated using voluntary exercise in aged animals (Leise *et al.*, 2013). In mice with a disrupted circadian system (*Vip–/–*; *Vipr2–/–*), the scheduling of wheel access for six hours every 24-hours improved the rhythms of behavior (Power *et al.*, 2010) and physiology (Schroeder *et al.*, 2012). Interestingly, the blunted molecular rhythms in SCN neurons of VIP-deficient mice were rescued by wheel access at some phases but not others. Studies suggest similar beneficial effects in humans. For example, long-term fitness training in the middle of the day, improved the consolidation of the sleep–wake cycle in older men (Someren *et al.*, 1997). Exercise during the afternoon or early evening improved self-reported sleep quality in older adults with insomnia (Reid *et al.*, 2010). Similar to studies in rodents, there may also be differential effects depending on the timing of exercise. Although both exercise in the morning and late afternoon improved cognitive abilities in aged individuals, late afternoon exercise improved more of these measures (Benloucif *et al.*, 2004). Unfortunately, in mice or men, the mechanisms mediating exercise's effect on the circadian system are not yet known.

23.5 Scheduled sleep

Neural connections between the SCN and brain regions that regulate arousal and sleep enable reciprocal regulation between circadian and sleep processes (Chapters 4 and 5). These functional interactions provide an opportunity for improving circadian rhythms by imposing a sleep schedule. While we are not aware of evidence for this in humans, there is some literature to support this hypothesis in mice. In a mouse model of HD (R6/2), both the sleep–wake cycle and gene expression rhythms in the SCN are disrupted (Chapter 21). Daily administration of alprazolam (a benzodiazepine) in these mice induced approximately four hours of sleep during the beginning of the light phase (Pallier *et al.*, 2007). The daily pharmacological imposition of sleep improved expression profiles of the clock gene *Per2* and of the circadian output gene *Prok2*. Importantly, this treatment improved health, cognitive and motor function, and prolonged survival. In a separate study, pharmacological control of both the sleep and wake cycle using alprazolam and modafinil, respectively, further improved cognitive function; however, the effects on the circadian system were not examined (Pallier and Morton, 2009). This work is beginning to provide the "proof of concept" that one way to fix a broken clock may be to impose a sleep schedule.

23.6 Pharmacological targeting of the circadian system

While behavioral or lifestyle changes are promising interventions aimed to stabilize the circadian system, these lifestyle changes may be difficult to impose under certain conditions of disease or societal pressures. Pharmacological targeting of the circadian system may one day be a potent means of modulating the circadian system to achieve various goals (Fig. 23.5).

Firstly, an ideal class of drugs should target the central clock and enhance SCN control of peripheral tissues. A potential target is the neuropeptide VIP (vasoactive intestinal polypeptide), which is required for synchronous gene expression and firing rate rhythms among the individual neurons of the SCN. This neuropeptide is reduced in the SCN of aged individuals and those with neurodegenerative disorders and likely contributing to circadian symptoms (Zhou *et al.*, 1995; van Wamelen *et al.*, 2013). Developing agonists for *Vipr2*, the dominant VIP receptor in the SCN, may help improve circadian symptoms by

Fig. 23.5 Behavioral or lifestyle changes as a means of fixing a broken circadian clock are promising interventions aimed to restore and stabilize the circadian system in a fixed LD environment. However, these lifestyle changes may be difficult to impose or ineffective with certain conditions. The development of pharmacological agents able to accelerate re-entrainment while maintaining synchrony within the body, even if the body is misaligned with the external environment, is a potential solution to minimize the consequences of disruptions to the circadian system.

enhancing neural synchrony and function. In mice, chronic infusion of a *Vipr2* agonist (BAY 55-9837) in the hypothalamus of wild-type animals was able to lengthen the circadian cycle *in vivo* (Pantazopoulos *et al.*, 2010). Effective circadian modulation by the *Vipr2* agonist warrants further study to determine possible benefits in circadian compromised animals.

Secondly, drugs able to modulate period or phasing of the central clock would help adjust the phase relationship of the endogenous rhythm relative to the LD cycle. Thirdly, drugs that directly entrain rhythms of peripheral tissues may help realign peripheral tissues under conditions of weak SCN signals. For example, circulating factors such as melatonin, cortisol and catecholamine can alter the molecular clock of peripheral tissues and phase dependently accelerate or delay realignment to a shifted LD cycle (Durgan *et al.*, 2005; Kiessling *et al.*, 2010; Pevet and Challet, 2011). Finally, designing drugs to acutely suppress the central clock may make the SCN easier to shift when followed by strong rhythm promoting cues. This approach may help the circadian system reset more rapidly to a new time zone or with an altered relationship to the LD cycle (Vitaterna *et al.*, 2006).

There is a growing number of promising drug targets for circadian modulation being developed. One of these drugs is an inhibitor of CK1δ. Application of this inhibitor lengthened the period of the circadian clock at both molecular and behavioral levels in wild-type animals. Daily administration rescued circadian deficits in the *Vipr2-/-* mouse by improving gene expression rhythms in the SCN and driving robust wheel-running rhythms (Meng *et al.*, 2010). This treatment also improved wheel-running behavior in wild-type animals housed under constant light conditions, which renders most animals arrhythmic. This finding is quite exciting, as it demonstrates the ability of pharmacological agents to entrain and strengthen the circadian system despite the aberrant presence of light, which would be highly beneficial for shift workers. The CK1δ inhibitor may be a possible drug target for advanced sleep phase syndrome caused by improper turnover of PER2, as the inhibition of CK1δ may lengthen period and delay the phase of the circadian system (Xu *et al.*, 2007).

More recent work has demonstrated the circadian modulating effects of a synthetic REV-ERB agonist (Meng *et al.*, 2008; Kumar *et al.*, 2010; Solt *et al.*, 2012; Trump *et al.*, 2013). *Rev-erb* (alpha and beta) is a rhythmic component of the molecular clock and is a negative regulator of *Bmal1* transcription. A single dose of the REV-ERB ligand applied in constant darkness at the normal peak time of REV-ERB expression (CT 6) altered the molecular clock in the SCN and suppressed wheel-running activity for one day. These effects were weaker when animals were placed in an LD cycle. The impact of chronic treatment on the SCN was not examined. Outside of the SCN, REV-ERB ligand injection shifted the timing of the molecular clock in the liver. Consistent with *Rev-erb*'s role in metabolism, the agonist altered the expression profile of metabolic genes in the liver, skeletal muscle, and white adipose tissue. Long-term administration of the agonist continued to modulate metabolic gene expression in the liver that ultimately resulted in weight loss in diet-induced obese mice as well as in leptin-deficient mice. The REV-ERB ligand was also shown to modulate the immune system, which is closely regulated by the circadian system (Gibbs *et al.*, 2012). These studies demonstrate effective manipulation of the molecular clock and physiological outputs by pharmacologically altering REV-ERB levels. Continuing studies will shape its potential as a therapeutic target.

An activator of the NAD-dependent deacetylase *Sirtuin-1* gene is another chemical agent having modulatory effects on the molecular clock (Bellet *et al.*, 2013). *Sirt1* is a sensor of the cellular metabolic state and adapts metabolic output with the energy needs of a cell. It is also thought to mediate information between the circadian system and metabolism, making *Sirt1* a potential target for circadian modulation. SIRT1 enzymatic activity is rhythmic in part by its direct association with the clock genes *Bmal1* and *Clock* (Nakahata *et al.*, 2008). Reducing *Sirt1* levels, using a liver-specific *Sirt1*-KO, altered clock gene expression rhythms in the liver, demonstrating SIRT1s regulation of the clock properties. The use of a synthetic activator to drive expression of *Sirt1* for multiple weeks caused a depression in *Per2* and *Dbp* expression in the liver brought about by changes in the levels of histone acetylation and disruption of promoter binding activity of CLOCK and BMAL1. These studies support the idea that manipulation of metabolic genes is a means to modulate the molecular clock and circadian behavior. Currently, the *Rev-erbα* and *sirtuin1* agonists appear to be disruptors of the molecular clock and could be used to "prime" the circadian system to allow for an incoming circadian signal to quickly re-entrain and shift rhythms throughout the body. Future studies may determine a correct timing and dosage of drug administration that will help boost circadian function.

Finally, the circadian system controls the timing of arousal (Chapter 5) through the regulation of the electrical activity in a network of neurotransmitter systems, including cell populations expressing norepinephrine (locus coeruleus), serotonin (raphe), histamine (tubelomammiary nucleus) and orexin/hypocretin (hypothalamus). Theoretically blocking any of these arousal systems will help induce or maintain sleep and, as described above, a pharmacologically-induced sleep schedule could well drive a circadian cycle. Orexin plays a critical role in promoting arousal and the loss of these neurons is associated with the sleep disorder narcolepsy (Mieda and Sakurai, 2012; Mahlios *et al.*, 2013). The discovery and characterization of this peptidergic system has created the opportunity for new classes of drugs, including hypnotics (orexin receptor antagonists) and stimulants (orexin receptor agonists). A number of these agents are under development with the work on dual orexin 1 and 2 receptor antagonists (DORAs) being the furthest along (Gotter *et al.*, 2012; Uslaner *et al.*, 2013; Riemann and Spiegelhald, 2014). These compounds are generating a lot of excitement, as they raise the possibility of new treatments for sleep and circadian disorders without some of the cognitive impairments observed with GABA-modulators (benzodiazepine-like), which are presently the main treatments for insomnia. Of course, we do not yet understand the potential side effects of these DORA drugs and whether they offer significant benefits over the "Z-class" drugs (zaleplon, zolpidem, zopiclone, and eszopiclone) that are presently so widely prescribed. Past experience, which has seen us welcome new sleeping aids with great enthusiasm (e.g., chloral hydrate or barbiturates) only to see the negatives appear later with widespread use, suggests that we take a cautious approach.

High-throughput screens are identifying new pharmacological targets that would allow measurable temporal control of the molecular clock. By utilizing luciferase-based readouts in cell cultures, thousands of drugs are being screened for their ability to change the amplitude, period and phase of clock gene rhythms. The large array of molecules that have so far been identified interact with the molecular clock using different pathways, which is promising from a pharmacological standpoint because it expands the possibility of designing drugs with more precise effects on the circadian system with minimal side effects (Chen *et al.*, 2012). We do not know much about the chemical identity of the clock modulators but cyclin-dependent kinase inhibitors (CKIs) were reported to lengthen period as expected.

Particularly intriguing is the class of compounds that was reported to restore the amplitude of damped clocks and could be a useful countermeasure against dampened circadian oscillations in aging and neurodegenerative diseases. In another high-throughput screen, a CRY agonist (KL001) was demonstrated to stabilize CRY protein, which lengthened period and depressed the amplitude of PER2 driven bioluminescence rhythms in culture (Hirota *et al.*, 2012). Similar to the REV-ERB ligand, KL001 altered metabolic gene expression in hepatocytes cultures. The multitude of potential chemical substances identified by high-throughput screens presents a challenge in advancing only the most promising targets. Time and resources will have to be invested to determine the effects of potential drugs in different tissue types, their effects on multi-oscillatory systems and, most importantly, whether drugs have measurable benefits on physiology and health.

23.7 Conclusions

Good health requires an intact circadian system that temporally organizes physiological and cellular processes throughout the body. This drives higher levels of activity during the day and promotes sound sleep at night. Disruption of this timing system causes a breakdown of the sleep–wake cycle that negatively impacts our health, leading to more serious diseases. Aging as well as neurological and psychiatric disorders challenge the proper functioning of the circadian system, which may worsen disease pathology. Even for healthy individuals, modern living creates work schedules that do not fit with our biology, resulting in inappropriate light exposure and mealtimes that disrupt the quality of our sleep – all factors which challenge our circadian system. Defenses against a "broken clock" include adopting a strategy of temporally structured light exposure, meals, and exercise. Pharmacological manipulations will need to be targeted to the specific goal, for example, aligning peripheral organs, enhancing the amplitude of the central clock or even suppressing the central clock during travel or shift work. There is still so much more to be done in order to understand the interactions between the circadian system and disease and how best to address and target dysfunction. With the growing prevalence of sleep and circadian dysfunction in the modern world, this direction of research is truly worth pursuing.

References

Adidharma W., G. Leach, and L. Yan. 2012. Orexinergic signaling mediates light-induced neuronal activation in the dorsal raphe nucleus. *Neurosci* 220:201–207.

Ancoli-Israel S., J.L. Martin, D.F. Kripke, *et al.* 2002. Effect of light treatment on sleep and circadian rhythms in demented nursing home patients. *J Am Geriatr Soc* 50:282–289.

Ancoli-Israel S., P. Gehrman, J.L. Martin, *et al.* 2003. Increased light exposure consolidates sleep and strengthens circadian rhythms in severe Alzheimer's disease patients. *Behav Sleep Med* 1:22–36.

Antoch M.P. and R.V. Kondratov. 2010. Circadian proteins and genotoxic stress response. *Circ Res* 106:68–78.

Atkinson G., B. Edwards, T. Reilly, and J. Waterhouse. 2007. Exercise as a synchroniser of human circadian rhythms: an update and discussion of the methodological problems. *Eur J Appl Physiol* 99:331–341.

Barion A. and P.C. Zee. 2007. A clinical approach to circadian rhythm sleep disorders. *Sleep Med* 8:566–577.

Bedrosian T.A., A. Galan, C.A. Vaughn, *et al.* 2013. Light at night alters daily patterns of cortisol and clock proteins in female Siberian hamsters. *J Neuroendocrinol* 25(6):590–6.

Bellet M.M., Y. Nakahata, M. Boudjelal, *et al.* 2013. Pharmacological modulation of circadian rhythms by synthetic activators of the deacetylase SIRT1. *Proc Natl Acad Sci USA* 110(9):3333–3338.

Benedetti F. 2012. Antidepressant chronotherapeutics for bipolar depression. *Dialogues Clin Neurosci* 14:401–411.

Benloucif S., L. Orbeta, R. Ortiz, *et al.* 2004. Morning or evening activity improves neuropsychological performance and subjective sleep quality in older adults. *Sleep* 27:1542–1551.

Benshoff H.M., G.C. Brainard, M.D. Rollag, and G.R. Lynch. 1987. Suppression of pineal melatonin in Peromyscus leucopus by different monochromatic wavelengths of visible and near-ultraviolet light (UV-A). *Brain Res* 420:397–402.

Boutrel B. and G.F. Koob. 2004. What keeps us awake: the neuropharmacology of stimulants and wakefulness-promoting medications. *Sleep* 27:1181–1194.

Burgess H.J., K.M. Sharkey, and C.I. Eastman. 2002. Bright light, dark and melatonin can promote circadian adaptation in night shift workers. *Sleep Med Rev* 6:407–420.

Buxton O.M., S.A. Frank, M. L'Hermite-Balériaux, *et al.* 1997. Roles of intensity and duration of nocturnal exercise in causing phase delays of human circadian rhythms. *Am J Physiol* 273:E536–542.

Buxton O.M., C.W. Lee, M. L'Hermite-Baleriaux, *et al.* 2003. Exercise elicits phase shifts and acute alterations of melatonin that vary with circadian phase. *Am J Physiol Regul Integr Comp Physiol* 284:R714–724.

Câmara Magalhães S., C. Vitorino Souza, T. Rocha Dias, *et al.* 2005. Lifestyle regularity measured by the social rhythm metric in Parkinson's disease. *Chronobiol Int* 22:917–924.

Castillo C., P. Molyneux, R. Carlson, and M.E. Harrington. 2011. Restricted wheel access following a light cycle inversion slows re-entrainment without internal desynchrony as measured in Per2Luc mice. *Neurosci* 182:169–176.

Chang A.-M., N. Santhi, M. St Hilaire, *et al.* 2012. Human responses to bright light of different durations. *J Physiol* 590:3103–3112.

Chellappa S.L., R. Steiner, P. Oelhafen, *et al.* 2013. Acute exposure to evening blue-enriched light impacts on human sleep. *J Sleep Res* 22(5):573–580.

Chen Z., S.-H. Yoo, Y.-S. Park, *et al.* 2012. Identification of diverse modulators of central and peripheral circadian clocks by high-throughput chemical screening. *Proc Natl Acad Sci USA* 109:101–106.

Cuesta M., J. Aungier, and A.J. Morton. 2014. Behavioral therapy reverses circadian deficits in a transgenic mouse model of Huntington's disease. *Neurobiol Dis* 63:85–91.

Czeisler C.A. 2013. Perspective: casting light on sleep deficiency. *Nature* 497:S13.

Dallmann R. and N. Mrosovsky. 2006. Scheduled wheel access during daytime: A method for studying conflicting zeitgebers. *Physiol Behav* 88:459–465.

Dhillon S. and M. Clarke. 2014. Tasimelteon: first global approval. *Drugs* 74:505–511.

Duffy J.F. and C.A. Czeisler. 2009. Effect of light on human circadian physiology. *Sleep Med Clin* 4:165–177.

Durgan D.J., M.A. Hotze, T.M. Tomlin, *et al.* 2005. The intrinsic circadian clock within the cardiomyocyte. *Am J Physiol Heart Circ Physiol* **289**:H1530–1541.

Eastman C.I., E.K. Hoese, S.D. Youngstedt, and L. Liu. 1995. Phase-shifting human circadian rhythms with exercise during the night shift. *Physiol Behav* **58**:1287–1291.

Fonken L.K., T.G. Aubrecht, O.H. Meléndez-Fernández, *et al.* 2013. Dim light at night disrupts molecular circadian rhythms and increases body weight. *J Biol Rhythms* **28**:262–271.

Frank E., S. Hlastala, A. Ritenour, *et al.* 1997. Inducing lifestyle regularity in recovering bipolar disorder patients: Results from the maintenance therapies in bipolar disorder protocol. *Biol Psychiatry* **41**:1165–1173.

Freeman G.M., R.M. Krock, S.J. Aton, *et al.* 2013. GABA networks destabilize genetic oscillations in the circadian pacemaker. *Neuron* **78**:799–806.

Friedman L., J.M. Zeitzer, C. Kushida, *et al.* 2009. Scheduled bright light for treatment of insomnia in older adults. *J Am Geriatr Soc* **57**:441–452.

Friedman L., A.P. Spira, B. Hernandez, *et al.* 2012. Brief morning light treatment for sleep/wake disturbances in older memory-impaired individuals and their caregivers. *Sleep Med* **13**:546–549.

Gibbs J.E., J. Blaikley, S. Beesley, *et al.* 2012. The nuclear receptor REV-ERBα mediates circadian regulation of innate immunity through selective regulation of inflammatory cytokines. *Proc Natl Acad Sci USA* **109**:582–587.

Gotter A.L., A.J. Roecker, R. Hargreaves, *et al.* 2012. Orexin receptors as therapeutic drug targets. *Prog Brain Res* **198**:163–188.

Hardeland R., A. Coto-Montes, and B. Poeggeler. 2003. Circadian rhythms, oxidative stress, and antioxidative defense mechanisms. *Chronobiol Int* **20**:921–962.

Hirota T., J.W. Lee, P.C. St John, *et al.* 2012. Identification of small molecule activators of cryptochrome. *Science* **337**:1094–1097.

Houben T., T. Deboer, F. van Oosterhout, and J.H. Meijer. 2009. Correlation with behavioral activity and rest implies circadian regulation by SCN neuronal activity levels. *J Biol Rhythms* **24**:477–487.

Jung C.M., S.B.S. Khalsa, F.A.J.L. Scheer, *et al.* 2010. Acute effects of bright light exposure on cortisol levels. *J Biol Rhythms* **25**:208–216.

Kalsbeek A., R.A. Cutrera, J.J. Van Heerikhuize, *et al.* 1999. GABA release from suprachiasmatic nucleus terminals is necessary for the light-induced inhibition of nocturnal melatonin release in the rat. *Neurosci* **91**:453–461.

Khalsa S.B.S., M.E. Jewett, C. Cajochen, and C.A. Czeisler. 2003. A phase response curve to single bright light pulses in human subjects. *J Physiol* **549**:945–952.

Kiessling S., G. Eichele, and H. Oster. 2010. Adrenal glucocorticoids have a key role in circadian resynchronization in a mouse model of jet lag. *J Clin Invest* **120**:2600–2609.

Kumar N., L.A. Solt, Y. Wang, *et al.* 2010. Regulation of adipogenesis by natural and synthetic REV-ERB ligands. *Endocrinology* **151**:3015–3025.

Leise T.L., M.E. Harrington, P.C. Molyneux, *et al.* 2013. Voluntary exercise can strengthen the circadian system in aged mice. *Age* **35**(6):2137–2152.

Lewy A.J., T.A. Wehr, F.K. Goodwin, *et al.* 1980. Light suppresses melatonin secretion in humans. *Science* **210**:1267–1269.

Lieverse R., E.J.W. Van Someren, M.M.A. Nielen, *et al.* 2011. Bright light treatment in elderly patients with nonseasonal major depressive disorder: a randomized placebo-controlled trial. *Arch Gen Psychiatry* **68**:61–70.

Liu A.C., W.G. Lewis, and S.A. Kay. 2007. Mammalian circadian signaling networks and therapeutic targets. *Nat Chem Biol* **3**:630–639.

Lucas R.J., G.S. Lall, A.E. Allen, and T.M. Brown. 2012. How rod, cone, and melanopsin photoreceptors come together to enlighten the mammalian circadian clock. *Prog Brain Res* **199**:1–18.

Magnusson A. and D. Boivin. 2003. Seasonal affective disorder: an overview. *Chronobiol Int* **20**:189–207.

Mahlios J., A.K. De la Herrán-Arita, and E. Mignot. 2013. The autoimmune basis of narcolepsy. *Curr Opin Neurobiol.* **23**(5):767–73.

Maywood E.S., N. Mrosovsky, M.D. Field, and M.H. Hastings. 1999. Rapid down-regulation of mammalian period genes during behavioral resetting of the circadian clock. *Proc Natl Acad Sci USA* **96**:15211–15216.

Maywood E.S., E. Fraenkel, C.J. McAllister, *et al.* 2010. Disruption of peripheral circadian timekeeping in a mouse model of Huntington's disease and its restoration by temporally scheduled feeding. *J Neurosci* **30**:10199–10204.

Meng Q.-J., E.S. Maywood, D.A. Bechtold, *et al.* 2010. Entrainment of disrupted circadian behavior through inhibition of casein kinase 1 (CK1) enzymes. *Proc Natl Acad Sci USA* **107**:15240–15245.

Meng Q.J., A. McMaster, S. Beesley, *et al.* 2008. Ligand modulation of REV-ERBalpha function resets the peripheral circadian clock in a phasic manner. *J Cell Sci* **121**:3629–3635.

Mieda M. and T. Sakurai. 2012. Overview of orexin/hypocretin system. *Prog Brain Res* **198**:5–14.

Miyazaki T., S. Hashimoto, S. Masubuchi, *et al*. 2001. Phase-advance shifts of human circadian pacemaker are accelerated by daytime physical exercise. *Am J Physiol Regul Integr Comp Physiol* **281**:R197–205.

Monk T.H., S.R. Petrie, A.J. Hayes, and D.J. Kupfer. 1994. Regularity of daily life in relation to personality, age, gender, sleep quality and circadian rhythms. *J Sleep Res* **3**:196–205.

Nakahata Y., M. Kaluzova, B. Grimaldi, *et al*. 2008. The NAD+-dependent deacetylase SIRT1 modulates CLOCK-mediated chromatin remodeling and circadian control. *Cell* **134**:329–340.

Pallier P.N. and A.J. Morton. 2009. Management of sleep/wake cycles improves cognitive function in a transgenic mouse model of Huntington's disease. *Brain Res* **1279**:90–98.

Pallier P.N., E.S. Maywood, Z. Zheng, *et al*. 2007. Pharmacological imposition of sleep slows cognitive decline and reverses dysregulation of circadian gene expression in a transgenic mouse model of Huntington's disease. *J Neurosci* **27**:7869–7878.

Pantazopoulos H., H. Dolatshad, and F.C. Davis. 2010. Chronic stimulation of the hypothalamic vasoactive intestinal peptide receptor lengthens circadian period in mice and hamsters. *Am J Physiol Regul Integr Comp Physiol* **299**:R379–385.

Pevet P. and E. Challet. 2011. Melatonin: both master clock output and internal time-giver in the circadian clocks network. *J Physiol Paris* **105**:170–182.

Power A., A.T.L. Hughes, R.E. Samuels, and H.D. Piggins. 2010. Rhythm-promoting actions of exercise in mice with deficient neuropeptide signaling. *J Biol Rhythms* **25**:235–246.

Reebs S.G. and N. Mrosovsky. 1989. Effects of induced wheel running on the circadian activity rhythms of Syrian hamsters: entrainment and phase response curve. *J Biol Rhythms* **4**:39–48.

Reid K.J., K.G. Baron, B. Lu, *et al*. 2010. Aerobic exercise improves self-reported sleep and quality of life in older adults with insomnia. *Sleep Med* **11**:934–940.

Riemann D. and Spiegelhalder K. 2014. Orexin receptor antagonists: a new treatment for insomnia? *Lancet Neurol* **13**(5):441–443.

Riemersma-van der Lek R.F., D.F. Swaab, J. Twisk, *et al*. 2008. Effect of bright light and melatonin on cognitive and noncognitive function in elderly residents of group care facilities: a randomized controlled trial. *JAMA* **299**:2642–2655.

Royer M., N.H. Ballentine, P.J. Eslinger, *et al*. 2012. Light therapy for seniors in long term care. *J Am Med Dir Assoc* **13**:100–102.

Ruger M. and F.A.J.L. Scheer. 2009. Effects of circadian disruption on cardiometabolic system. *Rev Endocr Metab Disord* **10**:245–260.

Rutten S., C. Vriend, O.A. van den Heuvel, *et al*. 2012. Bright light therapy in Parkinson's disease: an overview of the background and evidence. *Parkinsons Dis* **2012**:1–9.

Sakamoto K. and N. Ishida. 2000. Light-induced phase-shifts in the circadian expression rhythm of mammalian Period genes in the mouse heart. *Eur J Neurosci* **12**:4003–4006.

Schmidt K.P., W.K. Koehler, G. Fleissner, and B. Pflug. 1990. Locomotor activity accelerates the adjustment of the temperature rhythm in shiftwork. *J Interdisipl Cycle Res* **21**:243–245.

Schmidt T.M., S.-K. Chen, and S. Hattar. 2011. Intrinsically photosensitive retinal ganglion cells: many subtypes, diverse functions. *Trends Neurosci* **34**:572–580.

Schroeder A.M., D. Truong, D.H. Loh, *et al*. 2012. Voluntary scheduled exercise alters diurnal rhythms of behaviour, physiology and gene expression in wild-type and vasoactive intestinal peptide-deficient mice. *J Physiol* **590**:6213–6226.

Sheward W.J., E.S. Maywood, K.L. French, *et al*. 2007. Entrainment to feeding but not to light: circadian phenotype of VPAC2 receptor-null mice. *J Neurosci* **27**:4351–4358.

Solt L.A., Y. Wang, S. Banerjee, *et al*. 2012. Regulation of circadian behaviour and metabolism by synthetic REV-ERB agonists. *Nature* **485**(7396):62–68.

Someren E.J.W.V., C. Lijzenga, M. Mirmiran, and D.F. Swaab. 1997. Long-term fitness training improves the circadian rest-activity rhythm in healthy elderly males. *J Biol Rhythms* **12**:146–156.

Spengler M.L., K.K. Kuropatwinski, M. Comas, *et al*. 2012. Core circadian protein CLOCK is a positive regulator of NF-κB-mediated transcription. *Proc Natl Acad Sci USA* **109**:E2457–2465.

Szántóová K., M. Zeman, A. Veselá, and I. Herichová. 2011. Effect of phase delay lighting rotation schedule on daily expression of per2, bmal1, rev-erbα, pparα, and pdk4 genes in the heart and liver of Wistar rats. *Mol Cell Biochem* **348**:53–60.

Trump R.P., S. Bresciani, A.W.J. Cooper, *et al*. 2013. Optimized chemical probes for REV-ERBα. *J Med Chem* **56**:4729–4737.

Uslaner J.M., S.J. Tye, D.M. Eddins, *et al.* 2013. Orexin receptor antagonists differ from standard sleep drugs by promoting sleep at doses that do not disrupt cognition. *Sci Transl Med* **5**:179ra44.

Van Someren EJ. 2000. Circadian and sleep disturbances in the elderly. *Exp Gerontol* **35**:1229–1237.

Van Wamelen D.J., N.A. Aziz, J.J. Anink, *et al.* 2013. Suprachiasmatic nucleus neuropeptide expression in patients with Huntington's disease. *Sleep* **36**:117–125.

Viola A.U., L.M. James, L.J.M. Schlangen, and D.-J. Dijk. 2008. Blue-enriched white light in the workplace improves self-reported alertness, performance and sleep quality. *Scand J Work Environ Health* **34**:297–306.

Vitaterna M.H., C.H. Ko, A.-M. Chang, *et al.* 2006. The mouse Clock mutation reduces circadian pacemaker amplitude and enhances efficacy of resetting stimuli and phase-response curve amplitude. *Proc Natl Acad Sci USA* **103**:9327–9332.

Welsh D., G.S. Richardson, and W.C. Dement. 1988. Effect of running wheel availability on circadian patterns of sleep and wakefulness in mice. *Physiol Behav* **43**:771–777.

Willis G.L., C. Moore, and S.M. Armstrong. 2012. A historical justification for and retrospective analysis of the systematic application of light therapy in Parkinson's disease. *Rev Neurosci* **23**:199–226.

Wirz-Justice A., M. Terman, D.A. Oren, *et al.* 2004. Brightening depression. *Science* **303**:467–469.

Wright K.P. Jr, A.W. McHill, B.R. Birks, *et al.* 2013. Entrainment of the human circadian clock to the natural light-dark cycle. *Curr Biol* **23**:1554–1558.

Xu Y., K.L. Toh, C.R. Jones, *et al.* 2007. Modeling of a human circadian mutation yields insights into clock regulation by PER2. *Cell* **128**:59–70.

Yamadera H., T. Ito, H. Suzuki, *et al.* 2000. Effects of bright light on cognitive and sleep–wake (circadian) rhythm disturbances in Alzheimer-type dementia. *Psychiatry Clin Neurosci* **54**:352–353.

Yamanaka Y., K. Honma, S. Hashimoto, *et al.* 2006. Effects of physical exercise on human circadian rhythms. *Sleep Biol Rhythms* **4**:199–206.

Young K.W. and C.E. Greenwood. 2001. Shift in diurnal feeding patterns in nursing home residents with Alzheimer's disease. *J Gerontol A Biol Sci Med Sci* **56**:M700–706.

Yu X., D. Rollins, K.A. Ruhn, *et al.* 2013. TH17 cell differentiation is regulated by the circadian clock. *Science* **342**:727–730.

Zhou J.N., M.A. Hofman, and D.F. Swaab. 1995. VIP neurons in the human SCN in relation to sex, age, and Alzheimer's disease. *Neurobiol Aging* **16**:571–576.

Zisberg A., N. Gur-Yaish, and T. Shochat. 2010. Contribution of routine to sleep quality in community elderly. *Sleep* **33**:509–514.

Index

Circadian Medicine, First Edition. Edited by Christopher S. Colwell.
© 2015 John Wiley & Sons, Inc. Published 2015 by John Wiley & Sons, Inc.